W0112646

Second Edition

Textbook of Physiology

P Sathya MBBS, MD, DGO
Professor of Physiology
Institute of Physiology and Experimental Medicine
Madras Medical College
Chennai, Tamil Nadu

Viji Devanand MBBS, MD
Professor and Head
Department of Physiology
Stanley Medical College
Chennai, Tamil Nadu

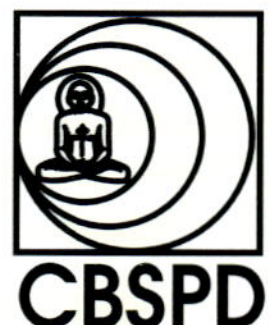

CBS Publishers & Distributors Pvt Ltd

New Delhi • Bengaluru • Chennai • Kochi • Kolkata • Lucknow • Mumbai
Hyderabad • Jharkhand • Nagpur • Patna • Pune • Uttarakhand

Disclaimer

Science and technology are constantly changing fields. New research and experience broaden the scope of information and knowledge. The authors have tried their best in giving information available to them while preparing the material for this book. Although, all efforts have been made to ensure optimum accuracy of the material, yet it is quite possible some errors might have been left uncorrected. The publisher, the printer and the authors will not be held responsible for any inadvertent errors, omissions or inaccuracies.

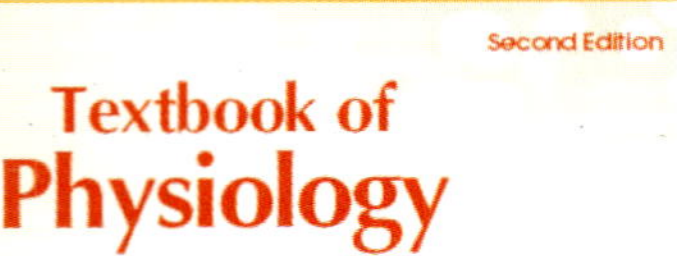

ISBN: 978-93-88108-39-3

Copyright © Authors and Publisher

Second Edition	2019
Reprint	2022
First Edition	2013
Reprint	2016

All rights reserved. No part of this book may be reproduced or transmitted in any form or by any means, electronic or mechanical, including photocopying, recording, or any information storage and retrieval system without permission, in writing, from the authors and the publishers.

Published by Satish Kumar Jain and produced by Varun Jain for

CBS Publishers & Distributors Pvt Ltd

4819/XI Prahlad Street, 24 Ansari Road, Daryaganj, New Delhi 110 002, India

Ph: 011-23289259, 23266861, 23266867 Website: www.cbspd.com

Fax: 011-23243014 e-mail: delhi@cbspd.com; cbspubs@airtelmail.in.

Corporate Office: 204 FIE, Industrial Area, Patparganj, Delhi 110 092, India

Ph: 011-4934 4934 Fax: 011-4934 4935 e-mail: publishing@cbspd.com; publicity@cbspd.com

Branches

- **Bengaluru:** Seema House 2975, 17th Cross, KR Road, Banasankari 2nd Stage, Bengaluru 560 070, Karnataka, India
  Ph: +91-80-26771678/79 Fax: +91-80-26771680 e-mail: bangalore@cbspd.com
- **Chennai:** 7, Subbaraya Street, Shenoy Nagar, Chennai 600 030, Tamil Nadu, India
  Ph: +91-44-26680620, 26681266 Fax: +91-44-42032115 e-mail: chennai@cbspd.com
- **Kochi:** 42/1325, 1326, Power House Road, Opp KSEB, Power House, Ernakulum Kochi 682 018, Kerala, India
  Ph: +91-484-4059061-65,67 Fax: +91-484-4059065 e-mail: kochi@cbspd.com
- **Kolkata:** 147, Hind Ceramics Compound, 1st Floor, Nilgunj Road, Belghoria, Kolkata-700056, West Bengal, India
  Ph: +033-25633055, 033-25633056 e-mail: kolkata@cbspd.com
- **Lucknow:** Basement, Khushnuma Complex, 7 Meerabai Marg (Behind Jawahar Bhawan),Lucknow-226001, UP, India
  Ph: +0522-4000032 e-mail: tiwari.lucknow@cbspd.com
- **Mumbai:** PWD Shed, Gala no 25/26, Ramchandra Bhatt Marg, Next to JJ Hospital Gate no. 2, Opp. Union Bank of India, Noorbaug, Mumbai-400009, Maharashtra, India
  Ph: 022-66661880/89 e-mail: mumbai@cbspd.com

Representatives

- Hyderabad 0-9885175004
- Jharkhand 0-9811541605
- Nagpur 0-9421945513
- Patna 0-9334159340
- Pune 0-9623451994
- Uttarakhand 0-9716462459

Printed at Nutech Print Services, Faridabad, Haryana, India

Preface to the Second Edition

Our sincere thanks to all the readers for their valuable suggestions, feedback and support for the first edition.

To meet the changing needs of its many readers, we have come up with the 2nd edition of the book which contains a wealth of new updates in the field of physiology.

This edition represents an extensive revision of the chapters of the first edition with technical corrections, updates and clarifications in certain areas which will make this edition more lucid and palatable to students.

A note on eminent scientists who have contributed to physiology has been added in this edition.

A sound knowledge of physiology for first year MBBS students is an essential basis for an effective clinical practice in future, so we have covered every topic in physiology from both examination and clinical point of view along with an insight into the pathophysiology of diseases by comparing normal processes in the body with the abnormal.

The first edition of this book has been well-received, both by MBBS students and paramedical students throughout the country and been through several printings. We have strived to improve the book along the lines suggested by our readers.

It is our hope and expectation that this book will provide an effective learning experience and reference resource for both students and medical practitioners.

P Sathya
Viji Devanand

Preface to the First Edition

Physiology is an interesting but vast subject in MBBS course. Every first year MBBS student faces a challenging time while studying this subject due to the old-fashioned and stoic language of the physiology textbooks. The aim of this book is to provide the undergraduate students a clear idea of physiology in a simple language with updated information and easy illustrations.

This book is primarily written for the first year MBBS students and also for the students of paramedical courses. It may be used as reference and study for any science student studying physiology. It is sincerely expected that this book will prove useful to all the undergraduate medical students as well as the students of allied health sciences and nursing, and BSc/MSc (physiology).

P Sathya
Viji Devanand

Acknowledgments

We sincerely thank Dr MR Renuka Devi (Associate Professor of Physiology, Sree Balaji Medical College, Chennai); Dr M Arifath (Associate Professor of Physiology, Adhiparasakhti Medical College, Mezhmaruvathur); Dr D Balanaganandhini (Associate Professor of Physiology, Tanjore Medical College, Tanjore); Dr A Anitha (Associate Professor of Physiology, Chengalpet Medical College, Chengalpet); and Dr Senthil Kumari, Dr B Anitha, Dr A Chandra (Assistant Professors of Physiology, Kilpauk Medical College, Chennai) for their contribution, motivation, guidance and never-ending support and also for helping and directing us towards the completion of the book in time.

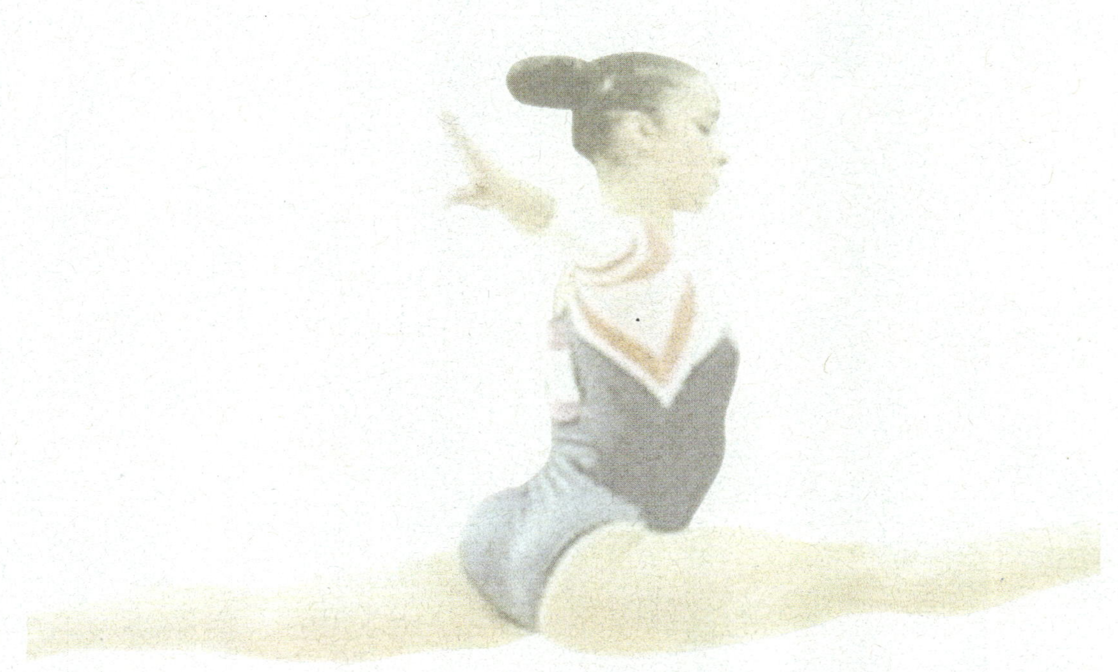

Contents

6. CARDIOVASCULAR SYSTEM

7. RESPIRATORY SYSTEM

8. EXCRETORY SYSTEM

12. SPECIAL SENSES

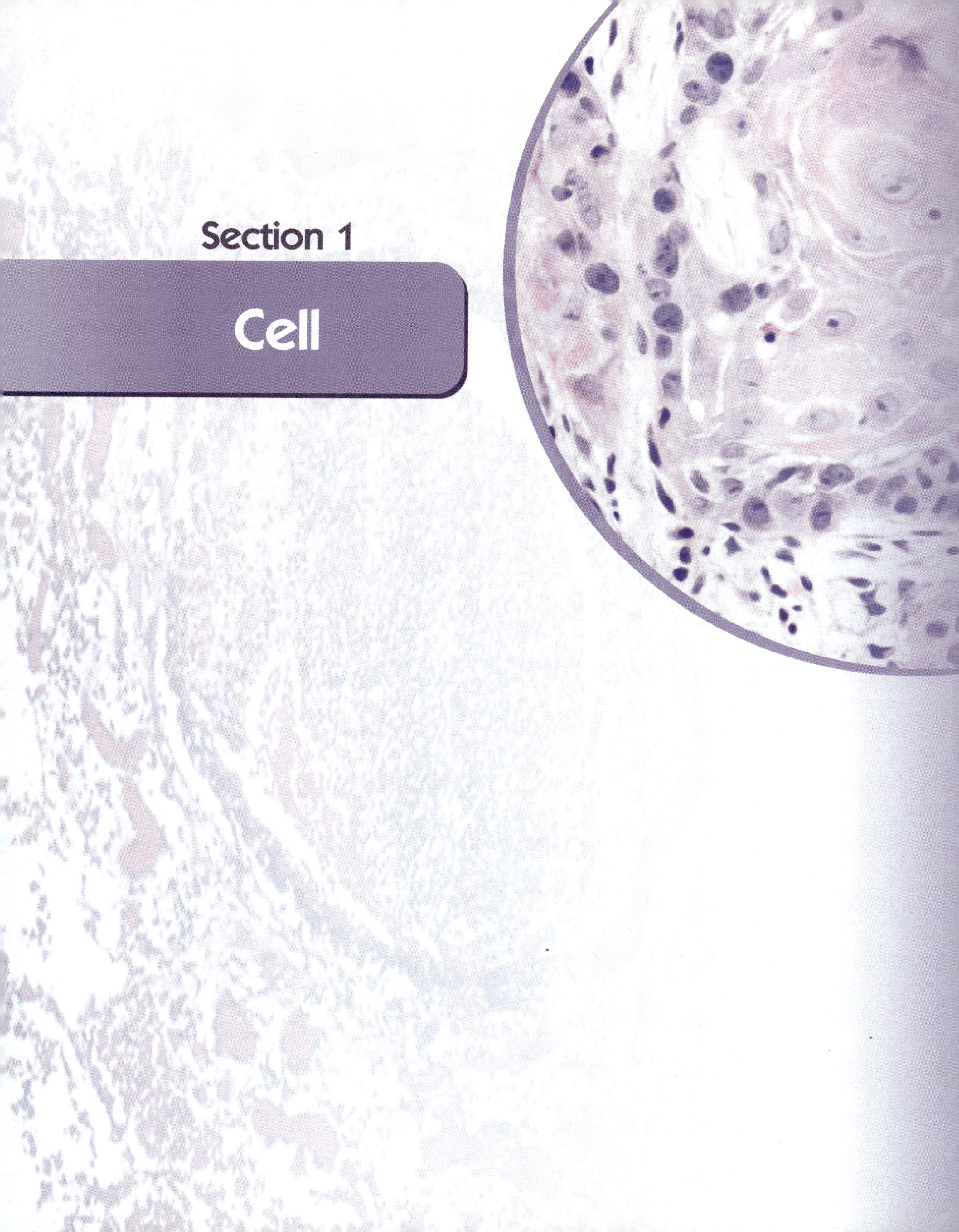

Section 1

Cell

1. CELL

INTRODUCTION

All living organisms on earth are made up of cells. Cells are small compartments that hold all of the biological equipment necessary to keep an organism alive and successful on earth (Fig. 1.1). The main purpose of a cell is to organize all the functions of the body.

STRUCTURE OF A CELL AND ITS ORGANELLES

The two major parts of a cell are the nucleus and the cytoplasm. The cytoplasm is made of cytosol and organelles. Cytosol is the fluid that fills the cytoplasm. Cell organelles are suspended in it. Organelles are highly organized physical structures. The nucleus is separated from the cytoplasm by a nuclear membrane and the cytoplasm is separated from the surrounding fluids by a cell membrane (Fig. 1.1).

CELL MEMBRANE

Structure

Cell membrane is like a big plastic bag with some tiny holes. Cell membrane surrounds the cell and is made of lipids and proteins. It is semi permeable, allowing some substances to pass through it and excluding others. The selective permeability of the cell membrane is due to presence of regulated ion channels and other transport proteins embedded in it. The structure of a cell membrane varies from one place to other depending on the function, but they share some common features.

Cell membrane is about 7.5 nm thick and is made up of proteins and phospholipids. The phospholipids make the plastic bag and the proteins are found around the holes and help movement in and out the cell.

Phospholipids Component of the Cell Membrane (Fig. 1.2)

Phospholipids make up the lipid bilayer and the major phospholipids are phosphatidylcholine and phosphatidylethanolamine. The head end of each phospholipids molecule is made of phosphate and is soluble in water and is called as the hydrophilic end. The tail end is the fatty acid portion which is insoluble in water and is called as the hydrophobic end. The hydrophobic ends of the bilayer are repelled by water of the ECF and ICF but are attracted to each other and line up in the centre. The hydrophilic end covers the side which is in contact with water (Fig. 1.2).

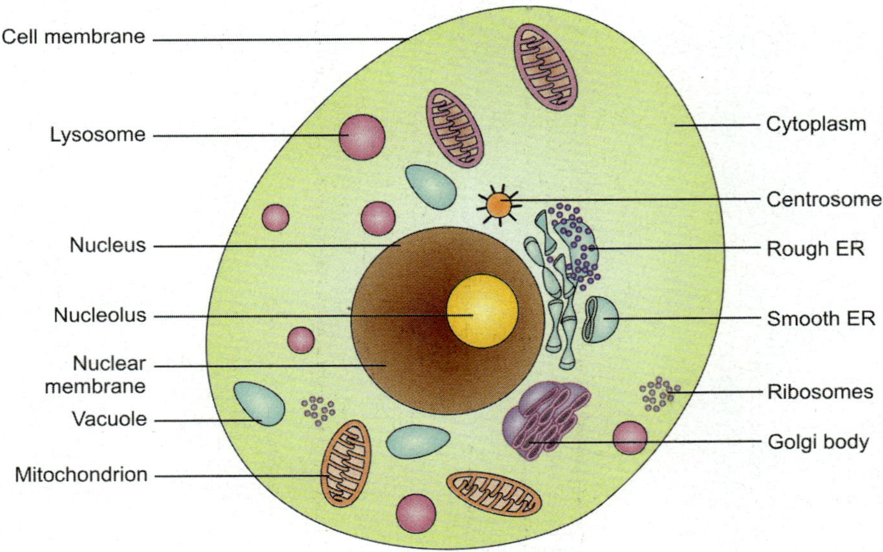

Fig. 1.1: Structure of cell

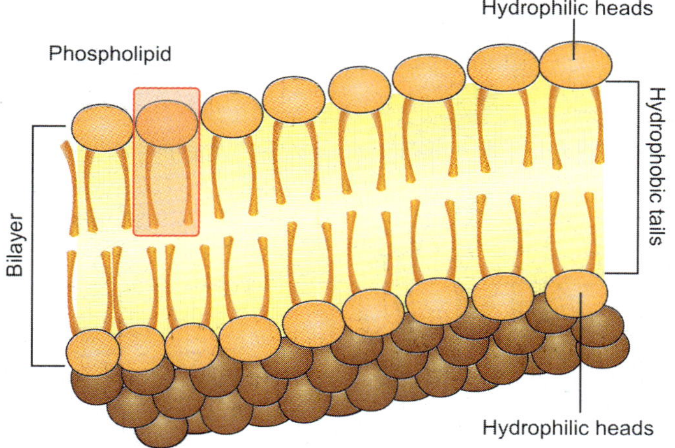

Fig. 1.2: Phospholipid component of cell membrane

The lipid bilayer is a fluid and fluidity depends on cholesterol molecule, and therefore, portions of the membrane can flow from one point to another.

Protein Component of the Cell Membrane

There are three types of proteins in the cell membrane namely (Fig. 1.3):

1. *Peripheral proteins:* They are not bonded as strongly to the membrane but just sit on the surface of the membrane either inside or outside anchored with a few hydrogen (H) bonds.
2. *Integral proteins:* They are embedded in the hydrophobic (middle) layer of the membrane.
3. *Transmembrane proteins:* They cross the membrane through and through and act as pathways for ions and molecules by either functioning as pump which actively transports ions, as carrier proteins and still some as ion channels.

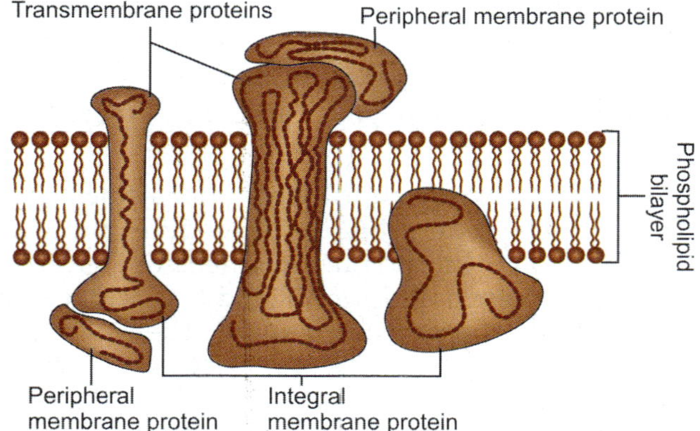

Fig. 1.3: Protein component of cell membrane

Functions of the Cell Membrane

1. The cell membrane protects the cytoplasm and the organelles. It acts as a barrier permitting only some substances to pass through it.
2. Integral proteins give stability to the cell membrane.
3. Peripheral proteins seated on the outer surface of the cell membrane act as receptors for neuro-transmitters and hormones. They also function as antigens.
4. Some proteins function as cell adhesion molecules that anchor cells to their neighbours or to basal lamina.
5. Transmembrane proteins act as carrier proteins and channels for the transport of ions, glucose and other water soluble substances.
6. The lipid bilayer helps in the transport of lipid soluble substances like oxygen and carbon dioxide which is vital for cell metabolism.

CELL ORGANELLES (Fig. 1.4)

Mitochondria

Structure: It is a sausage-shaped structure. It is made up of outer and inner membranes and the latter is folded to form selves called cristae onto which oxidative enzymes are attached. The inner cavity of the mitochondria is filled with matrix that contains large quantities of dissolved enzymes that are necessary for extracting energy from nutrients. Both these enzymes work in harmony to cause oxidation of nutrients and release of energy. Mitochondria are self-replicate.

Function: It synthesizes a high energy ATP (adenosine triphosphate) and the same is transported out of the mitochondria to the other areas of cell to be utilized for performing cellular functions.

Applied physiology: Sperm contributes no mitochondria to zygote, hence any disease related to mitochondria is purely maternal.

1. Mitochondrial diseases comprise those disorders that in one way or another affect the function of the mitochondria or are due to mitochondrial DNA. Mitochondrial diseases take on unique characteristics

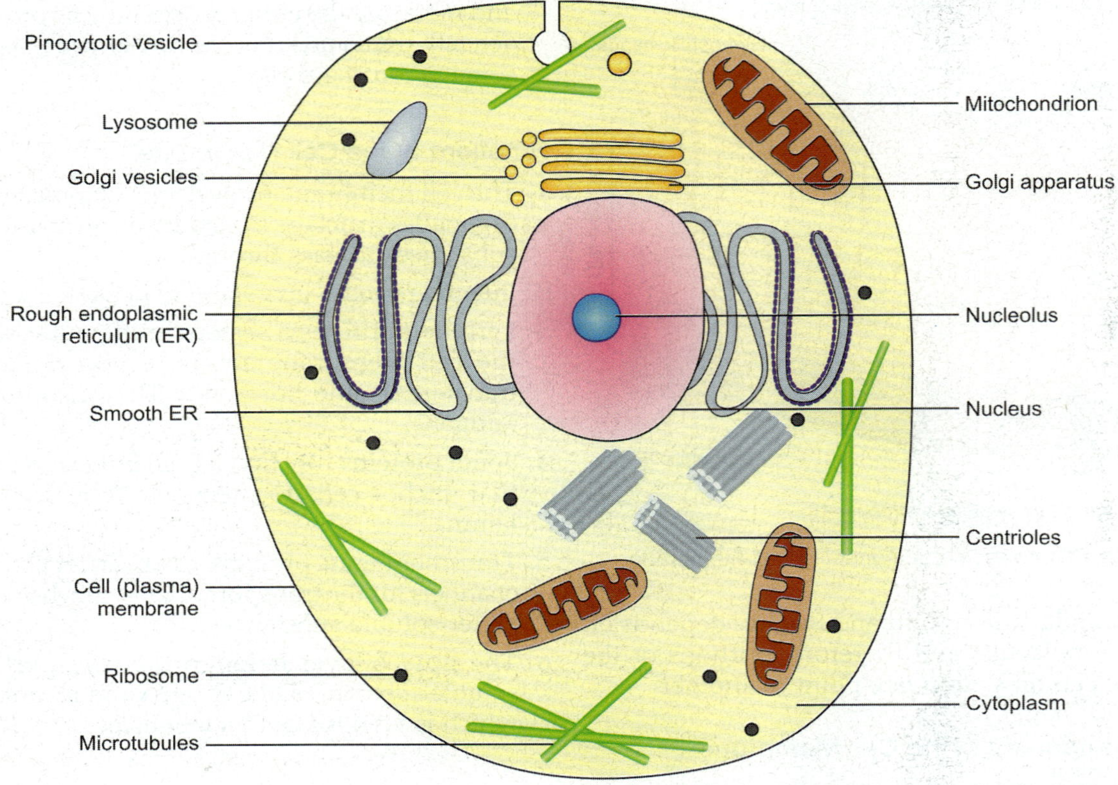

Fig. 1.4: Anatomy of animal cell

both because of the way the diseases are often inherited and because mitochondria are so critical to cell function. The subclass of these diseases that have neuromuscular disease symptoms are often referred to as a mitochondrial myopathy.

2. Leber's hereditary optic neuropathy causes multiple sclerosis and visual loss.

Endoplasmic Reticulum (ER)

Structure: It is a network of sacs and the outer limb of the sac is continuous with the nuclear membrane. It is of two types namely Rough endoplasmic reticulum with ribosomes on it which gives it the rough appearance and the smooth endoplasmic reticulum. The rough ER is abundant in cells which synthesizes protein. A modification of this in the skeletal and cardiac muscle is called as sarcoplasmic reticulum.

Functions

1. The rough endoplasmic reticulum is the site of protein synthesis.
2. Smooth endoplasmic reticulum is the site of steroid synthesis wherever necessary.
3. Smooth ER helps in detoxification of toxic substances and neutralization of hormones and noxious substances.

Golgi Apparatus

Structure: Each Golgi apparatus consists of 5–7 membranous sacs which are flattened sacs. It has two ends. The vesicle pinched off from the ER fuses with one end and exit via the other end after processing.

Functions

1. It is the distribution and shipping departments for the cell's chemical products. It modifies proteins and fats built in ER and prepares them for digestion. ER vesicles pinch off from ER and fuse with Golgi apparatus to be processed there. Then they are released as lysosomes and secretory vesicles from Golgi apparatus.
2. Packaging of secretory products into secretory granules.

3. Incorporation of carbohydrates into the newly synthesized proteins to form glycoproteins.

Lysosomes

Structure: They are membrane bound vesicles pinched off from Golgi apparatus. It contains proteases, lipases and amylases.

Function: Lysosomes provide an intracellular digestive system that allows the cell to digest damaged cellular structures, unwanted matter and food particles with the help of these digestive enzymes.

Applied physiology: Like other genetic diseases, individuals inherit lysosomal storage diseases from their parents. Although each disorder results from different gene mutations that translate into a deficiency in enzyme activity, they all share a common biochemical characteristic, i.e. all lysosomal disorders originate from an abnormal accumulation of substances inside the lysosome. Lysosomal storage disorders are caused by lysosomal dysfunction, usually as a consequence of deficiency of a single enzyme required for the metabolism of lipids, glycoproteins (sugar containing proteins) or so-called mucopolysaccharides. They are:

1. Fabry's disease
2. Tay-Sachs disease
3. Gaucher's disease, etc.

Peroxisomes

Structure: They are membrane bound vesicles formed by budding off from smooth ER. They contain oxidative enzymes such as oxidases and catalases.

Functions

1. They function mainly to detoxify poisonous substances.
2. They breakdown the excess fatty acid.

Nucleus

Structure: It is the information and administrative center of the cell. The nucleus is made up of chromosomes that is made up of DNA molecules (deoxyribonucleic acid). Each DNA molecule is made up of genes that carry complete blueprint of all the heritable species. The unit of heredity is the genes which are present on the chromosomes that form the largest part of nucleus. Nucleus is surrounded by nuclear membrane which is a double layer membrane, the outer layer of which is continuous with the membrane of rough ER, and therefore, there is continuous space with ER. The nucleus of most cells contains nucleolus that is rich in RNA which is the site of synthesis of ribosomes. The nucleoli are prominent in growing cells.

Functions

1. Nucleoli synthesize ribosome that is needed for protein synthesis.
2. Nucleus controls cell division.
3. Messenger RNA from the nucleus has codon for the synthesis of protein.

CYTOSKELETON

It is unique to eukaryotic cells. It is a dynamic three-dimensional structure that fills the cytoplasm. This structure acts like muscle and skeleton for movement and stability of a cell. The primary types are micro-filaments, microtubules and intermediate filaments (Fig. 1.5).

Microfilaments: These are fine thread like protein fibers, 3–6 nm in diameter. They are composed predominantly of a contractile protein called actin. They carry out

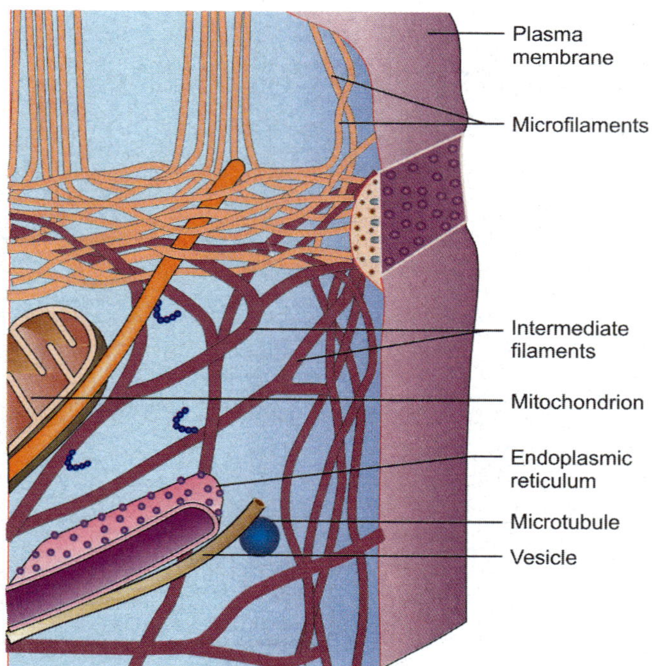

Fig. 1.5

1

cellular movement including gliding, contraction and cytokinesis.

Microtubules: They are cylindrical tubes, 20–25 nm in diameter. They are composed of protein tubulin and act as a scaffold to determine cell shape and provide "tracks" for cell organelles and vesicles to move on. They also form spindle fibers for separating chromosomes during mitosis. When arranged in geometric patterns inside flagella and cilia, they are used for locomotion.

Applied physiology: Since microtubules help in organelle movement, any drug that binds with microtubule and makes them stable can prevent organelle movement which can help in cancer treatment.

Intermediate filaments: They are about 10 nm diameter and provide tensile strength for the cell.

MOLECULAR MOTORS

They are biological molecular machines that are essential for movement in living organisms, i.e. to move proteins, organelles from one to other part of cell. Protein based molecular motors use the chemical free energy released by the hydrolysis of ATP in order to perform mechanical work. Some examples of biologically important molecular motors are as follows.

Cytoskeleton Motors

They are classified as (Fig. 1.6):

Microtubule Based

Kinesin and Dynein

1. Kinesin moves cargo inside the cell along microtubules.
2. Dynein produces the axonemal beating of cilia and flagella. It also transports materials along proton gradient inside microtubules towards the cell nucleus.

Actin Based

Myosin I–V: Myosin forms cross-bridges to actin filaments and the myosin heads move to generate force. This produces movement ranging from contraction of villi to skeletal muscle contraction.

Nucleic Acid Motors

RNA polymerase transcribes RNA from a DNA template.

DNA polymerase turns single-standard DNA into double-standard DNA.

Topoisomerase reduces super coiling of DNA.

Rotary Motors

ATP synthase generates ATP using the mitochondria.

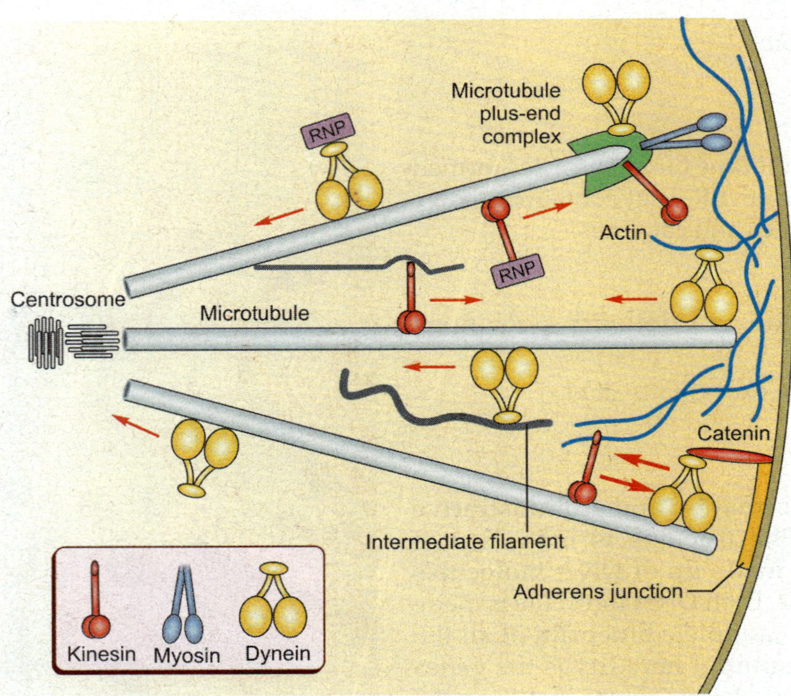

Fig. 1.6: Cytoskeleton motors

PROTEIN SYNTHESIS

Protein synthesis is the process in which cells build proteins. It is a multi-step process (Fig. 1.7).

Step 1

Transcription: The first step in protein synthesis is the transcription of a messenger RNA (mRNA) from a nuclear DNA gene in the nucleus. Here the double helix nuclear DNA is unzipped by the enzyme helicase, leaving single nucleotide chain open to be copied. RNA polymerase reads the DNA strand and synthesizes a single strand of messenger RNA. The mRNA then leaves the nucleus through nuclear pores and migrates into cytoplasm and functions as codons. Codon is a unit of three adjacent nucleotides along a DNA or messenger RNA molecule that designates a specific amino acid to be incorporated into a polypeptide. The order of the codons along the DNA or messenger RNA determines the sequence of the amino acids in the polypeptide. There is an initiation codon which always initiates an amino acid sequencing and a stop codon which stops the polypeptide chain with that amino acid when a ribosome scans through it.

Step 2

Translation: This takes place in rough ER. It is the process of converting the mRNA codon sequences into an amino acid polypeptide chain. This involves sub steps namely: (a) Amino acid activation, (b) Initiation, (c) Elongation and (d) Termination.

a. *Amino acid activation:* Each type of amino acid combines with specific RNA called transfer RNA (tRNA) which has anticodon, which is a sequence of three adjacent nucleotides in tRNA designating a specific amino acid that binds to a corresponding codon in mRNA during protein synthesis. Thus it

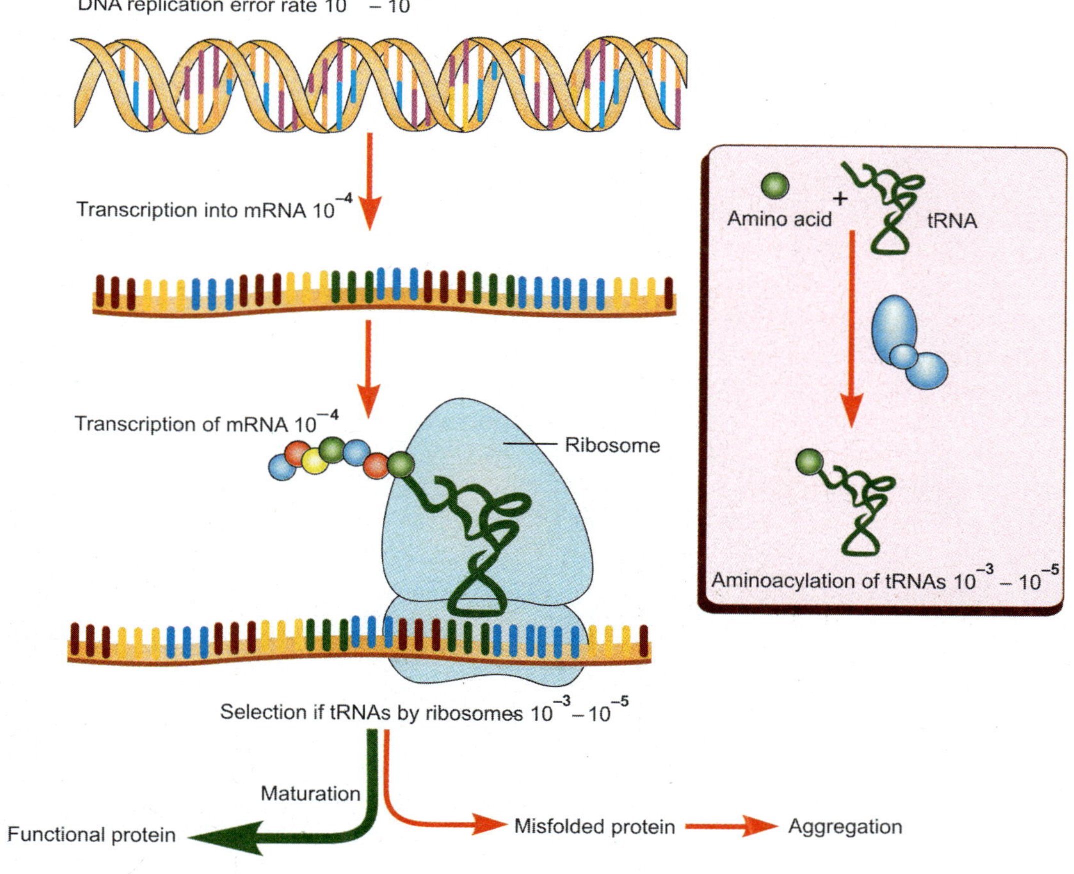

Fig. 1.7: Protein synthesis

forms tRNA-amino acid complex which recognizes a particular codon on the mRNA and can deliver the appropriate amino acid to appropriate place in the chain of new protein.

b. *Initiation:* A ribosome attaches to the mRNA and starts to read the codons of the mRNA.

c. *Elongation:* tRNA-amino acid complex brings the corresponding amino acid, in contact with the mRNA molecule in the ribosome where the anticodon of the tRNA attaches temporarily to its specific codon of the mRNA as the ribosome reads mRNA thus lining the amino acid in sequence.

d. *Termination:* Reading of final mRNA codon stops at stop codon which ends the synthesis of peptide chain.

The polypeptide chain buds off from rough ER and fuses with Golgi apparatus.

Step 3

Post-translational modification and protein folding: This takes place in Golgi apparatus. Post-translation modification includes the formation of disulfide bridges (or) attachment of functional groups such as acetate, phosphate, various lipids and carbohydrates.

Finally during and after synthesis, polypeptide chains often fold to assume secondary and tertiary structures. This is known as protein folding.

Applied physiology: The regulation of protein synthesis plays an important role in transcription, in the control of gene expression. Once thought solely to act globally, translational control has now been shown to be able to control the expression of most genes specifically. Dysregulation of this process is associated with a range of pathological conditions, notably cancer and several neurological disorders, and can occur in many ways. These include alterations in the expression of initiation factors and mutations in regulatory mRNA sequence. Translational control is increasingly open for study in both fresh and fixed tissue, and this rapidly developing field is yielding useful diagnostic and prognostic tools that will hopefully provide new targets for effective treatments.

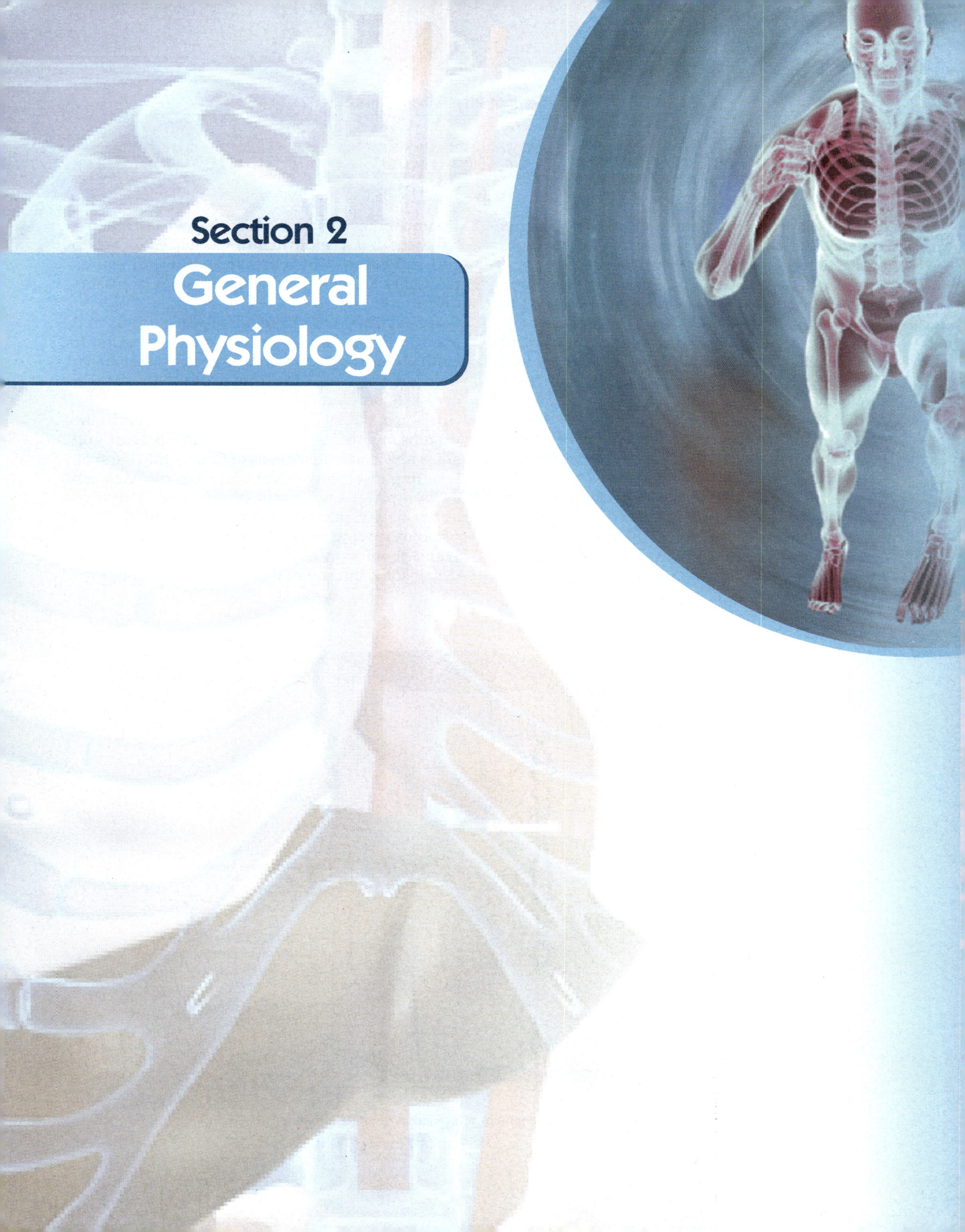

Section 2

General Physiology

2. INTERCELLULAR CONNECTION AND COMMUNICATION

2

Each cell is connected to adjacent cell and basal lamina by intercellular connection. There are various types of connections involved. They are (Fig. 2.1):

1. **Gap junctions** or nexus is a specialized intercellular connection which is an opening from one cell to another. It is large enough for cytoplasm to move from one cell to another and help for the movement of molecules. The diameter of channel is about 2 nm. Special transmembrane protein known as connexins join to form aqueous channel known as connexon. Connexon of one cell join with the connexon of the other cell to form the pore or gap. For example myocardial cell and visceral smooth muscle.
   Function: They permit rapid propagation of electrical activity from cell-to-cell.
   Applied physiology: Mutation in the gene for connexon causes X-linked form of Charcot-Marie-Tooth disease which causes peripheral neuropathy.
2. **Desmosomes:** They are also known as macula adherens. It is a cell structure specialized for cell to cell adhesion. They are spot like adhesions randomly arranged on the lateral sides of plasma membrane.
   Function: They help to resist shearing forces and are found in simple and stratified squamous epithelium. They act as linking proteins that attach the cell surface adhesion protein to keratin cytoskeleton filament.
   Applied physiology: If there is a genetic defect in the desmosomal protein, the skin can pull apart and allow abnormal movements of fluid within the skin, resulting in blisters called blistering disease such as pemphigus vulgaris. Blistering is due to abnormality in desmosome—keratin filament complex leading to breakdown in cell adhesion.
3. **Hemidesmosomes:** They appear similar to desmosome but rather than linking two cells, they

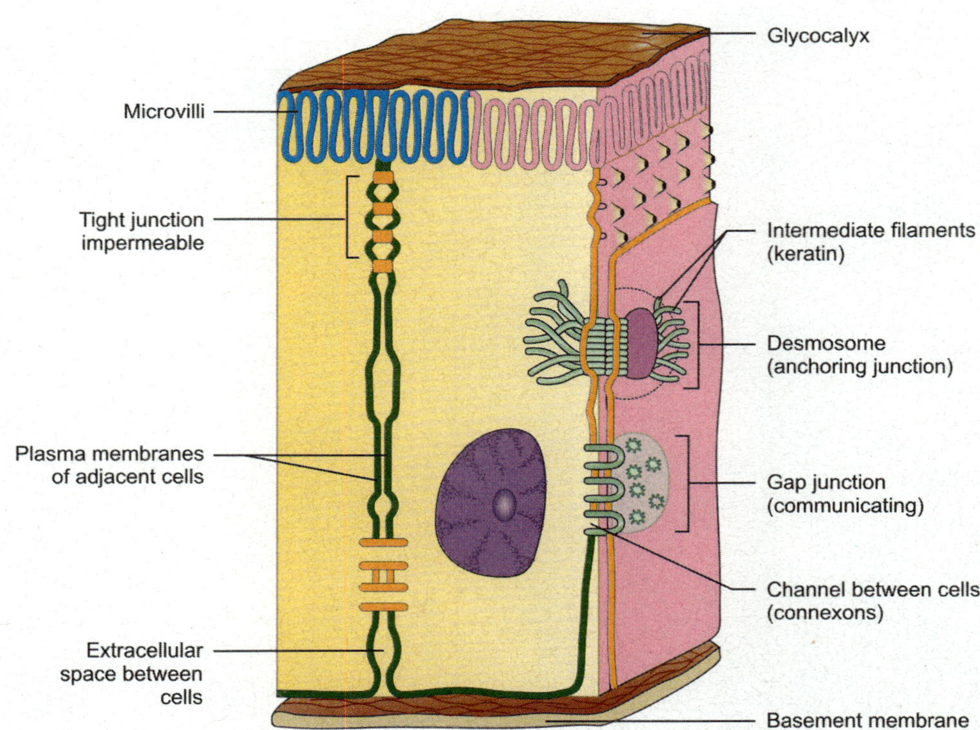

Fig. 2.1: Intercellular junctions in the mucosa of small intestine

attach cell to the extracellular matrix. They are asymmetrical and are found in epithelial cells, generally connecting basal surface of keratinocytes in the dermis of skin. For example, in teeth they attach junctional epithelium to the enamel.

4. **Tight junction:** They are otherwise called zonula occludens. They are tight areas between two cells whose membrane join together forming a virtually impermeable barrier to fluid. Tight junctions join together the cytoskeletons of adjacent cells. They are composed of a branching network of sealing strands, each strand acting independently from others. Therefore, the efficiency of the junctions in preventing ion passage increases exponentially with the number of strands.

   The main function is to:
   1. Hold cells together
   2. Maintain polarity
   3. Prevent passage of molecules and ions through the space between cells. For example, blood brain barrier in the brain, walls of renal tubules.

   Applied physiology: Mutation in the gene for tight junction leads to hereditary deafness.

INTERCELLULAR COMMUNICATION

Cells communicate with each other via chemical messengers. These messengers either bind with receptors on the surface of cell or cytoplasm or nucleus and trigger sequence of changes to bring about physiological effects. There are three basic types namely:

1. *Endocrine:* In which hormones and growth factors reach cells via blood circulation.
2. *Paracrine:* Here the products of cell diffuse to the neighboring cells.
3. *Autocrine:* The chemicals released from cell bind to receptors on the same cell and bring about effect.

There is an other variant apart from basic type which is present in the central nervous system. It is the **neural communication** in which neuro-transmitters are released at the synaptic junctions from nerve cells and act on the postsynaptic cell. An additional type called **juxtacrine communication** is identified which is a type of intercellular communication that is transmitted via oligosaccharide, lipid, or protein components of a cell membrane, and may affect either the emitting cell or the immediately-adjacent cells. It occurs between adjacent cells that possess broad patches of closely-opposed plasma membrane linked by transmembrane channels known as connexon. The gap between the cells can usually be between only 2 and 4 nm. Unlike other types of cell signaling (such as paracrine and endocrine), juxtacrine signaling requires physical contact between the two cells involved. Juxtacrine signaling has been observed for some growth factors, cytokine cellular signals.

3. TRANSPORT ACROSS CELL MEMBRANE

Introduction

Cell membrane acts as a barrier to most, but not all molecules. Cell membranes are semipermeable barrier separating the inner cellular environment from the outer cellular environment. Since the cell membrane is made up of a lipid bilayer with proteins attached on the surface and also passing through the cell membrane, there is possibility of transport across this membrane. All lipid soluble substances can easily and freely diffuse in and out, e.g. O_2 and CO_2. Whereas water soluble substances like ions, glucose and macromolecules should find a special way of transport with the help of integral and transmembrane proteins which act as binding sites, channels and gates to facilitate movement. Transport across cell membrane is classified as (Fig. 2.2).

1. Diffusion (passive transport)
2. Osmosis
3. Active transport
4. Vesicular transport.

DIFFUSION (PASSIVE TRANSPORT)

It is the net movement of a substance (liquid or gas) from an area of higher concentration to lower concentration without expenditure of energy is called diffusion (Fig. 2.3).

Diffusion can be further divided as follows:

1. Simple diffusion
2. Facilitated diffusion.

2

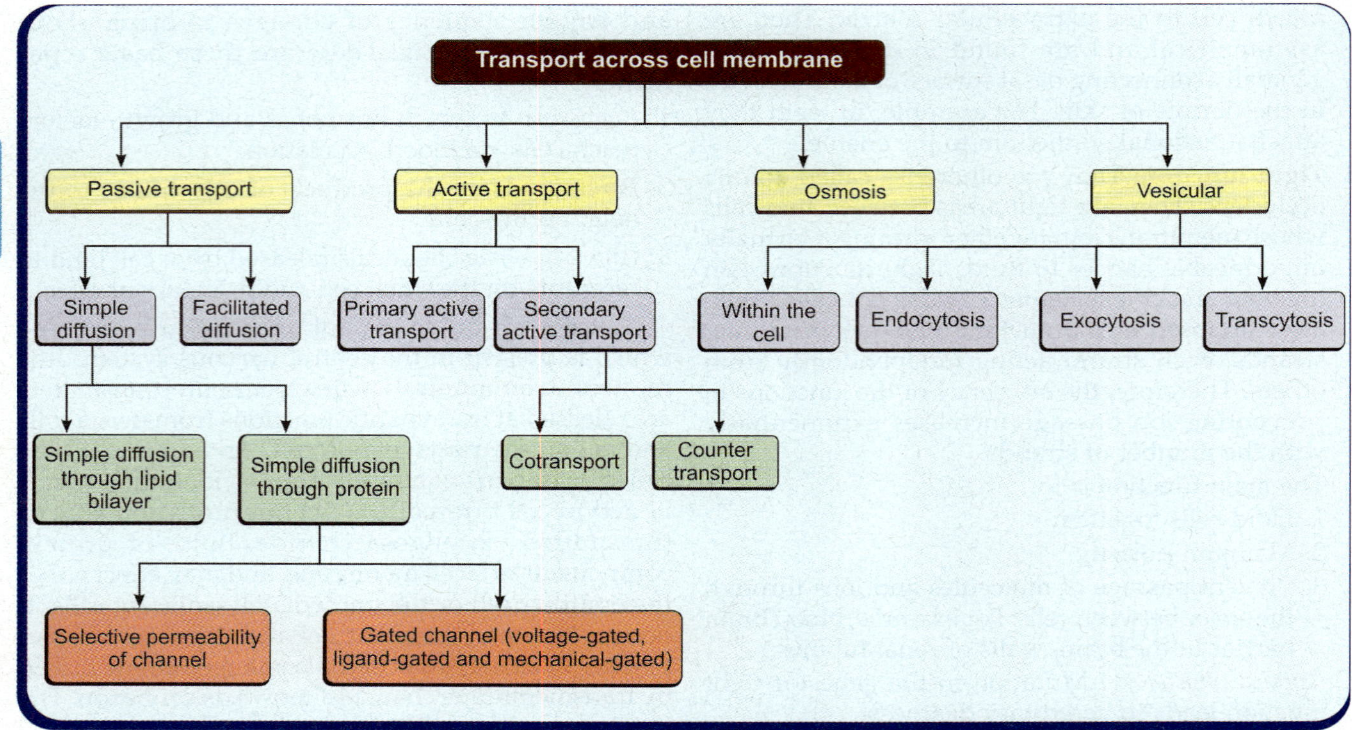

Fig. 2.2

Simple Diffusion

It is further classified into two categories:

1. Diffusion of lipid soluble substance through lipid bilayer.
2. Diffusion of lipid insoluble substance through protein channels.

Diffusion of lipid soluble substance through the lipid bilayer: Substance like oxygen and carbon dioxide and alcohols are highly lipid soluble and dissolve in the layer easily and diffuse through the membrane. The rate of diffusion is determined by the solubility of the substance. For example, exchange of gases in the lungs.

Diffusion of lipid insoluble substance through protein channels: This is possible through either selective permeability of protein channel or through gated channels.

Selective permeability of protein channel: This channel can permit only one type of ion to pass through it. The selectivity is due to diameter, shape and electrical charges along the inner surface of the channel. For example:

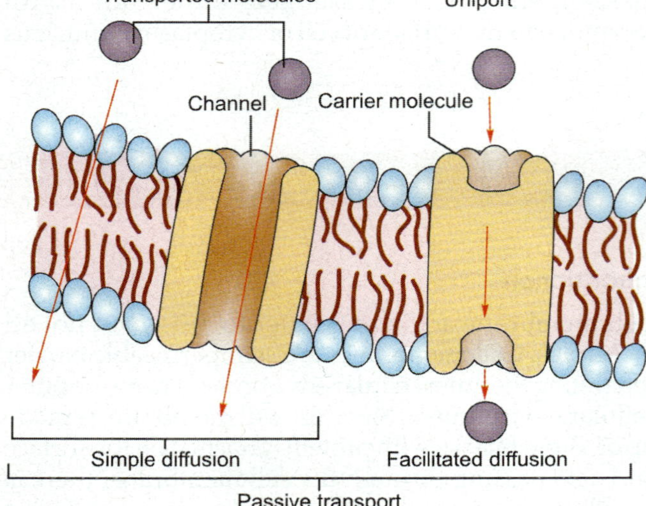

Fig. 2.3: Transport pathways through cell membrane and the basic mechanism of transport

a. *Sodium channels:* Sodium channel is a tetramer with a pore of 0.3 to 0.5 nm in diameter which is selective for sodium. It has strong negative charge on the inner surface which allows dehydrated sodium ion to diffuse in either direction from higher to lower concentration (Fig. 2.4).

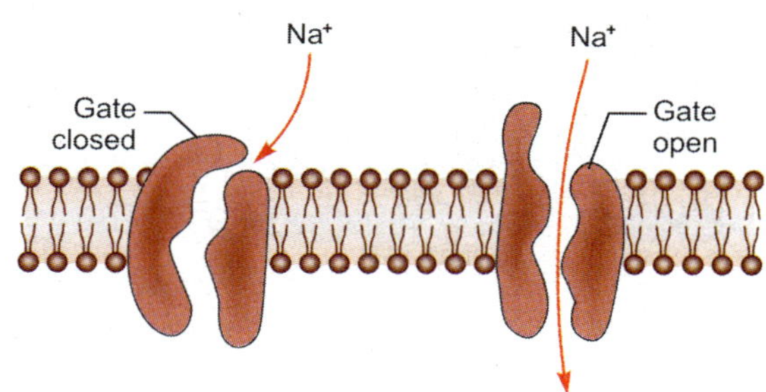

Fig. 2.4: Diffusion through protein channels

b. *Potassium channels:* It is selective for potassium. The pore of this channel is smaller than sodium channel and is not negatively charged. But hydrated form of potassium ion is smaller in size than sodium and all thus allows selectively permits potassium ion to diffuse (Fig. 2.5).

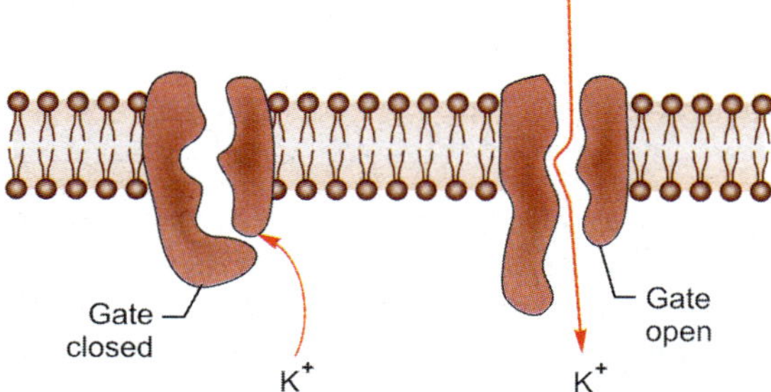

Fig. 2.5: Confirmational changes in protein molecules during gating of these channels

Diffusion through gated protein channels: A part of or projection from a protein channel behaves like a gate and can open or close in response to a change in voltage, ligand (chemical), mechanical stimuli like touch and stretch are called as voltage gated, ligand gated and mechanical gated channels respectively.

a. *Voltage-gated channels:* These channels open and close in response to change in electrical potential across the cell membrane.

   Example: Excitable cells like neurons and muscle cells. When the voltage across the membrane changes, the voltage-gated sodium channels open and allow flow of sodium ions into the cell which cause depolarization phase of action potential and outflow of potassium through voltage-gated potassium channel brings about repolarisation. This is basis of action potential in an excitable cell.

b. *Ligand (chemical) gated channel:* Some channels open in response to a chemical substance. They can be internal ligand, where binding side is on the cytosol side of channel (Fig. 2.6). For example, second messengers. There can also be external ligand which binds to a site on the extracellular side of the channel. For example: Neurotransmitters like acetylcholine, gamma-aminobutyric acid which transmits impulse in a synapse.

c. *Mechanical-gated channels:* They respond to mechanical stimulus and the deformation due to mechanical stimulus opens or closes the channel.

   Example: Pressure receptors when subject to pressure opens sodium channel and causes development of a receptor potential. This helps us to feel sense of pressure.

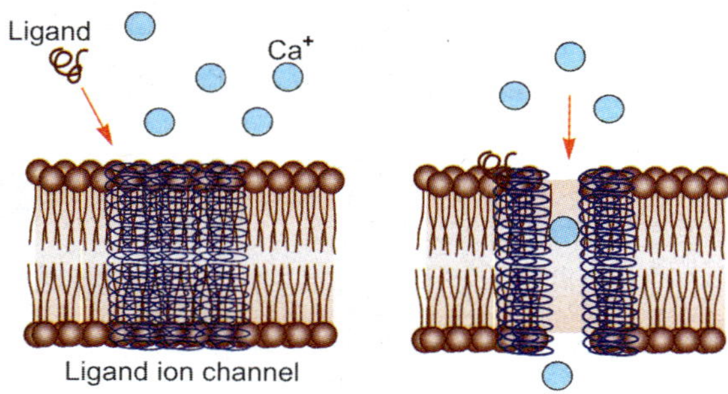

Fig. 2.6: Ligand-gated channels

Facilitated Diffusion

It is also called carrier mediated diffusion. Highly charged or big molecules which cannot pass through protein channels require carrier protein which facilitates the diffusion (Fig. 2.7). The carrier protein is selective for that particular substance. When a substance to be transported binds to a carrier protein on one side there is conformational change in the shape of the protein which carries the substance to the interior of the cell by opening to other side of membrane. It also obeys the law of diffusion (higher to lower concentration).

Example: Glucose transporters (GLUT) and amino acid transporters.

Factors that affect net rate of diffusion

Factors that are directly proportional to diffusion

1. Concentration gradient across the membrane
2. Electrical and pressure gradient across the membrane

2

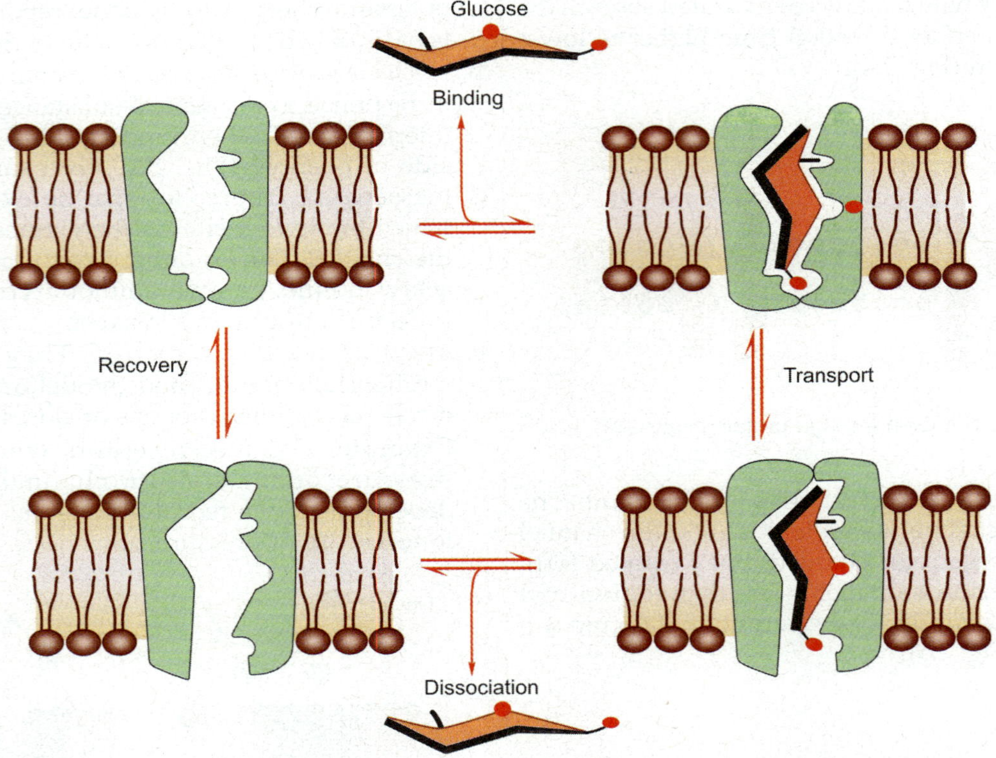

Fig. 2.7: Facilitated diffusion

3. Solubility of the substance
4. Body temperature
5. Permeability of cell membrane.

Factors that are inversely proportional to diffusion

1. Thickness of cell membrane
2. Size of ion/molecule.

Applied physiology: Local anesthetics act directly on gates of the sodium channel, making it difficult to open and thereby reducing excitability of the cell. The impulse fails to travel causing anesthesia.

Ion channel mutation is called as chanellopathies. They affect muscle and brain tissue mainly:

1. *Sodium channel disease:* Muscle spasm and Liddle's syndrome.
2. *Potassium channel disease:* Arrhythmia, seizures in newborn and inherited deafness.
3. *Chloride channel disease:* Kidney stones and cystic fibrosis.

OSMOSIS

Osmosis is net movement or diffusion of water molecules across a semipermeable membrane from a region of higher concentration to lower concentration of water (solvent) or in other words movement of water from a region of low concentration of solute (namely salts and electrolytes) to higher concentration of solute (Fig. 2.8).

Osmotic Pressure

If a pressure is applied to the sodium chloride solution, osmosis of water into the solution is stopped, reversed or slowed. The pressure required to stop osmosis is called as osmotic pressure. Osmotic pressure is determined by the number of particles per unit volume of fluid and not by the mass of the particle.

Osmolality and Osmolarity

A mole is gram molecular weight of substance. One osmole is equal to gram molecular weight of a substance divided by the number of particles in a solution. So osmolarity is the number of osmoles per liter of a solution. Osmolality is the number of osmoles per kg of solvent. Osmotically active substance are dissolved in the body water, so osmolarity is expressed as milliosmoles (mOsm) per liter of water.

2

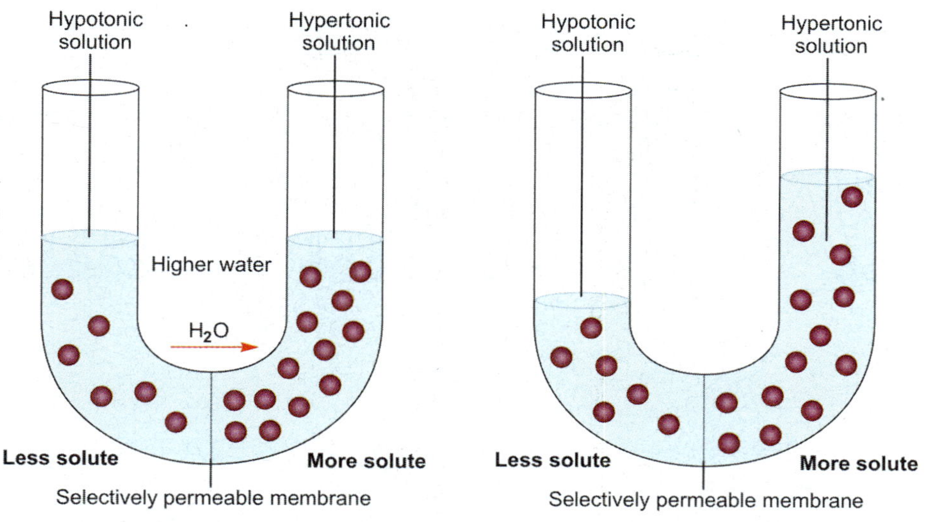

Fig. 2.8: Demonstration of osmotic pressure caused by osmosis at a semipermeable membrane

Colloid osmotic pressure: It is the pressure exerted by the colloids present in the solution.

Oncotic Pressure

The colloid osmotic pressure exerted by the plasma proteins is known as ***oncotic*** pressure.

Tonicity: It is the used to describe the osmolality of a solution relative to plasma. If a solution has same osmolality or increased or decreased osmolality as plasma it is said to be isotonic, hypertonic and hypotonic solution respectively.

Applied physiology: Any solution used for fluid replacement, the tonicity of the solution has to be considered depending on the clinical situation.

ACTIVE TRANSPORT

When a substance moves across the cell membrane against concentration or electrical gradient (uphill) with the expenditure of energy it is called active transport. The energy is obtained from the breakdown of high energy compounds like ATP. They are classified as primary and secondary active transport according to the source of energy utilized. The transporter involved here is also carrier protein. But it is different from that in facilitated diffusion. Here the carrier protein is capable of imparting energy to the transported substance to move against gradient.

Primary Active Transport

In the primary active transport, the energy is liberated directly from the break down of ATP and the carrier protein involved here is called as pump. The enzymes which catalyze the hydrolysis of ATP are called ATPases. Hence these pumps are called as ATPases.

Sodium Potassium Pumps or Sodium Potassium ATPases

Location: Almost all cells have Na^+ K^+ pumps especially in all excitable cells (Fig. 2.9).

Structure: It has two subunits namely α and β subunits. Separation of subunit eliminates activity but the function of β subunit is unknown. α subunit has:

a. Three receptor sites for binding sodium ion on the protein that protrudes to the interior of the cell.
b. Two receptor sites of potassium ions on the outside of the cell.
c. One site of ATPase enzyme which is near to the binding site for sodium.

Mechanism of action: The function is to pump out excess Na^+ from the intracellular fluid and to draw in K^+ into the cell. Since there are 3 sites for Na^+ and 2 sites for K^+, the pump gets activated only when three Na^+ ion and two K^+ ion attaches to the interior and exterior surface of the cell respectively. For every three sodium ions expelled out of cell, two potassium ions are drawn in. Thus, there is a net loss of positive charge (ion) out of the cell, which initiates osmosis of water out of the cell as well as prevents any cell from swelling.

The above mechanism also creates positivity outside the cell but leaves a deficit of positive ions inside the cell. Therefore the Na^+ K^+ pump is said to

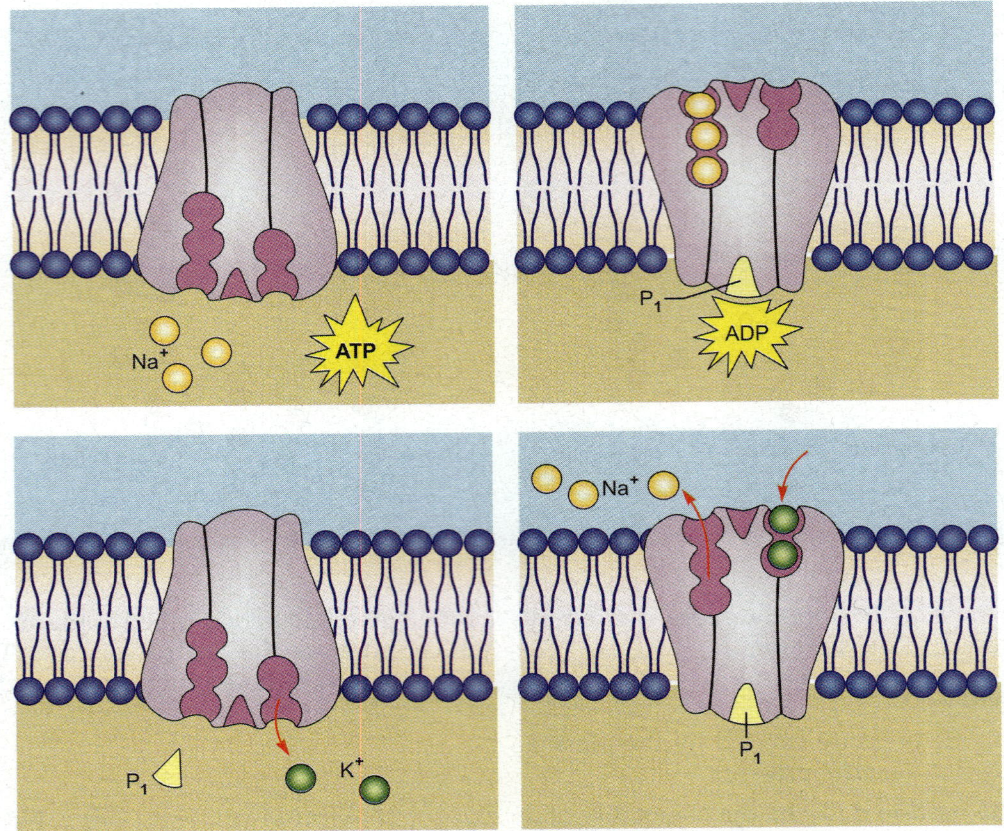

Fig. 2.9: Primary active transport

be electrogenic because it creates an electrical potential across the cell membrane as it pumps. This is required for genesis of resting membrane potential (RMP) which is the membrane potential across the cell membrane at rest.

Functions

1. It controls the volume of the cells
2. Maintains resting membrane potential.

Applied physiology: Digitalis is a drug used in management of congestive cardiac failure. It inhibits sodium potassium pump. This causes increase in ICF sodium. This decreases calcium efflux through sodium calcium antiport by decreasing sodium influx. This finally increases calcium concentration in the myocardial cells which increases myocardial contractility.

Hydrogen Potassium ATPases

Location: Gastric glands of stomach and distal convoluted tubules of nephron.

Functions

1. In parietal cells of the gastric glands it transports hydrogen ions. At the secretory end of these cells hydrogen is pumped into stomach along with chloride ions to form hydrochloric acid which is the main composition of gastric juice.
2. Intercalated cells in the distal tubules of the nephron pumps hydrogen ions for the formation of urine and controls pH in the body.

Secondary Active Transport

In some places, due to active transport of Na^+ out of cells by Na^+ K^+ pump, a large concentration gradient of sodium usually develops with high concentration outside than inside. This gradient stores free energy which is used to transport other substances like glucose and amino acid and other ions against their concentration gradient. The energy spent is not directly due to hydrolysis of ATP but stored energy due to primary active transport. Secondary active

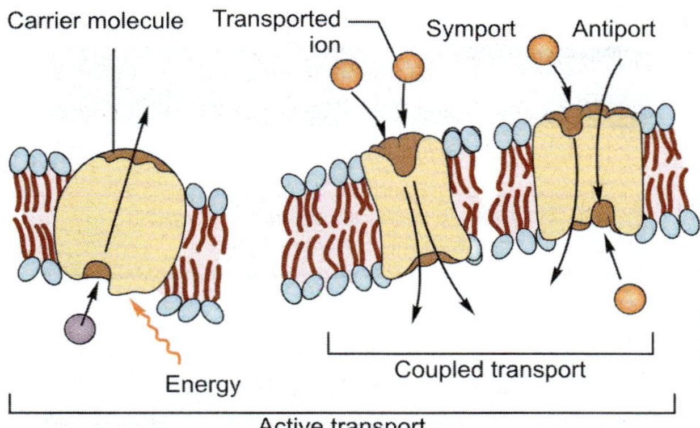

Fig. 2.10: Secondary active transport

transport is of two types: (a) Cotransport, (b) Counter transport (Fig. 2.10).

- *Cotransport:* Otherwise called symport. Here sodium and other substance that is be transported moves in the same direction.

  For example: Sodium glucose cotransport in proximal convoluted tubule of nephron: Here carrier protein undergoes conformational change and ready for transporting only when sodium and glucose attaches to it and both moves in same direction. The energy is obtained from the stored energy due to sodium transport by Na^+ K^+ pump on the basolateral membrane of the tubule. This creates a high concentration gradient for sodium ion inside the tubular cell. Thereby the stored energy due to the gradient is used for sodium as well as glucose transport along with it along the luminal side of the tubule.

- *Counter transport:* Otherwise called antiport. Here sodium and other substances to be transported move in the opposite direction.

  For example: Sodium calcium antiport in myocardial cells.

2

Vesicular Transport

They are classified as:

1. Vesicle transport within the cell
2. Endocytosis
3. Exocytosis
4. Transcytosis

Vesicle Transport within the Cell

Vesicles that help in transport of proteins from one organelle to the other within the cell have protein coats namely caveolin, clathrin 1, clathrin 2 and so on. These protein coats are specific for transport to specific organelle. A particular protein on vesicle will latch with its corresponding pair protein on the target so that vesicle makes sure that it docks to the correct destination. In general, vesicle move along microtubule motors like dynamin (Fig. 2.11).

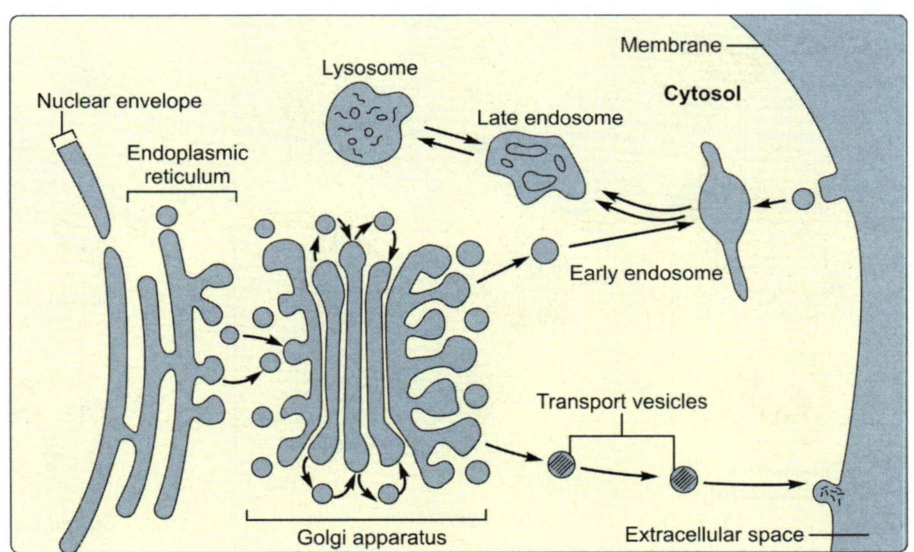

Fig. 2.11: Vesicle transport within the cell

2

Endocytosis

Endocytosis and exocytosis can also be considered under vesicle transport because this type of transport occurs by forming vesicle. Endocytosis is a process by which substance are engulfed by the cells. For example: Bacteria and dead tissue engulfed by WBC (Fig. 2.12).

- Receptor mediated endocytosis: Endocytosis can also be specific if it is receptor mediated called as receptor mediated endocytosis (Fig. 2.13). Here the molecule or ligand attach to the specific receptor on the cell membrane, which are present in pits called clathrin pits on the cell membrane. Clathrin molecules have three legs radiating from a central point that surrounds the endocytic vesicle and is pinched off into the cytoplasm. Once vesicle is formed, clathrin falls off and reutilized. The vesicle then reaches the target (Fig. 2.14). For example: Vitamins, transferrin and cholesterol entry into the cell.

Exocytosis

It is a reverse pinocytosis where substances synthesized within the secretory cells are secreted out of the cell. The secretory vesicle moves to the inside of the cell membrane and fuses with them. The contents are extruded and vesicle membrane becomes a part of cell membrane (Fig. 2.15). For example, release of neurotransmitters.

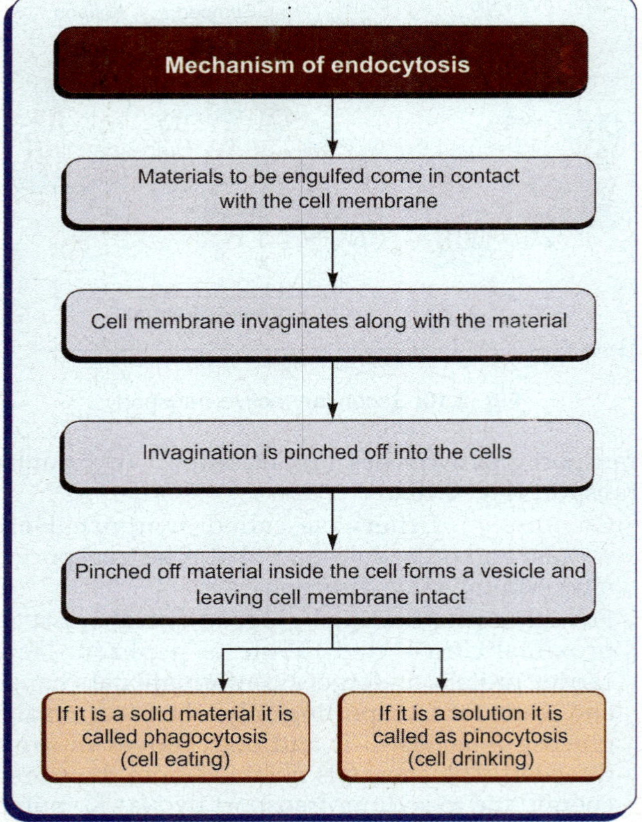

Fig. 2.12

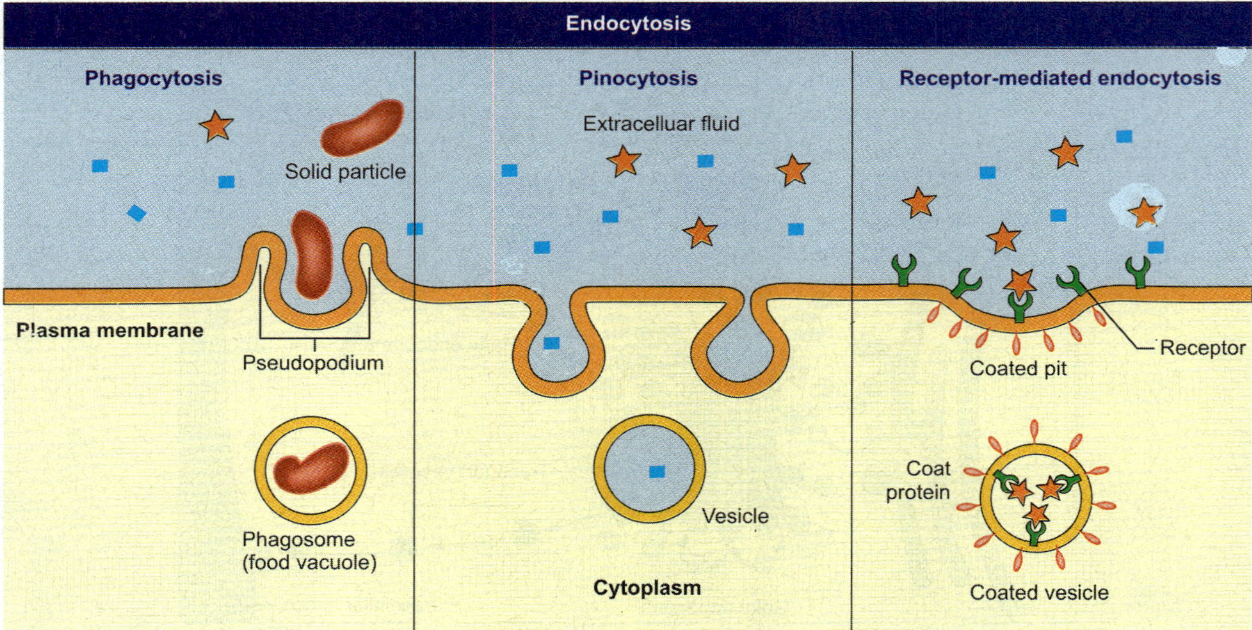

Fig. 2.13: Endocytosis

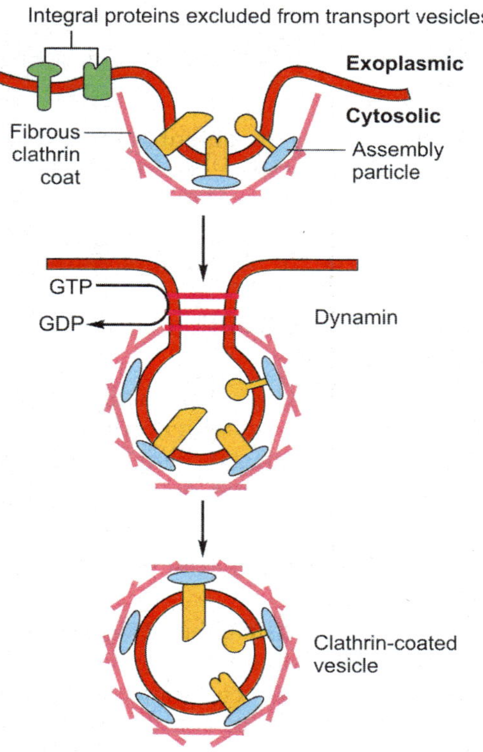

Fig. 2.14: Clathrin-mediated endocytosis

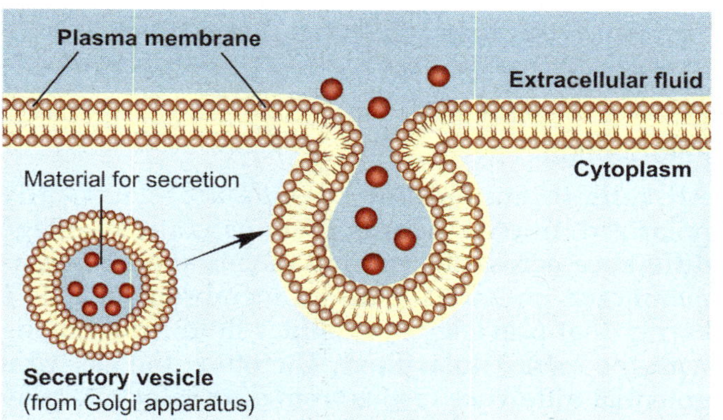

Fig. 2.15: Process of exocytosis

Both endocytosis and exocytosis maintains cell membranes surface area.

Transcytosis

It is otherwise called as *cytopempsis*. The mechanism involves the endocytosis of the vesicle at one side of the membrane and exocytosis at the opposite side. The binding site of the vesicle has caveolin coated pits. For example, transport of nutrients across endothelial cells of blood vessels to the interstitial fluid (Fig. 2.16).

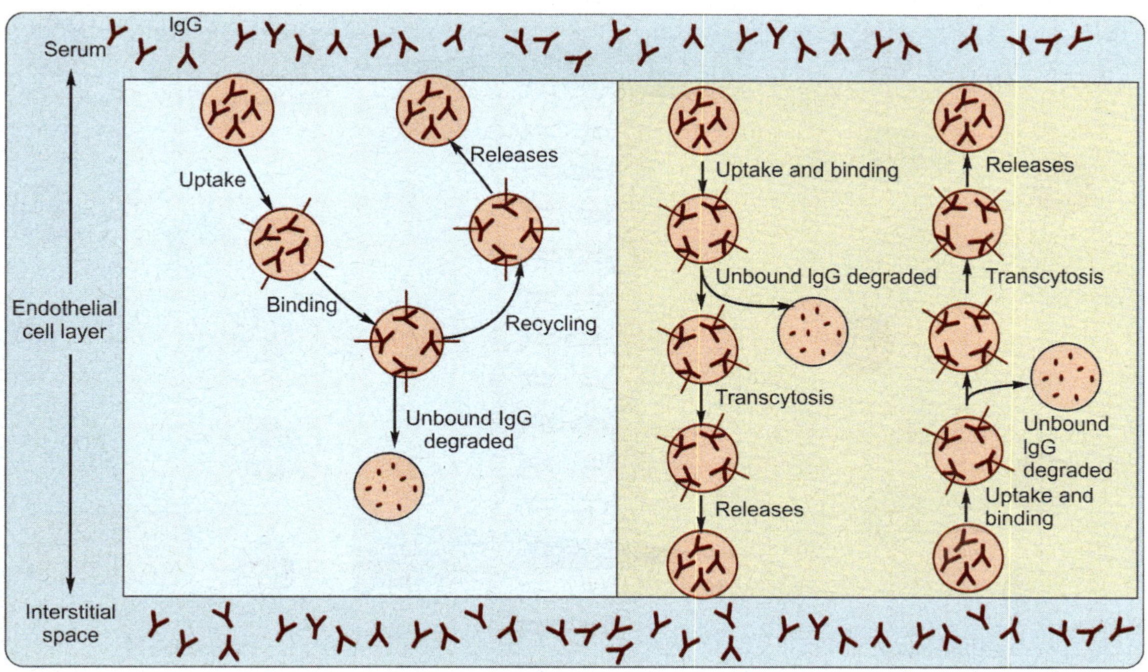

Fig. 2.16: Process of transcytosis

4. MEMBRANE POTENTIAL

2

Introduction

All cells in animal body tissue are electrically polarized, in other words they maintain a voltage difference across the plasma membrane known as membrane potential. The cell membrane acts as a barrier that prevents intracellular fluid from mixing with the extracellular fluid. Therefore, the electrical potential difference results from a complex interplay between protein structures embedded in the membrane called ion pumps and ion channels. Membrane potential is classified as:

1. Resting membrane potential
2. Action potential
3. Graded potential.

GENESIS OF RESTING MEMBRANE POTENTIAL

The membrane potential across the cell membrane when the cell is at rest is called resting membrane potential (RMP). We always express RMP by comparing ICF potential to ECF potential keeping ECF potential to be zero. For example: RMP for large nerve fibre is –90 mV. That is the potential inside the fiber is 90 millivolts more negative than the ECF potential. The nerve cell at this state is said to be in polarized state. RMP in a cell is generated due to two reasons: (a) Simple diffusion, (b) Sodium potassium pump.

Contribution of Simple Diffusion to the Genesis of RMP

Simple diffusion through protein channels like sodium and potassium channels, which allows movement down the concentration gradient is influenced by factors such as size, charge on surface of protein, hydration of the ion, etc. (Fig. 2.17).

Biophysical basis for membrane potential caused by simple diffusion alone.

a. *Gibbs-Donnan effect:* The Gibbs-Donnan effect (also known as the Donnan effect, Donnan law, Donnan equilibrium, or Gibbs-Donnan equilibrium) is a name for the behavior of charged particles near a semipermeable membrane which sometimes fail to distribute evenly across the two sides of the

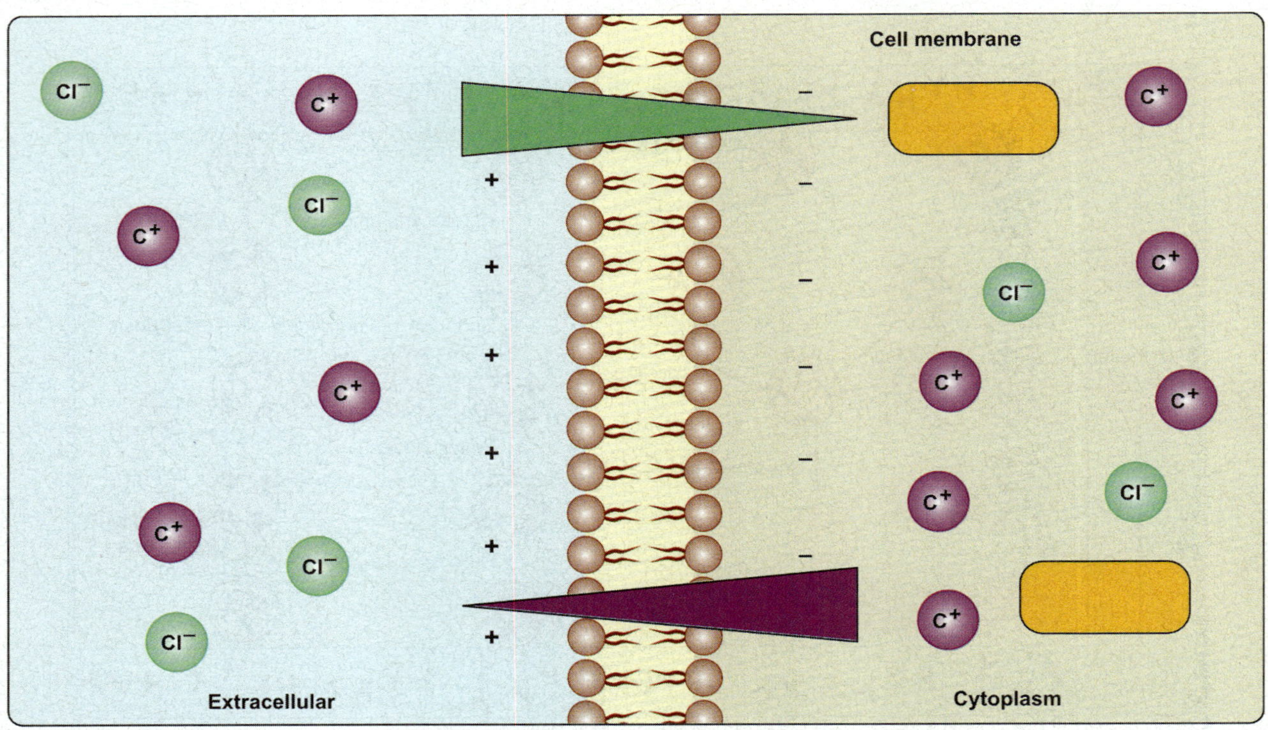

Fig. 2.17: Simple diffusion

membrane. The usual cause is the presence of a different charged substance that is unable to pass through the membrane and thus creates an uneven electrical charge. In the body, it is the Gibbs-Donnan effect of intracellular negatively charged protein forms the basis of the negative resting membrane potential. If it was not for the electrogenic activity of Na/K ATPases the resting membrane potential would be even more negative. This forms the basis for equilibrium potential of ions.

b. *Equilibrium potential and Nernst equation:* Particular ion will flow across a membrane from the higher concentration to the lower concentration (down a concentration gradient), causing a current. However, this creates a voltage difference across the membrane that opposes the movement of ions. When this voltage reaches the equilibrium value, the two balances (concentration gradient and the voltage) and the flow of ion stops. The voltage at which the flow of the ion stops is called the equilibrium potential of that ion. The equilibrium potential for any ion can be calculated by a equation called Nernst equation. Equilibrium potential for potassium is –94 mV, equilibrium potential for sodium is +61 mV. For example: Equation for calculating the equilibrium potential for potassium is as follows:

$$\text{Eeq K}^+ = \frac{\text{RT ln}[\text{K}^+]\text{o}}{\text{zF}[\text{K}^+]\text{i}}$$

Where

- Eeq K^+ is the equilibrium potential for potassium in volts
- R is the gas constant
- T is the absolute temperature
- Z is the number of elementary charge of the ion
- F is Faraday constant
- $[K^+]$ o is ECF concentration of potassium
- $[K^+]$ i is ICF concentration of potassium
- RT is a constant and the value is calculated as 61 and formula can be written as
- ZF

$$\text{Eeq} = +61 \log \frac{\text{Concentration of the ion in ICF}}{\text{Concentration of the ion in ECF}}$$

c. *Goldman-Hodgkin-Katz equation:* If membrane is permeable to only one ion, the membrane potential is the equilibrium potential of that ion. But in reality, animal cell is permeable to many ions. So the membrane potential has to be calculated taking equilibrium potential of all ions into consideration. Hence, membrane potential depends on:

1. Polarity of electric charge of each ion
2. Permeability of membrane
3. Concentration of ion in ICF and ECF.

The major ions involved in generating membrane potential are sodium, potassium and chloride. Membrane potential can be calculated from Goldman-Hodgkin-Katz equation

$$\text{Eeq} = -61 \log \frac{(\text{C Na}^+ \text{ i PNa}^+) + (\text{Ck}^+ \text{i Pk}^+) + (\text{CCl}^- \text{ o PCl}^-)}{(\text{C Na}^+ \text{ o PNa}^+) + (\text{Ck}^+ \text{o Pk}^+) + (\text{CCl}^- \text{ i PCl}^-)}$$

Where P is permeability of the cell membrane to the ion. Due to the negative charge of chloride ion, the concentration of chloride in ECF is written in the numerator.

Note: At rest the cell membrane is 100 times more permeable to potassium diffusion than sodium because the hydrated form of potassium is smaller in size compared to that of hydrated form of sodium ion. This is reason why RMP will be close to equilibrium potential of potassium.

Contribution of Sodium Potassium Pump for the Genesis of RMP

It is an electrogenic pump which pumps three Na^+ to ECF and two K^+ to ICF against concentration gradient leaving a net deficient of one positive ion on the inside, which causes a negative voltage inside the cell membrane. Let us calculate the RMP of the large nerve fiber:

i. The resting membrane potential of large nerve fiber, if potassium alone is considered as permeable is –94 mV which is calculated from Nernst equation.
ii. The RMP if sodium alone is considered will be +61 mV.
iii. But actually RMP is due to both sodium and potassium which can be calculated from Goldman equation to be –86 mV, which is nearest to equilibrium potential of potassium.
iv. But still we have –4 mV left to get –90 mV as RMP in large nerve fiber. What it is due to? It is due to the sodium potassium pump which leaves negativity inside the cell contributing to –4 mV by pumping an extra positive charge outside the cell.
v. So totally –86 mV and –4 mV negativity inside the cell is due to simple diffusion and active

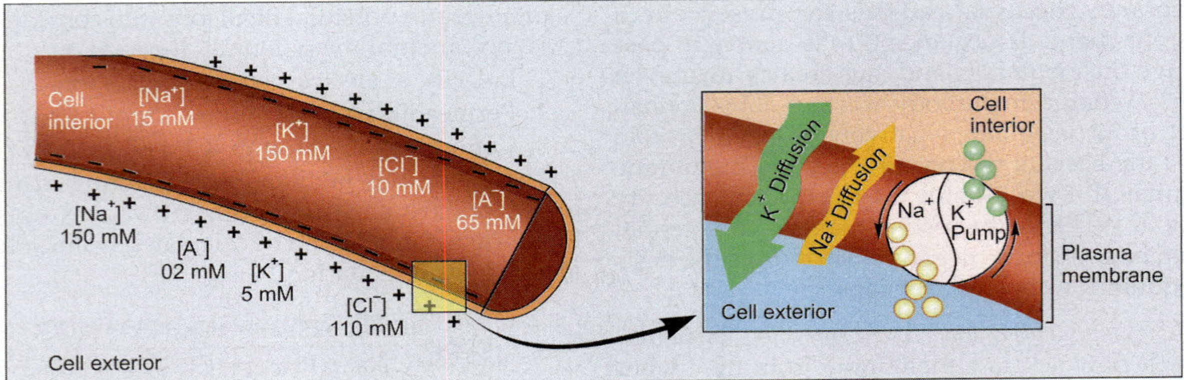

Fig. 2.18

transport respectively which contributes to –90 mV RMP in large nerve fiber.

Note: For calculating RMP in a muscle, calcium ion should also be considered for calculating Goldman equation (Fig. 2.18).

ACTION POTENTIAL (AP)

An action potential is a short lasting event in which the electrical membrane potential of cell rapidly rise and fall after sufficient strength of a stimulus is applied (during action). This occurs in excitable cell like neurons and muscle cell. In neurons, they play a central role in cell to cell communication (Fig. 2.19). In muscle cell, AP is the first step in chain of events leading to contraction.

The stages of action potential:

1. *Resting (polarized) stage:* This is the membrane potential before the stimulus, i.e. RMP and the membrane is said to be polarized.
2. *Depolarization stage:* After the sufficient stimulus to an excitable cell, there occurs a change in voltage which opens the voltage gated sodium channel, (Sodium permeability is more than potassium during action in contrast to what it is at rest) allowing tremendous flow of positively charged sodium ions through voltage gated sodium channels by simple diffusion to the interior of cell. The membrane potential which was negative compared with outside, now rapidly shifts to positive side due to flow of positive charge sodium ion. This shift from negative to positive potential is called as depolarization (i.e. polarized to depolarized state).
3. *Repolarization stage:* The gated channel is open only 1/10000th of a second. Within a few 10000th of a second the sodium channels begin to close. But the voltage for opening potassium channel is attained, and therefore, voltage gated potassium channel opens. Since K^+ is more inside, the potassium flows tremendously to the outside of the cell (Fig. 2.20). This rapid diffusion of K^+ which is also a positive charge to outside of the cell, re-establishes the negative RMP. This stage is called repolarization stage. After a fraction of second the gated potassium channel closes.

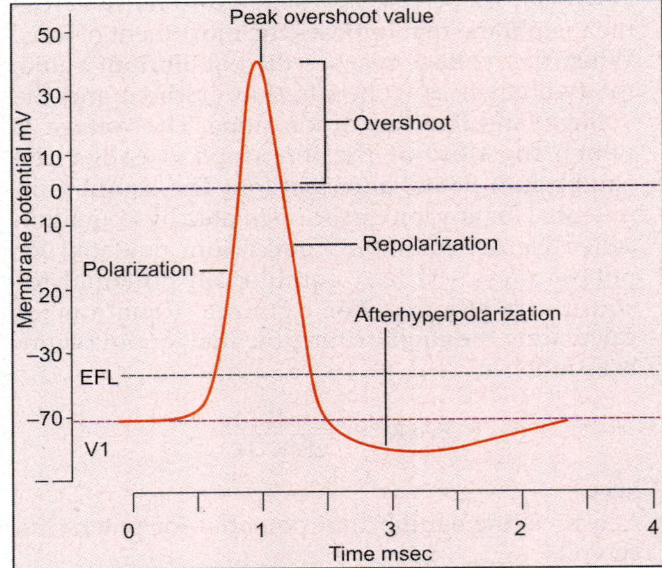

Fig. 2.19: Monophasic action potential

The ionic basis with an example of action potential in a large nerve fiber is explained in Chart 2.1

Propagation of Action Potential

An action potential elicited at any one point on an excitable membrane usually excites the adjacent portion of the membrane, resulting in propagation of

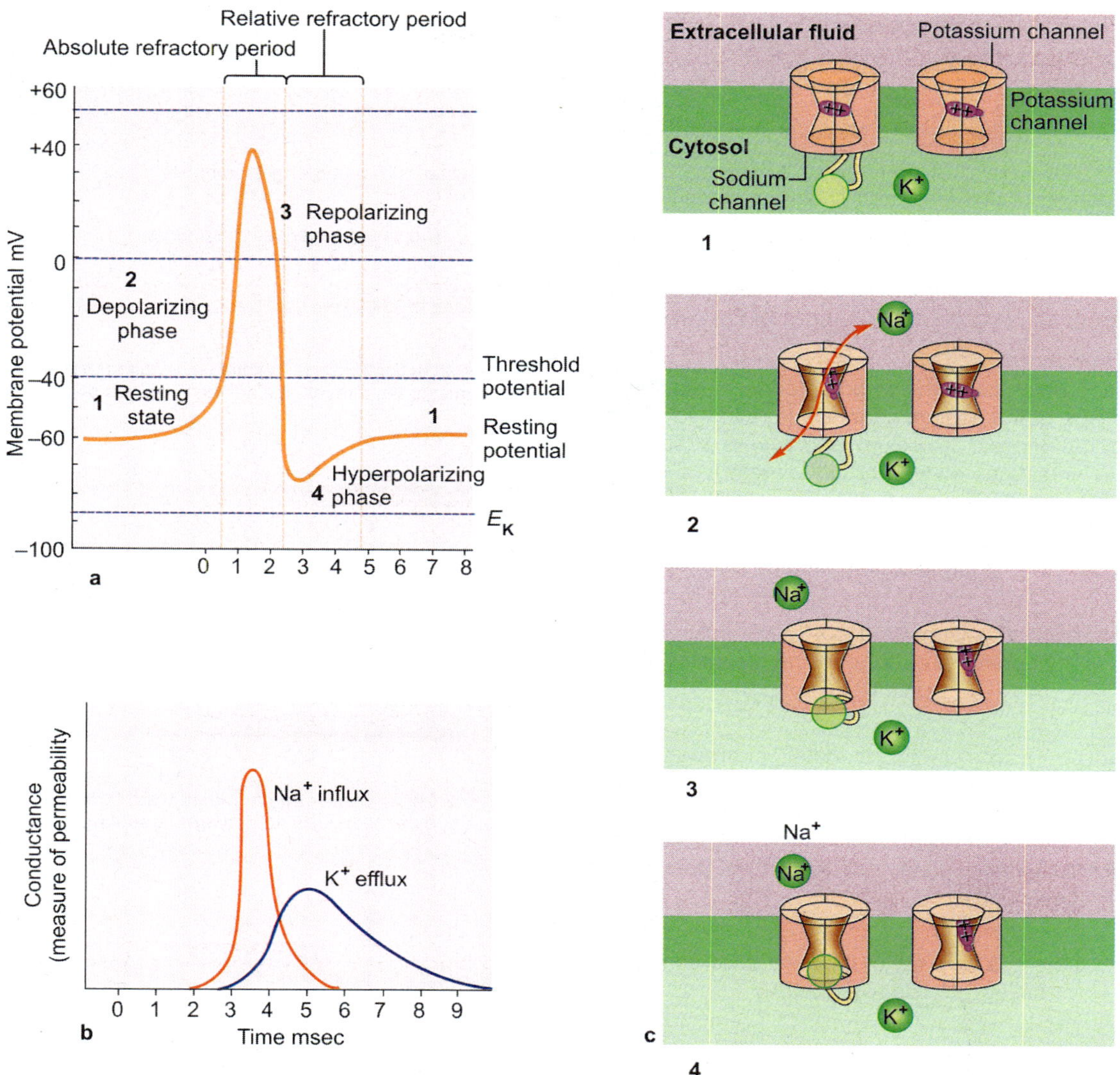

Figs 2.20a to c: (a) Diagram expanded to show the events; (b) Changes in sodium and potassium conductance during the course of an action potential; (c) Ionic fluxes during the action potential

action potential over the membrane. The local change in potential is carried inwards to several millimeter of adjacent membrane in both the directions, which slowly opens more Na^+ channel. This newly depolarized area in the same manner propagates the action potential. This transmission of depolarization process is called an impulse (Fig. 2.21).

Saltatory Conduction

The need for fast transmission of electrical signals in nervous system results in myelination of neuronal axons. Myelin sheath around axons is separated by intervals known as nodes of Ranvier. In saltatory conduction, an action potential at one node of Ranvier caused inward current that depolarize the membrane at the next node, provoking a new action potential, the AP hops from node to node because myelin offers resistance in internodal intervals (Fig. 2.22). The significance of this is that

1. The conduction of AP is faster.
2. The energy is conserved, which otherwise requires lot of energy if it travels through the entire neuron.

2

Chart 2.1

RMP nerve fibre is –90 mV (resting stage)
↓
Sufficient strength of a stimulus is applied
↓
Opening of voltage-gated sodium channel
↓
Sodium flows slowly from outside to inside through these channels thereby slowly decreasing the negativity inside the cell to –50 mV to –70 mV (threshold potential)
↓
Once firing potential or threshold potential is reached, more voltage gated sodium channels is recruited which causes rapid inflow of sodium (sodium permeability increases by 500 to 5000 times)
↓
The voltage inside the cell shoots up to +35 mV. This is depolarization stage
↓
Inactivation of sodium gate at +35 mV occurs, but this is voltage required for opening the potassium gates
↓
Potassium pours from inside to outside through these channel because ICF potassium is more than ECF concentration of potassium. There is rapid fall of potential. This event brings back the potential towards negativity. This is repolarization stage (sharp rise and fall of potential is called spike potential)
↓
At the end there is slow fall of potential towards RMP called **afterdepolarization**
↓
Potassium channel is slow to close, so there is extra outflow of the potassium ion to the ECF
↓
More negativity than RMP is created called **afterhyperpolarization**
↓
Here comes Na^+ K^+ pump which is re-establish RMP

Note: There will be some extra flow of K^+ ions outside the cell because they are very slow to close. This causes afterhyperpolarization. The gates will not reopen until the membrane potential returns to the original RMP. This is possible only with the help of Na^+ K^+ pump which helps to re-establish the RMP

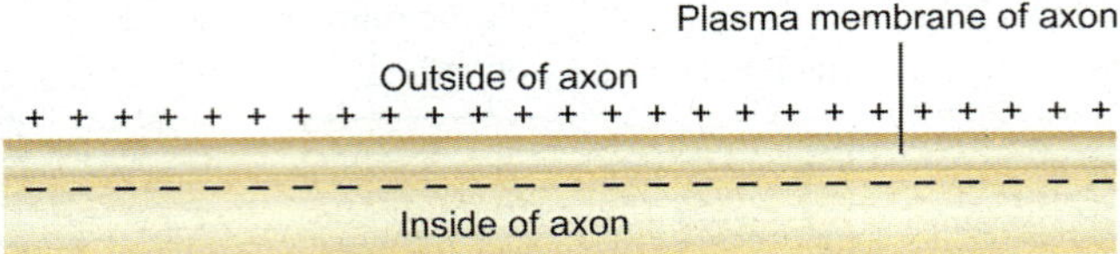

1. At the start the membrane is completely polarized.

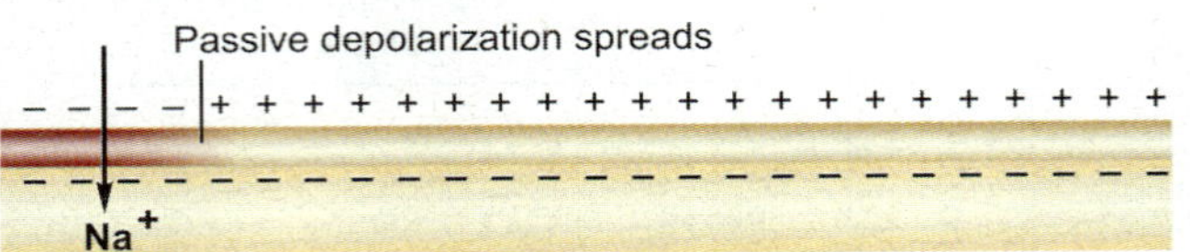

2. When an action potential is initiated, a region of membrane depolarizes. As a result, the adjacent regions become depolarize.

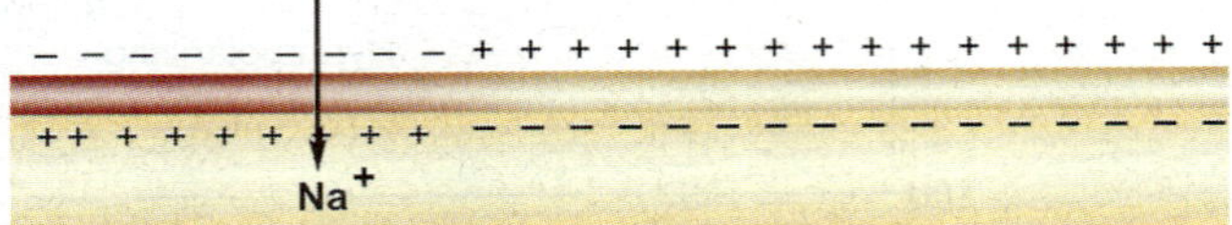

3. When the adjacent region depolarized to its threshold, action potential starts there.

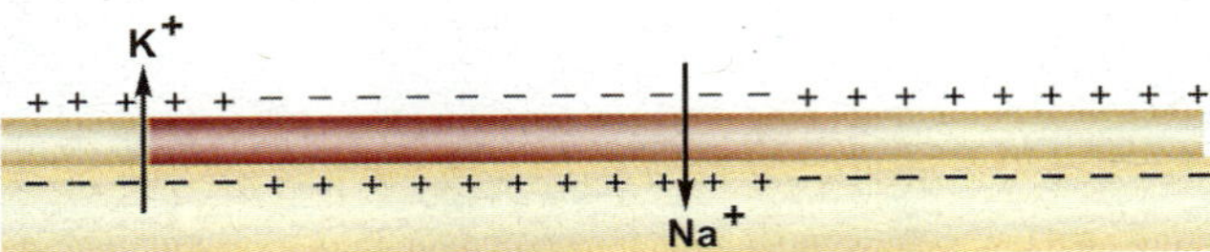

4. Repolarization occurs due to the outward flow of K^+ ions. The depolarization spreads forward, repeating the process.

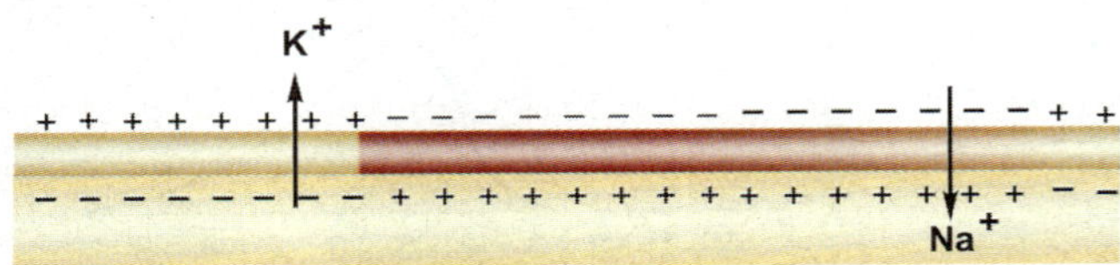

5. Depolarization spreads forward, repeating the process.

Fig. 2.21

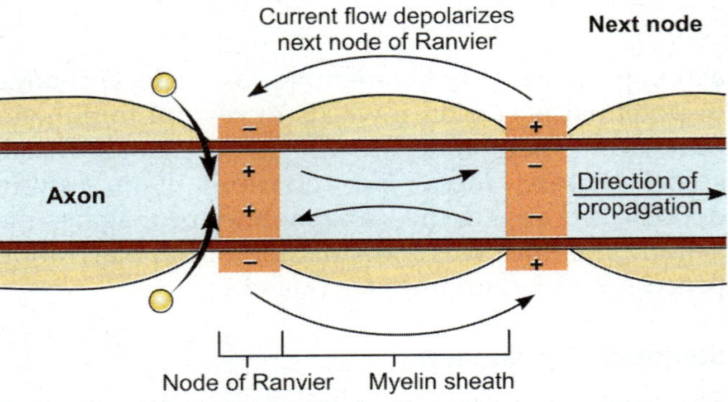

Fig. 2.22: Saltatory conduction

Properties of Action Potential

1. *All-or-none law:* States that a threshold or sub-threshold stimulus capable of producing action potential will produce the maximum possible amplitude of action potential or will not produce an action potential if the stimulus is subthreshold. In other words, large strength do not create large action potential, therefore, action potential are said to be all-or-none.
2. *Refractory period:* It is the period during which excitability of excitable tissue to second stimulus is decreased. It is divided into (Fig. 2.23):
   - *Absolute refractory period (ARP):* It is the period during which even a second strongest stimulus cannot produce an action potential. The period extends from firing level to one-third of repolarization stage of first action potential. This is responsible for unidirectional conduction of action potential in axon.

     Reason: Inactivation of sodium gates.
   - *Relative refractory period (RRP):* It is the period during which a stronger than normal stimulus can produce action potential. It extends from one-third of repolarisation stage to after depolarization.

     Reason: The excitability is increased but threshold is decreased, so you need stronger stimulus.
3. *Strength–duration curve:* This is a curve plotted to show the relationship of action potential with strength of a stimulus and duration of stimulus. A stimulus must be of adequate intensity and duration to evoke a response. If it is too short, even a strong pulse will not be effective. A long pulse below certain strength will evoke only a local non-propagated response (Fig. 2.24).

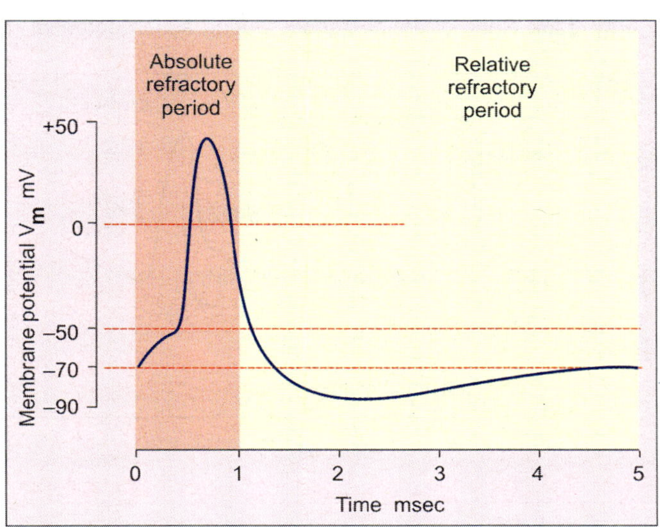

Fig. 2.23: Nerve action potential

Rheobase

It is the minimum threshold strength which can produce a action potential.

Chronaxie

It is duration for which twice the rheobase strength has to be applied to produce an action potential. It is the measure of excitability of the tissue. Chronaxie is inversely proportional to excitability.

Variations in Action Potential in other Tissues

- **Plateau in action potential:** For example, in cardiac muscle. This type action potential happens in cardiac muscle. The stages are:
  1. *Resting phase*
  2. *Depolarization phase:* Due to rapid sodium influx through voltage-gated sodium channel which is same as nerve action potential, but it is followed by
  3. *Plateau phase:* The membrane is held at high voltage for a few milliseconds prior to being repo-

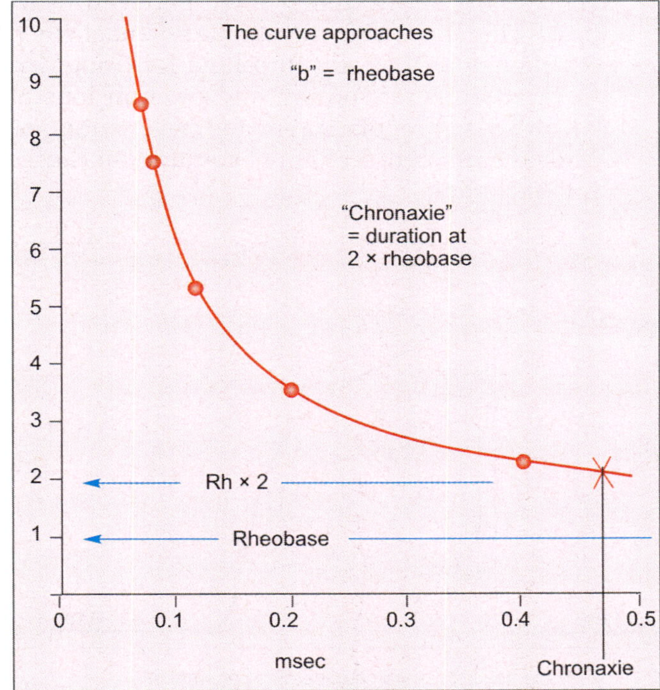

Fig. 2.24: Strength–duration curve

2

larized. This is due to two reasons: (a) voltage-gated calcium sodium channel, which is slow to open causing slow inflow of calcium and sodium, (b) voltage-gated potassium channel are slow to open which causes slow outflow of potassium, and therefore, potential remains in positivity for some time. This delays the return of membrane potential to resting level.

4. *Repolarization phase:* Due to rapid outflow of potassium through K^+ channels and closing of slow calcium sodium channel which returns the action potential to resting level.

- **Pacemaker potential:** For example, cardiac pacemaker and smooth muscle (Fig. 2.25).

The cardiac pacemaker cells of the sinoatrial node in the heart provide a good example. They have self induced rhythmical action potential without any stimulus. This is due to spontaneous excitability. This is attributed to two reasons:

1. The resting membrane potential of pacemaker cells is between –55 mV to –60 mV. It is very close to the threshold potential which makes the cells to depolarize easily.
2. The resting sinoatrial nodal cells have sodium leaking channel called funny channels that are already open to sodium. Without any stimulus, the sodium leak to the inside of the pacemaker cell causes a slow rising RMP between heart beats. This slow rising membrane potential when reaches –40 mV attains threshold for firing due to rapid entry of sodium and calcium ions at –40 mV. After repolarization the cycle continues. Thus the inherent leaking of sodium ion causes self-excitation.

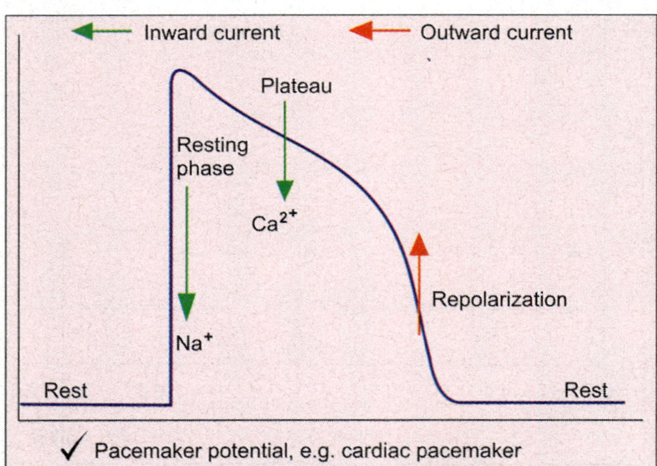

Fig. 2.25: Action potential in a ventricular muscle fiber

GRADED POTENTIAL

It is the localized change (depolarization or hyperpolarization) in the potential difference across a cell surface membrane. A strength of the graded potential varies with the intensity of the stimulus and causes local flows of current which decrease with distance from the stimulus point (Fig. 2.26). Graded potentials are given different names according to their function (Fig. 2.27). The membrane potential at any point in a cell's membrane is determined by the ion concentration differences between the intracellular and extracellular areas and by the permeability of the membrane to each type of ion. The ion concentrations do not normally change very quickly (with the exception of calcium,

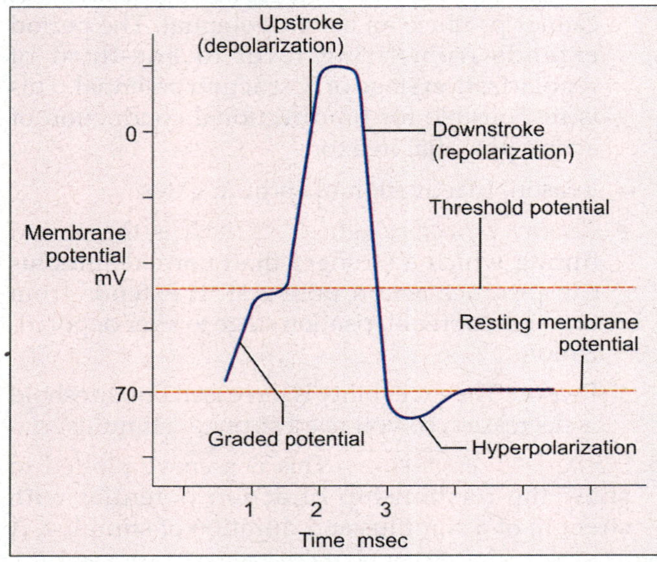

Fig. 2.26: Ratio of conductances during action potential

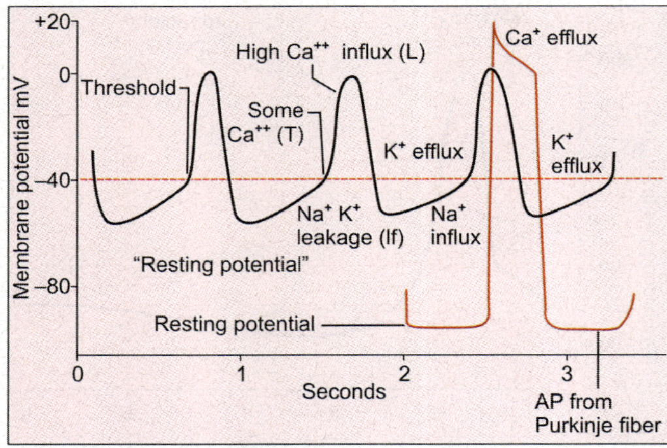

Fig. 2.27: Rhythmical action potentials similar to those recorded in the rhythmical control of the heart

where the baseline intracellular concentration is so low that even a small inflow may increase it by orders of magnitude), but the permeability can change in a fraction of a millisecond, as a result of activation of ligand-gated or voltage-gated ion channels. The change in membrane potential can be large or small, depending on how many ion channels are activated and what type they are. Changes of this type are referred to as graded potentials, in contrast to action potentials, which have a fixed amplitude and time course. Graded membrane potentials are particularly important in neurons, where they are produced by synapses: a temporary rise or fall in membrane potential produced by activation of a synapse is called a postsynaptic potential.

Comparison of Graded Potentials and Action Potentials

Characteristics	*Graded potentials*	*Action potentials*
Origin	Arise mainly in dendrites and cell bodies	Arise at trigger zones and propagate along axon
Types of channels	Chemical, mechanical, or light	Voltage-gated ion channels
Conduction	Not propagated, localized, thus permit communication over a few mm	Propagated, thus permit communication over long distances
Amplitude	Depends on strength of stimulus; varies from less than 1 mV to more than 50 mV	All-or-none, typically 100 mV
Duration	Longer, ranging from msec to several minutes	Shorter, ranging from 0.5–2 msec
Polarity	May be hyperpolarizing, depolarizing.	Always consist of depolarizing phase followed by repolarising phase and then return to resting membrane potential
Refractory period	No	Yes

5. HOMEOSTASIS

Human homeostasis refers to the body's ability to physiologically regulate its internal environment (milieu interior) to ensure its stability in response to fluctuation. Each body system contributes to the homeostasis of other system and of the entire organism. A disruption within one system generally has consequences for several additional body systems. Here are some examples of how various systems contribute to maintenance of homeostasis (Figs 2.28 and 2.29).

NERVOUS SYSTEM

- Nervous system along with the endocrine system serves as the primary control center of the body working below the consciousness.
- Hypothalamus of brain is the body's "thermostat". Humans are homeothermic and our cell metabolism functions only in a narrow range of temperature. Certain physiological mechanisms are activated by heat and cold to bring our body temperature to normal. The sensor is situated in the hypothalamus.
- Hypothalamus regulates the pituitary gland to release various hormones that control metabolism and development of the body.
- Nervous system regulates blood pressure, heart rate, respiration and gastrointestinal movement and secretion.

ENDOCRINE SYSTEM

Endocrine system consists of glands which secrete hormone into the blood stream. Each hormone has an effect on target tissue, which regulates metabolism and development of most body cells and system.

- Calcium homeostasis is by parathormone, calcitonin and vitamin D
- Glucose homeostasis is by insulin and glucagon secreted by endocrine pancreas.

SKIN

It is involved in protecting the body from invading microbes:

- Regulating body temperature through sweating and vasodilatation.
- Synthesizes vitamin D, which helps in calcium homeostasis.

2

SKELETAL SYSTEM

- It forms the structural framework for the human body. Bone and muscular system aid in posture and locomotion.
- Bones serve as mineral reserves.
- Bone synthesizes red blood cells and white blood cells.

LYMPHATIC SYSTEM

- Cardiac muscle pumps blood throughout the body
- Voluntary muscle (skeletal muscle) helps in walking skilled movements, etc.

CARDIOVASCULAR SYSTEM

It plays role in:

- Transporting nutrients, gases, hormones throughout the body by pumping blood through aorta.
- It maintains blood and tissue volume.
- Absorbs fatty acids and triglycerides.
- Defends the body against invading microbes.

RESPIRATORY SYSTEM

- Along with cardiovascular system it provides oxygen to cell for cellular metabolism and removes carbondioxide.
- Maintains blood pH by excreting carbon dioxide.

DIGESTIVE SYSTEM

Supplies regular supply of energy and nutrients by absorbing organic substances, vitamins, ions and water, which is needed by our body.

URINARY SYSTEM

- Toxic nitrogenous wastes accumulate as proteins and nucleic acid are broken down and used for

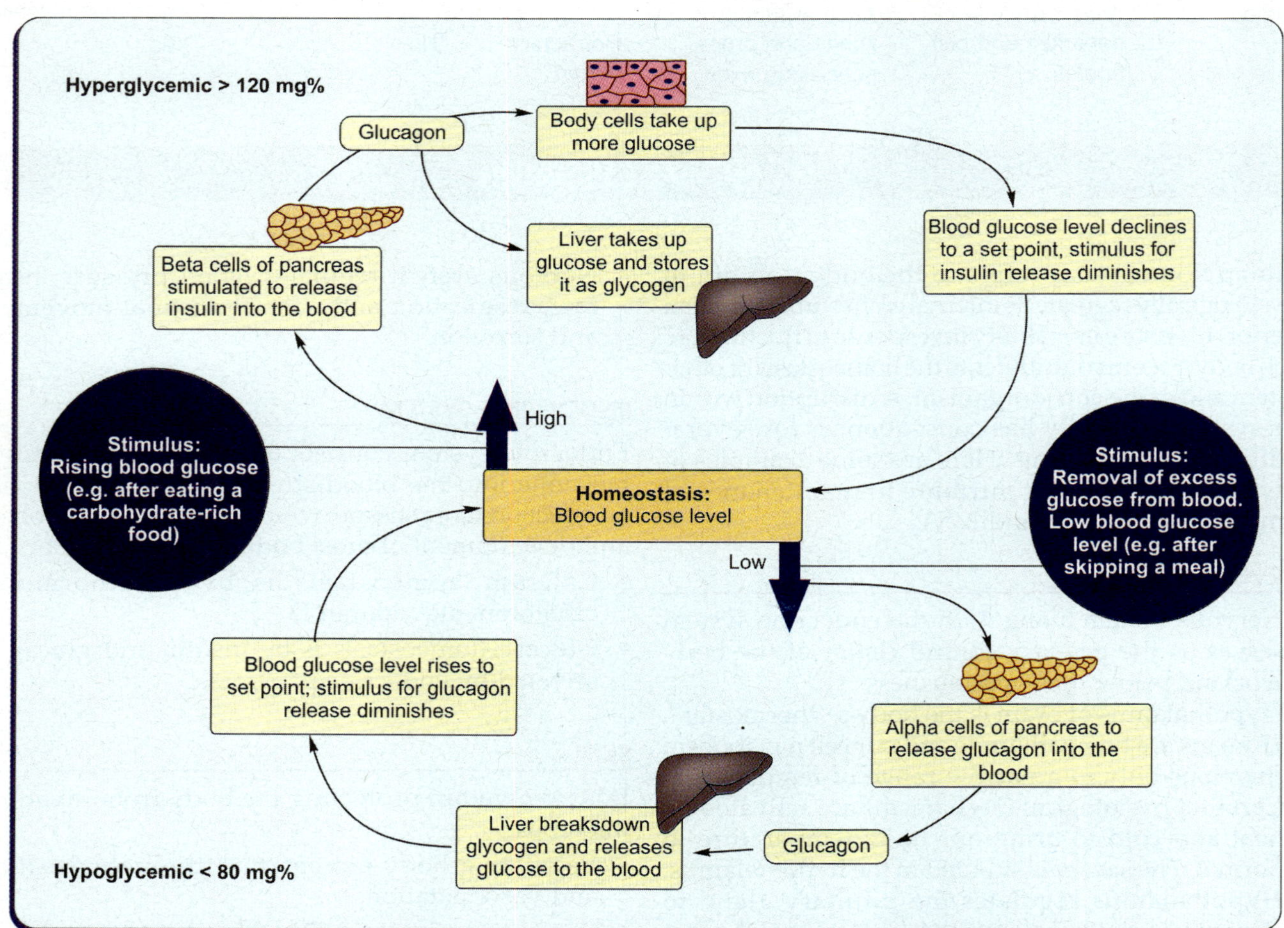

Fig. 2.28: Homeostasis

other purposes. The kidney gets rid the body of these wastes.

- Also maintains blood volume and therefore regulates blood pressure.
- Renal tubules secrete erythropoietin that stimulates RBC production.
- Maintains acid-base homeostasis by gaining or losing acid and base in the urine.

REPRODUCTIVE SYSTEM

- It maintains the species.
- Sex hormones also have additional effect on other body systems.

HEMOSTASIS

It is the process by which bleeding is arrested by stimulating the clotting mechanism.

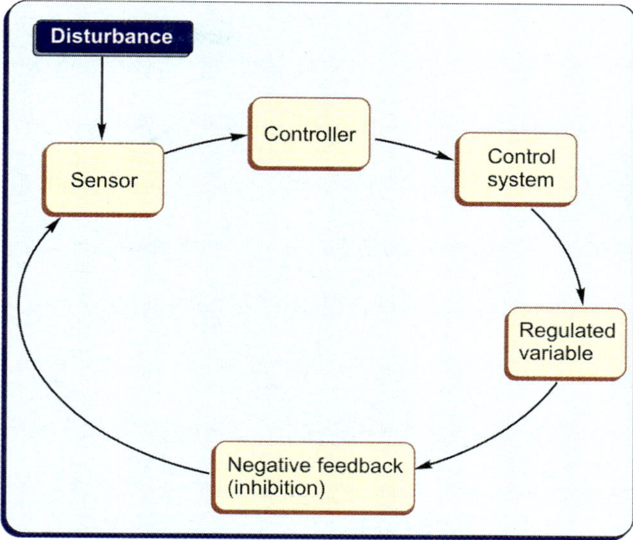

Fig. 2.29: Feedback inhibition

Control Mechanism in Homeostasis

All homeostatic control mechanisms have at least three interdependent components for the variable being regulated (Fig. 2.28). The receptor is the sensing component that monitors and responds to changes in the environment. When the receptor senses a stimulus, it sends information to a control center, the component that sets the range at which a variable is maintained. The control center determines an appropriate response to the stimulus. In most homeostatic mechanisms, the control center is the brain. The control center then sends signals to an effector, which can be muscles, organs or other structures that receive signals from the control center. After receiving the signal, a change occurs to correct the deviation by either enhancing it with positive feedback or depressing it with negative feedback (Fig. 2.29). For example, glucose homeostasis.

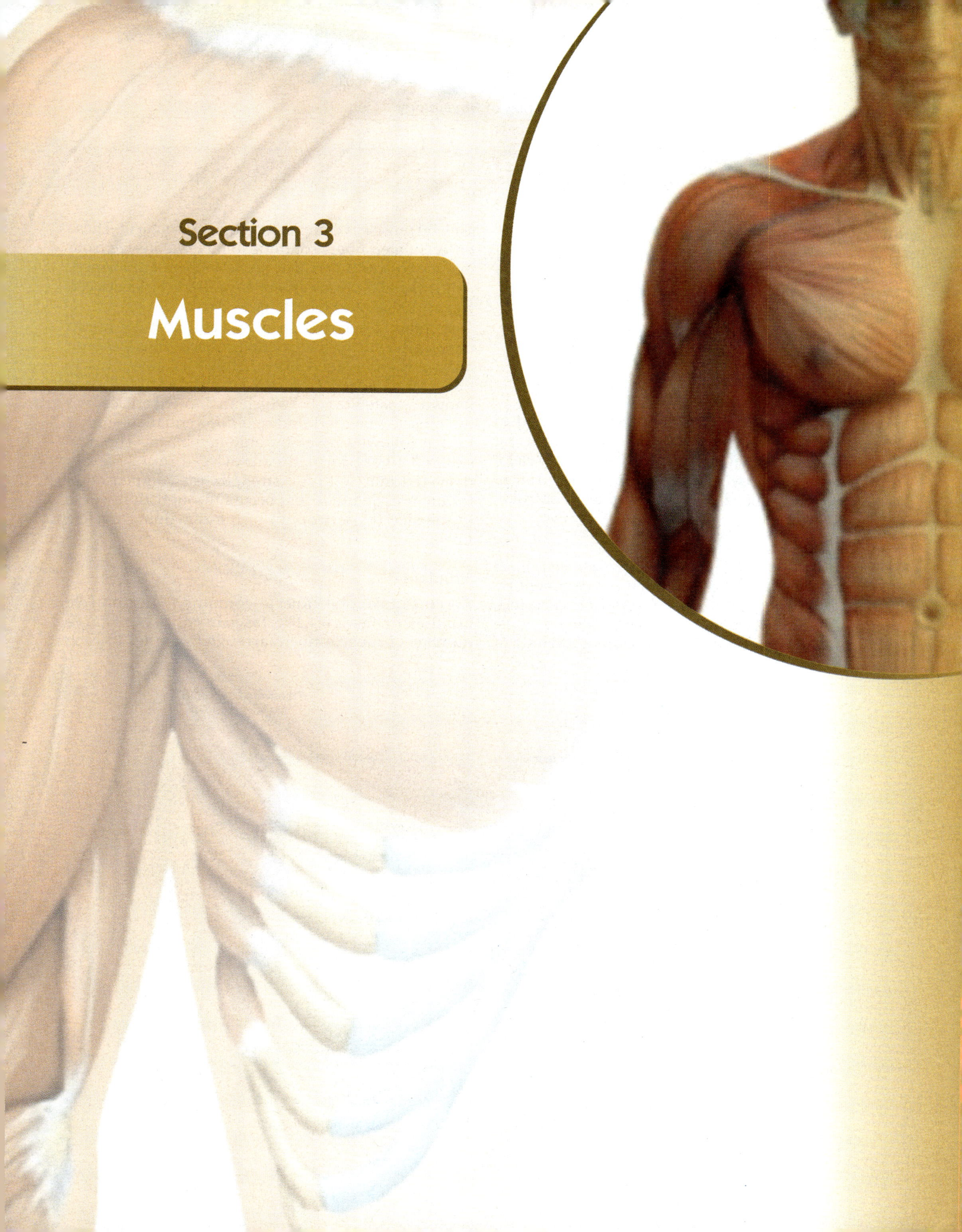

Section 3

Muscles

3

6. SKELETAL MUSCLE

Introduction

Three types of muscle tissue can be identified based on the basis of structure, contractile proteins and control mechanisms—skeletal muscle, smooth muscle and cardiac muscle. The skeletal muscle constitutes about 40% of body weight and another 10% by smooth and cardiac muscle.

Organization

Skeletal muscle, as the name implies, is attached to bone, and its contraction is responsible for supporting and moving the skeleton. The contraction of skeletal muscle is initiated by impulses from the neuron to the muscle and is usually under voluntary control.

Development

Muscle fiber is the single skeletal muscle cell. Each muscle fiber is formed during fetal development by the fusion of a number of undifferentiated, mononucleated cells known as myoblasts, into a single cylindrical, multinucleated cell. The differentiation of skeletal muscle is completed at the time of birth. These differentiated fibers continue to increase in size from infancy to adulthood, but no new fibers are formed. Adult skeletal muscle fibers have diameters between 10 and 100 m, and length up to 20 cm.

If there is destruction of skeletal muscle due to injury after birth, the existing muscle fibers cannot replace the damaged fibers. However, new muscle fibers are formed from the undifferentiated cells known as satellite cells, which are located adjacent to the muscle fiber and undergo differentiation similar to that followed by embryonic myoblasts. The new skeletal fibers formed cannot restore a severely damaged muscle to full strength, the compensation for the muscle tissue loss occurs through an increase in the size (hypertrophy) of the remaining muscle fibers.

Structure (Fig. 3.1)

A typical skeletal muscle contains many muscle bundles or fascicles.The fascicle consists of large number of muscle fibers arranged parallel to each

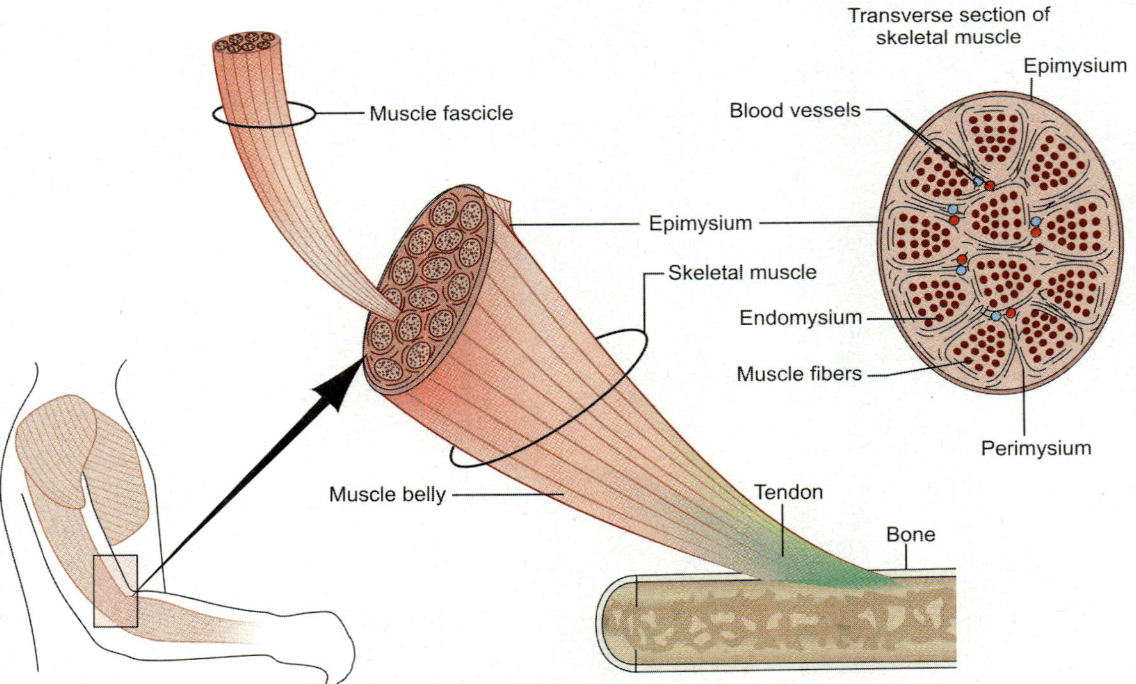

Fig. 3.1: Organisation of skeletal muscle from gross to molecular level

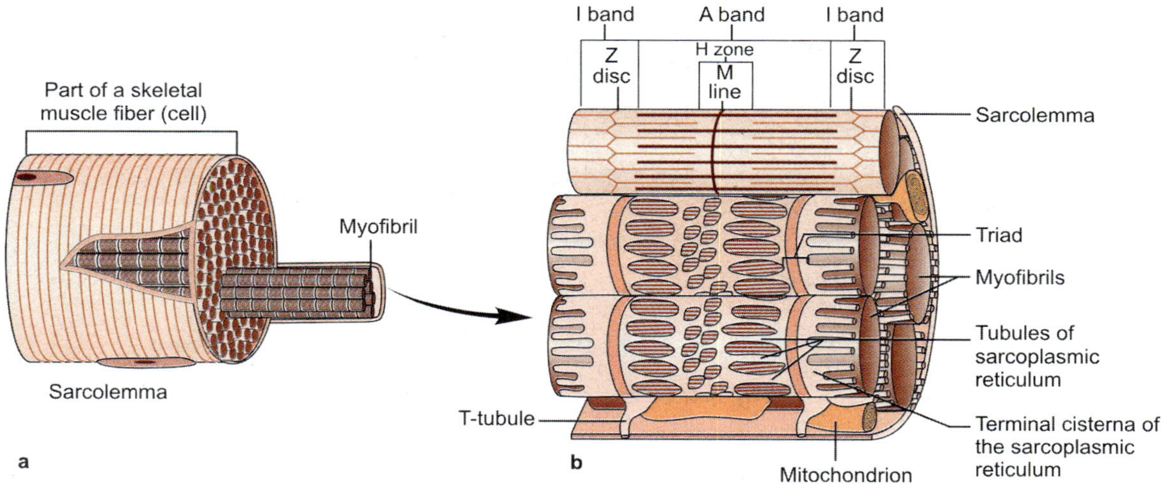

Figs 3.2a and b: (a) Muscle fiber; (b) sarcotubular system

other. The connective tissue layer around the skeletal muscle is called epimysium, connective tissue layer covering each fascicle is called perimysium and the covering for each muscle fiber is called endomysium. The blood vessels and nerve supply to the muscle are present within perimysium. Muscles are usually linked to bones by bundles of collagen fibers known as tendons (Fig. 3.1).

The structural unit of muscle is muscle fiber that is a single muscle cell (myocyte). Sarcolemma is the cell membrane of myocytes and sarcoplasm is the cytoplasm of myocytes. There are no syncytial bridges between the cells. The muscle fibers are made up of myofibrils of 1 m in diameter and 1 to 4 cm in length depending upon the muscle fiber length. Each myofibril consist of many thick and thin filaments made up of contractile proteins.

Muscle Fiber

The presence of striations on the skeletal muscle is due to alternate light and dark bands throughout the length of the fiber (Fig. 3.2).

- The dark band is also called A band (anisotropic to polarized light), contains the thick (myosin) filaments.
- In centre of each A band is a lighter H-zone, where thin filaments do not overlap the thick filaments.
- The light band is also called I band (isotropic to polarized light), contains the thin (actin) filaments.
- The light band is divided by the narrow dark Z line.
- A transverse M line is seen in the middle of the H band.

Sarcomere

The structural and functional unit of muscle fiber is the sarcomere. It is defined as the portion of muscle fibril between two successive Z lines. Each myofibril may contain hundreds or thousands of sarcomere that are joined end to end. The average length of sarcomere is 2 m (Fig. 3.3).

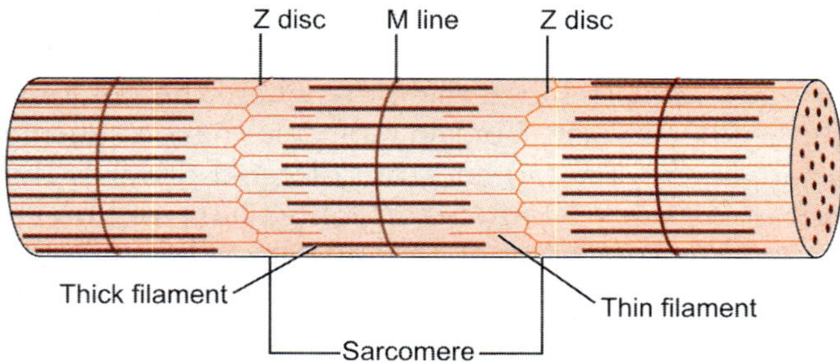

Fig. 3.3: Myofibril showing arrays of thick and thin filaments

Skeletal Muscle Proteins

- *Contractile proteins:* Myosin and actin (Fig. 3.4)
- *Regulatory proteins:* Troponin and tropomyosin
- *Attachment proteins:* Titin, nebulin, alpha actinin and dystropin.

Contractile Proteins

Myosin

The thick filaments in the muscle is made up of myosin-II (MW 480,000) which as two heavy chains and four light chains. Heavy chains are coiled together

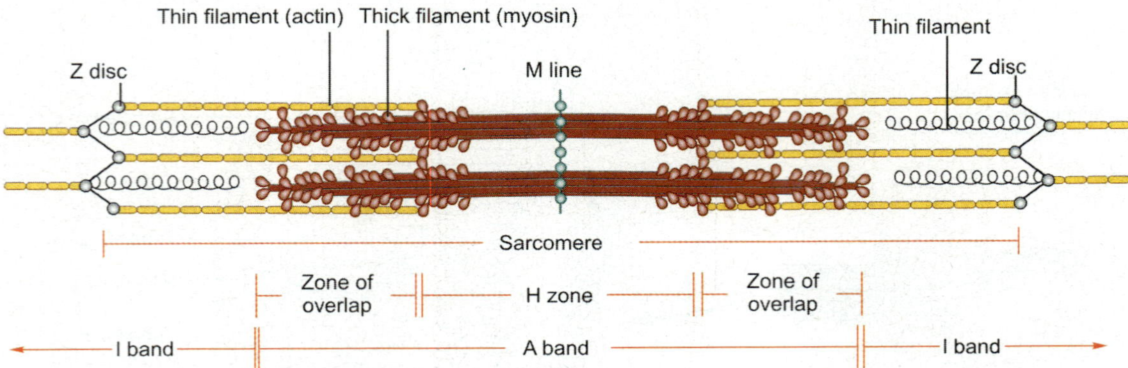

Fig. 3.4: Sliding of actin on myosin

to form double helix. One end of this helix forms a two globular protein mass called the head of myosin. The other end of the helix forms the tail of myosin (Figs 3.5 and 3.6).

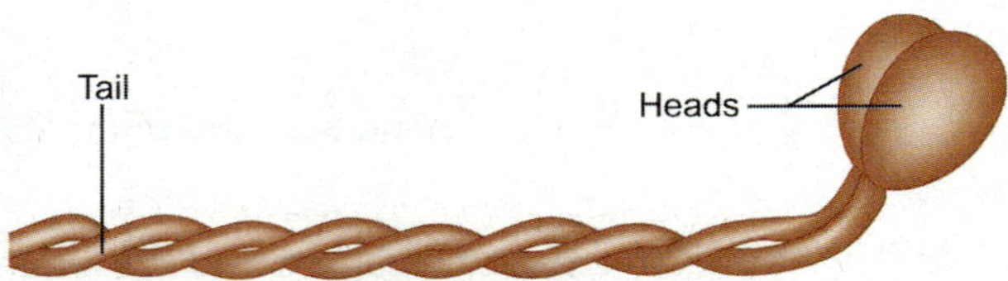

Fig. 3.5: Myosin molecule

Myosin head: Each myosin head is made up of amino terminal portions of one heavy chain forming complex with two light chains, one alkali and one regulatory. The myosin head has two binding sites: one for actin and one for ATP. The myosin head is stabilized by alkali chain and the ATPase activity is regulated by the regulatory chain.

Myosin tail: The tail of each myosin molecules lies along the axis of thick filament and the two globular heads extend out to the sides, forming the cross-bridges. Myosin hinge region is where the tail joins the head of myosin. Myosin molecules have a specific arrangement, the tail ends are directed towards the center of thick filaments creating bare region in the middle consisting of only myosin tails, while the globular heads point away from both sides of the tail (Fig. 3.7).

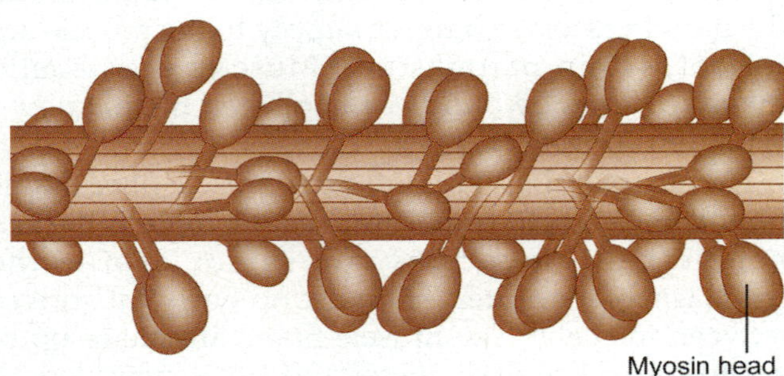

Fig. 3.6: Combination of myosin molecules to form a myosin filament

Actin

The thin filaments are made up of actins. It is a double helix made up of F-actin, which is formed by polymerization of G-actin. Nebulin is the cytoskeleton protein which extends along the length of the F-actin and plays a role in regulation of the length of the thin filament.

Each actin monomer contains binding sites for myosin, tropomyosin, troponin I and other actin monomers. Each thin filament contains 300–400 actin molecules and 40–60 tropomyosin molecules. Once the Ca^{2+} ions binds to troponin during contraction, the tropomyosin molecules move away exposing binding sites for myosin (Fig. 3.8).

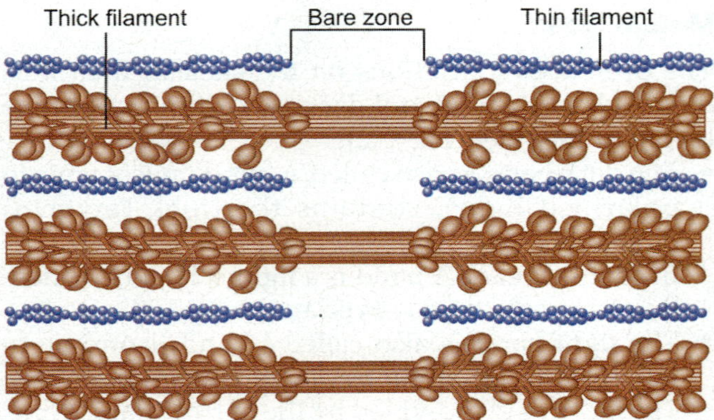

Fig. 3.7: Relation of myosin to actin in an individual sarcomere and functional unit of muscle

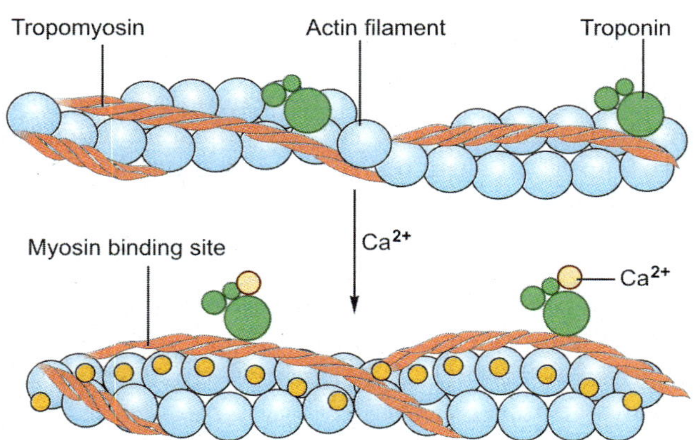

Fig. 3.8: Actin filament with 2 helicle strands of troponin and tropomyosin

Regulatory Proteins

Tropomyosin

It is a rod shaped molecule (MW 70,000), with a double helix pattern, with a length approximately equal to seven actin monomers and located in the groove between two chains of actin. In a relaxed muscle each tropomyosin molecules cover seven active sites on actin and prevent the interaction between the actin and myosin.

Troponin

It is a complex of three proteins:

- *Troponin T:* (MW 30,000) it binds the troponin complex to tropomyosin.
- *Troponin I:* (MW 22,000) it binds the troponin complex to actin. It is called I because it inhibits the binding of myosin to actin by blocking the myosin binding site on actin.
- *Troponin C:* (MW 18,000) it binds with calcium.

Anchoring Proteins

Titin

It is the large, elastic, cytoskeleton protein extending from the Z line to the M line. It prevents the overextension of the thick filaments and hence maintains the A band in the center.

Nebulin

It is the large, filamentous protein extending along the length of the thin filaments. It stabilizes the length of actin filament during muscle contraction.

Actinin

It anchors the thin filaments to Z lines.

Dystrophin

It is a rod like protein that connects actin to the membrane protein beta-dystroglycan, which in turn is connected to the extracellular matrix protein laminin through alpha-dystroglycan.The force from the contractile system is transferred to the extra-cellular region with the help of dystrophin. Muscular dystrophy is a genetic disease where dystrophin is disrupted, which leads to muscle degeneration, weakness and even death.

Desmin

It binds Z lines to plasma membrane.

Sarcotubular System

Sarcotubular system is the membranous structures which surrounds the myofibrils. It is made up of a transverse tubular system (T system) and a longitudinal sarcoplasmic reticulum (L system) (Figs 3.2 and 3.9).

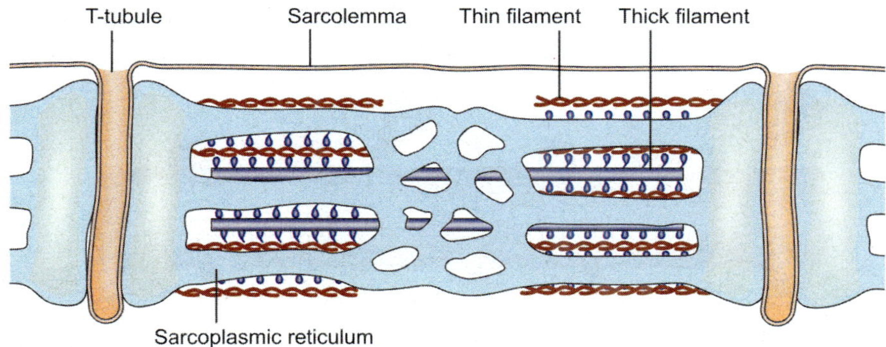

Fig. 3.9: Sarcoplasmic reticulum with its transverse tubules showing thick and thin filaments

3

T-tubules, also called sarcotubules are tubular extensions of the sarcolemma. They penetrate to the center of the muscle fiber at the junctions of A and I band.The lumen of the T-tubules is filled by the surrounding extracellular fluid (Fig. 3.9).

Longitudinal sarcoplasmic reticulum in the skeletal muscle corresponds to the endoplasmic reticulum found in other cells. It has an elongated portion in the middle and dilated region at both ends known as lateral sacs or terminal cisternae, which lie in close contact with T-system at the A-I junctions. At these points the arrangement of T-tubule membrane with a cistern of sarcoplasmic reticulum on either side is called as triad. This plays an important role in transmission of cell membrane action potential to all the fibrils in the muscle. The sarcoplasmic reticulum is an important store of Ca^{2+} and also participates in muscle metabolism.

Functions of Sarcotubular System (Fig. 3.10)

1. Action potential is transferred from muscle surface into the muscle cell.
2. Calcium release is regulated during muscle contraction.

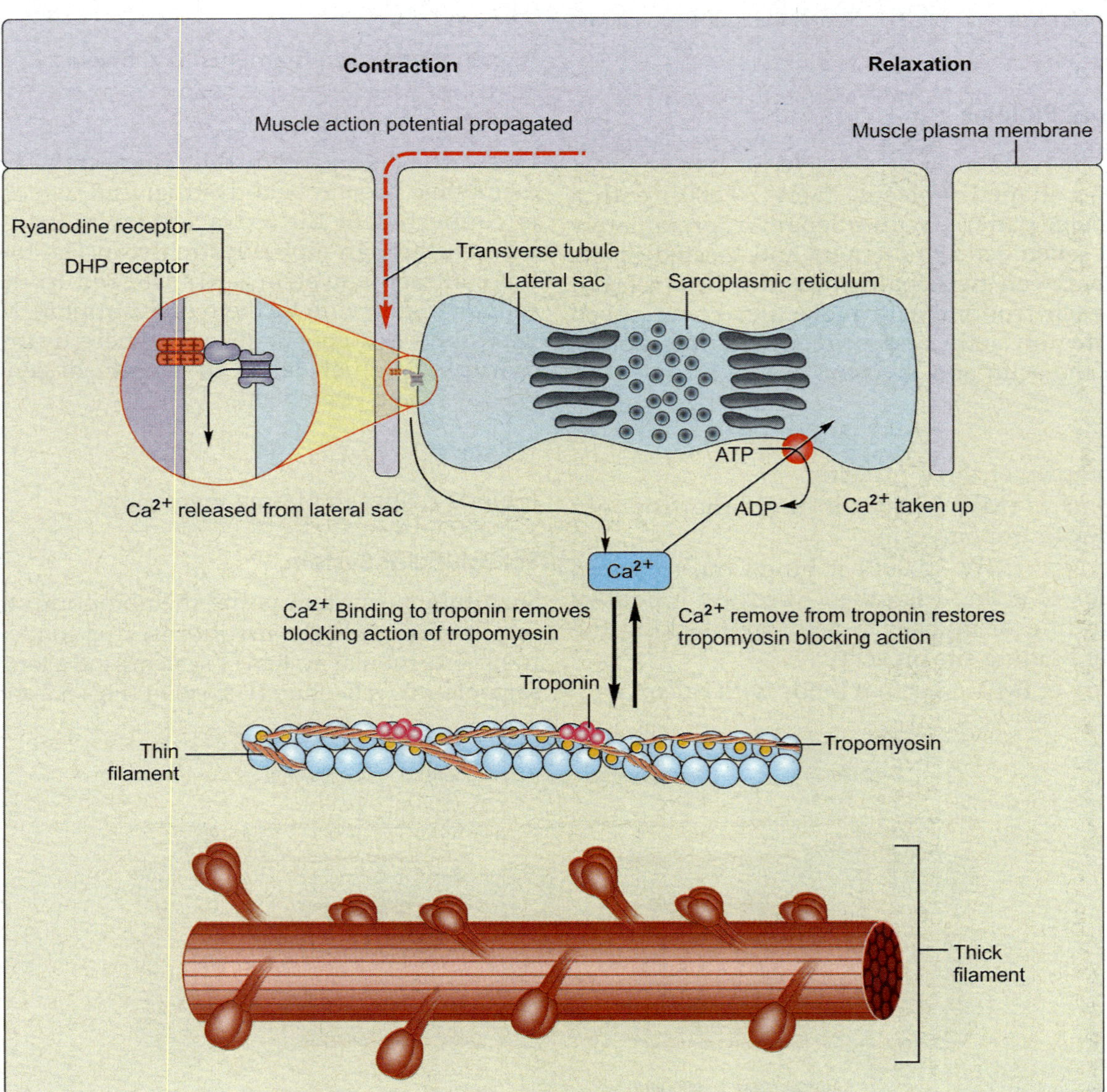

Fig. 3.10: Relation of T-tubules to the sarcoplasmic reticulum in Ca^{2+} transport

3. Sarcoplasmic reticulum stores the calcium.
4. Reuptake of calcium by sarcoplasmic reticulum through Ca^{2+} ATPase pumps, ensures the muscle relaxation.

Receptors in Sarcotubular System

1. *Dihydropyridine (DHP) receptor:* It is a protein present on the T-tubule. It is a modified voltage sensitive calcium channel.
2. *Ryanodine receptors:* It is present on the terminal cisternae membrane that faces the T-tubule. They act as calcium release channels (Fig. 3.10).

Role of Sarcotubular System in Muscle Contraction and Relaxation

Action potential arrives at T-tubules and gets transmitted inside
↓
Opens the voltage gated calcium channels in DHP receptor
↓
Conformational changes in ryanodine receptor, leads to release of calcium into sarcoplasm
↓
Calcium binds to troponin C to cause muscle contraction
↓
Autoactivation of Ca^{2+} ATPase channels pumps calcium from sarcoplasm to SR
↓
Decrease in sarcoplasmic calcium concentration causes muscle relaxation

Excitability of Skeletal Muscle

The transmission of impulse across neuromuscular junction leads to end plate potential (EPP), when an EPP reaches a threshold level, it produces an action potential which travels over the muscle fiber surface and into the muscle fiber along the T tubule system.

Contraction of Skeletal Muscle

The sequences of events by which an action potential in the plasma membrane of a muscle fiber leads to cross-bridge activity is known as excitation-contraction coupling.

Molecular basis of Muscle Contraction

The sliding filament theory or ratchet theory was given by AF Huxely and HE Huxely in 1954 to explain how actin filaments slide over the myosin filaments forming the actin-myosin complex during muscular contractions. This is brought about by repeated cycle of formation of cross-bridges. Changes produced in sarcomere are (Fig. 3.11)

- I: Bandwidth decreases
- H: Zone disappears
- Z: Lines moves closer
- A: Bandwidth remains constant
- Sarcomere length shortens.

Steps of Cross-bridge Cycling

Major steps involved in cross-bridge cycling in a contractile muscle

Motor neuron stimulation
↓
Propagation of action potential in the motor neuron
↓
Neuromuscular transmission
↓
EPP leads to muscle excitation
↓
Propagation of action potential along the T-tubules and into the muscle fiber
↓
Release of Ca^{2+} ions from sarcoplasmic reticulum
↓
Ca^{2+} attaches to troponin
↓
Movement of tropomyosin uncovers myosin binding sites on actin
↓
Binding of cross-bridge to actin
↓
Sliding of thin filaments over thick filaments
↓
Initiation of muscle contraction
↓
ATP binds to cross-bridge
↓
Affinity of myosin to actin is lost
↓
Dissociation of cross-bridge occurs
↓
Hydrolysis of ATP causes cross-bridge to gain energy and affinity for actin

Contraction is the continuous cycling of cross-bridges (Fig. 3.12). The process of cross-bridge cycling

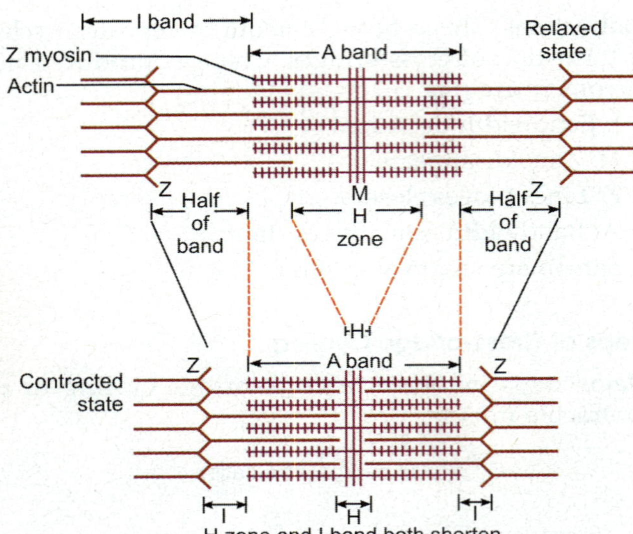

Fig. 3.11: Sliding of action on myosin

starts when free calcium is available and attaches to troponin. ATP is not required to form the cross-bridge linking to actin but is required to break the link with actin. Every time a cross-bridge completes a single cycle, one ATP is hydrolyzed. This provides energy for the mechanical aspects of contraction that is active shortening and/or development of active tension.

Cross-bridge cycling continues (contraction continues) until there is either:

- Withdrawal of Ca^{2+} or decrease level of Ca^{2+} due to re-entry of Ca^{2+} into sarcoplasmic reticulum through Ca^{+}ATPase pumps
- When ATP is depleted, this occurs after death. Absence of dissociation leads to Rigor mortis.

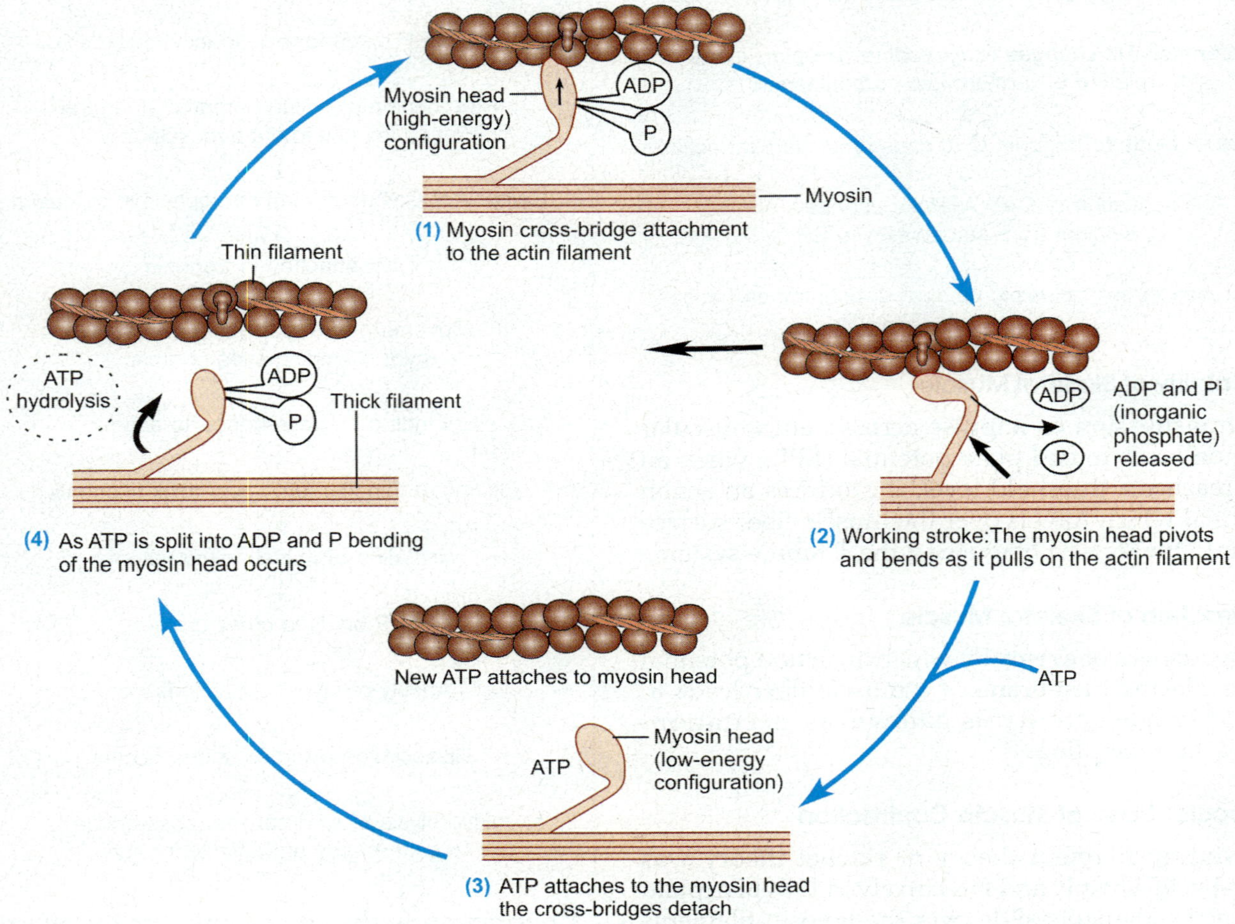

Myosin head (high-energy) configuration
ADP
P
Myosin
(1) Myosin cross-bridge attachment to the actin filament

ADP
ADP and Pi (inorganic phosphate) released
P
(2) Working stroke: The myosin head pivots and bends as it pulls on the actin filament

ATP
New ATP attaches to myosin head
ATP
Myosin head (low-energy configuration)
(3) ATP attaches to the myosin head the cross-bridges detach

Thin filament
ATP hydrolysis
ADP
P
Thick filament
(4) As ATP is split into ADP and P bending of the myosin head occurs

Fig. 3.12: Power stroke of myosin in skeletal muscle

Steps in Muscle Relaxation

Active transport Ca^{2+} ions into the longitudinal sarcoplasmic reticulum
↓
Ca^{2+} ions concentration in the sarcoplasm decreases
↓
Removal of Ca^{2+} ions from troponin-C
↓
Troponin-tropomyosin complex, covers the active sites on actin
↓
Myosin cross-bridge cycle stops
↓
Muscle relaxes

Energy Source for Muscle Contraction

Contraction of muscle requires lots of energy. The immediate source of energy is ATP and ultimate source is intermediate metabolism of carbohydrate and lipids.

ATP stored in the muscle undergoes hydrolysis to provide energy for muscle contraction. Re-synthesis of ATP is necessary since the ATP stored in the muscle gets depleted in about 3 seconds. Muscle fiber can re-synthesize ATP from ADP during contraction in three ways:

1. Phosphorylation of ADP by creatine phosphate
2. Glycolysis
3. Oxidative metabolism

Changes during Muscle Contraction

- The resting pH of muscle is alkaline (7.3) and during contraction due to dephosphorylation of ATP to ADP, the pH becomes acidic.
- Thermal changes occur during different phases of contraction:
  1. *Resting heat:* It is the heat generated when the muscle is at rest. It is the external manifestation of basal metabolic process of the muscle.
  2. *Initial heat:* It is the heat generated in excess to the resting heat during muscle contraction.
  3. *Recovery heat:* It is the heat generated in excess to the resting heat after the cessation of muscle contraction.
  4. *Relaxation heat:* It is the extra heat produced during relaxation of isotonically contracted muscle.
- *Fenn effect:* The heat produced is directly proportional to the work done. When work done is more the ATP used will also be more.

Types of Contractions

Isometric Contraction (iso = same, metric = length)

- In this type of contraction the length of the muscle remains same but tension increases.
- Work done = force × distance. Hence in isometric contraction there is no movement produced or no external work is done.
- *Example:* Contraction of muscles which help in maintaining posture against gravity and contraction of arm muscles when trying to push a wall.
- During isometric contraction there is maximum load on cardiovascular system and blood pressure increases. Hence, isometric exercise is not recommended for heart patients.

Isotonic Contraction (iso = same, tonic = tone or tension)

- In this type of contraction the tension in the muscle remains same and the length decreases.
- In isotonic contraction, since the length decrease, external work is done.
- *Example:* Contraction of leg muscles while walking and running, contractions of muscles while lifting a weight.
- During isotonic contraction the work load on cardiovascular system is less and blood pressure increase is less. Hence, isotonic exercises are recommended for heart patients.

Properties of Skeletal Muscle

1. Excitability
2. Single muscle twitch
3. Refractory period
4. Tonicity
5. Factors affecting contractile response
6. Fatigue

Excitability

Skeletal muscle gets excited when a threshold stimulus is given through its nerve or directly on the muscle. The strength duration curve, which gives the relation between strength and duration of stimulus, can be used to measure the excitability (Fig. 3.13)

- The minimum strength of stimulus required to excite the muscle is called rheobase.
- The duration to apply minimum strength of stimulus to get rheobase is called utilization time.

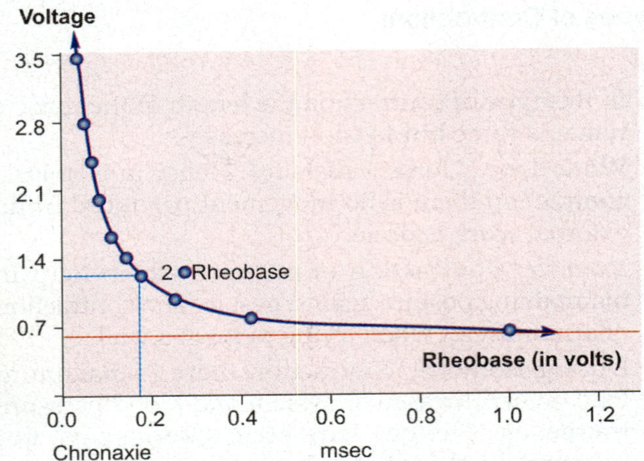

Fig. 3.13: Strength–duration curve

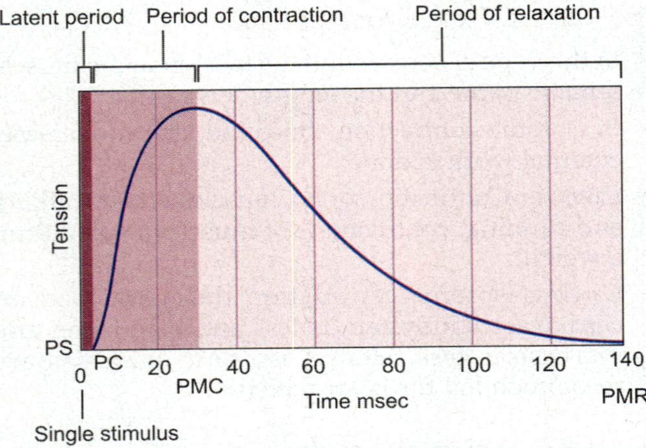

Fig. 3.14: Simple muscle curve

- The duration to get a response when double the rheobase strength of stimulus is used is called Chronaxie. This is used to assess the excitability of tissue. When the chronaxie is less, the excitability of the tissue is more and when the chronaxie more, the excitability of the tissue less.

Single Muscle Twitch

The typical contractile response of skeletal muscle to a single stimulus is known as single muscle twitch or simple muscle twitch (Fig. 3.14). The total duration of the twitch is 0.1 sec, and shows three phases:

1. *Latent period (LP):* The time interval between the point of stimulus (PS) and the point of start of contraction (PC) is called Latent period. This brief time gap for contraction to occur after stimulation is due to:
   - Time taken by the impulse to travel from point of stimulation to NMJ
   - Time taken by neuromuscular transmission
   - Time taken for excitation-contraction coupling and time taken to develop muscle tension
   - Time taken by inertia of recording lever.
2. *Contraction phase:* It is the duration of muscle contraction from the point of start of contraction (PC) to the point of maximum contraction (PMC).
3. *Refractory period* of skeletal muscle is 3 m/sec.

Relaxation Phase

It is the duration when the muscle is stretched back to its original length; it is from the point of maximum contraction (PMC) to point of maximum relaxation (PMR).

Tonicity

The muscle normally remains in partial state of contraction, due to reflex activity initiated from the receptors in the muscles. Tonicity of muscle is assessed by the resistance offered by the muscle during passive movement. (hypotonia = decrease in muscle tone, hypertonia = increase in muscle tone).

Factors Affecting Contractile Response

a. *Strength of stimulus:* There is no contractile response with subthreshold stimulus and the contractile response remains constant with threshold, maximal and supramaximal stimulus. Hence, single muscle fiber obeys all-or-none law.

b. *Frequency of stimulus*

Stair case effect or treppe or wave summation: Occurs when the next successive stimulus falls after complete relaxation phase of the previous twitch. Due to the beneficial effect of previous twitch, each successive twitch has increase force of contraction (Fig. 3.15).

Incomplete tetanus or clonus: Occurs when the next successive stimulus falls on the relaxation phase of the previous twitch.The succeeding contraction obtained will be superposed over the previous twitch due to incomplete summation of waves (Fig. 3.15).

Complete tetanus: Occurs when the next successive stimulus falls before relaxation phase. The muscle remains in sustained contraction due to complete summation effect (Fig. 3.15).

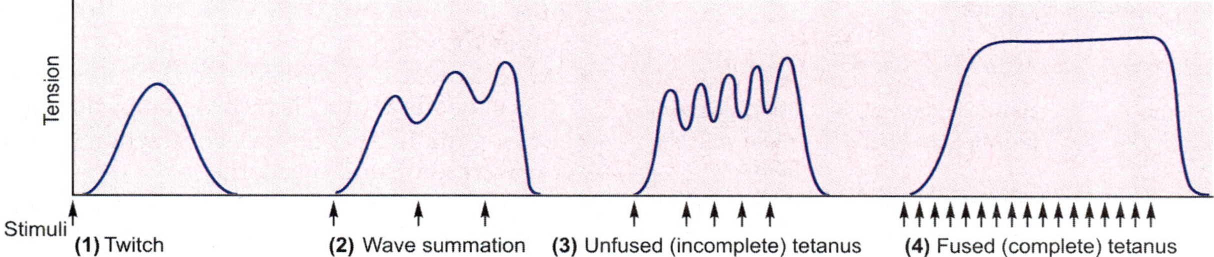

Fig. 3.15: Genesis of tetanus

c. *Load on muscle*

Preload (free load): Is the load acting on the muscle in relaxed state; this causes the muscle to stretch and develop passive tension, which increases the force of muscle contraction.

Afterload: The load acting on the muscle after the beginning of muscular contraction. The afterload opposes the force produced by muscle contraction; hence the work done by afterloaded muscle is less than preloaded muscle.

d. *Length–tension relationship* (Fig. 3.16)

The tension that a muscle develops when stimulated to contract isometrically is called the total tension and the tension a muscle develops when stretched is called passive tension. The difference between the two values at any length is the tension actually generated by contractile process is called active tension (Fig. 3.16). There is a direct relation between length and tension of the muscle, i.e. as the length of the muscle is increased, the tension also increases. This relation is called Starling's law. The force of contraction is directly proportional to the initial length within physiological limits.

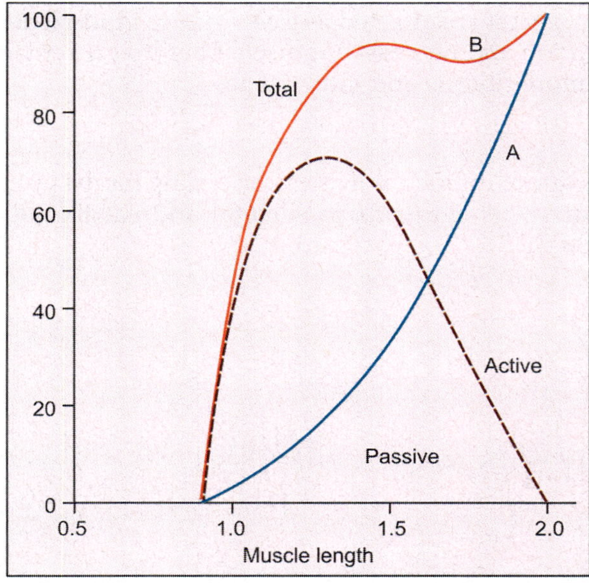

Fig. 3.16: Length–tension relationship for human triceps muscle

e. *Effect of temperature*

Moderate (40°C)	*Low (5°C to 10°C)*	*High (above 50°C)*
Increase in amplitude of muscle curve	Decrease in amplitude of muscle curve	Heat rigor occurs: Coagulation of muscle proteins leads to stiffness and shortening of muscle
Increase in isotonic shortening of muscle occurs due to decrease in internal visco-elastic resistance	Reversible, after re-warming excitability is regained	Irreversible phenomenon

- Cold rigor occurs following exposure to cold and is a reversible phenomenon.
- Calcium rigor occurs due to increase in calcium concentration and is a reversible phenomenon.

Fatigue

When the muscle is repeatedly stimulated, it loses its excitability and gradually becomes less excitable and finally fails to respond to stimuli. This phenomenon is called fatigue. This is a temporary reversible physiological state, after rest, the muscle will respond to stimuli. In intact body the first site of fatigue is synapse (CNS), and then the neuromuscular junction and lastly the muscle. Various factors like rate and amount of work, condition of the body, type of muscle, blood supply and motivation influences fatigue.

Types of Skeletal Muscles

Characteristics	*Type I*	*Type II*
Other names	Slow, oxidative, red muscle fibers	Fast, glycolytic, white muscle fibers
ATP production main source	Oxidative phosphorylation	Glycolysis
Glycolytic capacity	Low	High
Glycogen content	Low	High
Glycolytic enzyme activity	Low	High
Oxidative capacity	High	Low
Mitochondria	Many	Few
Capillaries	High	Low
Myoglobin content	High (red muscle)	Low (white muscle)
Rate of fatigue	Slow (fatigue resistant)	Fast (easily fatiguable)
Myosin: ATPase activity	Low	High
Fiber diameter and motor unit	Small	Large
Type of movements	Adapted for tonic contraction, i.e. for posture maintenance	Adapted for phasic contractions, i.e. fine and skilled movements

3

Electromyography (EMG)

The technique (machine) of recording the electrical activity of the motor nerve and muscle is called electromyography and the record obtained is called electromyogram (Fig. 3.17). The basis of EMG is the motor unit potential (MUP), it is the potential changes recorded in contracting muscle.

- At rest there is complete electrical silence and no spontaneous activity is recorded muscles are silent.
- During minimal voluntary contraction there is one or two motor unit discharge.
- During progressive increase in voluntary contraction, there is a recruitment pattern with moderate force of contraction.
- During maximal contraction, many motor units are recruited and EMG gives a normal interference pattern.

Abnormal Recording

- **Fasciculation potentials:** Resemble MUPs and represent involuntary contraction of single motor unit. Seen in lower motor neuron type of lesions.
- **Fibrillation potentials:** Spontaneous contractions of denervated individual muscle fiber. The waves have short duration and low amplitude.

Applied Physiology

Muscular Dystrophy (MD)

It includes a variety of degenerative muscle diseases that are due to mutations in the genes coding for the various components of the dystrophinglycoprotein complex. The commonest MD is Duchenne muscular dystrophy (pseudohypertrophic MD), is an X-linked hereditary disease that affects mostly male children. Characterized by progressive muscle weakness and enlargement of affected muscles, due to gradual degeneration and necrosis of muscle fiber that is replaced by more fibrous and fatty tissue.

Myopathies

It is due to mutations in the gene coding for the protein desmin, which leads to skeletal and cardiac myopathies.

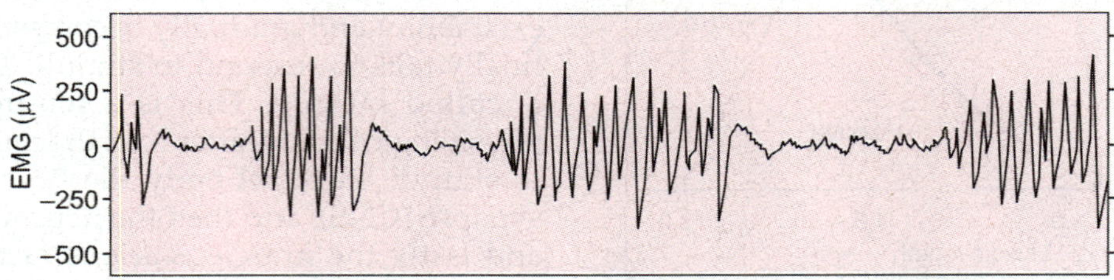

Fig. 3.17: Electromyograph from human biceps and triceps during flexion and extension of elbow

Myotonia

In a condition where the muscle relaxation is prolonged after voluntary contraction. This occurs due to abnormal genes, which leads to malfunction of Na^+ or Cl^- channels.

Dystonia

Means faulty contraction of muscle.

Muscle Cramp

In a painful condition due to involuntary tetanic contraction of skeletal muscle. This occurs due to a very high rate of generation of nerve action potential due to electrolyte imbalance in ECF surrounding nerve fibers and muscle due to dehydration or over exercise.

Muscle Sprain

It occurs due to overstretching or forced extension of an active muscle during sports activity or physical labor. Usual symptoms are pain, soreness, weakness and swelling. Treatment includes rest and immobility, ice packs and drugs to relieve pain.

3

7. NEUROMUSCULAR JUNCTION

Introduction

Neuromuscular junction (NMJ) is the junction between a motor neuron and a muscle fiber, through which action potential from the neuron is transmitted to the muscle fiber (Figs 3.18 and 3.19).

Structure

The structure of NMJ can be broadly divided into three parts:

1. Presynaptic
2. Synaptic cleft
3. Postsynaptic portions.

Presynaptic Portion

- Motor neurons that have their cell bodies in the anterior horn of spinal cord or brainstem innervate the skeletal muscle. Motor neuron axons are myelinated and are the largest diameter axons in the body.

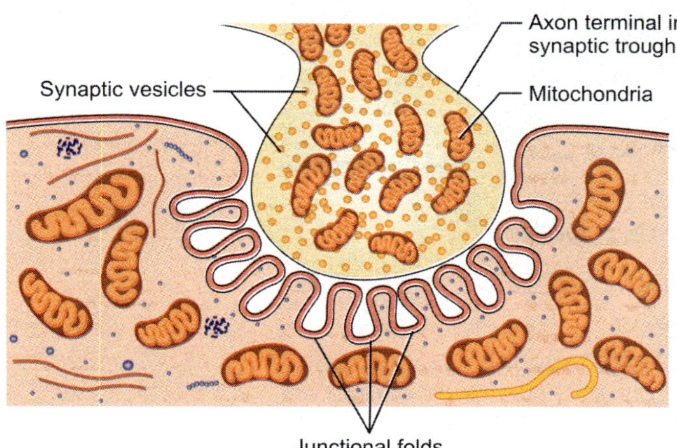

Fig. 3.18: Neuromuscular junction

- As the motor neuron axon approaches the skeletal muscle fiber it loses its myelin sheath and divides into number of fine branches (terminal axons) which end in small swellings (knobs) called terminal buttons, at the center of muscle fiber in the groove (synaptic trough) but outside the muscle fiber membrane (Fig. 3.1).
- Each muscle fiber is supplied by one motor neuron terminal. The motor neuron plus the muscle fiber it innervates is called as motor unit.
- Terminal buttons (synaptic knobs) contains plenty of mitochondria and neurotransmitter vesicles. The acetylcholine (ACh) is synthesized in mitochondria and stored in vesicles.
- The vesicles are clustered around a specific point called active zone, where voltage-gated Ca^{++} channels are present and mediate ACh release.

Synaptic Cleft

- This is gap between the terminal button and muscle fiber (50–100 nm wide).
- The basement membrane of muscle fiber in the cleft contains the enzyme acetylcholinesterase, which hydrolyzes ACh into acetate and choline.

Postsynaptic Portion (End Plate Membrane)

- The muscle fiber plasma membrane that lies directly under terminal axon portion is known as the end plate membrane (motor end plate).

- The endplate membrane is thrown into several folds called junctional folds, which contains nicotinic type of ACh receptors at their crests.

Mechanism of the Neuromuscular Transmission

Arrival of motor neuron action potential, depolarizes the membrane of terminal buttons
↓
Activation and opening of voltage-gated calcium channels, leads to calcium influx in axon terminal
↓
Movement of ACh vesicles to inner surface of presynaptic membrane
↓
Vesicles fuse to the membrane and release ACh into synaptic cleft by exocytosis
↓
ACh diffuses across synaptic cleft and bind to the ACh receptors on the motor end plate
↓
Binding of ACh causes Na^+ influx and K^+ efflux, producing a local depolarization of the motor end plate known as end plate potential (EPP)
↓
EPP is nonprogressive, but when critical level of –60 is reached, generates action potential
↓
Spread of action potential in both the direction along muscle fiber to the T-tubules
↓
Excitation–contraction coupling occurs, which leads to muscle contraction (Fig. 3.19)

Miniature End Plate Potential (MEPP)

Even at rest the motor neuron has spontaneously occurring potentials of minute amplitude (0.4 mV) lasting for a few milliseconds due to ACh release randomly from the nerve terminal. This is called miniature endplate potential.

Drugs acting at Neuromuscular Junction

Neuromuscular Blockers

1. *Botulinum toxin:* It blocks neuromuscular transmission by preventing the release of ACh from the terminal buttons of nerve ending. This toxin is derived from the bacteria *Clostridium botulinum.*
2. *Curare:* Prevents neuromuscular transmission by competitive inhibition. It binds to the ACh receptors on postsynaptic membrane and hence ACh released fails to bind with the receptor and so no endplate potential is developed.

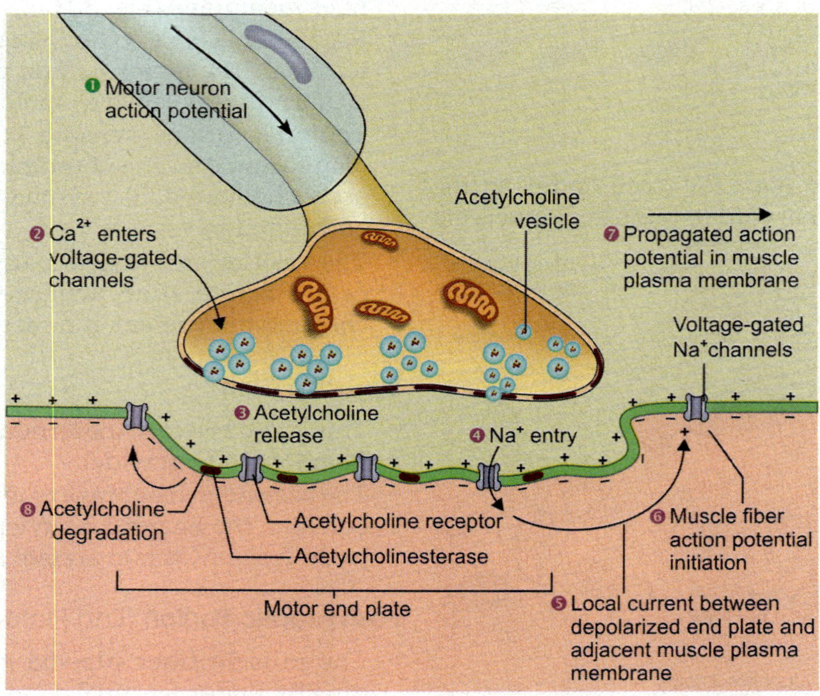

Fig. 3.19: Events of neuromuscular junction that leads to action potential in muscle fiber plasma membrane

3. *Bungarotoxin:* Found in the venom of snakes, blocks the neuromuscular transmission by binding to ACh receptors.
4. *Succinylcholine and carbamylcholine:* It blocks the neuromuscular transmission by keeping the muscle in depolarized state. It acts like ACh and depolarize the postsynaptic membrane, but these are not destroyed by ACh esterase and hence muscle remains in depolarized state for long time.

Neuromuscular Stimulators

1. *Drugs having ACh like action:* Carbachol and nicotine, both are not destroyed or destroyed little by ACh esterase. So they cause muscle spasm due to repeated stimulation and continuous action of muscle.
2. *Drugs that inactivate ACh esterase:* Neostigmine and physostigmine stimulate neuromuscular junction by inactivating acetylcholinesterase.

Disorders at Neuromuscular Junction

Myasthenia Gravis

It is an autoimmune disorder affecting the neuromuscular junction. It occurs in about 1 in every 20,000 persons. In this disease antibodies are produced against the ACh receptors on motor endplate and they are destroyed. Hence, ACh released is unable to bind with the ACh receptor to produce adequate EPP to excite the muscle fiber. So, the transmission of signals from the nerve fiber to muscle does not occur, leading to paralysis of the involved muscle. If the disease is intense, patient dies due to paralysis of respiratory muscle. It is treated by neostigmine, physostigmine and di-isopropyl fluorophosphates (DIFP).

Lambert-Eaton Myasthenic Syndrome

It is a presynaptic disorder of neuromuscular junction, where autoantibodies are produced against voltage-gated Ca^{++} channels. This leads to decrease in calcium influx in terminal knob, and decreases the release of ACh. Upper limb muscular weakness is seen in this disease.

8. SMOOTH MUSCLE

Structure

Smooth muscle cells are spindle-shaped (2 to 10 m diameter and 50 to 400 m in length), have single nucleus and are capable of cell division. They lack cross striations and hence the name smooth muscle (Fig. 3.20).

They contain actin and myosin filament and contract by sliding filament mechanism. The actin filaments take their origin from dense bodies in the cytoplasm which are functionally similar to Z lines in skeletal muscle (Fig. 3.20). Actin filaments contain actin and tropomyosin, but troponin is absent. Sarcoplasmic reticulum is present but poorly developed. T-tubules are absent, and hence, triads are absent.

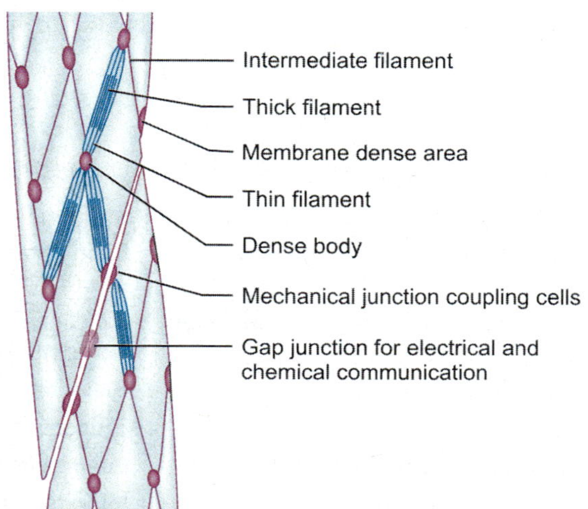

Fig. 3.20: Structure of smooth muscle

Mechanism of Smooth Muscle Contraction

Contraction of smooth muscle occurs by sliding mechanism. Ca^{2+} ions are responsible for excitation-contraction coupling. Calcium binds to calmodulin, a calcium binding protein present in the cytoplasm. This calcium-calmodulin complex binds to another cytosolic protein, myosin light-chain kinase, thereby activating the enzyme for cross-bridge formation. In smooth muscle cross-bridge cycling is controlled by calcium-regulated enzyme that phosphorylates myosin, instead of actin filaments that regulates cross-bridge cycling in skeletal muscle.

3

Smooth Muscle Contraction

Increase cytosolic Ca^{2+}
↓
Ca^{2+} binds to calmodulin
↓
Ca^{2+} – calmodulin complex binds to myosin light-chain kinase
↓
Myosin light-chain kinase uses ATP to phosphorylate myosin cross-bridges
↓
Phosphorylated cross-bridges bind to actin filaments
↓
Cross-bridge cycling produces tension and shortening of smooth muscle

Factors Influencing Smooth Muscle Contractile Activity

- Spontaneous electrical activity in plasma membrane of smooth muscle cell
- Neurotransmitters released by autonomic nervous system
- Hormones
- Stretch
- Changes in chemical composition of ECF surrounding the cell (paracrine agents, acidity, oxygen, osmolarity and ion concentration).

Characteristics of Muscle Cells

Characteristics are listed below.

Types of Smooth Muscle

Two types:

1. *Single-unit smooth muscle:* Also called as visceral smooth muscle, since they are present in the walls of hollow viscera such as gastrointestinal tract, uterus, urinary bladder and respiratory tract.

   Features
   - Has a low resistance bridge (gap-junctions) between individual muscle cells and function in a syncytial fashion.
   - Have own rhythmic contractility myogenic tone that is independent of nerve supply.
   - Contraction is also stimulated by stretching.
   - Contractile activity is also controlled by hormones and local tissue factors.

2. *Multi-unit smooth muscle:* Made up of multiple individual units without interconnecting bridges, i.e. non-syncytial in nature. These are located in most blood vessels, epididymis, vas deferens, iris, ciliary body and piloerector muscles.

   Features
   - Multiple individual units of muscle fibers each innervated by a single nerve ending.
   - No spontaneous contractions, i.e. no pacemaker activity.

Skeletal muscle	*Cardiac muscle*	*Smooth muscle*
Striated	Striated	Nonstriated
Actin and myosin form sarcomeres	Actin and myosin form sarcomeres	Actin and myosin not organized into sarcomeres
Sarcolemma lacks functional complexes between fibers	Junctional complexes between fibers including gap junctions	Gap junctions
Each fiber innervated	Electrical syncytium	Electrical syncytium
Troponin to bind calcium	Troponin to bind calcium	Calmodulin to bind calcium
High ATPase activity (fast muscle)	Intermediate ATPase activity	Low ATPase activity (slow muscle)
Extensive sarcoplasmic reticulum	Intermediate sarcoplasmic reticulum	Limited sarcoplasmic reticulum
T-tubules form triadic contacts with reticulum at A-I junctions	T-tubules form dyadic contact with reticulum near Z lines	Lack T-tubules
Somatic nerve supply	Autonomic nerve supply	Autonomic nerve supply
Pacemaker potential: Absent	Pacemaker potential: Present	Pacemaker potential: Absent in multi-unit and present in single-unit type smooth muscle

- Gap junctions are absent; hence the excitation remains localized within the motor unit.
- Does not respond to stretching.

Properties of Smooth Muscle

1. *RMP:* It ranges from –50 to –70 mV. The peculiarity of this RMP is it is highly unstable.
2. *Sinusoidal wave:* The instability of RMP can be recorded from the longitudinal muscles of stomach and intestine. This is known basic electrical rhythm (BER).
3. *Action potential (AP):* Three types of AP occur in visceral smooth muscle:
   a. Spike potential
   b. Spike potential initiated by slow wave rhythm
   c. Action potential with plateau
   d. Tonic contraction of the muscle without any AP.

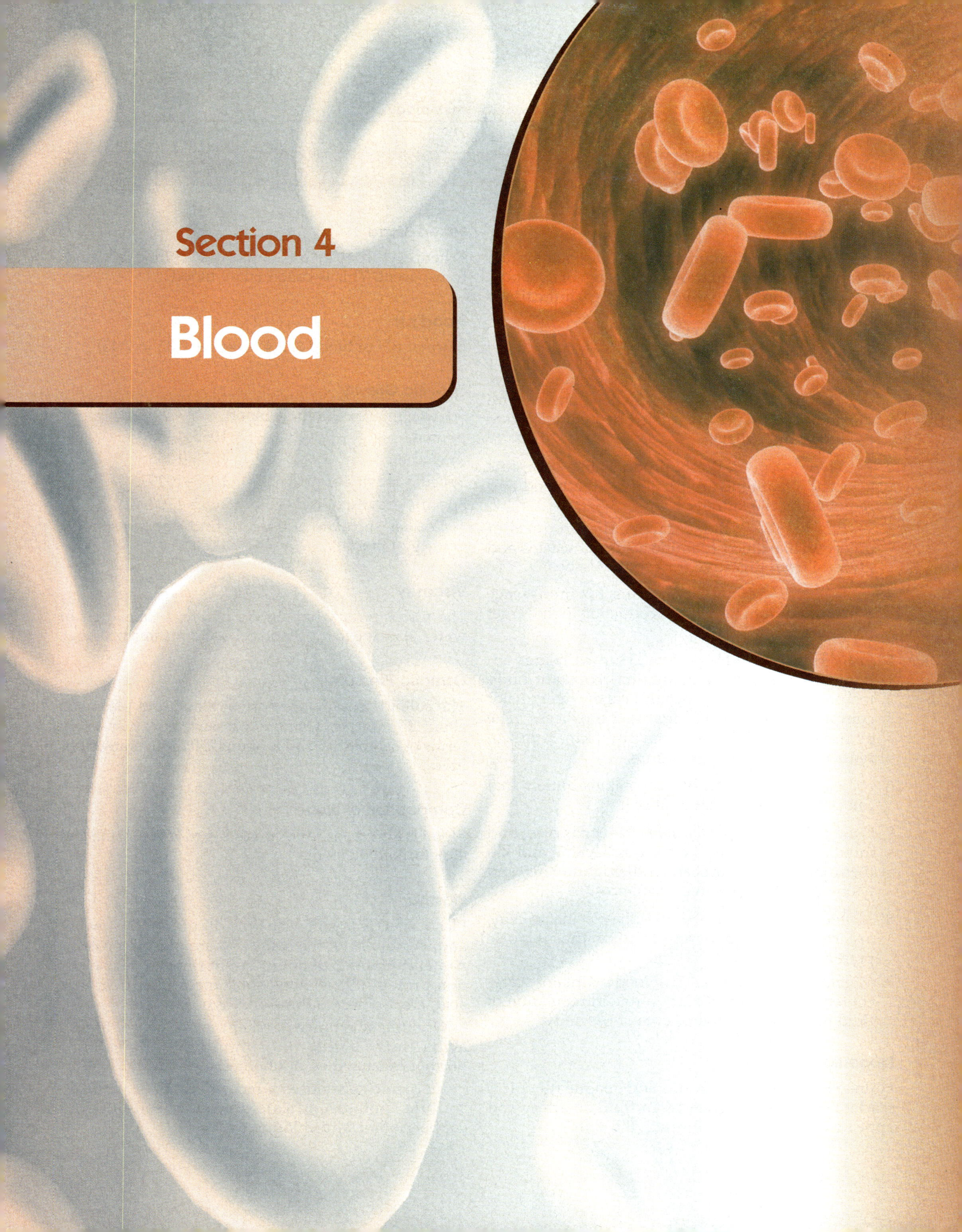

Section 4

Blood

4

9. COMPOSITION AND FUNCTIONS

Introduction

Blood is a fluid that circulates in the vascular system and forms most efficient transport system of the body. When circulation is impaired, it will impair the tissue functions.

Functions of Blood

1. *Transport of respiratory gases:* Hemoglobin conveys oxygen from the lungs to tissues. The carbon dioxide from tissues are carried by hemoglobin to the lungs and exhaled.
2. *Excretory functions:* Waste products like urea, uric acid and creatinine are carried by the blood and removed by the kidney.
3. *Transport of food:* Blood carries the products of digestion like glucose, amino acids, fatty acids and glycerol from digestive tract to the tissues.
4. *Transport of hormones:* Various hormones are transported from the site of production to the target tissues.
5. *Regulation of body temperature:* Human beings are homeothermic. They maintain a constant body temperature. The high specific heat of water, major component of blood helps in the process. The evaporation of water from the skin helps in reducing the body temperature.
6. *Regulation of blood pH:* Blood contains buffers that can prevent the alteration of pH.
7. *Role in defense mechanism:* Neutrophils and monocytes fight with the various bacteria and kill them. Blood transports antibodies, antitoxins, and lysins that are protective substances.
8. *Maintenance of osmotic pressure:* The plasma proteins are responsible for maintaining the osmotic pressure of blood.
9. *Maintenance of water balance:* Blood maintains water content of tissues and plays a role in regulation of fluid in various compartments of the body.

Properties of Blood

Human blood is thick, viscous and opaque fluid. It is scarlet red in colour when taken from an artery and appears blue when seen through the skin.

Laked Blood

When erythrocytes are hemolysed, blood becomes transparent. This is called laked blood.

Blood pH

Normal pH of blood is 7.4 (range is 7.35 to 7.45)

Specific Gravity

Specific gravity of whole blood

In men	1055–1060
In women	1050–1055
Specific gravity of plasma	1025–1029
Specific gravity of red cells	1085–1100

Copper sulphate is used to find out the specific gravity of blood.

Viscosity

The viscosity of whole blood is 3 to 4 times that of water. It is due to the blood cells and plasma proteins.

Osmotic Pressure

The colloid osmotic pressure of blood and plasma is about 25 mm Hg. Osmotic pressure is expressed in terms of osmolarity and is about 290 milliosmoles per liter.

Composition of Blood

Blood is a complex fluid consisting of 55% plasma and 45% formed elements.

Plasma

Plasma is a clear yellowish fluid. It contains 91% water and 9% solids. Of the solids 7% are plasma proteins namely albumin, globulin, and fibrinogen. It also has non-protein nitrogenous substances like urea, uric acid, creatinine, xanthine and hypoxanthine.

Organic substances present are glucose, amino acids, fatty acids, phospholipids, cholesterol, hormones, enzymes, antibodies, etc.

Inorganic substances which form about 0.9% are sodium, potassium, calcium, magnesium, iron, copper, iodine and chloride.

Formed Elements

Formed elements consist of RBC, WBC and platelets. The hematocrit can be determined by packed cell volume. Heparinized blood is taken in a hematocrit tube and rotated rapidly at 3000 revolutions per minute. The lower portion of packed red cell mass is called packed cell volume (or) PCV. Normal PCV is 45%. WBC and platelets appear as thin layer of buffy coat.

Normal PCV

In men	45–50%
In women	40–45%
In newborn	54%

Packed cell volume less than the normal means anemia. Along with PCV if hemoglobin is reduced it is a good clue for diagnosis of severity of anemia. PCV well above normal indicates polycythemia.

Decrease in PCV

Physiological
- Pregnancy
- Excess water intake

Pathological
- Anemia
- Hyperaldosteronism

Increase in PCV

Physiological
- High altitude
- Newborn
- Excess sweating

Pathological
- Congenital heart disease
- Emphysema
- Polycythemia
- Hemoconcentration, e.g. vomiting.

4

10. PLASMA PROTEINS

Plasma contains proteins namely:
- Serum albumin 3.5–5 gm%
- Serum globulin 2.0–3.5 gm%
- Fibrinogen 0.2–0.3 gm%

Plasma protein fraction are separated into serum albumin, serum globulin, alpha 1, alpha 2, beta, and gamma globulins by the technique of electrophoresis. In serum electrophoresis, fibrinogen is not seen, as serum does not contain fibrinogen. Other globulins are protease inhibitors alpha 1 antitrypsin, alpha 2 macroglobulin, several transport proteins, coagulation factors, anti-thrombin hormone binding proteins, lipoproteins and complement components.

Methods to detect tiny amounts of proteins are
- Radioimmunoassay
- Enzyme linked immunosorbent assay (ELISA).

Functions of Plasma Proteins

1. *Colloid osmotic pressure:* Plasma colloid osmotic pressure is due to albumin. Hence albumin has a role in:
   - Fluid exchange between blood and tissue fluids
   - Regulation of blood volume
   - Water balance
2. *Viscosity:* Plasma proteins give viscosity to blood and this contributes to the peripheral resistance a factor in the maintenance of blood pressure.
3. *Acid-base balance:* Proteins act as buffer and hence regulate the acid base balance.
4. *Clotting of blood:* Fibrinogen, prothrombin, and factor V, VIII, etc. are essential for clotting of blood.
5. *Immune substances:* The gamma globulins react with antigens present on microorganisms. These gamma globulins give passive immunity.
6. *Protein store:* When a person is fasting, plasma proteins serve as a reservoir on which the body can depend on for some time.
7. *Rouleaux formation:* Fibrinogen and globulin fraction help in rouleaux formation thus helping in erythrocyte sedimentation rate.

Formation of Plasma Proteins

Albumin, globulin, fibrinogen and prothrombin are formed in liver. The antibodies (gamma globulin) are formed by plasma cells and B lymphocytes. Proteins of food help in the formation of plasma proteins.

Albumin globulin ratio (A:G ratio) is 3:2. This albumin globulin ratio is reversed in cirrhosis, kidney diseases like nephritis, nephrosis, etc.

Decrease in albumin

Reduced intake, liver diseases, and when albumin escapes into tissue spaces.

Increase in globulin

Liver disease, multiple myeloma, acute nephritis, leukemias, and tuberculosis.

Increase in fibrinogen: Pregnancy, menstruation, tissue injuries of various type, acute infectious diseases, and malaria.

Decrease in fibrinogen: Hepatectomy and liver diseases. All fractions of plasma proteins are reduced in haemorrhage.

11. BLOOD VOLUME

4

Average healthy male has 5 liters of blood. Normal blood volume is 60–80 ml/kg body weight. Blood volume is less in children. It increases gradually to adult value by 18 years.

Methods of Measurement of Blood Volume

Blood volume can be estimated using a non-toxic dye.

Characteristics of an Ideal Dye

- Dye must not diffuse too rapidly out of the blood stream.
- Must colour the plasma but it must not be absorbed by the cells of blood
- Dye must not cause hemolysis
- Dye must mix evenly throughout plasma

Evans blue or T-1824 satisfies all these criteria.

Method of Estimation of Blood Volume

Blood sample is collected before the dye is injected intravenously. Dye is injected intravenously and blood samples are collected at 10, 20, 30, 40, 50 minutes interval after the injection. Concentration of dye in the plasma is measured by a photoelectric colorimeter and from the value, plasma volume can be calculated. The hematocrit value of the blood sample before injecting the dye gives relative volumes of plasma and corpuscles. From this the total volume of blood can be calculated.

The amount of dye injected = 10 mg

Concentration in plasma = 0.4 mg/100 ml plasma

$$\text{Plasma volume} = \frac{\text{Amount of dye injected}}{\text{Concentration of the dye in 100 ml}} \times 100$$

$$= \frac{10 \times 100}{0.4}$$

$$= 2500 \text{ ml}$$

Total blood volume is calculated from this by knowing the hematocrit value of the blood. If hematocrit is 45%

$$\text{Total blood volume} = \frac{\text{Plasma volume}}{\text{100-hematocrit}} \times 100$$

$$= \frac{2500}{100-45}$$

$$= \frac{2500 \times 100}{55}$$

$$= 4545 \text{ ml}$$

The other methods used to measure the blood volume are:

Radiotracer Method

Radioiodine tagged albumin is injected intravenously and sufficient time is allowed for mixing. Radioactivity is determined by an appropriate counter.

Red Cell Marking Method

RBCs are labeled with radioactive iron, radioactive chromium or radioactive phosphorus.

Conditions Causing Reduction in Blood Volume

Hemorrhage: Loss of whole blood causes reduction in total blood volume.

- *Burns:* Plasma is exuded from burned surface causing reduction in blood volume.
- *Dehydration:* Loss of water due to diarrhea and vomiting causes decrease blood volume.
- *Anemia:* Decrease in blood cells causes decrease in blood volume.
- *Posture:* Erect posture for 30 minutes cause a reduction in blood volume as fluids leak from vessels of lower limbs into extracapillary tissues.

Regulation of Blood Volume

Exchange of fluid between blood and tissue fluids: When blood volume is increased, capillary hydrostatic pressure is increased and plasma colloid osmotic pressure is decreased. This causes movement of fluid from the blood vessel into tissue space.

When blood volume is decreased, capillary hydrostatic pressure is decreased and osmotic pressure is increased, drawing fluid from tissue space into vascular space.

Hormones regulating blood volume

- Angiotensin II
- Aldosterone
- Vasopressin

Thirst

When water content of body is low, thirst is felt due to stimulation of thirst center in hypothalamus. When the person drinks water, blood volume and water content are restored.

Erythrocyte Sedimentation Rate

The rate at which the red cells settle is called erythrocyte sedimentation rate (ESR) (Fig. 4.1).

ESR is measured by depth in millimeter at the end of one hour.

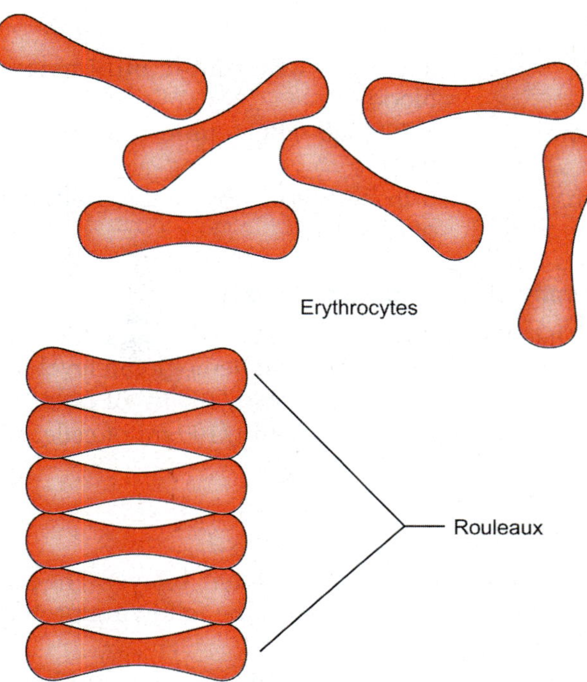

Fig. 4.1: Erythrocyte sedimentation rate

Erythrocyte sediment is due to the formation of rouleaux (red cells piling up like coins).

Uses of ESR

ESR gives additional information in diagnosing a disease. It also helps in determining the prognosis of a disease.

Methods

ESR is determined by:

- Westergren's method
- Wintrobe's method

Normal Values

Men	1 to 10 mm/hr
Women	4 to 15 mm/hr

Increase in ESR

Menstruation, pregnancy, acute bacterial septicemia, tuberculosis, rheumatic fever, pelvic inflammatory disease, malignant tumors, anemia and trauma.

Decrease in ESR

Allergy, sickle cell anemia and acholouric jaundice.

Factors that Determine ESR

Concentration of fibrinogen (increase in fibrinogen increases ESR).

Concentration of gamma globulin (increase in gamma globulin increases ESR).

Serum albumin (decrease in albumin increases ESR).

Other Factors Influencing ESR

- Viscosity of plasma
- Specific gravity
- Size of RBC

C-Reactive Protein

C-Reactive protein is a better alternative to ESR. Normal value is less than 1 mg/100 ml of blood. It is synthesized in liver. Its rise occurs within 6 hours and follows the course of the disease.

Increase in CRP

- Inflammation
- Tissue trauma

12. RED BLOOD CORPUSCLES

Red blood corpuscles (RBCs) also known as erythrocytes, contains hemoglobin, hence red in color (Fig. 4.2a).

Special Features of RBC

RBCs are:

- Biconcave disc-shaped
- Mature red cell have
  - No nucleus
  - No endoplasmic reticulum
  - No mitochondria
  - No centriole
  - No ribosome
- Glucose can be transported into the red cell without insulin.

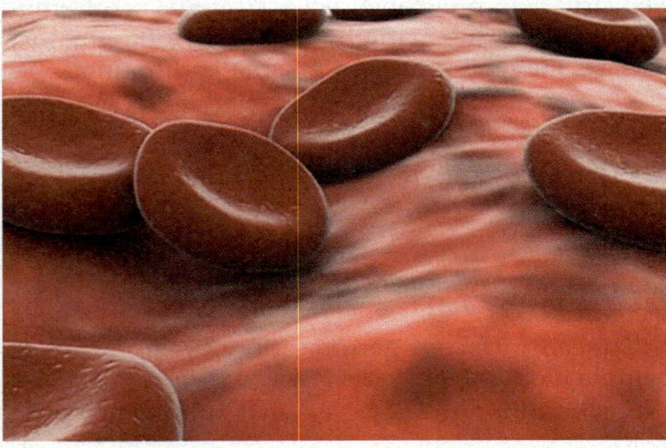

Fig. 4.2a: Red blood cells

Advantages of Biconcavity of RBC

1. Biconcavity increases the surface area of RBC, which facilitates the diffusion of O_2
2. RBC can squeeze itself into the capillary more easily.

Basic Functions of RBC

1. Transport of oxygen and carbon dioxide.
2. *Maintenance of pH of blood:* Hemoglobin in RBC acts as an acid-base buffer.
3. *Determination of blood group:* Blood group antigens present on the surface of the RBC help in determination of blood group.

Shape and Size

Functional morphology

Shape	Biconcave disc
Size	Diameter is 7.8 micrometer Thickness is 2.5 micrometer at thickest point and 1 micrometer at the center.
Surface area	120–140 μm^2

Volume

80 μm^3 (Fig. 4.2b)

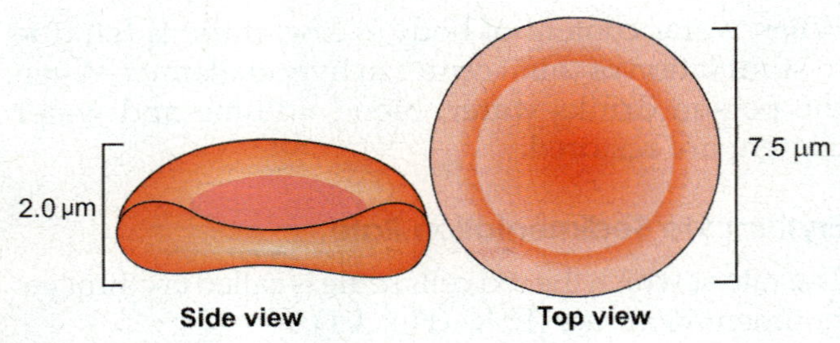

Fig. 4.2b

Normal Count

Men	5,200,000 RBC/cubic millimeter of blood.
Women	4,700,000 RBC/cubic millimeter of blood.
Birth	6 to 7 million RBC/cubic millimeter of blood.

Quantity of Hemoglobin in Cells

RBC has the ability to concentrate hemoglobin up to 34 gm/100 ml of cells. Normal hemoglobin level in

Men	15 gm of hemoglobin/100 ml of cells.
Women	14 gm of hemoglobin/100 ml of cells.

RBC-Structure

Cell Membrane

RBC cell membrane is a lipoprotein bilayer. The inner side of the cell membrane has the following proteins.

1. Actin
2. *Spectrin:* Both are contractile proteins and help in keeping up the shape of RBC.

Absence of spectrin leads to hereditary spherocytosis. Spherocytes (Fig. 4.2c) are RBCs smaller and denser than normal RBCs.

3. *Glycophorin:* It is a protein in RBC cell membrane and contains blood group antigens.

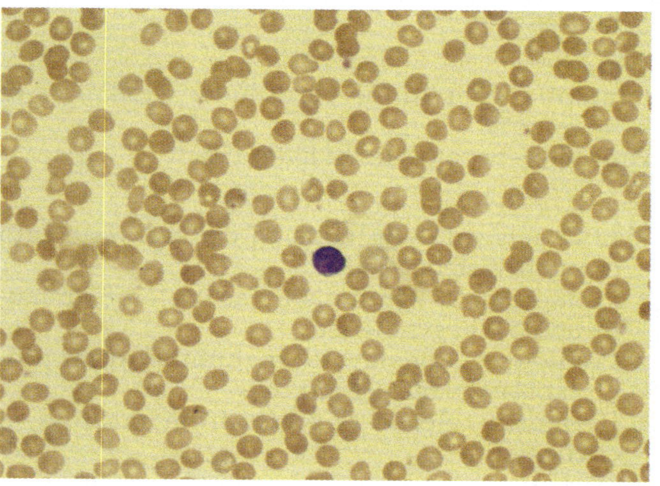

Fig. 4.2c: Spherocytes

Cell Contents

Water	60–63%
Hemoglobin	34%
Others	3–6%

Production of Red Blood Cells

Embryonic life	Yolk sac
Mid-trimester	Liver, spleen and lymph nodes
Last trimester and after birth	Bone marrow
Up to 5 years	Bone marrow of all bones
6–20 years	Red bone marrow of long bones and membranous bones
After 20 years	Shaft of humerus and tibia gets deposited with fat. Proximal end of these bones produce RBC. Flat bones like sternum, ribs, iliac and vertebrae produce RBC.

Genesis of RBC

1. *Pleuripotent hematopoietic stem cells (PHSC):* These cells are capable of forming any kind of blood cell.
2. *Committed stem cells:* PHSC become committed to a particular line of cells called committed stem cells.
3. *Colony forming unit:* Erythrocyte (CFU-E): committed stem cells that produce erythrocytes is called colony forming unit-erythrocyte.
4. *Proerythroblast:* 15–20 μm in size. First cell that can be identified belonging to red blood cell series (Fig. 4.3). It divides multiple number of times to form basophil erythroblast.

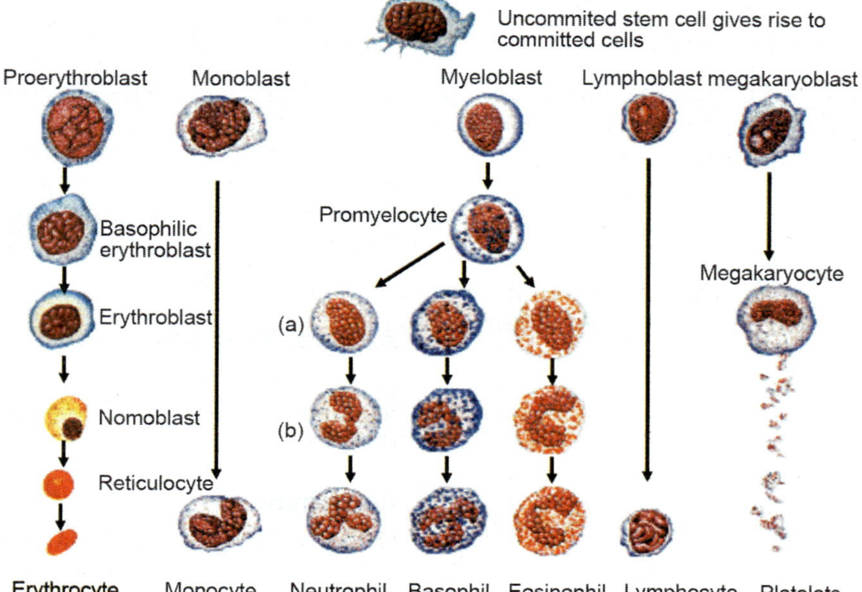

Fig. 4.3: Genesis of RBC

5. *Basophil erythroblast (early normoblast):* 12–16 µm in size. These cells stain with basic dyes. Hemoglobin is absent.
6. *Polychromatophil erythroblast (intermediate normoblast):* 10–14 µm in size. Hemoglobin appears in this stage. It has basophilic cytoplasm with acidophilic hemoglobin.
7. *Orthochromatic erythroblast (late normoblast):* 8–10 µm in size. Hemoglobin increases. Acidophilic cytoplasm with basophilic nucleus.
8. *Reticulocyte:* About 1% of total red cells are reticulocytes. 7.5 µm in size. Also called as young red cells. With Brilliant cresyl blue, RNA appears as reticulum.

   Nucleus condenses and gets extruded from the cell.

   Endoplasmic reticulum is reabsorbed. Remnants of Golgi apparatus, mitochondria, and few other cytoplasmic organelles are present. Reticulocyte response: anemic persons on treatment show increased release of reticulocytes in response to therapy. This is called as reticulocyte response.
9. *Mature erythrocyte:* Reticulocyte by the process of diapedesis pass from bone marrow into blood capillaries.

   Basophilic materials disappear in 1 to 2 days and mature erythrocytes are formed. Because of short life their concentration is less than 1%.

FACTORS NECESSARY FOR ERYTHROPOIESIS

Growth Inducers and Differentiation Inducers

Growth inducers: Multiple proteins that induce growth and reproduction of different stem cells are called growth inducers, e.g. interleukin-3.

Differentiation inducers: They cause one type of committed stem cells to differentiate into one or more steps in final blood cells.

Hypoxia-reduced oxygen levels results in growth induction, differentiation and production of erythrocytes.

Hormones

Erythropoietin

Erythropoietin is a glycoprotein hormone with a molecular weight of 34,000.

Function: To regulate erythropoiesis.

Stimulus for erythropoietin (EPO) secretion occurs, in:

- High altitude
- Cardiopulmonary disorders.

Other factors that stimulate EPO secretion are
- Epinephrine
- Norepinephrine
- Prostaglandins.

Site of formation of EPO

Interstitial cells in the peritubular capillaries of kidneys: 85%

Perivenous hepatocytes of liver: 15%

Actions of erythropoietin
- EPO acts on stem cells to differentiate into committed stem cells.
- Promotes 'Hb' synthesis by acting on 8 amino-levulinic acid synthetase.
- Promotes every stage of maturation from pro-normoblast to mature red cells.
- Promotes release of RBCs from marrow to circulation.

Half-life of EPO: 5 hours

Effect of EPO on erythropoiesis

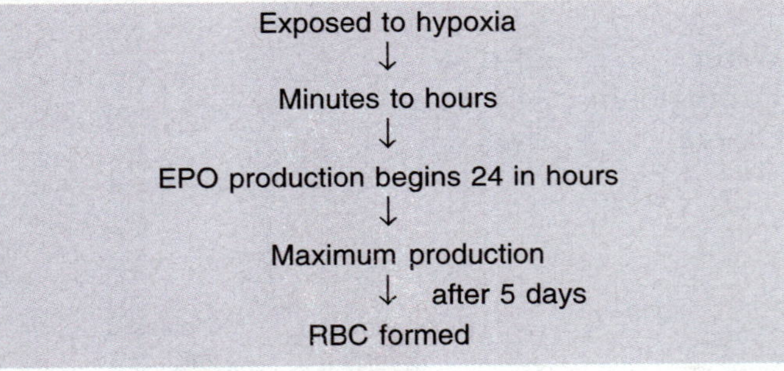

EPO activates hematopoietic stem cells in bone marrow, to become proerythroblast. EPO also speeds up each step in the production of new red cells. Production continues as long as a person remains in low oxygen state.

Applied Physiology

Renal failure: When both kidneys fail, the person becomes anemic as kidneys produce 90% of EPO (Fig. 4.4).

Androgens

Males have higher RBC count than females because androgens are potent stimulators of:
- Erythropoietin production
- Erythropoiesis.

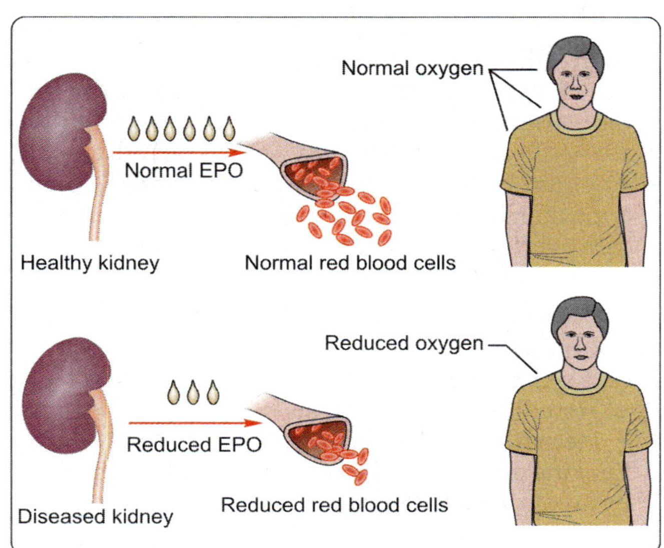

Fig. 4.4: Role of EPO in erythropoiesis

Estrogens

Estrogens have inhibitory effect on erythropoiesis.

Thyroxine

Thyroxine deficiency leads to anemia.

Hypofunction of Adrenal Cortex and Pituitary Gland

Leads to mild-to-moderate anemia:

i. *Nutritional factors:* First class proteins are necessary for globin formation.

ii. *Minerals:* Iron, copper, cobalt and zinc are necessary for erythropoiesis. Iron is necessary for haem production.

iii. *Vitamins:* Vit B_{12}, vit C, and folic acid
Vit C: Promotes iron absorption from the gut.
Vit B_{12} and folic acid are necessary for synthesis of DNA.

Maturation of Red Cells

Maturation of red cells is by:

- Vitamin B_{12}
- Folic acid

Thymidine triphosphate forms one of the essential building blocks of DNA.

Maturation Failure

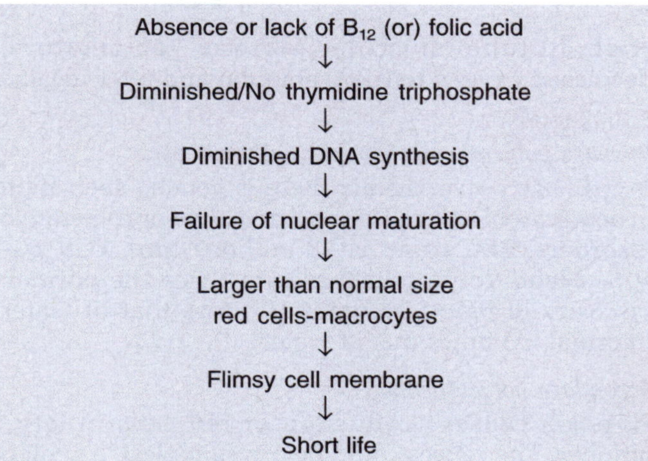

Intrinsic Factor of Castle

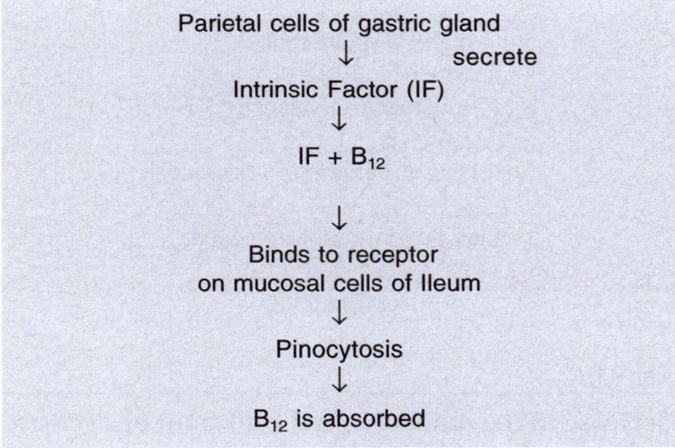

Applied Physiology

Absence of IF leads to maturation failure caused by lack of B_{12}. This condition is called pernicious anemia.

FOLIC ACID (PTEROYLGLUTAMIC ACID)

Folic acid is necessary for DNA synthesis. Absence of folic acid causes failure of maturation.

Variations of RBC

In Number

Increase in number of red cells is called polycythemia. It may be:

- Physiological
- Pathological

Cause

Physiological

High altitude, muscular exercise, temperature, decreased oxygen tension, emotion and after meals.

Pathological

Primary polycythemia (or) polycythemia vera

In primary polycythemia there is genetic aberration in hemocytoblastic cells. It occurs in myeloproliferative disorders. RBC count is >8 million/mm^3, PCV 60–70%, blood volume increases to twice the normal, viscosity of blood becomes 10 times that of water (Normal = 3 times that of water).

4

Secondary polycythemia

Hypoxia causes production of red cells in large number. The causes could be physiological, e.g. high altitude, pathological, e.g. congenital heart disease.

Effects of polycythemia on circulatory system

Polycythemia
↓↓↓
Increase in viscosity
↓
Increase in peripheral resistance
↓
Increase in arterial pressure
↓
Hypertension

ANEMIA

Decrease in the number of red cell count or decrease in the quantity of hemoglobin leading to decrease in oxygen carrying capacity is called anemia.

Classification of Anemia

Morphological Classification

- *Normocytic normochromic:* Size and hemoglobin content of RBC is normal, e.g. haemorrhage (Fig. 4.5a).
- *Microcytic hypochromic:* RBCs are smaller in size and pale, e.g. iron deficiency anemia (Fig. 4.5b).
- *Macrocytic (or) megaloblastic:* RBCs are larger in size and hemoglobin is less, e.g. B_{12} (or) folic acid deficiency (Fig. 4.5c).

Etiological Classification

- *Nutritional deficiency:* Anemia is due to deficiency of iron, folic acid, vitamin B_{12}, vitamin C and proteins.
- *Aplastic anemia:* Marrow failure with reduction in stem cell number occurs in aplastic anemia. It occurs due to exposure to radiation, excessive X-ray, and industrial chemicals (Fig. 4.5d).
- *Hemolytic anemia:* Red cells are destroyed quickly. Anemia occurs due to excess hemolysis of RBC and bone marrow tries to compensate by increasing red cell production. When hemolysis is more than production, hemolytic anemia occurs.

Causes of hemolytic anemia

Congenital

1. Red cell membrane defect:
   - Hereditary spherocytosis
   - Hereditary elliptocytosis.
2. Enzyme defect, e.g. glucose-6-phosphate deficiency, pyruvate kinase deficiency.

Hemoglobin abnormalities: Sickle cell anemia, thalassemia.

Acquired

Erythroblastosis fetalis
Infection, e.g. malaria
Drugs and chemicals, e.g. dapsone.

Investigations

Reticulocyte count is high, plasma bilirubin is increased.

Sickle Cell Anemia

Common among blacks in West Africa and America. Abnormal hemoglobin called "Hb-S" is present in these people. The defect occurs in 6th position of β-chain of hemoglobin. Instead of glutamic acid, valine is present in sickle all anemia. Hypoxia causes this hemoglobin to precipitate into long crystals in RBC called tectoids. These tectoids causes sickling of red cells (Fig. 4.5e).

Microcytic Hypochromic Anemia

Pathophysiology

1. Defective iron absorption
2. Decreased transferring in blood

↓
Less of iron to form 'Hb'
↓
Decreased hemoglobin synthesis
↓
Decreased cell volume
↓
Small sized cell:
microcytes with pale colored RBC: hypochromic

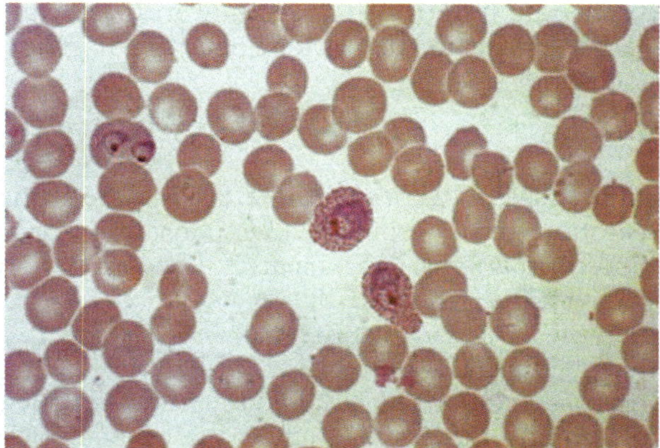

Fig. 4.5a: Normocytic normochromic cells

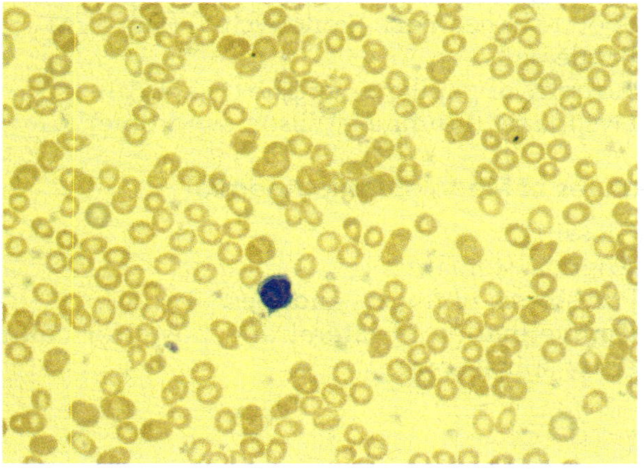

Fig. 4.5b: Microcytic hypochromic cells

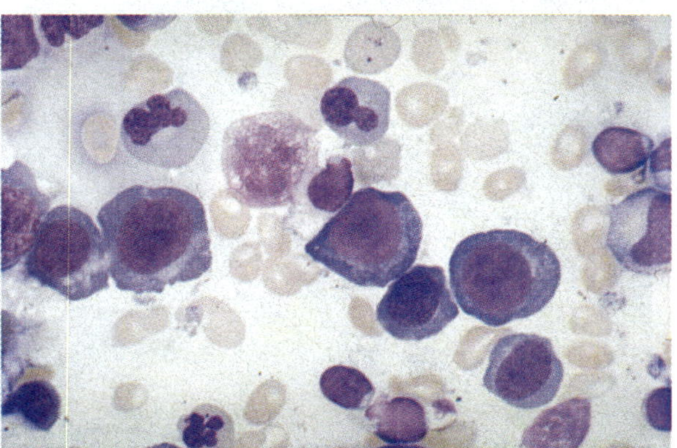

Fig. 4.5c: Megaloblastic red cells

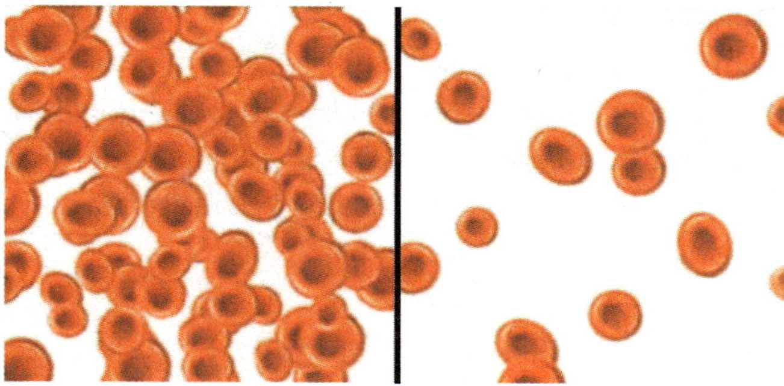

Fig. 4.5d: Few red cells in aplastic anemia

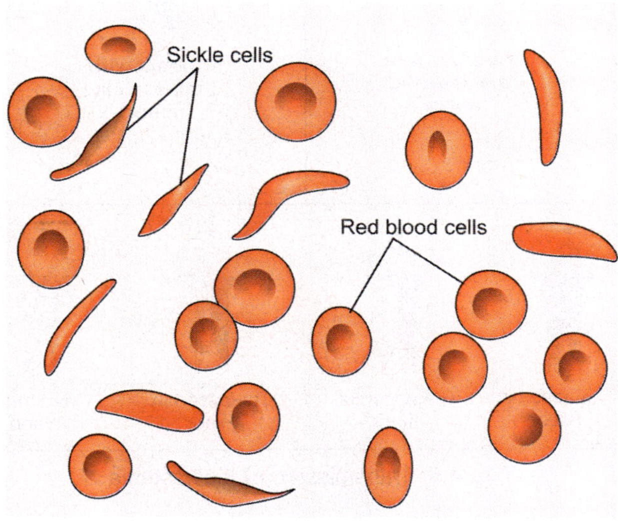

Fig. 4.5e: Sickle shaped red cells

Sickle Cell Crisis

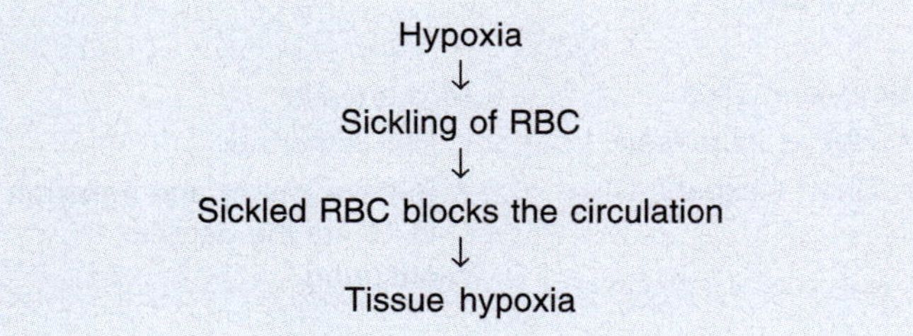

Sickle cell crisis leads to death within few hours. Sickle cell trait is the heterozygous state of sickle cell anemia. People with sickle cell trait are resistant to *Plasmodium falciparum* malaria. Treatment includes hydroxyurea and bone marrow transplantation.

Thalassemia

In thalassemia there is:

- Defect in synthesis of globin part of hemoglobin
- Defect in α-chain synthesis is α-thalassemia
- Defect in β-chain synthesis is β-thalassemia
- β-thalassemia can be:
  - β-thalassemia major
  - β-thalassemia minor (Fig. 4.6)

A parent with thalassemia minor

A parent with thalassemia minor

Thalassemia major

Thalassemia minor

Thalassemia minor

Normal blood

Fig. 4.6: Transmission of thalassemia

β-thalassemia major	*β-thalassemia minor*
• Less common	• More common
• Homozygous transmission	• Heterozygous transmission
• Complete absence of β-chain ↓	• Partial absence ↓
Severe anemia	Mild anemia
• HbF is increased	• HbF is normal
• Short lifespan: 17	• Survive longer and trans-mit to 18 yrs the gene to offspring

Blood Loss Anemia

In acute haemorrhage, body replaces the fluid portion of plasma in 1 to 3 days. This leads to normocytic normochromic anemia. Replacement of RBC takes 4–6 weeks.

In chronic blood loss, intestinal mucosa cannot absorb adequate iron, leading to microcytic hypochromic anemia.

Symptoms

Anemia causes weakness, fatigue, lassitude, dyspnoea on exertion and palpitation. Compensatory changes that occur in anemic persons are:

- Tachycardia
- Increased cardiac output
- Redistribution of blood flow
- Increased content of 2, 3, DPG: that favors oxygen release into the tissues to meet the tissue hypoxia.
- Hemic murmur: A nonconducted systolic murmur is heard at the apex.

Features of Iron Deficiency Anemia

- Pallor (seen in conjunctiva)
- Spoon-shaped nails (koilonychia) (Fig. 4.7a)
- Brittle nails
- Atrophy of papilla in tongue (Fig. 4.7b)
- Dysphagia (Plummer-Wilson syndrome).

Features of Megaloblastic Anemia

- Glossitis
- Angular stomatitis
- Paresthesia of fingers and toes.

Demyelination of lateral and posterior column fibers of spinal cord.

Investigations

- Hemoglobin estimation
- RBC count
- Peripheral blood smear
- Red cell indices

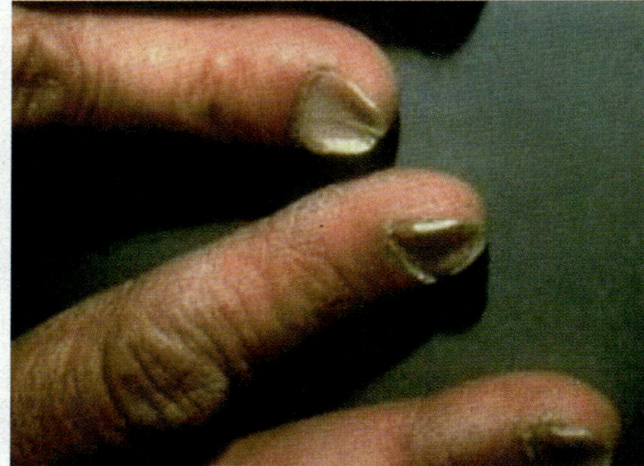

Fig. 4.7a: Koilonychia—in iron deficiency anemia

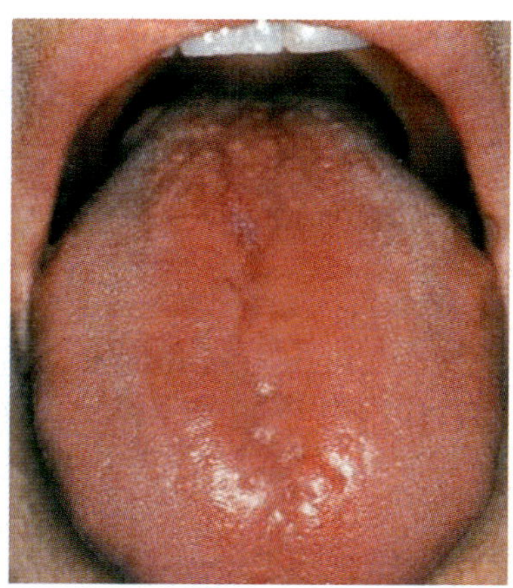

Fig. 4.7b: Atrophy of papilla in anemia

- Reticulocyte count
- If necessary, bone marrow smear
- Estimation of iron content in serum
- Serum iron binding capacity.

Treatment

Treatment depends on the severity of anemia.

Severe anemia is treated by giving packed cell transfusion. This will prevent volume overload and hence congestive cardiac failure.

Mild and moderate anemia are treated by giving iron and B_{12}.

I. *Nutritional factors:* First class proteins are necessary for globin formation.

II. *Minerals:* Iron, copper, cobalt and zinc are necessary for erythropoiesis.

i. Iron is necessary for haem production

ii. Iron deficiency is due to:

a. Inadequate intake

b. Inadequate absorption

c. Excess loss

d. Hookworm infestation.

III. *Vitamins:* Vit B_{12}, vit C, folic acid.

Vit C: Promotes iron absorption from the gut.

B_{12} and folic acid are necessary for synthesis of DNA.

4

13. HEMOGLOBIN

- Hb is an oxygen binding protein
- Molecular weight of 'Hb': 68,000
- It carries respiratory gases.

Normal values

- Birth up to 23 gm/dl
- Adult female 12–14 gm/dl
- Adult male 15–17 gm/dl

Functions of Hemoglobin

- *Transport of oxygen from lungs into tissue:* O_2 is loosely and reversibly bound to 'Hb'.
- *Transport of carbon dioxide from tissues to lungs*
  - Carboxyhemoglobin is formed rapidly than oxyhemoglobin.
- Hemoglobin plays an important role as blood buffer. It is 6 times more potent than plasma proteins.
- *Structure of hemoglobin* (Fig. 4.7c)
- Hemoglobin is a spherical molecule with molecular weight of 64,500.

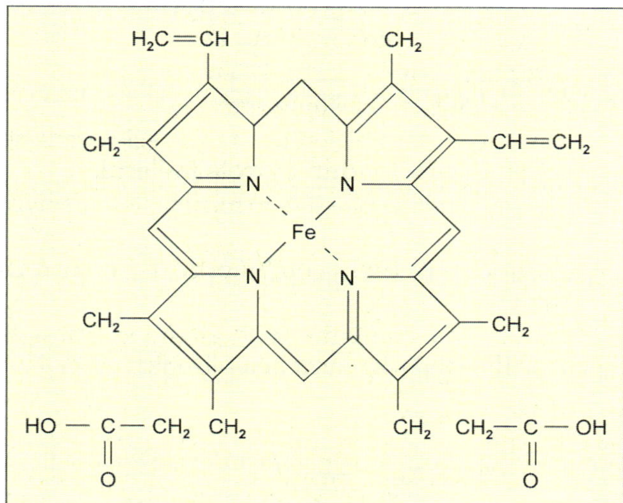

Fig. 4.7c: Structure of hemoglobin

- Hemoglobin molecule has 2 parts:
  - Heme
  - Globin

Heme

- Heme is made up of iron and protoporphyrin
- Iron is in ferrous form
- Fe^{++} is attached to N^- atom of each.

PYRROLE RING

Protoporphyrin

The 4 pyrrole rings are linked together by methane bridges to form protoporphyrin.

CH CH
CH CH
NH

Pyrrole ring

Globin

- There are 4 polypeptide chains in each Hb molecule.
- Normal adults have HbA
- HbA has 2 alpha-chains: each with 141 amino acid
  2 beta-chain: each with 146 amino acids.

  So, HbA is 2,2.

Synthesis of Hemoglobin

Synthesis of hemoglobin occurs in 4 steps:

i. 2 succinyl CoA + 2 glycine → pyrrole
ii. 4 pyrrole → protoporphyrin IX
iii. Protoporphyrin IX + Fe → heme
iv. Heme + globin → hemoglobin
   - Succinyl CoA formed in Kreb's cycle combines with glycine to form pyrrole molecule.
   - 4 pyrrole molecules join to form protoporphyrin IX.
   - Protoporphyrin IX combines with iron to form heme.
   - Each heme combines with globin synthesized by ribosomes to form hemoglobin.

Each Hb molecule has

- 4 Hb chain
- Each Hb chain has 1 Fe atom
- Each Fe atom loosely binds with 1 molecule of oxygen (8 oxygen atoms)

1 gm of Hb combines with 1.34 ml of oxygen.
In men: 15.5 gm Hb + 1.34 ml O_2 = 21 ml of oxygen.
In women: 14 gm Hb + 1.34 ml of O_2 = 18.5 ml.

Physiological Varities of Hb

Hb embryo	Gower 1, Gower 2, hemoglobin Portland
Hb F (fetal)	$\alpha_2\gamma_2$
Hb A (adult)	$\alpha_2\beta_2$
HbA_2	$\alpha_2\delta_2$

- Adult hemoglobin
  In adults: 98% of hemoglobin is $\alpha_2\beta_2$.
  2% of adult Hb is $\alpha_2\delta_2$

Fetal Hemoglobin

- HbF is present in fetal RBC.
- By the end of 1st year of child's life, fetal hemoglobin almost disappears and adult Hb appears.

Destruction of Hb

- RBCs are destroyed by reticuloendothelial system, particularly the spleen.
- Hb is released into plasma.
- Hb is degraded by RES to form
  - Iron
  - Globin
  - Porphyrin

  Iron is stored in the body as ferritin and hemosiderin.

Porphyrin gets converted into green pigment called biliverdin which in turn gets converted into bilirubin.

Globin is used in the resynthesis of Hb.

Applied Physiology

Defect in globin synthesis:

- Sickle cell anemia
- Thalassemia

Defect in synthesis of heme:

- Porphyrias
- Increased activity of amino levulinic acid leads to increased synthesis of porphyrins.
- Porphyrias may be inherited or acquired.
- Symptoms include photosensitivity and psychosis.

Hemoglobin Complexes

- *Oxyhemoglobin:* (HbO_2)
  Oxygen combines with hemoglobin to form oxyhemoglobin and the combination is loose and reversible.
- Glycosylated hemoglobin
  - Glucose gets attached to chain of HbA to form glycated hemoglobin (GHb).

- GHb must not exceed 6%
- GHb above 6% indicates poor control of blood sugar in diabetes mellitus.

- *Methemoglobin:* It is combination of NO with Hb. Normally, small amount of methemoglobin is present. Methemoglobinemia occurs in smokers, drugs, e.g. dapsone (antileprosy drugs).
  - Sulphemoglobin
  - Glycosylated hemoglobin
- Reduced hemoglobin
- Carboxyhemoglobin
- Carbaminohemoglobin

IRON METABOLISM

Requirement of Iron

Iron in needed to form:
Hemoglobin, myoglobin, cytochromes, cytochrome oxidases, peroxidase and catalase.

Total Body Iron

Total iron content of our body is 6 g.

Distribution of Iron

- Hemoglobin 65%
- Myoglobin 4%
- Various forms of Fe compound 1%
- Combination with transferrin 1%
- Stored in liver 15 to 30%

Absorption of Iron from Intestinal Tract

- Iron is absorbed from duodenum (2nd part)
- Iron can be absorbed only as ferrous form: Fe^{+++}
- Liver forms a betaglobulin called "apotransferrin".
- Iron combines with apotransferrin to form transferrin.

By the process of pinocytosis, transferrin containing 'Fe' is absorbed into epithelial cells.

- From the enterocytes, it is released into blood capillaries to form plasma transferrin.

Transport of Iron

Transferrin is the transport form of iron. Iron is bound loosely to transferrin and released in any tissue as per need.

Storage Form of Iron

Iron is stored in the liver and bone marrow as:

- Ferritin
- Hemosiderin

Regulation of Total Body Iron

Body is saturated with iron
↓
Decreased iron absorption from intestines

Iron stores are depleted
↓
Iron absorption ↑ increased by 5 times

Daily Loss of Iron

Human beings excrete 0.6 milligrams of iron each day into feces.

Menstrual loss of iron = 1.3 mg/day.

When blood loss is more peripheral smear shows—microcytic hypochromic picture:

- Hb content is less
- MCV: <75 u^3 (unit)
- MCH: <25 picograms
- Total Fe binding capacity (TIBC) is increased.

14. THE LEUKOCYTES

Introduction

WBC or leukocytes are body's protective system. They have the ability to "Seek out and destroy" the foreign invader. Thus, they protect us from bacteria, virus, fungus and parasite.

Classification

see next column

Leucocytes (Fig. 4.8)

Granulocytes (contain granules)	*Agranulocytes (do not contain granules)*
Polymorphonuclear	
• Neutrophils	• Lymphocytes
• Eosinophils	• Monocytes
• Basophils	

Concentration of Various WBC in Blood

- Polymorphonuclear neutrophils 55–60%
- Polymorphonuclear eosinophils 2–3%
- Polymorphonuclear basophils 0–1%
- Monocytes 4–5%
- Lymphocytes 30–35%

Functions of WBC

- Ganulocytes and monocytes protect the body against the invading organism by phagocytosis
- Lymphocytes are responsible for immunity.

4

Staining of WBC

Peripheral smear is stained by Leishman's stain a variant of Romanowsky's stain. It helps to identify the different types of WBC. Other variants of Romanowsky's stain.

- Giemsa's
- Jenner
- Wrights

Concept of Pools

There are three different pools, where the different types of WBC are seen.

Marrow Pool

90% of neutrophils are in marrow pool, i.e. red bone marrow.

Blood pool

3% of neutrophils are in blood pool.

Tissue pool

7% of neutrophils are in tissue pool.

Blood pool

It is further divided into:

- Circulating pool (in flowing blood)
- Marginal pool (adhering to vascular margin)

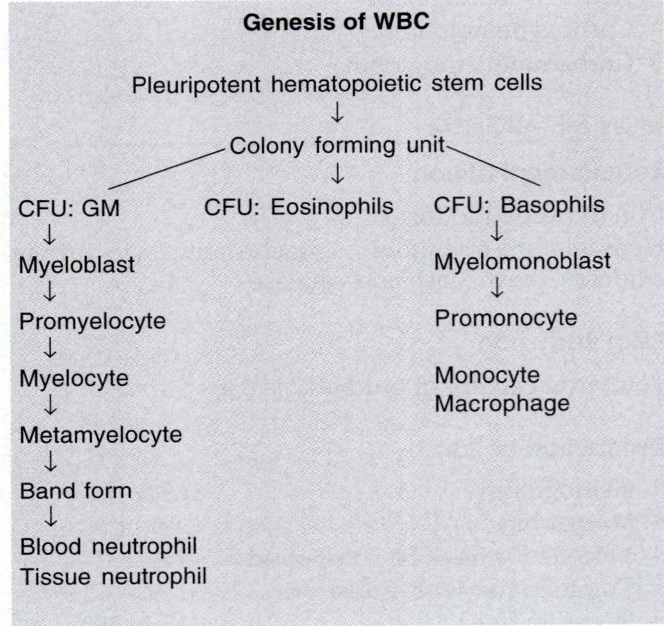

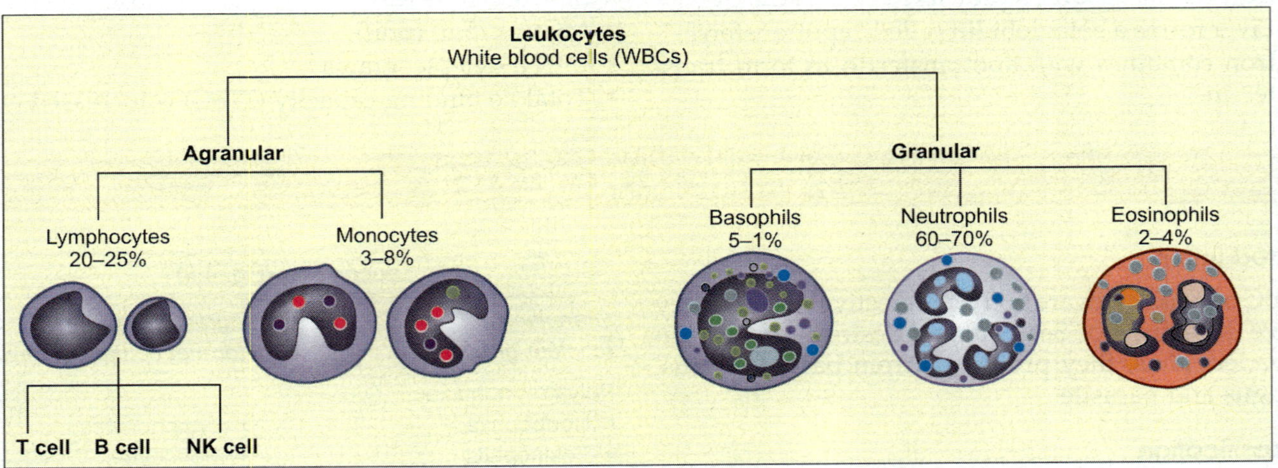

Fig. 4.8: Leukocytes (WBCs)

- Development of granulocyte through various series is called myeloid series.
- Process of granulopoieses takes 12 days.
- More than 3 times granulocytes are stored in bone marrow.

Formation of Lymphoid Series

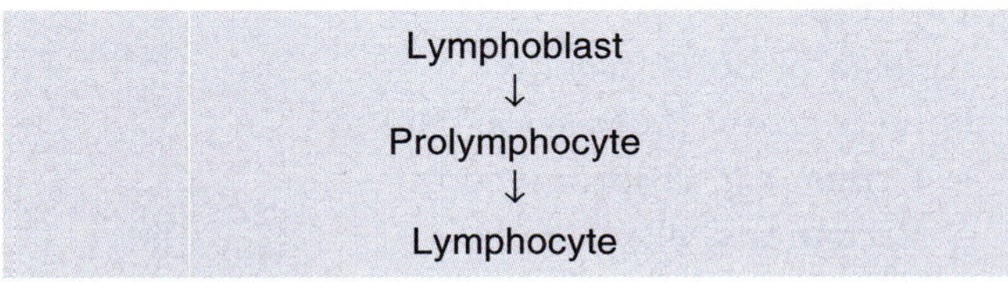

Regulation of Leucopoiesis

- *Colony stimulating factor:* Cytokines that stimulate the formation of different types of granulocytes are called colony stimulating factor. They are:
  - G-CSF (granulocyte CSF)
  - M-CSF (monocyte CSF)
  - GM-CSF (granulocyte monocyte CSF)
- *Interleukins:* Interleukins are cytokines that stimulate lymphocyte formation.

Neutrophils

Diameter	10–14 μm
Cytoplasm	Fine pinpoint granules. These granules contain glycosidase, sulphatase, phosphatase, nuclease and peroxidase (Fig. 4.9a).

Nucleus

- *Young neutrophils:* Single horseshoe shaped nucleus
- *Mature neutrophils:* 2 to 6 lobes
- Nuclei are connected by chromatin filament.

Functions

- 1st line of defense
- Neutrophils function by the process of phagocytosis.

Phagocytosis

- Phagocytosis is also called as "cell eating". Various steps in phagocytosis (Fig. 4.9b) are:
  1. *Margination:* The process of attachment of neutrophils to the capillary endothelium is called margination. Cell adhesion molecules are present on the endothelial surface that helps the neutrophils in margination.
  2. *Diapedesis:* Marginated neutrophils squeeze through intercellular spaces in blood vessel and pass out.
  3. *Chemotaxis (Chemo-chemical, Taxis-movement):* Movement of neutrophils towards the chemical substance present at the site of inflammation is called chemotaxis.

     Substances that mediate chemotaxis are called chemokines. Some of the chemokines are C5, leukotriene B4, and cytokines.
  4. *Opsonization:* Process of coating of bacteria by opsonin, by which bacteria becomes tasty for

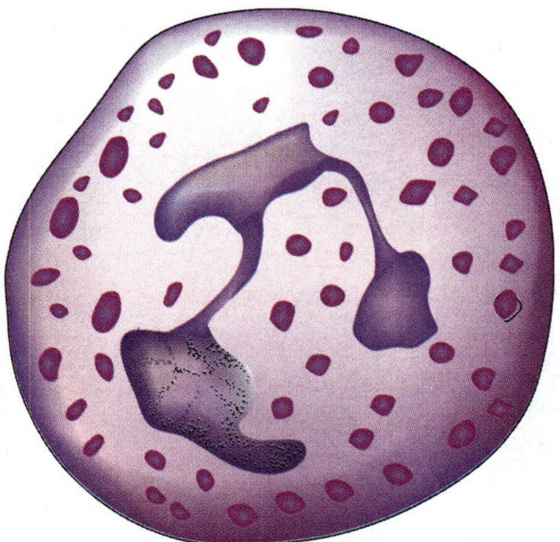

Fig. 4.9a: Neutrophils

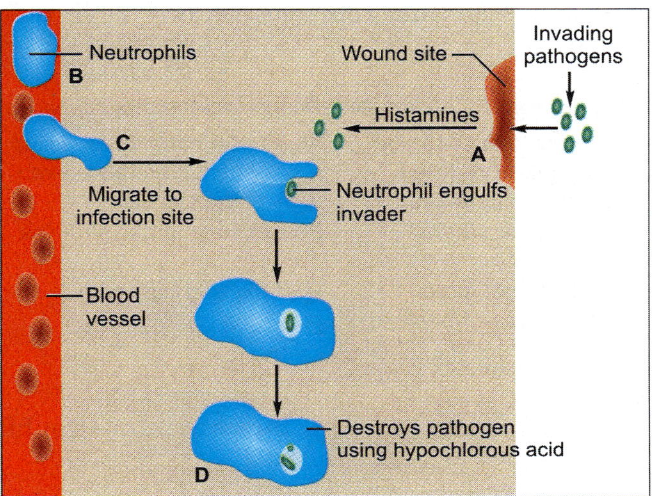

Fig. 4.9b: Phagocytosis by neutrophil

phagocytosis is called opsonization, e.g. IgG opsonin.

Engulfment

- Pseudopodia are put out in all direction.
- Pseudopodia meet each other and fuse to form phagocytic vesicle.
- Single neutrophil can phagocytize 3–20 bacteria before it dies.

Degranulation

Proteolytic enzymes present in neutrophils digest the bacteria.

4

In macrophages, lipases and digest the bacteria.

Phagocytosis by Macrophage

- Monocytes in blood when they enter into tissue, become macrophages.
- They phagocytize around 100 bacteria.
- Lipases digest the bacterial wall.
- Oxidizing agents that help in killing the bacteria are:
  - Superoxide
  - Hydrogen peroxide
  - Hydroxyl ions
- Enzyme myeloperoxidase is also a powerful bacterial agent.

Applied Physiology

Tubercle bacilli are resistant to killing effects of neutrophils and macrophages leading to chronic disease.

Phagocytosis by neutrophils	*Phagocytosis by macrophages*
• 3–20 bacteria are killed	About 100 bacteria are killed
• Neutrophils are killed during phagocytosis	Macrophages are alive even after phagocytosis
• Phagocytize smaller particles	Phagocytize larger particles
• Particles: Not more than the size of bacteria	Bacteria and malarial parasites

Variation in Neutrophil Count

Neutrophilia (>15,000/mm^3): Increase in neutrophil count is called as neutrophilia.

Physiological

Newborn, exercise and emotion.

Pathological

- Pyogenic bacterial infections
- Acute rheumatic fever
- Burns
- Myocardial infarction.

Neutropenia (< 2500/mm^3)

- Typhoid
- Aplasia of bone marrow
- Bone marrow depression due to:
  - Drugs, e.g. chloromycetin
  - Radiations, e.g. X-rays.

Arneth Count

Counting the number of lobes in neutrophils and expressing it as % of cells with different number of lobes is called Arneth count or Cooke's Arneth count.

Shift to left: (N1 + N2 + N3)

Indicates hyperactive bone marrow.

Shift to right: (N4 + N5)

Indicates hypoactive bone marrow.

Eosinophils

Diameter	10–14 µm
Cytoplasm	Acidophilic
	coarse granules (Fig. 4.10)

Granules contain major basic protein, eosinophilic cationic protein, lyophospholipase, aryl sulphatase and histaminase.

Nucleus: Bilobed connected by chromatin strand.

Functions: Eosinophils are weak phagocytes. They act as parasiticide and larvicide by releasing hydrolytic enzymes and highly reactive forms of oxygen.

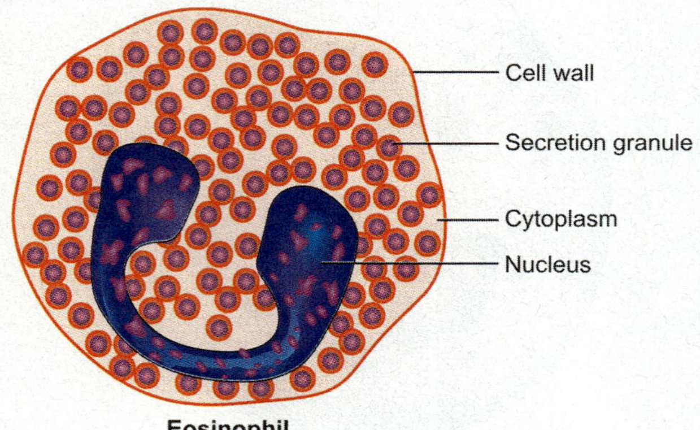

Fig. 4.10: Eosinophil

Role of Eosinophils in Allergy (Lungs and Skin)

Basophils and mast cells release
↓
Eosinophilic chemotactic factor
↓
Eosinophils migrate towards allergic tissue
↓
Detoxify inflammation inducing substances
↓
Destroy the allergen–antibody complexes
↓
Prevents spread of local inflammatory process

Eosinophilia

Allergy, asthma, hay fever, skin diseases, e.g. urticaria, eczema, parasitic infection, e.g. round worm, hookworm, tapeworm.

Eosinopenia

- ACTH and steroid therapy
- Stress

Lymphocytes

Lymphocytes are agranular cells. There are small and large lymphocytes.

Small Lymphocytes

Size	8 µm in diameter
Cytoplasm	Very thin rim of cytoplasm is seen
Nucleus	Large nucleus staining deeply with basic dyes
Function	Responsible for immunity of a person

Large Lymphocyte

They are younger form of lymphocytes

Size	10 µm in diameter
Cytoplasm	Clear blue cytoplasm
Nucleus	Oval or kidney shaped nucleus.

Basophils (Fig. 4.11a)

Size	10–14 µm
Cytoplasm	Basophilic cytoplasm is full of granules-coarse in nature and blue black in color. Granules contain: Heparin, histamine, 5-hydroxytryptamine (serotonin).
Nucleus	It has 2 lobes connected by a strand. It is spectacle shaped.

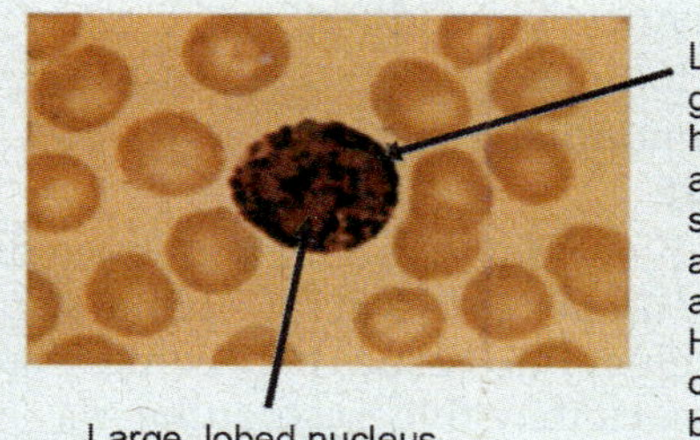

Fig. 4.11a: Basophils

Function	Mild phagocytosis plays a role in allergic reaction release heparin that prevents clotting.
Basophilia	Viral infections Allergic reactions Chronic myeloid leukemia
Basopenia	Steroid therapy Drug induced reaction.

Monocytes (Fig. 4.11b)

Size	18–25 µm, largest of the leukocytes
Cytoplasm	Clear without granules
Nucleus	Horseshoe or kidney shaped and is situated eccentrically.
Functions	1. Role in defense by phagocytosis. 2. Role in tumor immunity: From blood these cells enter into tissues to form tissue macrophages (60 to 80 µm in size).

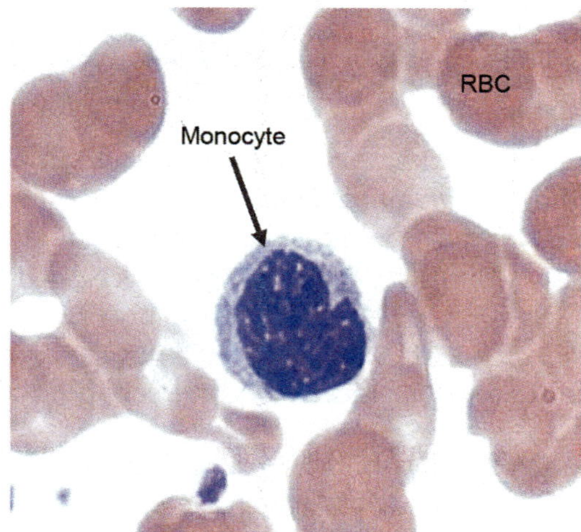

Fig. 4.11b: Monocytes

3. Monocytes produce
   Cytokines
   Hemopoietic factors
   TNF

They circulate in blood for 72 hours and leave the blood and enter into tissues to blood for 72 hours and leave the blood and enter into tissues to become tissue macrophages. In tissues they live for months.

Monocytosis

- Increase in monocyte
- Certain bacterial infections, e.g. tuberculosis
- Infectious mononucleosis
- Monocytic leukemia.

4

Monocytopenia

- Decrease in monocytes
- Occurs in hypoplastic marrow.

Mast Cells

- Located outside the capillaries in the body.
- Mast cells liberate heparin into blood. This prevents blood coagulation.

Mast cells in allergic reaction

Antigen + antibody IgE
↓
Mast cells rupture
↓
Release of histamine, serotonin, bradykinin, SRS—of anaphylaxis, lysosomal enzymes, heparin cause
↓
Local vascular and tissue reactions
↓
Responsible for allergic manifestations

INFLAMMATION

When injury occurs to the tissues by

Bacteria, trauma, chemical, heat or some other way, multiple substances are released to produce local reaction called inflammation.

Inflammation is characterized by

- Vasodilatation of local blood vessels (Redness or Rubor).
- Increased permeability of capillaries and leakage of fluid into interstitial space.
- Clotting of fluid due to leakage of fibrinogen from capillaries.
- Migration of granulocytes and monocytes into tissues.
- Swelling of tissue cells (tumor).

Inflammatory changes—clinically are

- Rubor: Redness
- Tumor: Swelling
- Calor: Heat
- Dolor: Pain
- Loss of function

Physiologically, steps of inflammation are

- Vasodilation
- Leukocyte emigration
- Chemotaxis
- Phagocytosis

  Inflammation causes "Walling off" effect. This effect delays the spread of infection.

Strepotococcal infection	*Staphylococcal infection*
• Walling off occurs slowly • Greater tendency to spread	• Walled off rapidly • Prevented from spreading to other parts

Various Lines of Defense

Tissue macrophage: First line of defense

When an organism enters the body, the tissue macrophages enlarge in size and move towards the site of infection forming the 1st line of defense. For example alveolar macrophages in lungs, microglia in brain, and histiocytes in skin.

Neutrophils: Second line of defense

Within 1 hour after the entry of the organism, neutrophils invade the inflamed area. The step involved are:

- Margination
- Diapedesis
- Chemotaxis
- Phagocytosis.

Second macrophage invasion: 3rd line of defense

Along with neutrophils, monocytes enter into circulation. Monocytes need 8 hours to swell and acquire tremendous lysosomes and become macrophages. Now, macrophages can phagocytize more bacteria.

Increased production of granulocyte and monocyte by bone marrow: 4th line of defense

Bone marrow starts producing more number of granulocyte and monocytes. It takes 3–4 days for the bone marrow to form new cells and release them into blood.

LEUKEMIA

Leukemia is a malignant disease of white blood cells. There is uncontrolled production of white blood cells with plenty of immature cells.

Classification

Depending on cell type, leukemia can be classified as

- Lymphocytic leukemia
- Myeloid leukemia.

Depending on the time duration, leukemia can be classified as

- Acute leukemia
- Chronic leukemia.

In lymphocytic leukemia, there is uncontrolled production of lymphoid cells.

In myeloid leukemia, granulocyte and its precursors are increased. Myeloid leukemia can be:

- Neutrophilic leukemia
- Eosinophilic leukemia
- Basophilic leukemia
- Monocytic leukemia.

Leukemia can be

- Well differentiated
- Undifferentiated

In well differentiated type, the disease will have a chronic course over 10–20 year.

In undifferentiated type, the disease will have acute course and often leads to death within few months if untreated.

Causes of Leukemia

- Ionizing radiation, cytotoxic drugs, mutations and immune deficiency states.
- Extramedullary hematopoieses takes place leading to enlargement of liver, spleen and lymph nodes. Leukemic cells of bone marrow invade the surrounding bone leading to bone pain and a tendency to fracture easily.
- Bleeding tendency such as purpura , epistaxis and gum bleed occurs. Diagnosis is not obvious and is uncovered by laboratory investigations.

  Peripheral smear shows blast cells (Fig. 4.12).
- Anemia and thrombocytopenia occurs (leading to bleeding).

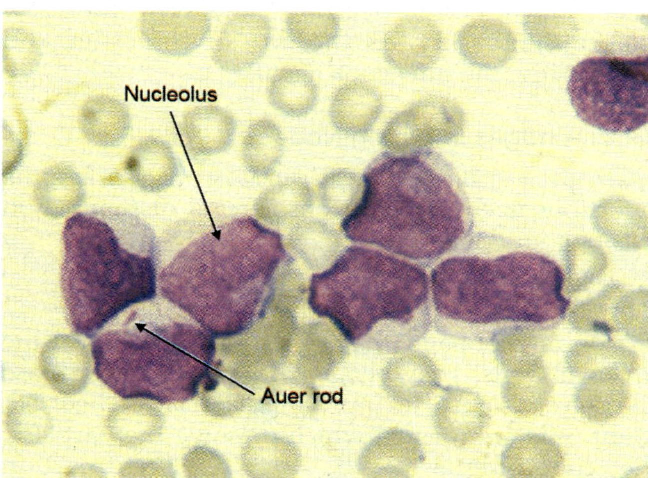

Fig. 4.12: Blast cells in leukemia

Leukopenia

Decrease in the number of WBC count leaves the body unprotected against disease.

Causes are irradiation, X-ray or gamma rays and exposure to drugs and chemicals.

Treatment with antibiotics and blood transfusion will improve the condition.

15. RETICULOENDOTHELIAL SYSTEM

Definition

The combination of monocytes, macrophages and fixed tissue macrophages with specialized cells in the bone marrow, spleen and lymph nodes is called reticuloendothelial system (RES).

RES is also called as *monocyte-macrophage system.*

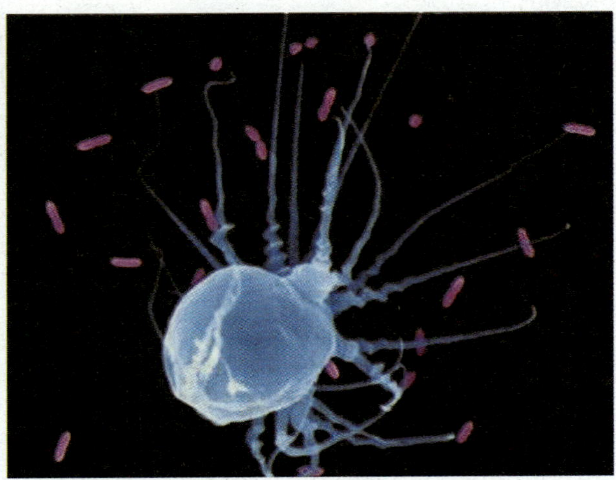

Fig. 4.13a: Alveolar macrophage

Tissue Macrophges in Skin and Subcutaneous Tissues (Histiocytes)

When an infection begins in the skin, the local macrophages invade the site of infection and phagocytise the infectious agent.

Macrophages in Lymph Nodes

Macrophages lining lymph sinuses phagocytize the infectious agent and prevent general dissemination throughout the body.

Alveolar Macrophages in Lungs

Tissue macrophages (Fig. 4.13a) are present in the alveolar walls. They phagocytise, digest and release the digestive particles into lymph. If it is not digested, giant cells are formed which dissolve the particles, e.g. tuberculous bacilli, silica dust and carbon particles.

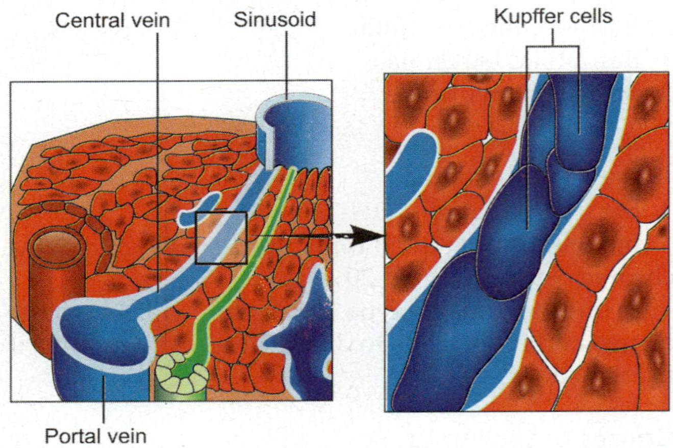

Fig. 4.13b

Macrophages in Liver Sinusoides

Tissue macrophages in liver (Fig. 4.13b) are called Kupffer cells. They form an effective particulate filtration system. So, no bacteria can enter from portal blood into systemic circulation.

Kupffer cells can phagocytize single bacterium in less than 1/100th of a second.

Macrophages of Spleen and Bone Marrow

Macrophages are trapped in the reticular meshwork of spleen and bone marrow. When blood passes through the spleen, it phagocytizes the unwanted debris in blood. Old and abnormal blood cells are destroyed.

16. BLOOD GROUPS

Blood transfusion in earlier days led to the death of recipients. In 1901, Landsteiner demonstrated that human beings could be classified into four groups depending on antigens presents on red cell surface.

ABO SYSTEM

Two agglutinogens were found on surface of red cell. If agglutinogen A is present on red cell surface, it is blood group A. It is further divided into A1 and A2.

If B agglutinogen is present on the surface of red cell, it is blood group B.

If A and B agglutinogen are present on the red cell surface, it is blood group AB. It is further divided into A1B and A2B.

If no agglutinogen is present on the red cell surface, it is O blood group (Fig. 4.14).

Blood group	*Antigen on RBC*	*Antibody in plasma*
Blood group A	Antigen A	Antibody B
Blood group B	Antigen B	Antibody A
Blood group AB	Antigen AB	No antibody
Blood group O	No antigen	Antibody AB

AGGLUTINOGEN (ANTIGEN)

Agglutinogen are inherited as Mendelian dominant. Agglutinogen A and B first appear in the sixth week of fetal life. They are complex oligosaccharides. Red cell surface has 'H' antigen which is the precursor of A and B antigen. In blood group O, this 'H' antigen persist.

Marathi speaking people around Mumbai were reported to have RBC that had

No H antigen
No A antigen
No B antigen

This blood group is called as "Bombay blood group" and symbolized as Oh. Since the RBC have neither H, nor A or B antigen, on their red cell surface, their serum contains all three agglutinins (antibody A, B, AB). So, if they need blood transfusion, only Bombay blood group must be given.

Secretors

Agglutinogen of ABO group are present not only on the RBC surface but also on salivary glands, pancreas,

	Group A	Group B	Group AB	Group O
Red blood cell type				
Antibodies present	Anti-A	Anti-B	None	Anti-A and Anti-B
Antigens present	A antigen	B antigen	B and B antigens	None

Fig. 4.14: ABO system

kidney, liver, lungs and testis. They are water soluble and present in gastric juice, saliva and other body fluids of 80% people. They are called as secretors.

Nonsecretors

The agglutinogens of nonsecretors are confined to the red cells.

Agglutinin (Antibody)

Antibody A and antibody B present in the serum are IgM type and hence do not cross the placenta.

Concentration of agglutinin is negligible at birth. It increases gradually and reaches a peak at 10 years. This is caused by entry of antigen A and B via food and bacteria.

4

Landsteiners Law

If an antigen is present on the surface of RBC, the corresponding antibody will be absent in plasma.

If an antibody is present in the plasma, the corresponding antigen will be absent on the surface of RBC.

Determination of Blood Group

To determine the blood group of an individual, a suspension of red cells is made in isotonic saline. A drop of red cell in saline is taken on a slide and a drop of antisera A, antisera B is placed over the blood (contains antibody).

If agglutination occurs with antisera A, then the blood group is A.

If agglutination occurs with antisera B, then the blood group is B.

If agglutination occurs with antisera A and antisera B then the blood group is AB.

If agglutination does not occur with antisera A or B then the blood group is O.

Inheritance of ABO Blood Groups

ABO genes are located in the ninth pair of human chromosomes. A child's blood group is determined by two genes received from the parents.

If the child is O → the father cannot be AB

If the child is AB → the father cannot be O

If the child is A and mother is B or O → the father cannot be B or O

If the child is B and mother is A or O → the father cannot be A or O

Rh Typing

There are several varities of Rh antigens, e.g. C, D, E. D is the most common antigen present and is highly immunogenic. It is the presence or absence of D agglutinogen that determines whether a person is Rh positive or negative. If D agglutinogen is present, a person is Rh (D) positive. If D agglutinogen is absent, a person is Rh (D) negative. There is no naturally occurring antibody for Rh (D) antigen. Two conditions where Rh antibodies are formed are:

a. When Rh negative person receives Rh positive blood.
b. Erythroblastosis fetalis.

Erythroblastosis Fetalis

Erythroblastosis fetalis is a disease of fetus and newborn due to development of Rh incompatibility between mother and fetus. If Rh –ve mother, carries Rh +ve fetus, (father Rh +ve), during severance of cord, Rh –ve fetal red cell enter into maternal circulation. First baby is not affected. Mother starts producing Rh antibodies against fetal red cells. During the second pregnancy, the preformed antibodies in the mother cross the placenta and enter into fetus causing hemolysis of fetal RBC. As a result of hemolysis the newborn develops:

a. Anemia due to hemolysis
b. Erythroblasts in peripheral blood as the body tries to replace hemolyzed RBC
c. Jaundice within 24 hours of birth
d. *Kernicterus:* Elevated serum bilirubin crosses the blood brain barrier and fix to the basal ganglia leading to the disturbance in motor activities
e. *Hydrops fetalis:* Grossly edematous fetus (Fig. 4.15).

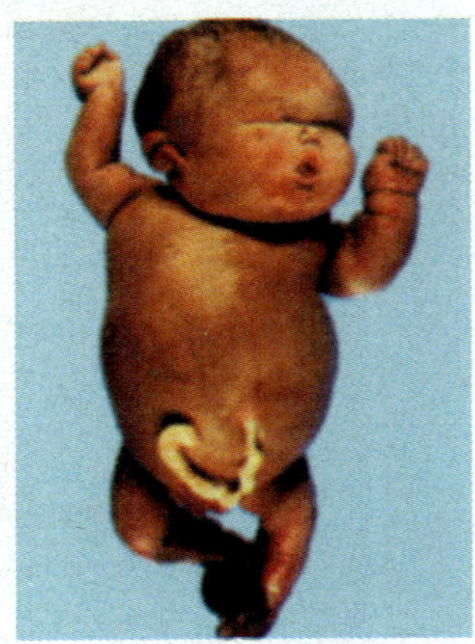

Fig. 4.15: Hydrops fetalis

Investigations

a. Blood grouping
b. Rh typing
c. Serum bilirubin
d. Peripheral blood smear
e. Reticulocyte count
f. Direct Coombs' test is positive in erythroblastosis fetalis.

Prevention and Treatment

Anti-D agglutinin is given as single dose to mother within 72 hours of delivery. This destroys the Rh +ve RBC of fetus in maternal circulation before they form antibodies.

Treatment of Baby

a. Phototherapy
b. Double exchange transfusion.

Minor Blood Groups

In 1927, Landsteiner with Levine found blood groups M, N and MN.

Other minor blood groups are Lutheran, Levis, Kidd, Duffy, etc.

MN blood group was used in disputed paternity. Now, DNA techniques are used in disputed paternity.

If child is M father cannot be N

If child is N father cannot be M

Gene for MN group is located in chromosome 4.

Uses of Blood Grouping

a. Before blood transfusion
b. In paternal disputes
c. Medicolegal case
d. Knowing susceptibility of disease.

BLOOD TRANSFUSION

Blood transfusion is a life saving measure and must be given only when it is absolutely essential.

Indications

- *Blood loss:* For example: Accidents, during surgery
- *Severe anemia:* In severe anemia, it is better to administer packed red blood cells to prevent volume overload.
- *Exchange transfusion:* Acute poisoning, e.g. carbon monoxide poisoning.

Criteria to Select a Donor

- Age: 18 to 60 years
- Hemoglobin >11 gm/dl
- PCV: Must be normal
- Exclude HIV, hepatitis, malaria and syphilis.
- Nonpregnant and nonlactating mother.

Precautions before Blood Transfusion

- Must be an absolute indication: Must be life saving.
- Cross-matching must be done.
- *Major cross-matching:* Donor's RBC is mixed with recipient's plasma.
- *Minor cross-matching:* Recipient's RBC is mixed with donor's plasma.
- For doubtful clumping, keep a drop of the sample on a cover slip and examine under a microscope.
- Blood bag must be checked:
  - Transfusion must be given at the rate of 100–200 ml/hour
  - Proper aseptic precautions must be taken.

Temperature for Storage

Blood is stored at 4 degree until it is required.

1 Unit of blood: 1 unit of blood is 450 ml of whole blood, 63 ml of anticoagulant and preservative made up of citrate, phosphate, dextrose, and adenine. Dextrose maintains the Na K pump.

Stored Blood

Blood can be stored at 4°C for 21 days. At the end of this period 70 to 80% of RBC is viable but not WBC or platelets:

- K^+ content of red cell is reduced
- Na^+ content of red cell is increased
- K^+ content of plasma is increased.

Effects of Mismatched Blood Transfusion

- Death can occur due to anaphylaxis
- Hemolysis of agglutinated red cells → hemolytic jaundice
- Hemoglobinuria
- Hemoglobin precipitates in renal tubules, blocking the tubules leading to acute renal failure.
- Circulatory overload → Congestive cardiac failure
- Agglutinated RBCs block the small blood vessels leading to shooting pain in lumbar region and precordium (Fig. 4.16a).

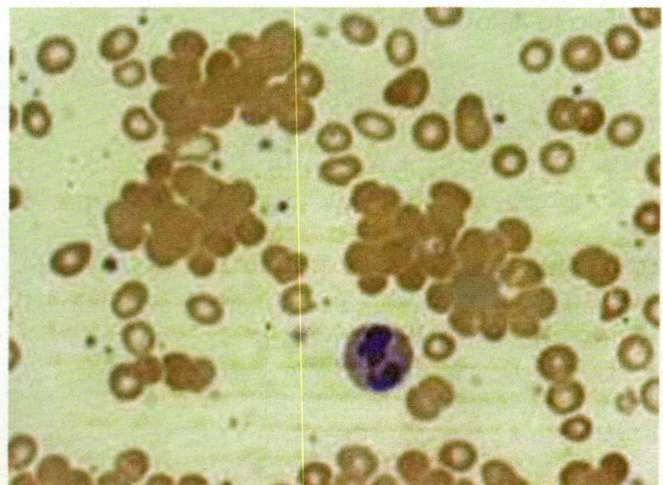

Fig. 4.16: Agglutinated red cells

Minor Transfusion Reactions

a. Fever, chills and rigor occurs due to pyrogens.
b. Allergic reactions like anaphylaxis, urticaria can occur.

Autologous Blood Transfusion

Blood can be withdrawn from a person and can be transfused into the same person during elective surgery. If iron rich diet is given, 1000–1500 ml of blood can be withdrawn over a three-week period.

Advantages

a. Transmission of AIDS and other blood borne infections can be avoided.
b. Incompatibility is NIL.

Blood Substitutes

Various blood substitutes are used where volume replacement is needed more urgently.

Plasma or Serum

- Plasma can be stored for many months
- Plasma is used in the treatment of burns and shock
- There is no need for cross-matching.

Colloid

Dextran is a colloid which gives proper osmotic equilibrium without causing untoward reactions.

Crystalloid

- Crystalloids do not remain in blood vessels.
- They are used in cases of fluid loss with hemoconcentration (dehydration).
- Intravenous mannitol solution is useful in relieving cerebral edema.

Blood Products

- *Fresh frozen plasma:* Can be obtained by freezing plasma to 30°C. FFP is used in clotting factor deficiency.
- *Plasma protein fraction:* PPF is used in hypoalbuminemia.
- *RBC concentrate:* Used in severe anemia.

Platelet Concentrate

Used in reduced platelet count with bleeding. Matching must be done for ABO and Rh groups as the concentrates are likely to contain some RBC.

17. IMMUNITY

Immunity is the ability of the body to defend against the invading agent. There are 2 types of immunity:

I. Innate immunity
   a. Nonspecific defenses
   b. Relatively specific defenses.

II. Acquired immunity (through infection)
   a. Active immunity
      Cellular immunity
      Humoral immunity
   b. Passive immunity (mother to fetus)
      IgG (through placenta)
      IgA (through breastfeeds).

Innate Immunity Includes

1. Lysozymes: Present in saliva and tears.
2. Cilia and mucus of bronchial passage.
3. Acid in stomach
4. Rapid pH change in duodenum
5. Body skin
6. Flushing of urinary tract
7. Low pH of vagina
8. In the blood certain chemical compounds destroy the foreign organism.
   a. *Lysozymes:* Dissolve the bacteria
   b. *Basic polypeptides:* Inactivate certain gram-positive bacteria.
   c. *Complement complex:* Destroy the organisms in various ways.
   d. *Natural killer cells:* Recognize and destroy foreign cells, tumor cells and some infected cells.

ACQUIRED IMMUNITY

The ability of the body to develop extremely powerful specific immunity against bacteria, viruses, toxins and even foreign tissues is called acquired or adaptive immunity.

Acquired immunity gives us extreme protection, e.g. botulinum toxin and tetanizing toxin.

Types of acquired Immunity

a. Cellular immunity
   i. Also called cell mediated immunity (or) T cell immunity.
   ii. In response to an antigen, T-lymphocytes are activated.
   iii. Acts against intracellular organisms, cancer cells, tumor cells, transplanted tissue.

b. Humoral immunity
   i. Also called as B cell immunity
   ii. In response to an antigen, B-lymphocytes are activated to form antibodies.
   iii. Acts against extracellular organisms, bacteria and antigens in fluids.

Immunity Initiated by Antigens

Antigens (Antibody Generators)

Antigens are high molecular weight proteins (> 8000) or polysaccharides that initiate acquired immunity.

Haptens

Haptens are low molecular weight (< 8000) proteins that can seldom act as antigens.

Epitopes

Epitopes are large molecules with antigenicity on their surface.

Role of Lymphocytes

Lymphocytes are essential for survival of human beings. Absence of lymphocytes or decrease in lymphocytes will result in death due to fulminating bacterial infection. Causes for decrease in lymphocytes:

a. Genetic
b. Radiation
c. Chemicals

Lymphocytes are extensively distributed in:

a. Lymph nodes
b. Spleen
c. Submucosal areas of GI tract
d. Thymus
e. Bone marrow

Two Types of Lymphocytes

a. T-Lymphocytes
b. B-Lymphcoytes

Lymphocytes are derived in embryo from pluripotent hematopoietic stem cells.

Lymphocytes that are destined to form T lymphocytes, migrate to thymus and preprocessed in thymus

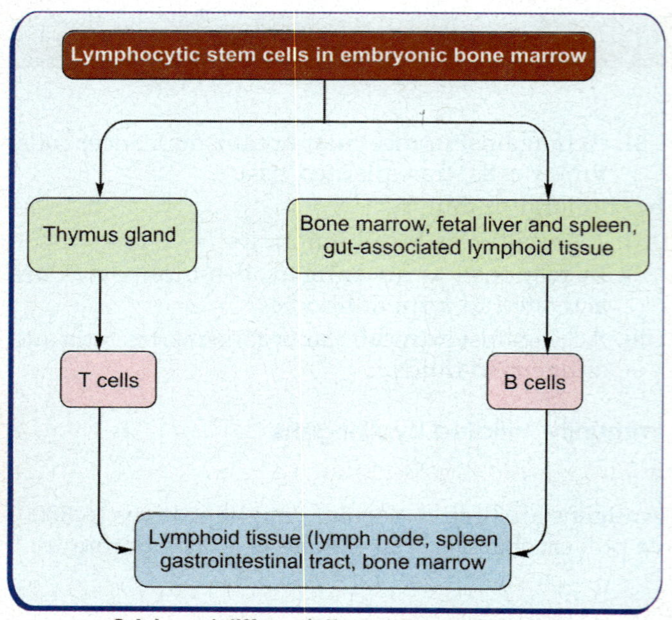

Origin and differentiation of cells and B cells

gland. They are called as T-lymphocytes to designate the role in thymus. They are responsible for cell mediated immunity.

B-Lymphocytes that are destined to form antibodies are preprocessed in liver during midfetal life and in bone marrow in late fetal life.

Preprocessing in Thymus

Each lymphocyte in thymus is specific for one antigen. So, thymus contains thousands of lymphocytes that are specific against thousands of antigens.

Thymus makes certain that any T-lymphocyte leaving the thymus will not react with any proteins (or) self antigens of bodies own tissues.

Time of Preprocessing

Preprocessing occurs shortly before birth of a baby or for few months after delivery.

Removal of thymus before birth can prevent development of cell mediated immunity. So, transplantation of heart and kidney will be tolerated and rejection is less likely.

Thymectomy
↓
No cell mediated immunity
↓
Transplanted organs like heart and kidneys are not rejected

Preprocessing in Liver and Bone Marrow

B-Lymphocytes destined to form antibodies are preprocessed in liver during midfetal life and in bone marrow in late fetal life and afterbirth.

Bursa of fabricius is the special preprocessing organ seen in birds. Since, this population of cells were first seen in birds these lymphocytes are called as B-lymphocyte. These B-lymphocytes form plasma cells which in-turn form antibodies.

Cloning of Lymphocytes

a. When specific type of antigen enter the body, specific lymphocytes get activated, and wildly reproduce to form tremendous number of duplicate lymphocytes called cloning of lymphocytes.
b. Gene code is present for millions of different types of antibodies.
c. Each clone of lymphocyte responds to single antigen.
d. Surface receptor protein present on the surface of T cell membrane is also specific for each antigen.

Types of Lymphocytes

T-Lymphocytes form 75% of circulating lymphocytes. They are made up of subsets of:

a. Helper T cells
b. Cytotoxic T cells
c. Suppressor T cells
d. Memory T cells
e. T cells that mediate hypersensitivity reaction.

Helper T cells (Th)

a. Most numerous of T cell subpopulation.
b. They release lymphocytes that cause growth and proliferation of cytotoxic T cells and suppressor T cells.
c. Stimulate memory cell formation.

Cytotoxic T Cells (Tc)

a. Kills virus invaded cells
b. Effective against parasites and bacteria, e.g. tubercle bacilli. They act by:
   i. Perforins formation
   ii. Release of cytotoxic substances into cells, e.g. malignant cells and foreign cells.

Memory Cells (Tm)

a. Memory cells remain dormant in the lymphocyte pool.

b. When the same antigen enters the body memory cells are activated and converted into more powerful effector T cells.

Suppressor T Cells (Ts)

a. Ts inhibit Th and Tc cells.
b. Ts cells also inhibit antibody formation thus preventing excess immunological response.

T Cells that Mediate Delayed Hypersensitivity Reaction (Td Cells)

Hypersensitivity reaction that occurs after 12 hours is called delayed hypersensitivity reaction. Intradermal tuberculin skin test is a good example of delayed hypersensitivity reaction.

CELLULAR IMMUNITY

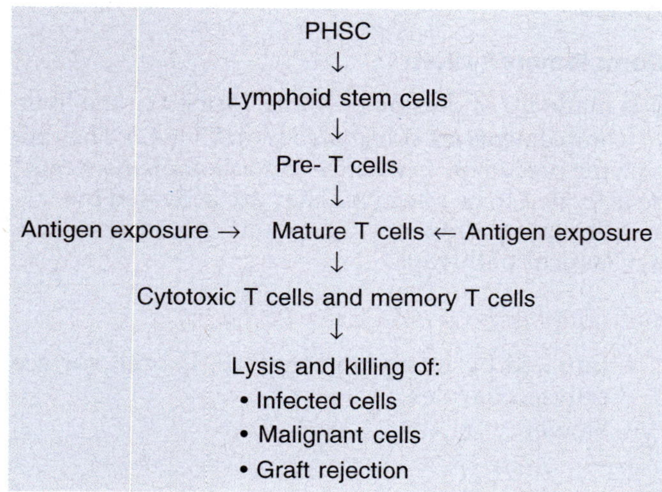

Other Cells Causing Immune Response

- Monocytes
- Eosinophils
- Neutrophils
- Basophils

Antigen Presenting Cells

Dendritic cells acting as antigen presenting cells.

The antigen is presented to the lymphocyte by antigen presenting cells (APC). The APC are:

- Macrophages
- Dendritic cells in lymph node and skin (Fig. 4.17a).
- Langerhans cells in (skin).

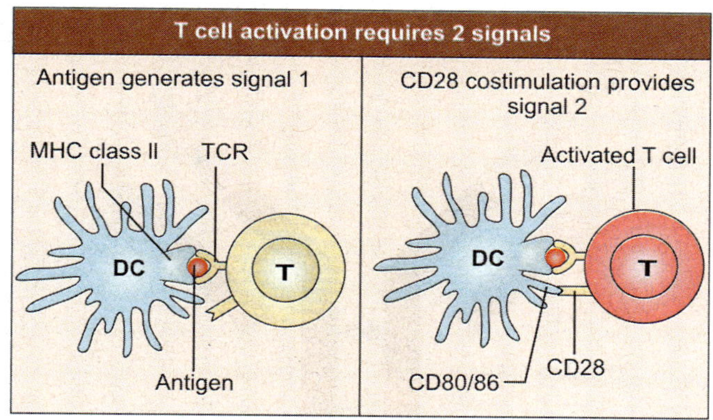

Fig. 4.17a

HUMORAL IMMUNITY

Formation of Antibodies by Plasma Cells

Entry of foreign antigen (Ag), causes the macrophages to phagocytize the antigens. Macrophages act as APC and present it to B-lymphocytes. These cells enlarge and form lymphoblast. These lymphoblast differentiate to form plasmablast and in turn plasma cells are formed. Mature plasma cells produce antibodies at an extremely rapid rate.

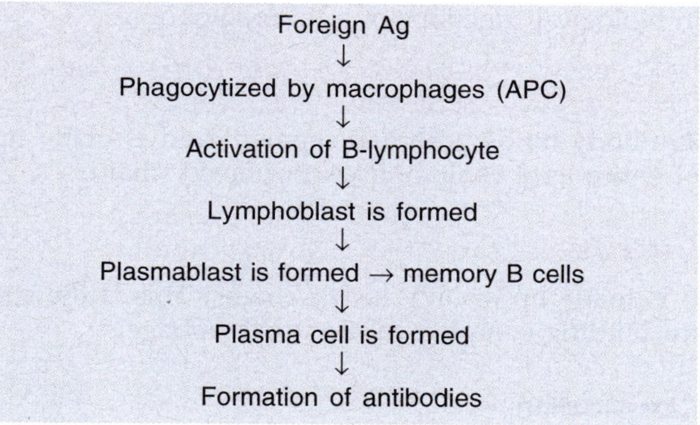

Immunoglobulins

Structure of immunoglobulin (Fig. 4.17b)

The antibodies are gammaglobulins called immunoglobulins. They form 20% of plasma proteins. Immunoglobulins are made up of 4 polypeptide chain.

- Two identical short light chains
- Two identical long heavy chains

They are linked by disulfide bond. Each chain has:

Variable Segment

The amino acid sequence is variable and forms a site for antigen binding.

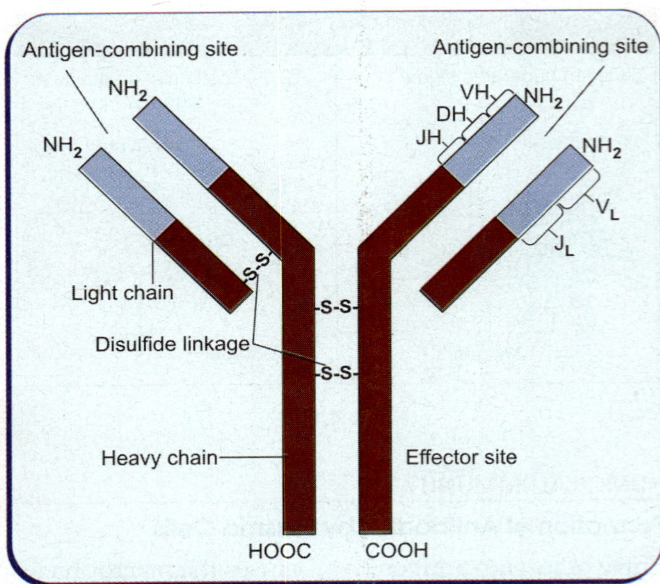

Fig. 4.17b: Structure of immunoglobulin

4

Constant Segment

The amino acid sequence is constant and is involved in biological functions of immunoglobulins.

Fab Segment

Antibody binds with Fab segment and is made up of entire light chain and part of heavy chain.

Fc-fragment

It is made up of only heavy chains. This is the site for binding complement and macrophage.

Classification

Based on the nature of heavy chains immunoglobulins are divided into five classes:

1. *Immunoglobulin G*

It is responsible for secondary antibody formation. IgG crosses the placenta. These antibodies help in opsonization, immunity against bacteria and toxins.

2. *Immunoglobulin A*

This antibody is present in the secretions of respiratory, gastrointestinal and genitourinary tract. Present in saliva, tears, and nasal secretion.

3. *Immunoglobulin M*

It is a macroglobulin responsible for primary antibody response. It cannot cross the placenta due to its large size.

4. *Immunoglobulin E*

It binds to mast cells and basophils and release chemical mediators.

5. *Immunoglobulin D*

It acts as receptor for antigens on B cells.

Immunoglobulins Act by

Agglutination: Clumping of antigen
Precipitation: Forming insoluble precipitate
Neutralization: Antibody covers the toxic site of antigen.
Lysis: Rupture of cell membrane.

Immunoglobulins are more effective by complement system.

Complement System

It is made up of plasma proteins, formed in the liver.

Complements are designated from C1 to C9. They are enzyme precursors in inactive form. Complement must be activated to be effective. They are activated by:

a. Alternate pathway
b. Classical pathway.

Alternate Pathway (Properdin Pathway)

i. Initiated by interaction by B, P, D with surface polysaccharides.
ii. Slower

Classsical Pathway

i. Initiated by antigen antibody complex.
ii. Rapid and efficient.

Classical pathway	*Alternate pathway*
Antigen-antibody complex	Surface polysaccharides of organism
(Activated by IgM and IgG)	(Activated by IgA and IgE)
↓	↓
C1 + C4 + C2	B, D, P
↓	↓
C3 activation	→ C3 ← C3 activation
	↓
	C3 b + C3 a (opsonization of organism)

Contd.

Contd.

Classical pathway	*Alternate pathway*
Causes chemotactic effect	→ C5 b (chemotactic effect) + C6,7,8,9 ↓ C5 b, 6,7,8,9 (causes lysis of organism by forming holes)

Cytokines and Lymphokines

Lymphokines are protein substances released by activated lymphocytes. They act as mediators of immune response.

Cytokines are protein substances released by endothelial cells, neuroglial cells and macrophages. They include:

- Interleukins
- Interferons
- Tumor necrosis factor.

Interleukins: Act as hemopoietic growth factor.
Interferons: They are products of virus infected cells.

Interferon alpha: Formed by neutrophils and macrophages.

Interferon beta: Formed by fibroblast and epithelial cells.

Interferon gamma: Formed by T-lymphocytes and NK cells.

Functions of Interferons

- Activate B cells
- Cause cell growth and cytotoxicity
- Expression of major histocompatible class I and II
- Used in the treatment of myeloid leukemia and leprosy.

Tumor Necrosis Factor

It is released by the macrophages and lymphocytes in response to infection and inflammation.

Functions

- It activates phagocytosis
- Causes necrosis of tumor cells.

IMMUNIZATION

Immunization is the process of preparing the body to fight against the disease.

Active Immunization

Active immunization is induced by the injection of vaccines containing antigens and thus producing antibodies to protect against the specific disease.

Live Attenuated Vaccines

Measles, mumps, oral polio vaccine and yellow fever vaccine.

Killed Vaccine

Typhoid and whooping cough.

Toxoid

Diphtheria, tetanus.

Passive Immunization

Administration of gammaglobulin obtained from human or animal (horse) that is already actively immunized. Passive immunity is further divided into:

Natural

Transmission of antibodies from mother to fetus, e.g. immunoglobulin G.

Artificial

This includes injection of previously prepared antibody to a person, e.g. immunoglobulin for rabies.

Allergy and Hypersensitivity

Hypersensitivity is defined as abnormal hyperimmune reaction to an agent. Hypersensitive reactions are classified as:

Type I	Anaphylactic reaction
Type II	Cytotoxic reaction
Type III	Antibody mediated reaction
Type IV	Cell mediated reaction
Type V	Stimulatory blocking reactions.

Immune Deficiency Diseases

Immune deficiency diseases occur when defense mechanism becomes defective.

Organisms that invade the body due to defective defense mechanism are called opportunistic organism. Immune deficiency can be:

- Congenital
- Acquired.

Congenital Immune Deficiency Disease

- Congenital diseases are inherited and occur due to defect in B cell.

- T cell or both, e.g. DiGeorge syndrome (absence of thymus).
- Severe combined immune deficiency syndrome (SIDS).

Acquired Immune Deficiency Syndrome

AIDS is due to human immunodeficiency virus.

Mode of Transmission

- Contaminated blood transfusion
- Contaminated needles
- Transmission from mother to fetus during pregnancy or delivery of baby
- Breastfeeding
- Unprotected sexual intercourse.

4

HIV activates the enzyme reverse transcriptase. This virus utilizes the enzyme and converts its own viral RNA into viral DNA. This viral DNA gets incorporated into host cell DNA and prevents the normal activities of host cell DNA. This increases the viral load inside the host body.

Incubation Period

Period between the entry of the organism and development of symptoms is called incubation period. For HIV the incubation period is 3 months to 3 years.

Symptoms

- Weight loss
- Chronic diarrhea
- Prolonged low grade fever
- Oral ulcer
- Fungal infection of tongue (oral candidiasis).

The common opportunistic infections are

- *Pneumocystis carinii pneumonia*
- Kaposi sarcoma
- Burkitts lymphoma.

Prevention

Avoid spread of disease to others by

- Screening of blood before transfusion
- Avoid sharing of needles
- If mother is positive for HIV, treatment with zidovudine will reduce infection to baby
- Avoid multiple sex partners
- Use of condoms

Autoimmune Disorders

Antibodies in a person reacts with self-antigens:

- *Rheumatic fever:* Streptococcal antigen has a molecular structure similar to structure of body's own self antigen.
- *Glomerulonephritis:* Person's antibodies react against basement membrane of glomeruli.
- *Myasthenia gravis:* Immunity against acetylcholine receptors of neuromuscular junction.
- *Lupus erythematosis:* Immunity against different body tissues causing extensive tissue damage and early death.

18. PLATELETS

Platelets also called as thrombocytes, are minute discs.

Size 2–4 μm

Shape Discoid, oval, or round in shape (Fig. 4.18a).

Platelet Membrane

- Platelet membrane is made up of glycoprotein and phospholipids.
- Glycoprotein: Repels vascular endothelium
- Phospholipids: That activate various stages.
- Platelet membrane has receptors for collagen, fibrinogen, ADP, von Willebrand factor (vWF).

Cytoplasm of Platelets

Cytoplasm of platelets contains:

- Actin, myosin, thrombosthenin that are contractile proteins.
- Endoplasmic reticulum and Golgi apparatus that synthesize various enzymes.
- *Mitochondria:* Synthesize ATP and ADP
- *Prostaglandin:* A local hormone synthesized by enzymes.
- Fibrin stabilizing factor
- Growth factor
- *Granules:* Cytoplasm contains granules like

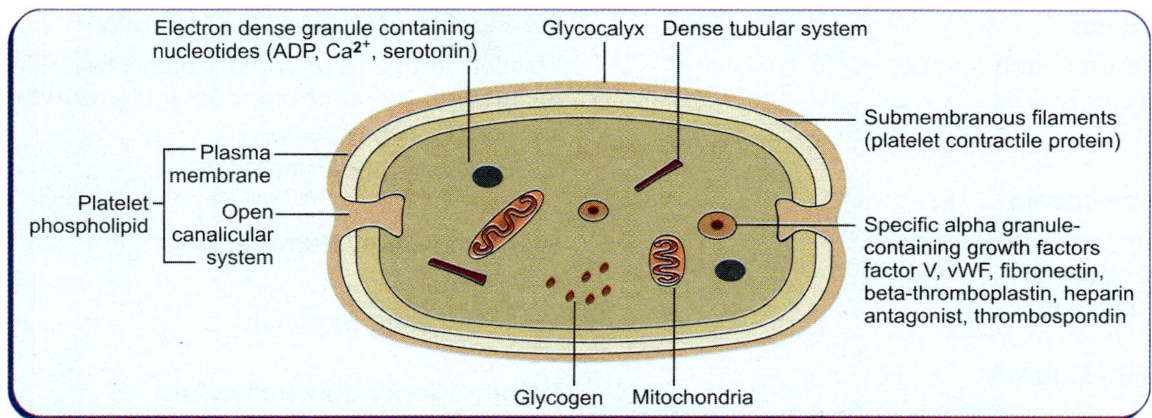

Fig. 4.18a: Ultrastructure of platelet

a. *Alpha granules:* Contain von Willebrand factor, fibrinogen and platelet derived growth factor.
b. *Dense granules:* Contain ATP, ADP, 5HT, non-protein substances.
c. Lysosomes

Microtubules: It is responsible for the shape of platelets.

Nucleus: Platelets have no nucleus, DNA, RNA and hence cannot reproduce.

Canaliculi

1. Open canaliculi
2. Closed canaliculi.

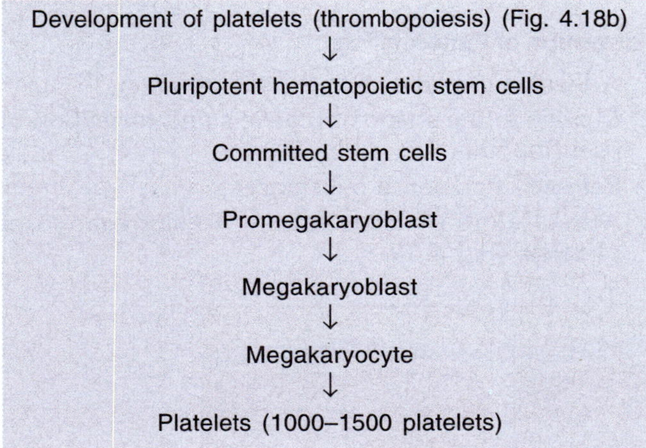

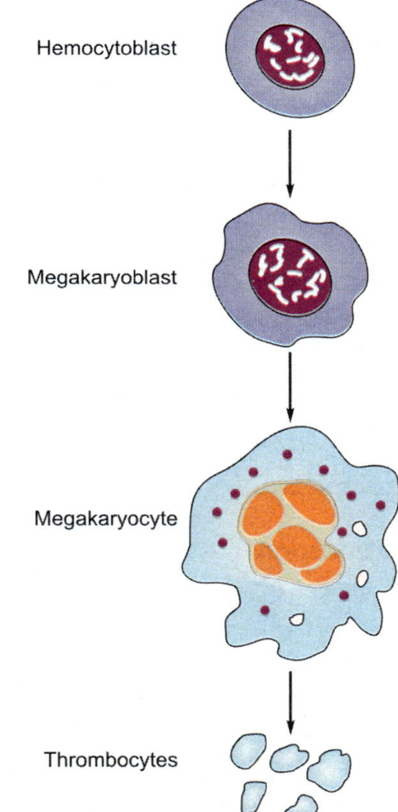

Fig. 4.18b

Lifespan

Lifespan of platelets is 8–14 days. After completing their lifespan they are destroyed in spleen. Factors controlling thrombopoiesis:

- *Colony stimulating factor:* Interleukin 1, 2, 6, 11
- *Thrombopoietin:* Produced by liver and kidney.

Count and Variations

Normal count:

- 1.5 lakhs to 3 lakhs
- 75% of platelets are in circulating pool.
- 25% of platelets are seen in spleen (reservoir of platelets).

Thrombocytosis

- After trauma and surgery
- Splenectomy
- Stress.

Thrombocytopenia

- Bone marrow depression
- Hypersplenism
- Viral infection.

Functions of Platelets

4

Hemostasis: Various steps that bring about hemostasis are:

- Platelet adhesion
- Platelet activation
- Platelet aggregation.

Blood Coagulation

ADP from platelets cause platelet activation and "Temporary hemostatic plug" formation.

Clot Retraction

Thrombosthenin causes clot retraction in a blood clot.

Phagocytic Function

Platelets can phagocytize:

- Carbon particles
- Viruses
- Immune complexes.

Storage and Transport

Platelets can store:

- Histamine
- 5-hydroxytryptamine.

Mechanism of Platelet Plug Formation

Platelets form part of primary hemostasis. Hemostasis means prevention of blood loss. It is of two types:

1. Primary hemostasis
2. Secondary hemostasis.

Events of Primary Hemostasis

- Vasoconstriction
- Platelet plug formation.

Events of Secondary Hemostasis

- Formation of blood clot
- Growth of fibrous tissue into blood clot.

VASOCONSTRICTION

Vasoconstriction (Fig. 4.19) is achieved after a blood vessel has been cut by:

- Local myogenic spasm
- Local autacoids from injured blood vessels and platelets
- Nervous reflexes initiated by pain nerve impulses from traumatized blood vessels
- Thromboxane A2 released from injured platelets are responsible for vasoconstriction of smaller vessels.

Formation of Platelet Plug

1. Adhesion of platelets to the site of injury.
2. Change in the shape of platelets and formation of pseudopods.
3. Release of chemical substances.
4. Attract more platelets leading to aggregation of platelets (Fig. 4.19).

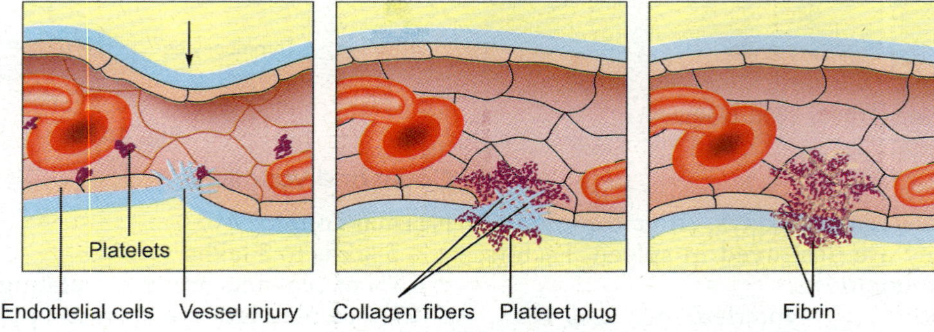

Fig. 4.19: Vasoconstriction, platelet aggregation and clot formation

I. Platelet Adhesion

When platelets come in contact with damaged vessels exposing collagen, the platelets adhere to the vessel. Platelets need a rough surface to adhere. Factors responsible for adhesion are:

- Adenosine diphosphate
- Thromboxane A2
- Calcium ions
- von Willebrand factor
- Collagen

II. Change in Shape of Platelets

On adhering to the collagen, platelets begin to swell and assume irregular forms with numerous pseudopods protruding from their surface.

Release of chemical substances: The contractile proteins namely actin, myosin, thrombosthenin within the platelets contract forcefully and release granules. These granules make the platelets to become sticky to each other and to collagen and von Willebrand factor that is from plasma.

Aggregation of Platelets

ADP and thromboxane act on nearby platelets to activate them and more number of platelets are recruited to form platelet plug.

First, a loose plug is formed. Then, subsequently fibrin threads are formed on the platelet plug thus converting the loose plug into an unyielding plug.

Importance of Platelet Plug

Platelet plugging is important for closing minute ruptures in very small blood vessels that occur multiple times a day. If the platelet count is less, thousands of small hemorrhages occur under the skin.

BLOOD CLOT

The clot is composed of a meshwork of fibrin threads running in all directions with blood cells, platelets and plasma.

Clot Retraction

After the clot is formed, within minutes, it begins to contract and usually express most fluid within 20–60 minutes. The fluid expressed is called serum. This serum cannot clot as it does not have fibrinogen and other clotting factors.

Platelet is essential for clot retraction. Failure of clot retraction is an indication of low platelet count. The contractile proteins namely actin, myosin, and thrombosthenin in platelets cause strong clot retraction.

As clot retraction proceeds, the injured blood vessel is pulled together and hemopoiesis is achieved.

Dissolution of Clot

Fibroblasts invade the clot and complete organization of the clot into fibrous tissue occurs in 1 to 2 weeks.

4

19. BLOOD COAGULATION

Mechanism of Coagulation

Procoagulants

Substances that promote coagulation are called procoagulants.

Anticoagulants

Substances that inhibit coagulation are called anticoagulants. Whether blood will or not will depend on the balance between these two groups of substances.

Clotting Factors in Blood

Clotting factor	*Synonyms*
Fibrinogen	Factor I
Prothrombin	Factor II
Tissue factor	Factor III
Calcium	Factor IV
Factor V	Proaccelerin; labile factor. Ac-globulin (Ac-G)
Factor VII	Serum prothrombin conversion accelerator, proconvertin: Stable factor

Contd.

Contd.

Clotting factor	*Synonyms*
Factor VIII	Antihemophilic factor A
Factor IX	Plasma thromboplastin component, Christmas factor, antihemophilic factor B
Factor X	Stuart Prower factor
Factor XI	Plasma thromboplastin antecedent
Factor XII	Hageman factor
Factor XIII	Fibrin stabilizing factor
Prekallikrein	Fletcher factor
High-molecular weight kininogen	Fitzgerald factor

4

Three essential steps in clotting are

i. Formation of prothrombin activator
ii. Conversion of prothrombin to thrombin
iii. Conversion of fibrinogen to fibrin by thrombin.

Formation of Prothrombin Activator

Prothombin activator is formed

a. When there is trauma to vascular wall and adjacent tissue
b. Trauma to blood
c. Contact of blood with damage endothelial cells or with collagen.

Prothrombin activator is formed in two ways

I. *By extrinsic pathway:* That begins with trauma to vessel wall and surrounding tissue.
II. *By intrinsic pathway:* That begins in blood itself.

Extrinsic Pathway for Clotting

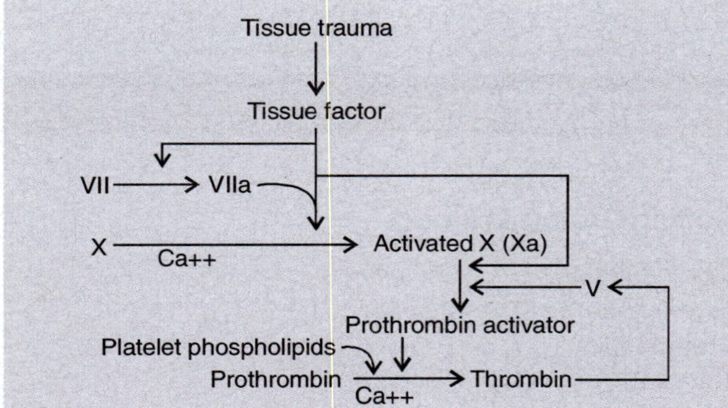

Step I: Traumatized tissue release, tissue factor or tissue thromboplastin.

Step II: Factor X is activated with the help of factor VII and tissue factor.

Step III: Activated Xa forms prothrombin activator, with the help of tissue factor and factor V.

Prothrombin activator converts prothrombin into thrombin in the presence of calcium.

Intrinsic Pathway

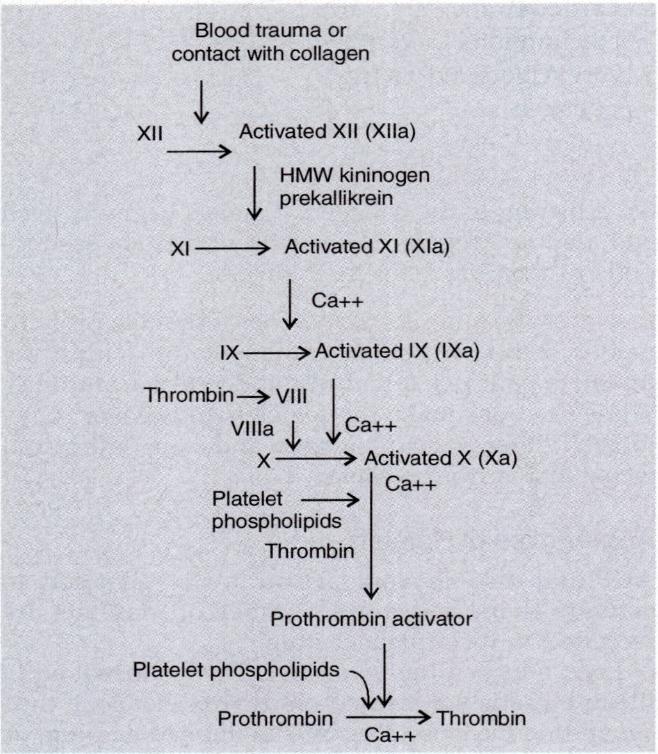

Intrinsic pathway begins with trauma to the blood itself or exposure of blood to collagen from traumatized blood vessel wall.

1. Blood trauma causes activation of factor XII and release of platelet phospholipids.

   Factor XII is disturbed when blood comes in contact with collagen and forms activated factor XII.
2. Activated factor XII causes activation of factor XI to form activated factor XI.
3. Activated factor XI causes activation of factor IX.
4. Activation of factor X occurs with the help of factor VIII, platelet phospholipids, factor 3.
5. Activated factor X forms prothrombin activator, in the presence of calcium, thrombin, and platelet phospholipids.
6. Prothrombin activator causes cleavage of prothrombin to form thrombin.

Formation of Fibrin

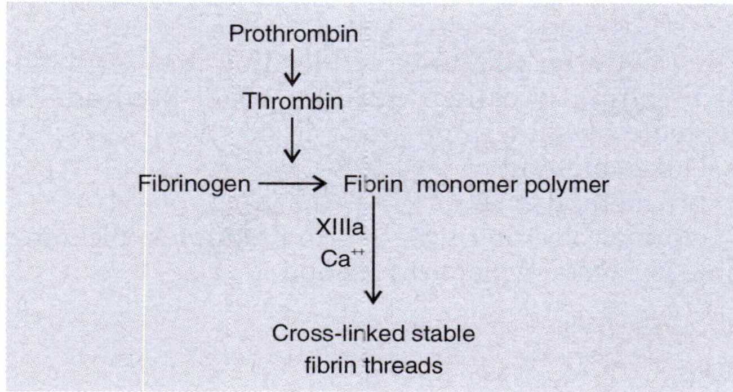

Difference between the Extrinsic and Intrinsic Pathway

Extrinsic pathway	*Intrinsic pathway*
Tissue factor initiates the extrinsic pathway	Contact of factor XII and platelets with collagen in vessel wall initiates the intrinsic pathway
Explosive: Once it is initiated it completes quickly. Clot formation within 15 seconds	Occurs much slowly requiring 1 to 6 minutes for clot formation

Prevention of Blood Clotting in Vascular System

The factors that prevent clotting in normal vascular system are:

- Smoothness of endothelial surface
- A layer of glycocalyx on the endothelium
- *Thrombomodulin:* A protein that binds with thrombin
- *Protein C:* That inactivates factors V and VIII thus acts as anticoagulant.

Anticoagulants in Blood

Anticoagulants in blood remove the thrombin from the blood. The most powerful anticoagulants are:

Fibrin fibers formed during the clotting process.

Antithrombin III or antithrombin-heparin cofactor.

90% of thrombin formed becomes absorbed to fibrin. This helps to prevent spread of thrombin into the remaining blood. 10% of thrombin binds with antithrombin III that further blocks the effect of thrombin.

Velocity of Circulation

When the blood moves with reduced velocity thrombus is formed.

Prostacyclins

- Prostacyclins inhibit aggregation
- Promote vasodilation
- If a clot is formed inspite of all these factors, it is removed by plasmin.

Heparin

Heparin is a powerful anticoagulant. It is produced by mast cells in precapillary tissue and basophils in the blood. Heparin acts by combining with antithrombin III thus removing thrombin from the blood. Heparin along with antithrombin also removes the clotting factors XII, XI, X, IX. Lungs and liver receive many embolic clots. Heparin produced by mast cells in the liver and lungs prevent further growth of clot. Clinically, heparin is used in the dose of 1 mg/kg by injection. It increases clotting time to 30 minutes. Duration of action is for 4 hours. Heparin is destroyed by heparinase enzyme.

Coumarin

Coumarin derivatives like warfarin are oral anticoagulants. They reduce levels of prothrombin factors VII, IX, X.

It acts by competing with vitamin K for reactive sites. Coagulation is not blocked immediately. Normal coagulation returns in 1–3 days after discontinuing the drug.

Hemophilia

Hemophilia is a bleeding disorder affecting the males exclusively. It is a X-linked disorder. Hemophilia is caused by deficiency of factor IX. Females are "Carriers of hemophilia". They do not suffer from the disease because one of the X chromosome will have appropriate gene. Factor VIII has 2 components:

- Large component
- Small component.

Deficiency of small component of factor VIII is called "classical hemophilia" or "hemophilia A". Deficiency of large component of factor VIII is called von Willebrand disease. Deficiency of factor IX is called "hemophilia B" or "Christmas disease". Severe and prolonged bleeding can occur after a minor surgical procedure like tooth extraction lasting for days. People with classic hemophilia are treated with purified factor VIII.

4

Thrombocytopenia

Thrombocytopenia means presence of reduced number of platelets in blood. People with thrombocytopenia bleed as hemophiliacs but the bleeding is from small vessels or capillaries. Small punctuate hemorrhages occur all over the body tissues causing purplish blotches giving the name thrombocytopenic purpura. If the cause for thrombocytopenia is unknown its known as idiopathic thrombocytopenia.

- Normal platelet count is 1,50,000 to 3,00,000/microliter
- Bleeding occurs when the count falls below 50,000/microliter
- Levels as low as 10,000/microliter is lethal in a person.

Thromboembolic Conditions

Thrombus: Abnormal clot formation in a vessel is called thrombus.

Embolus: When a thrombus moves within a blood vessel it is called embolus.

When a person is confined to bed for a long period, stasis of blood occurs. This causes intravascular clotting of blood. When the blood clot disintegrates from the vessel wall it moves freely to the right side of the heart and blocks the pulmonary arteries, leading to massive pulmonary embolism. If the clot is very large, it leads to immediate death.

Disseminated Intravascular Coagulation

Clotting occuring over a widespread area within the circulation is called disseminated intravascular coagulation (DIC).

DIC occurs in septicemia, where the bacterial toxin especially endotoxins activate coagulation mechanism.

Blood Coagulation Tests

Bleeding Time

Time between the onset of bleeding and stoppage of bleeding is called bleeding time. Methods to evaluate bleeding time are:

- Dukes method
- Ivy method.

Normal bleeding time is 1 to 5 minutes. Bleeding time is a test for platelet function.

Prolonged Bleeding Time

Prolonged bleeding time occurs in:

- Thrombocytopenia
- Thrombosthenia
- von Willibrands disease
- Drugs, e.g. aspirin
- Allergic purpura.

Indications for Bleeding Time

1. Prolonged bleeding after trivial injury.
2. Gum bleed, joint bleed and bleeding under the skin.
3. Before major and minor surgery.

Clotting Time

Time between the onset of bleeding till clot formation is called clotting time. It is done by:

- Capillary tube method.
- Normal bleeding time is 2–8 minutes.

Prolonged clotting time with normal bleeding time occurs in:

1. Hemophilia
2. Christmas disease
3. Deficiency of any clotting factor.

Prothrombin Time

Prothrombin time gives us an idea about the concentration of prothrombin in blood. Normal prothrombin time is 12 seconds.

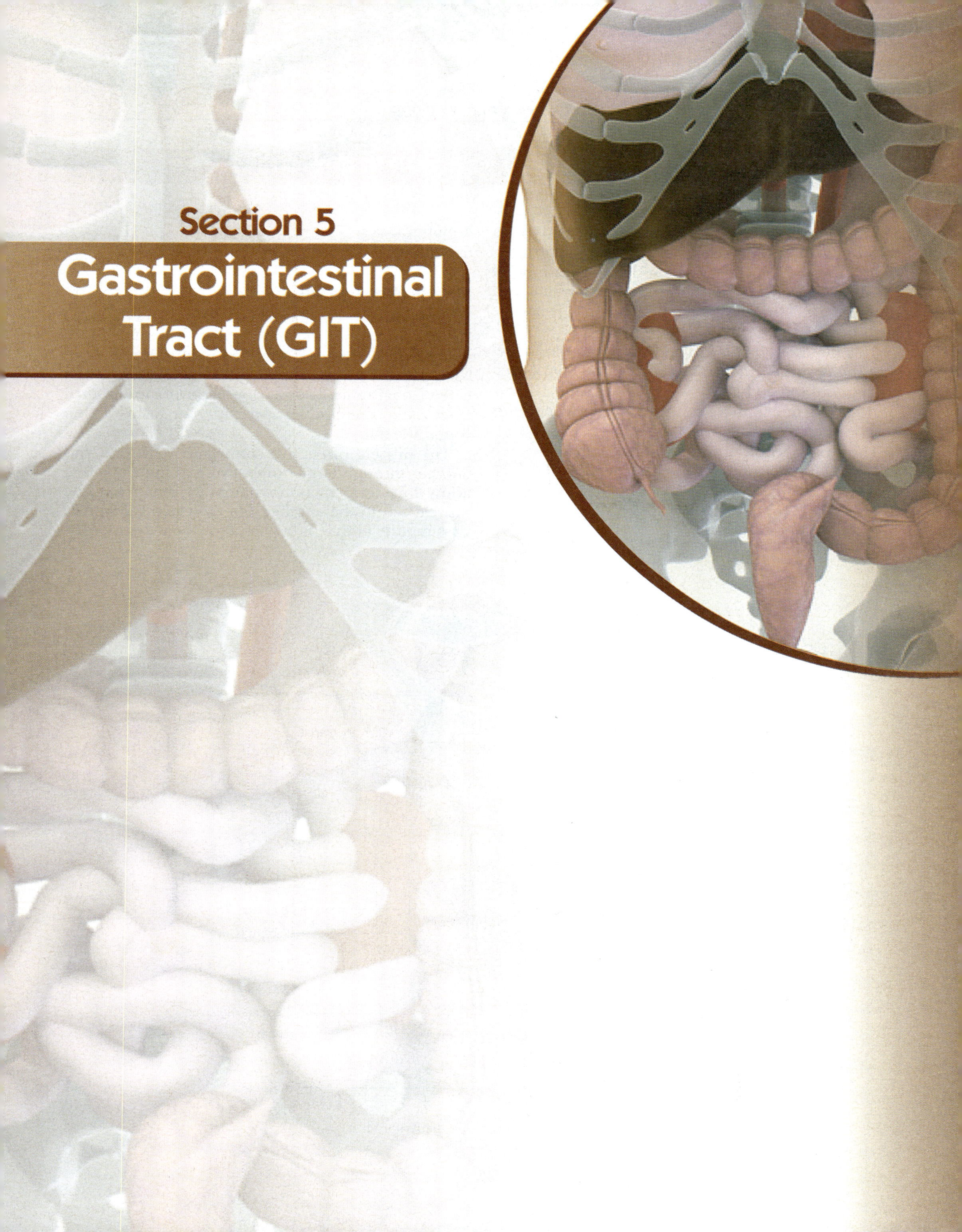

Section 5

Gastrointestinal Tract (GIT)

20. ORGANIZATION OF GIT

The alimentary tract (Fig. 5.1) provides the body with continuous supply of water, electrolytes and nutrients.

For these functions, the food must be moved through the length of the alimentary tract and digested into simpler substances so that it can be absorbed.

This requires adequate blood supply to the GIT so that the absorbed food materials can be distributed throughout the body.

All these functions are controlled by local, nervous and hormonal systems.

The cross section of the intestinal wall shows the following layers from outersurface inwards (Fig. 5.2):

5

1. Serosa
2. Longitudinal muscle layer
3. Circular muscle layer
4. Submucosa
5. Mucosa

Smooth Muscle of GIT

The smooth muscle fiber of GIT have a length of 200 to 500 micrometers and a diameter of 2 to 10 micrometers. They are arranged in bundles of about 1000 parallel fibers. The longitudinal muscle layers extend longitudinally down the length of the intestinal tract while the circular muscle layer forms a ring round the gut.

The muscle fibers are connected with one and another through large number of gap junctions that allow low resistance movement of ions from one muscle cell to the another. So, the electrical signals pass rapidly both length wise and side ways rapidly.

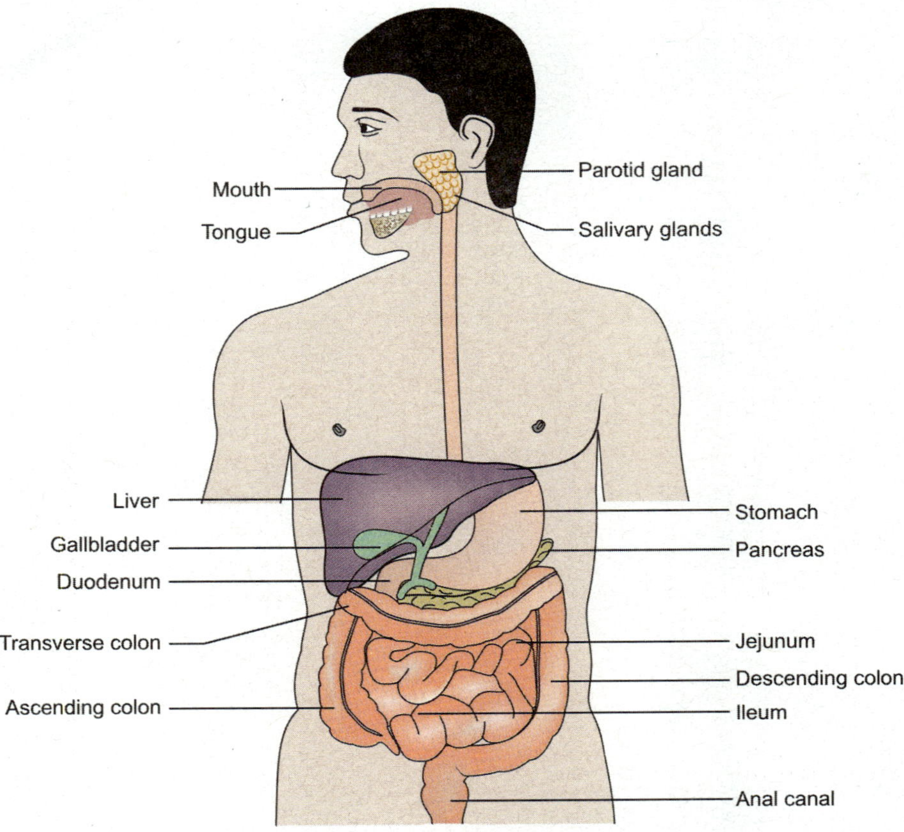

Fig. 5.1: Structure of the alimentary tract

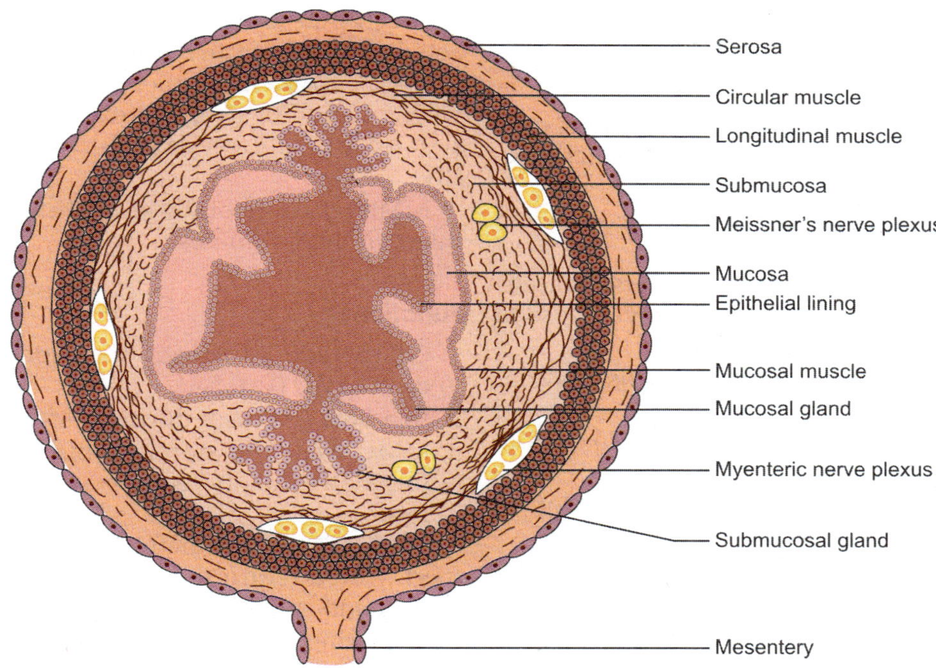

Fig. 5.2: Physiological anatomy of the GIT

Electrical Activity of Gastrointestinal (GI) Smooth Muscle (Fig. 5.3)

Two basic types of electrical waves:

1. Slow waves
2. Spikes

Voltage of RMP of GI smooth muscle can be made to change to different levels.

Slow Waves

Most GI contraction occur rhythmically and this is determined mainly by the frequency of slow waves of smooth muscle potential (Fig. 5.3).

- Intensity 5 to 15 millivolts
- *Frequency:* 3 to 12/min (3 in stomach,12 in duodenum and 8 to 9 in terminal ileum).
- Slow waves are not action potentials but are slow, undulating changes in the resting membrane potential.
- Slow waves caused by interaction between smooth muscle cells and specialized cells called interstitial cells of Cajal (electrical pacemaker of smooth muscle).
- Slow waves do not cause muscle contraction except in stomach.

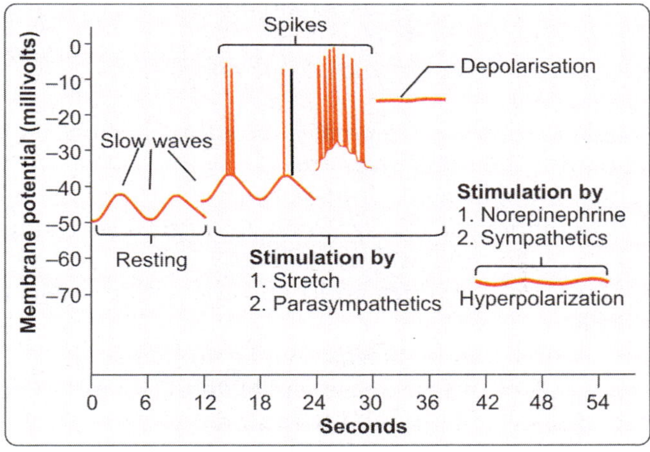

Fig. 5.3

- They cause spike potentials which evoke muscle contraction.

Spike Potentials

Initiate action potential. Occur automatically when resting membrane potential becomes more positive to –40 mV (normal resting membrane potential is between –50 and –60).

When slow wave peak reaches –40 millivolts, spike potentials occur.

BASIC ELECTRIC RHYTHM (BER)

- Membrane potential ranges from –65 to –45 millivolts.
- Basic electric rhythm is initiated by interstitial cells of Cajal, which are mesenchymal pacemaker cells.
- They have smooth muscle like features.
- They send long multiple branched processes into the intestinal smooth muscle.
- In the stomach and small intestine, interstitial cells of Cajal lie outer to circular muscle layer close to myenteric plexus.
- In the colon, it is present near submucosal border of circular muscle.
- There is descending frequency of pacemaker from stomach to the intestine.
- BER does not cause smooth muscle contraction.
- BER increases muscle tension.

Depolarization spike is due to large numbers of calcium influx and small amount of sodium influx (called calcium-sodium channels).

Factors that depolarize the membrane are:
1. Stretching the muscle
2. Stimulation by acetylcholine
3. Stiumulation by parasympathetic nerves secreting acetylcholine at their endings
4. Stimulation by specific GI hormones.

Repolarization due to potassium efflux. Factors that repolarize the membrane are:
1. Norepinephrine or epinephrine
2. Stimulation of the sympathetic nerves secreting norepinephrine at their endings

- Many polypeptides and neurotransmitters effect BER.
  - Acetylcholine increases spike and tension
  - Epinephrine decreases spike and tension
  - BER-rate: 4 per minute in stomach
    12 per min in duodenum
    8 per min in distal ileum
    9 per min in caecum
    16 per min in sigmoid

Functions of BER is to coordinate peristaltic and motor activity.

Contractions occur only during depolarization of the waves.

MIGRATING MOTOR COMPLEX (MMC)

The pattern of electrical and motor activity in GI smooth muscles becomes modified during fasting between digestion, so that cycles of smooth motor activity migrate from the stomach to the distal ileum.

MMC starts with a quiet period (phase I), continues with a period of irregular electrical and mechanical activity (phase II), ends with regular activity (phase III).

MMCs occur aborally at a rate of 5 cm/minute, at intervals of 90 minutes.

Functions

1. Gastric and pancreatic secretion increase during each MMC (Fig. 5.4)
2. Bile flow increases during MMC
3. MMC clear the stomach and small intestine of luminal contents to prepare for the subsequent meal.

MMCs stop immediately followed by ingestion of food, with a return to peristalsis and the other form of BER and spike potentials.

Migrating motor complexes from the stomach to the distal ileum occurring at a regular rate during fasting and completely inhibited by ingestion of meal, returining after meal at 90 minutes.

Neural Control of Gastrointestinal Function: Enteric Nervous System

The GIT has a nervous system of its own called the enteric nervous system (ENS). It extends from the oesophagus down to the anus, lying in the wall of the gut. There are about 100 million neurons in the ENS. It plays an important role in controlling the movements and secretions of the GI tract. The ENS is made up of two plexus:

1. *Auerbach's or myenteric plexus:* It is the outer plexus lying between the longitudinal and circular muscle layers. It mainly control GI movements.
2. *Meissner's or submucous plexus:* It lies in the submucosa. It controls the GI secretions and blood flow.

The extrinsic sympathetic and parasympathetic fibers connect to both the myenteric and submucous plexuses. The ENS can function autonomously but the sympathetic and parasympathetic can greatly enhance or inhibit GI functions.

The sensory nerve endings from the GI epithelium and gut wall send afferent fibers to both the plexuses of nervous sysem as well as to:

1. Prevertebral ganglia of the sympathetic nervous system.

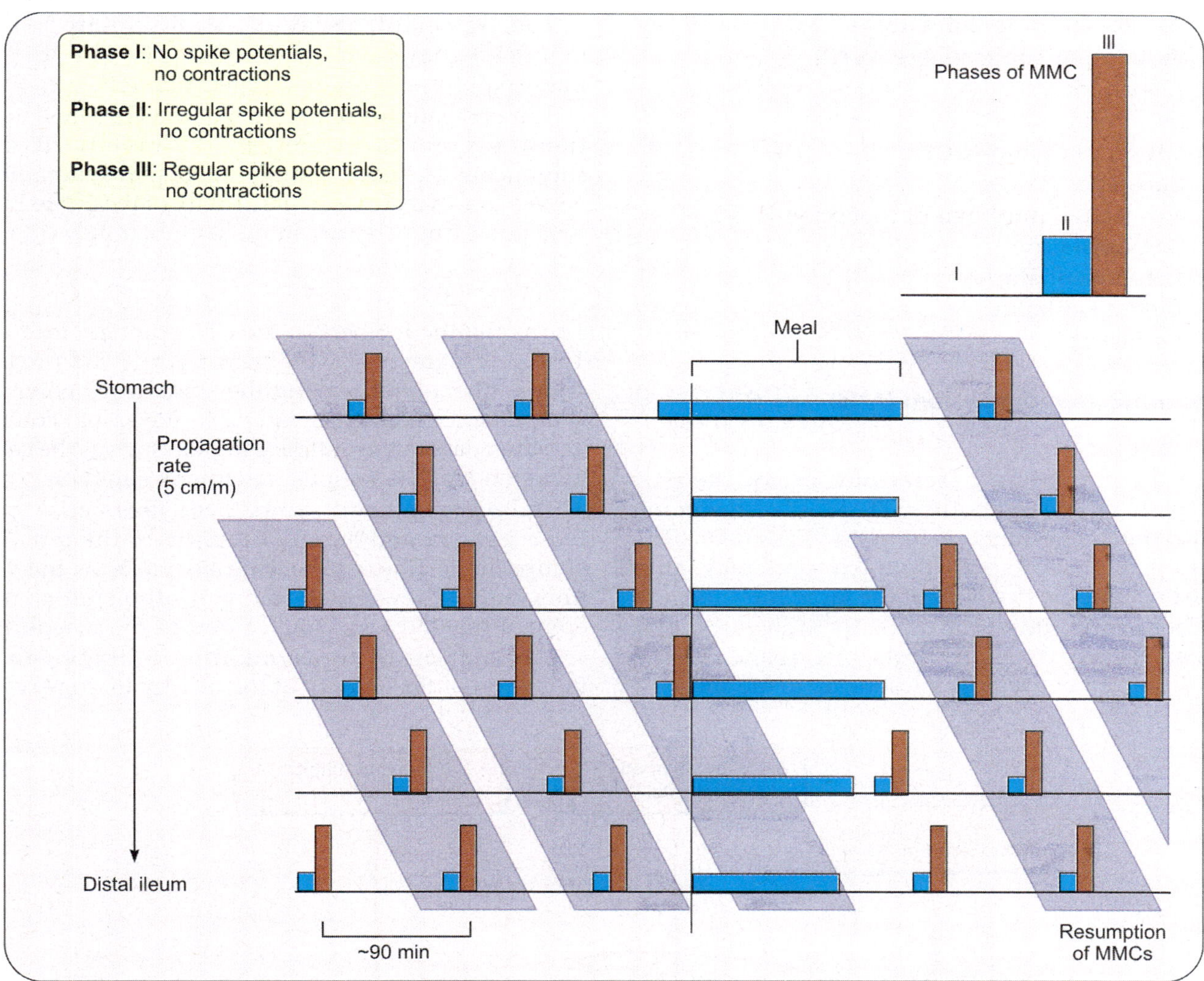

Fig. 5.4

2. Spinal cord
3. Vagus nerve all the way to the brainstem.

These sensory nerves can elicit local reflexes within the gut wall itself and other reflexes that are relayed to the gut from the prevertebral ganglia or the basal regions of the brain.

The stimulation of the myenteric plexus causes increase:

1. In the tone of the gut wall
2. In the intensity of rhythmic contractions
3. Increase rate of rhythm of contractions
4. Increase velocity of conduction of excitatory waves along the gut wall.

Myenteric plexus is not entirely excitatory but some of its neurons are inhibitory. These inhibitory fibers secrete vasoactive intestinal polypeptide (VIP): an inhibitory neurotransmitter. These inhibitory signals inhibit the intestinal sphincter muscles (e.g. pyloric sphincter) that impede the movements of food through successive segments of the GI tract.

The submucosal plexus controls the function of the inner wall of the intestine. Many signals originating from the GI epithelium are integrated in the submucosal plexus and this helps to control the local secretion, absorption, contraction of the submucous muscle and various degrees of infolding of GI mucosa.

Neurotransmitters in ENS

They include:

1. Acetylcholine (excitatory)

2. Norepinephrine (inhibitory)
3. Adenosine triphosphate (ATP)
4. Dopamine
5. Serotonin
6. Cholecystokinin (CCK)
7. Substance P
8. Vasoactive intestinal polypeptide (VIP)
9. Somatostatin
10. Leu-enkephalin
11. Met-enkephalin
12. Bombesin

Autonomic Nervous System (ANS) (Fig. 5.5)

1. *Parasympathetic Innervation*

Both the cranial and sacral outflow of the parasympathetic innervate the GIT. Most of the cranial parasympathetic fibers are from the vagus nerve. They supply the esophagus, stomach, pancreas, small intestine and the first half of the large intestine.

The sacral outflow from the S2, S3, S4 segments of the spinal cord pass through the pelvic nerves and innervate the distal half of the large intestine up to the anus.

The sigmoidal, rectal and anal regions receive extensive parasympathetic supply and this is important for execution of defecation reflex.

The postganglionic neurons of the GI parasympathetic system is located in the myenteric and submucous plexuses. Stimulation of parasympathetic nerves causes increase in the activity of the entire ENS, which in turn increases all the GI functions.

2. *Sympathetic Innervation*

The sympathetic fibers to the GIT originate from the T5 to L2 segments of the spinal cord. The preganglionic fibers after leaving the spinal cord enter the sympathetic chain lying lateral to the spinal column and then pass to the outline ganglion such as the celiac ganglion and the various mesenteric ganglion.

The postganglionic sympathetic fibers arise from these ganglia and supply all parts of the gut. The sympathetic fibers innervate all parts of the GIT uniformly. They secrete the neurotransmitter norepinephrine (NE) and small amounts of epinephrine.

Stimulation of the sympathetic fibers causes inhibition of the activity of the GIT by three ways:

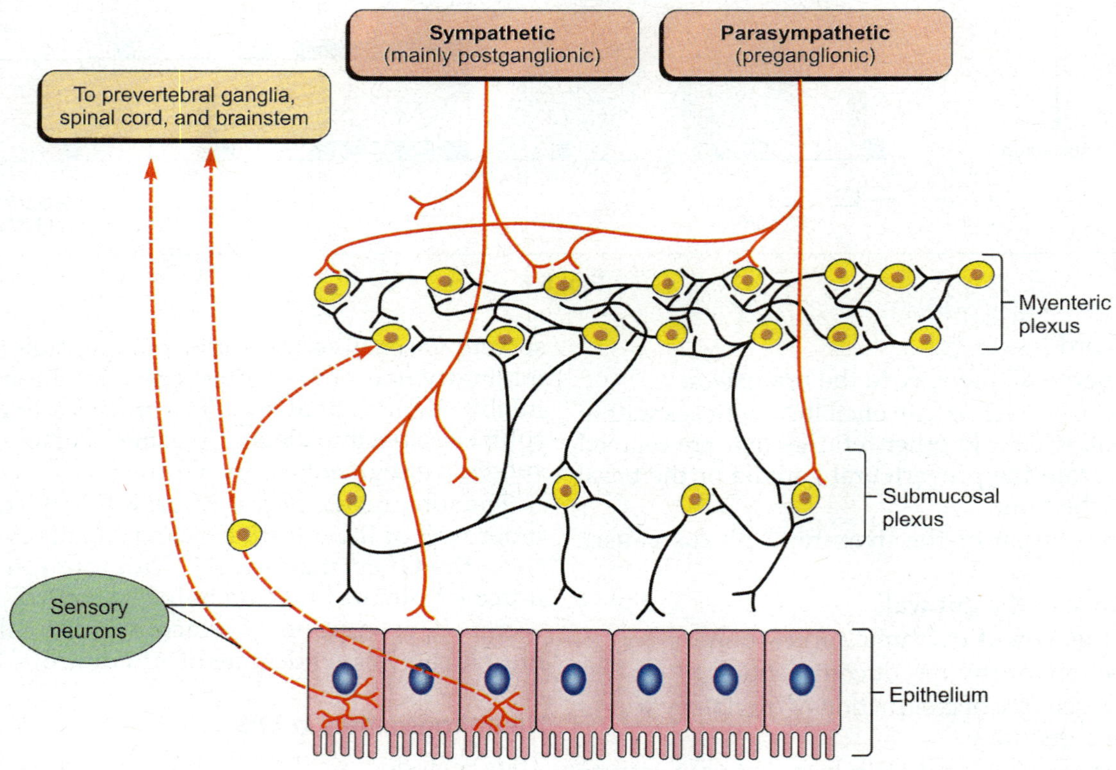

Fig. 5.5

1. By direct effect of secreted NE to inhibit intestinal tract
2. Smooth muscles (except the mucosal muscle which it excites)
3. By inhibitory of NE on the neurons of the ANS.

Afferents Sensory Nerve Fibers from the Gut

The neurons of the sensory nerve fibers may be located either in the ENS itself or in the dorsal root ganglia of the spinal cord. The sensory nerve fibers are stimuated by:

1. Irritation of the gut mucosa
2. Distension of the gut
3. Chemical substances in the gut

Stimulation of the fibers can cause either excitation or inhibition of GI movements or secretions.

GI Reflexes

There are three types of gastointestinal reflexes which help to regulate the GI functions:

1. *Reflex that are integrated entirely within the gut wall ENS:* These include reflexes that control GI secretions, peristalsis, mixing contractions and local inhibitory effects.
2. *Reflexes from the gut to the prevertebral sympathetic ganglia and back to the GIT:* These reflexes transmit signals: long distances to other parts of the GIT such as gastrocolic reflex which causes evacuation of the colon, enterogastric reflex which are signals from the colon and small intestine which inhibit the stomach secretions and motility.
3. Reflexes from the gut to the spinal cord of the brainstem and back to the GIT. These include:
   a. Reflexes from the stomach and duodenum via the vagus to the brainstem and back to the stomach; it controls the gastric motor and secretory activity.
   b. Pain reflexes that cause general inhibition of the GIT.
   c. Defecation reflexes that travel from the colon and the rectum to the spinal cord and back again to produce powerful colonic, rectal and abdominal contractions required for defecation.

Blood Supply

The splanchnic circulation supplies the GI system. All the blood that passes through the gut, spleen and pancreas then flows immediately to the liver by way of the portal vein. In the liver, the blood passes through the minute liver sinusoids and then leaves the liver through the hepatic vein that empty into the inferior vena cava of the general circulation. As the blood flows through the liver, the reticuloendothelial cells that line the liver sinusoids remove the bacteria and other toxic substances that might enter the blood from the GIT.

Factors Influencing the GI Blood Flow

The blood flow to each area of the GIT is directly related to the level of local activity. For example during active absorption of the nutrients, blood flow into the villi and the adjacent submucosa is increased by eight fold. During increased motor activity of the gut, the blood flow to the muscles is greatly increased.

1. Vasodilator substances are released from the mucosa of the GIT during the digestive process. These include peptide hormones like CCK, VIP, secretin and gastrin.
2. Gastrointestinal glands in the gut wall release two kinins-kallidin and bradykinin which are powerful vasodilators and increase the mucosal vasodilation during GI secretions.
3. Decrease oxygen concentration in the gut wall increases intestinal gut flow 50 to 100%. The increased mucosal and gut wall metabolic rate during gut activity reduces the oxygen concentration resulting in vasodilation.

Hypoxia also causes increase in adenosine which is also a powerful vasodilator.

Countercurrent Blood Flow in the Villi

The arterial flow into the villus and the venous flow out of the villus are in direction opposite to each other and the vessels lie in close apposition to each other. Because of this, much of the arterial oxygen diffuses out of the arterioles directly into the adjacent venules without being carried in the blood to the tip of the villi. About 80% of the oxygen takes this short circuit route. Under normal conditions, this shunting of oxygen from the arterioles to the venules is not harmful to the villi, but in diseased conditions (circulatory shock), the blood flow to the gut is greatly reduced and can cause ischemic death or disintegration of the entire villus.

21. SECRETIONS OF GIT

Introduction

The secretory glands of the GIT serve two primary functions:

1. The digestive enzymes are secreted from the mouth to the distal part of the ileum.

   The digestive secretions occur only in the presence of food and the quantity secreted in each segment is just sufficient for proper digestion.
2. The mucous glands secrete mucus which help in the lubrication and protection of various part of the alimentary tract.

Salivary Secretion

There are three pairs of salivary glands:
1. Parotid
2. Submandibular or submaxillary glands
3. Sublingual glands

Some minor salivary glands may be of mucous and serous types which are located in the buccal, labial and palatal areas.

Physioanatomy of Salivary Glands (Fig. 5.6)

- The parotid gland is the largest of the salivary gland and is located at the side of the face just below and in front of the ear.
- It weighs about 20 to 30 gm.
- It empties its secretion into the oral cavity via the Stensen's duct which opens in the upper second molar teeth.

Submandibular Gland

- It is located in the submaxillary triangle, medial to the mandible.
- It weighs 8 to 10 gm.
- It empties its secretion through the Wharton's duct which opens at the side of the frenulum of the tongue.

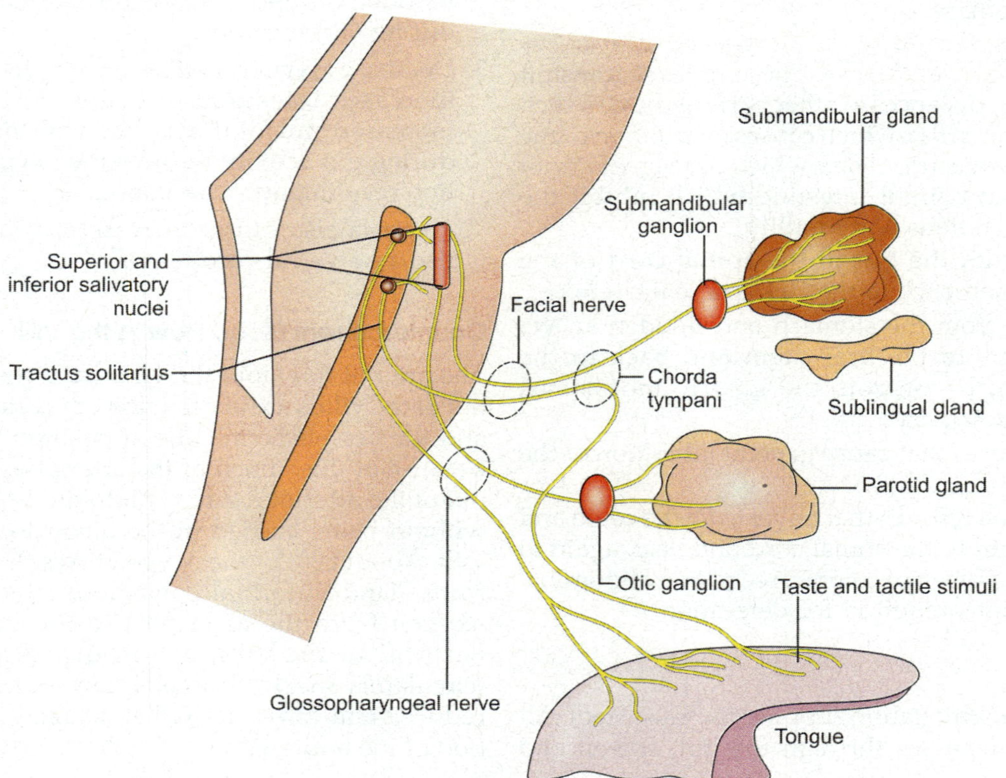

Fig. 5.6: Parasympathetic nerve supply of the salivary gland

Sublingual Gland

- It is the smallest gland, situated in the mucosa at the floor of mouth.
- It weighs 2 to 3 gm.
- It empties through 5 to 15 small ducts called the ducts of ravinus.

Classification of Salivary Glands

1. Serous Glands

- They are made up of serous cells
- Their secretion is mainly thin and watery and contains the enzyme ptyalin, e.g. parotid gland.

2. Mucus Glands

Their secretion are thick and viscus with a high mucin content, e.g. lingual, buccal and palatal glands.

3. Mixed Glands

They contain both serous and mucus cells, e.g. sublingual and submandibular gland.

Nerve Supply (Fig. 5.6)

Parasympathetic nerve supply

Superior salivary nucleus	Inferior salivary nucleus
↓	↓
Nervous intermedius of Wrisberg nerve	Glossopharyngeal
↓	↓
Geniculate ganglion	Tympanic branch
↓	↓
Facial nerve	Tympanic plexus
↓	↓
Chorda tympani	Lesser petrosal nerve
↓	↓
Lingual nerve	Otic ganglion
↓	↓
Submaxillary ganglion	Parotid gland
↓	
Sublingual and submandibular gland	

Composition of Saliva

1. *Volume:* 1000 to 1500 ml per day (1 ml per minute).
   Contributions by each gland
   Parotid 25%
   Submaxillary 70%
   Sublingual 5%
2. pH 6.35 to 6.85
3. Specific gravity 1.002 to 1.012.
4. *Tonicity:* Hypotonic to plasma
5. *Constituents*
   Water: 99%, Solids: 0.5%
   Solids: Organic and inorganic substances.

Organic Substances

a. Enzymes (ptyalin or salivary α-amylase, lysozyme (bactericidal), lingual lipase (lipolytic enzyme), kallikrein (proteolytic enzyme).
b. *Other organic substances:* Mucin, urea, uric acid, creatinine, free amino acids, blood group antigens.

Inorganic Substances

Cations: Sodium, potassium and calcium
Anions: Chloride, bicarbonate, phosphates and bromides.

Functions of Saliva

1. Digestive Function

Saliva contains ptyalin which helps in the digestion of starch into maltose.

Amylase acts in a neutral or mild acidic medium (pH of 6.5). Amylase digestion can continue in the stomach for half an hour until it is arrested by the high acidicity of the gastric contents. It is inactivated at a pH of 4.

2. Lubrication

Saliva contains mucin which helps in lubricating food. It helps in masticating food and facilitating in swallowing. It helps in protecting the oral mucosa.

3. Role in Speech

It aids in speech by facilitating movements of lip and tongue.

4. Cleansing and Protective Function

Lysozyme is an antibacterial agent.

IgA provides immunological defence against bacteria and viruses. Lactoferrin binds with iron and arrest bacterial multiplication.

5. Appreciation of Taste

Saliva keeps the mouth moist and acts as a solvent for the food and stimulates the taste bud.

6. Buffering Action

Buffers and proline rich proteins in saliva help to bind toxic tannin and maintains the oral pH at 7.0.

This protects the tooth enamel by preserving the calcium. It also helps to neutralize the gastric acid regurgitated into the esophagus and helps to relieve heart burn.

7. Excretory Function

It helps in the excretion of drugs like alcohol, morphine and inorganic ions like potassium, calcium, HCO_3^-, iodine and thiocyanate.

8. Regulation of Body Temperature

In animals like dogs, sweat glands are absent and salivation is accompanied by panting which forms a part of the physiological response to increase body temperature.

5

9. Regulation of Water Balance

When there is dehydration, salivary secretion is suppressed and drying up of mouth and pharynx causes sensation of thirst. This leads to drinking of water which helps in the restoration of fluid balance.

10. Middle Ear Pressure Adjustment

During swallowing of small amount of saliva at regular intervals, the pharyngeal end of eustachain tube is opened. This helps in the equilization of pressure on either side of the tympanic membrane.

Mechanism of Salivary Secretion

The acinar cells secrete potassium and bicarbonate by active process into the acinar lumen. Chloride is also secreted to maintain the electrical neutrality.

Due to the osmotic changes, water is drawn into the acinar lumen.

The salivary duct cells actively reabsorb Na^+, Cl^- and transfer K^+ and HCO_3^- into the saliva. The duct cells are impermeable to water and hence the final salivary secretion is hypotonic.

At rest, saliva contains more of K^+ and less Na^+, Cl^- and HCO_3^- compared to the plasma concentration. When the salivary flow increases, there is less time for ion exchange in the ducts and so saliva becomes less hypotonic. Na^+, Cl^-. and HCO_3^- concentration increases and K^+ concentration decreases.

Aldosterone increases the K^+ conc. and decreases the Na^+ conc. of the saliva.

Regulation of Salivary Secretion

Stimulation of parasympathetic nerves produces vasodilation of blood vessels of the salivary glands and stimulate secretion from acini.

Therefore, it causes profuse secretion of watery saliva with low content of organic material and protein. Atropine (parasympatholytic) reduces salivary secretion.

Sympathetic nerve stimulation causes secretion of small amounts of saliva rich in organic contents and mucus from the submandibular and sublingual glands.

Unconditioned Salivary Reflex

The presence of food in the mouth cause reflex secretion of saliva after a short latent period of 1 to 2 seconds.

Conditioned Salivary Reflex

This is an acquired reflex learned by association of some sensations with food: sight, smell or thought of food provokes salivary secretion even when food is not present. The receptors are the visual and olfactory receptors which are located outside the mouth. The cerebral cortex is involved in conditioned reflexes.

Applied Physiology

Hyposalivation

1. *Temporary:* Conditions like fever, fear and dehydration
2. *Permanent*
   a. Sialolithiasis due to formation of calculi in the salivary gland duct which obstructs the flow of saliva.
   b. Congenital aplasia or hypoplasia of the salivary glands.
   c. Bell's palsy: Paralysis of the facial nerve results in hyposalivation only on the paralyzed side.

Hypersalivation

It is also known as sialorrhea or ptyalism.

Physiological: Pregnancy

Pathological: Parkinsonism, irritant foci in the stomach, esophagus and pancreas.

Following an attack of encephalitis or epileptic seizures. Drugs used in the treatment of psychiatric disorders (cholinergic, adrenergic and histamine like drugs) iodides and mercuric salts.

Chorda Tympani Syndrome

Trauma to the chorda tympani nerve may result in the misdirected regeneration of severed peripheral nerve fiber which grow into the nerves innervating the sweat glands in the submental region. So, reflex excitation of the salivary centers lead to sweating on the affected side, i.e. gustatory sweating in the affected side. Auriculotemporal syndrome is also another such anomaly salivation.

Mumps: Viral infection of the parotid gland associated with fever and painful swelling of the gland, most commonly seen in children.

GASTRIC SECRETION

Gastric Glands

Types of Glands

1. *Mucus glands:* On the surface of the epithelium in most part of the GIT, there are billions of single cell mucus glands (mucus cells are goblet cells). They secrete mucus in response to local irritation of the epithelium.
2. *Crypts:* Many parts of GIT are lined by pits that are invagination of the epithelium into the submucosa, e.g. the crypts of Liberrkuhn in the small intestine which contain specialized secretory cells.
3. *Tubular glands:* These are located in the stomach and upper duodenum, e.g. oxyntic glands in the stomach secreting acid and pepsinogen.
4. *Complex glands:* For example, salivary glands, pancreas and the liver which provide secretions for digestion and emulsification of food.

Surface

Single layer of columnar epithelial cells. Surface mucosal cells.

Gastric pits or foveolae into which two or more gastric glands opens.

Total number of gastric glands: 35 million.

They are of three types:

a. Fundus or oxyntic glands
b. Cardiac glands
c. Pyloric glands.

Fundic or Oxyntic Glands

Elongated tubular glands. Have body and neck connected by isthumus. Have four type of cells:

1. Peptic, Chief, Zymogen Cells

Contains pepsinogen or zymogen granules which are precursors of pepsin: secrete pepsinogen.

2. Oxyntic Cells or Parietal Cells

Shape: Oval or pyramidal, mitochondria present granules are absent. The cells are scattered in between chief cells, mostly near the neck.

They are connected to the lumen of the gland by minute intracellular canaliculi which have microvilli. The function is secretion of hydrochloric acid (HCl) and intrinsic factor (IF).

3. Neck Mucus Glands

Present in the neck and also in the body of the gland. They contain secretory granules and secrete mucus.

4. Argentaffin Cells or Enterochromaffin Cells (ECL)

Are also present.

Cardiac Glands

Located near the cardioesophageal junction. They are short, branched, tortuous and contain mucus cells similar to those in the neck mucus glands. They open into short gastric foveolae.

Pyloric Glands (Antral Glands)

They constitue 1/5 of the total glands and are present in the pyloric antrum and pyloric canal. They are short, tortuous glands. They open into deep gastric pits. They contain mucus similar to that of surface mucus cells up to the isthumus, and lower down they resemble neck mucus cells. Few peptic and argentaffin cells are also present.

The G cells which secrete gastrin are also located here.

They are flask shaped with a broad base and a narrow apex which has microvilli. The gastic granules are located at the base.

Innervation

The glands are innervated by the sympathetic and the parasympathetic nerves.

COMPOSITION OF GASTRIC JUICE

Volume	2–3 liters
Specific gravity	1.006–1.009
pH	1–1.5 (can go to 2–3 in between meals)
Contains water	99%
Solids	1%

Organic solids
1. Pepsinogen
2. Rennin
3. Lipase
4. Gelatinase
5. Mucin
6. Carbonic anhydrase
7. Histamine
8. Intrinsic factor

Inorganic solids: Cations
1. Sodium
2. Potassium
3. Magnesium
4. Hydrogen
   - Anions
     - Chloride
     - Biphosphates
     - Sulphates

Mucosal Barrier

The acid in the gastric juice is highly concentrated and can cause tissue damage. This is prevented by the mucosal barrier formed by the mucus and the bicarbonate (HCO_3^-).

Mucus is made up of glycoprotein called mucin which forms a flexible gel coating the mucosa.

The surface mucosal cells also secrete bicarbonate which is trapped in the mucus gel so that the pH of 6–7 is established at the surface of the epithelial cells. HCl secreted by the gastric glands process this barrier by finger like channels, leaving the rest of the gel layer intact.

Factors stimulating mucus and bicarbonate secretion: Prostaglandins and local reflexes. Autodigestion of the surface epithelium is also prevented by the trefoil peptides in the mucosa. They have a three loop structure which looks like a three-leaf clover. They are of several types and are acid resistant.

Pepsinogen Secretion

The chief cells secrete pepsinogen: The inactive precursors of the pepsins in gastric juice. As soon as the pepsinogen comes in contact with HCl, it is activated to form active pepsin. Pepsinogen has a molecular weight of 42,500 and on splitting, it forms pepsin having a molecular weight of 32,000. Pepsin is active in a highly acid medium (pH 1.8–3.5). Above pH of 5, it is completely inactivated.

Functions of Pepsin

It is an active proteolytic enzyme.

HCl Secretion (Fig. 5.7)

When stimulated, the parietal cells secrete an acid solution that contains 160 millimoles of HCl per liter, which is almost isotonic with the body fluids.

The pH of this acid is 0.8, showing its extreme acidity. At this pH, the HCl concentration is about 3 million times as that of arterial blood.

Steps in the secretion of HCl acid (Fig. 5.7)

1. Chloride ion is actively transported from the cytoplasm of the parietal cells into the lumen of the canaliculus, and sodium ions are actively transported out of the canaliculus into the cytoplasm of the parietal cells. This creates a negative potential of –40 to –70 millivolts in the canaliculus, causing the diffusion of positively charged potassium cells and a smaller amount of sodium ions from the cell cytoplasm into the canaliculus. This results in the formation of KCl and a smaller amount of NaCl in the canaliculus.
2. Water becomes dissociated into hydrogen ions and hydroxyl ions in the cell cytoplasm. The hydrogen ions are then actively secreted in the canaliculus in exchange of potassium ions, which is catalysed by the H^+K^+ ATPase. Sodium ions are actively reabsorbed by a separate sodium pump. Since, most

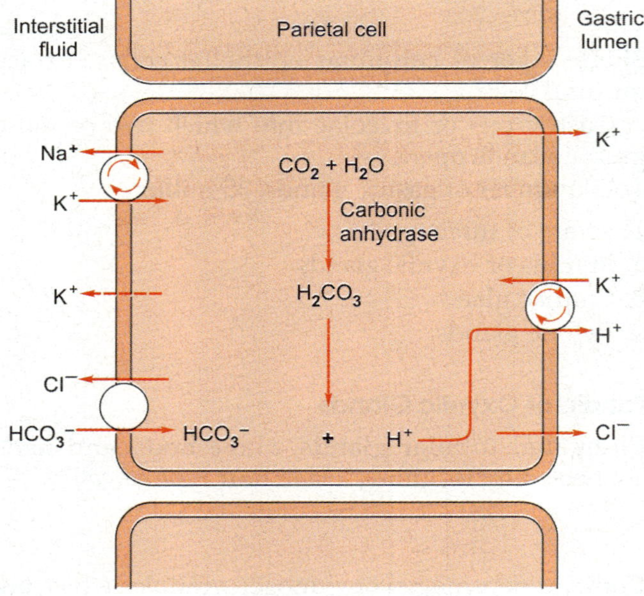

Fig. 5.7: Secretion of HCl

of the sodium and potassium are absorbed into the cells, hydrogen ions take their place in the canaliculus giving a strong solution of HCl in the canaliculus. The HCl is then secreted through the open end of the canaliculus into the lumen of the gland.

3. Water passes into the canaliculus by osmosis because of the extra ion secreted into the canaliculus. Thus, the final secretion contains water, HCl acid at a concentration of about 150 to 160 milli-equivalents/Liter (mEq/L), potassium chloride at a concentration of 15 mEq/L and a small amount of NaCl.
4. Finally, carbon dioxide, either formed during metabolism in the cells or entering the cell from the blood, combines under the influence of carbonic anhydrase with the hydroxyl ions (From Step 2) to form HCO_3 ions. This then, diffuses out of the cytoplasm into the ECF in exchange for chloride ions that enter the cell from the extracellular fluid and are later secreted into the canaliculus. Because of the efflux of HCO_3^- into the blood, the stomach has a negative respiratory quotient (RQ), i.e. the amount of CO_2 in arterial blood is greater than the amount in gastric venous blood. When gastric acid secretion is elevated after a meal, sufficient H^+ may be secreted to raise the pH of systemic blood and make the urine alkaline (postprandial alkaline tide).

Acid secretion is stimulated by histamine via H_2 receptors and by acetylcholine via M3 muscarinic receptors. Gastrin probably acts directly as well as via ECL cells. The H2 receptors increase intracellular CAMP via Gs, whereas the muscarinic receptors and the gasrtric receptors exert their effects by increasing intracellular free Ca^{++}.

Acid secretion is inhibited by prostaglandins-E series.

Secretion of Intrinsic Factor

The parietal cells also secrete intrinsic factor, a glycoprotein that binds with cyanocobalamin (vit B_{12}) and is necessary for its absorption from the small intestine. Other enzymes are:

Gelatinase: Which liquefies gelatin.

Gastric renin (chymosin): It is a milk clotting enzyme which curdles milk and converts caseinogen to whey protein and paracasein (absent in humans).

Gastric lipase: It is a weak fat splitting enzyme. It acts on finely emulsified fat present in milk, egg, yolk and triglycerides of butter fat. Its importance in fat digestion occurs in pancreatic insufficiency.

Regulation of HCl Secretion

Phases of gastric secretion: The gastric secretion is divided into three phases (Fig. 5.8)

1. Cephalic phase
2. Gastric phase
3. Intestinal phase.

Cephalic Phase

It begins even before the entry of food into the stomach.

Cause

a. Presence of food in the mouth which stimulates the taste receptors, reflexly activates the vagus nerve, stimulating gastric secretion. This is an unconditioned reflex.
b. Sight, smell and thought of food increases the gastric secretion. It is a conditioned reflex mediated via the vagus nerve.

The secretions in the cephalic phase is referred to as the appetite juice and is provoked by appetizing foods. This phase contributes to less than 10% of the gastric secretion during a meal. It causes a secretion of about 30 to 150 ml of gastric juice within a period of 20 minutes.

It sets in a latency of less than 5 minutes and the increase in secretion may last for half to two hours. During this phase, both HCl and pepsin secretion occur. Experimental evidence for cephalic phase: Sham feeding.

Gastric Phase

When food enters the stomach, further secretion of gastic juice occurs. More than 2/3 of the total gastric secretion occurs during this phase. The rate of secretion is lower than during the cephalic phase, but it continues for several hours as long the food remains in the stomach. It is mediated by both neural and hormonal influence. The nervous is the vagus and the hormone is the gastrin release from the pyloric antrum.

Gastric distension caused by food in the stomach produces secretion which is sustained as long as the distension continues. It sets up a local visceral reflex (vagovagal reflex). Even in the absence of vagal innervation, distension of the pyloric antrum by food as well as chemical stimulation of the antral mucosa

5

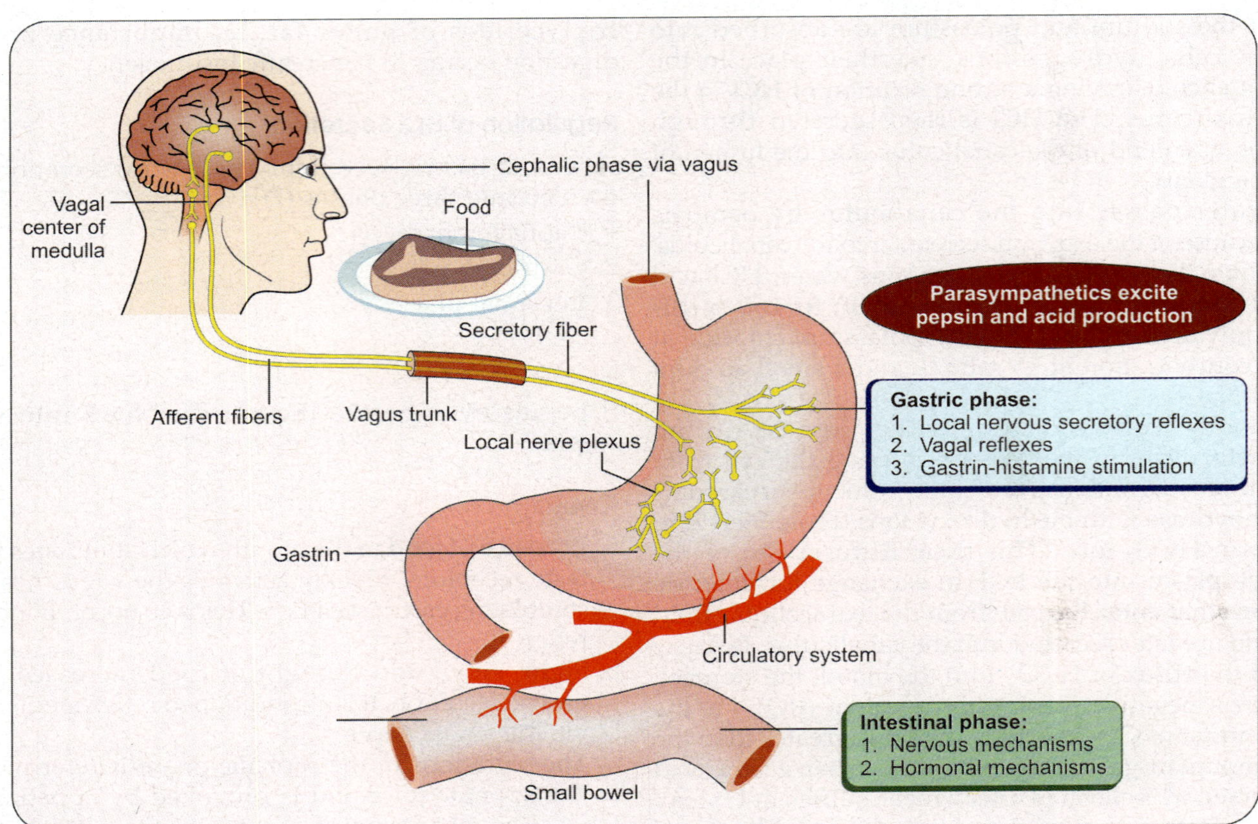

Fig. 5.8

5

by food like meat extracts and products of protein digestion evoke acid secretion.

Experimental Evidence

Pavlov showed that when food was placed in the stomach of a dog through a fistula, while it was asleep, thereby not allowing it to see it or smell it thus avoiding psychic stimulation, gastric secretions still occurred within 15 minutes.

Intestinal Phase

Begins with the entry of food products into the intestine. The rate of secretion is lower than the gastric phase. It commences about 2–3 hours after a meal and is maintained for 3 to 9 hours.

Mechanical distension of the intestine also elicits acid secretion in the stomach. Since food in the duodenum can induce secretion in a denervated gastric pouch, the hormonal mechanism (gastrin) is responsible for the intestinal phase.

Experimental Evidence

Pavlov showed that when the food substances or products of digestion was directly introduced into the duodenum (surgically separated from the stomach), evoked acid secretion in the stomach.

Gastric Function Tests

Tests used to assess the acid secretory functions of the stomach involves the collection of gastric secretions over a period of time.

The most suitable method used to collect gastric secretions is the Ryle's tube: which is a thin rubber tube, tip is blind and bulbous with weighted metal (which makes the tip radiopaque) and with numerous small perforations 2 cm from the tip.

In the tube, the cardiac and pyloric positions are marked from the incisor teeth. The patient is made to swallow the tubes, till the tip is in the most dependent part of the stomach, which is verified by fluoroscope.

1. Fractional Test Meal (FTM)

This is the oldest method. The amount of acid secreted in response is estimated by obtaining periodic fractions of the gastric contents.

After obtaining empty stomach sample following overnight fasted subject, the test meal is swallowed and 10 to 15 ml samples of the gastric contents collected at interval of 5 minutes for 2 and ¼ hour. The samples are analyzed for free and total acid by titrating against suitable indicators.

2. Histamine Test Meal (HTM)

Acid secretion in response to standard dose of histamine is measured following 12 hours fasting. Histamine is injected subcutaneously and the gastric juice is continuously aspirated for 60 minutes.

3. Augmented Histamine Test (AHT)

It is a modified histamine test, introduced by Kay. Large dose of histamine acid phosphate is administered to achieve maximal acid secretion. Basal acid output (BAO) are obtained for 1 hour. During this period, an antihistamine is administered to neutralize the effects of histamine. At the end of this period, histamine is injected subcutaneously and the gastric juice is collected at 15 minutes intervals for the next 60 minutes. This acid output is called the maximal acid output (MAO).

4. Pentagastrin Test

Pentagastrin, an analog of gastrin is used.

5. Insulin Test

After an overnight fast, the patient is intubated, fasting contents removed and the basal secretion of gastric acid is assessed for 60 minutes. Blood glucose is checked. Then 2 units/10 kg body weight of crystalline insulin is given intravenously, sufficient to reduce the sugar to 40 or 50 mg. Gastric contents are aspirated every 15 minutes for 2 to 4 hours. Blood samples are checked to prevent hypoglycemia.

Recent Advances Include

Barium meal: X-ray after swallowing a barium meal, gives information of break in the outline of the stomach, e.g. filling defect in tumors, or a projection in ulcers. Serial X-rays are useful for detecting motility disorders.

Endoscopy: Lesion can be visualized by passing a fiberoptic endoscope through the mouth into the esophagus. Biopsy done to rule out malignancy and removal of polyps also done by endoscopy.

Applied Aspects

Peptic Ulcer

Gastric and duodenal ulcer: Occur as a result of the breakdown of the mucosal barrier.

Infection with the bacterium *Helicobacter pylori* disrupts this barrier.

Drugs like aspirin, nonsteroidal anti-inflammatory drugs (NSAIDs) inhibit the production of prostaglandins and decrease the mucus and HCO_3^- secretion, resulting in mucosal ulceration.

Prolonged excess secretion of acid occurs in Zollinger-Ellison's syndrome as a result of gastrinomas, which causes peptic ulcer (Fig. 5.9).

5

Treatment

Inhibition of acid secretion with drugs such as cimetidine that blocks the H2 receptors on the parietal cells or omeprazole that inhibits H^+ K^+ ATPase.

H. pylori can be treated with antibiotics. Ulcers due to NSAIDs can be treated by stopping the drug or when it is not possible, prostaglandins agonist misoprostol can be given. Gastrinomas should be removed surgically.

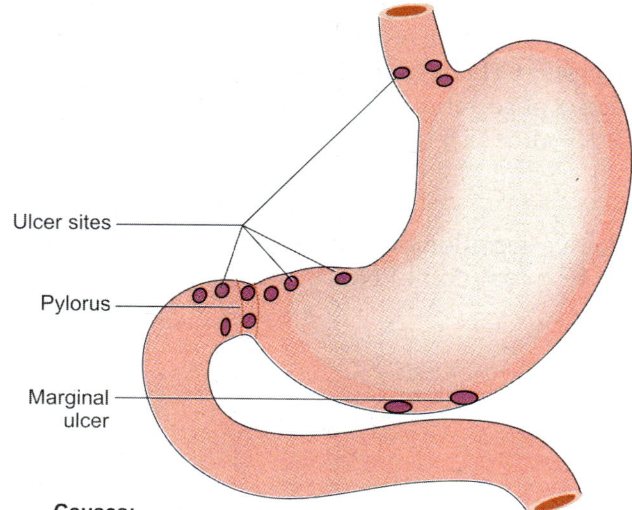

Fig. 5.9

Small Intestine: Secretions

Brunner's glands: They are compound mucus glands located in the wall of the duodenum. These glands secrete large amount of alkaline mucus in response to tactile or irritating stimuli on the duodenal mucosa, vagus stimulation and GI hormones, especially secretin.

Functions

1. To protect the duodenal wall from the highly acid gastric contents entering from the stomach.
2. The mucus also contains large quantities of HCO_3^- ions which along with the HCO_3^- from the pancreatic juice and bile neutralizes the HCl from the stomach.

Brunner's glands are inhibited by sympathetic stimulation. Such a stimulation in very excitable persons, leaves the duodenal bulb unprotected and is one of the factors that cause this area of the GIT to be the site of duodenal ulcer.

5

Secretion by Intestinal Digestive Juice: By the Crypts of Liberkuhn

The Crypts of Liberkuhn lies over the entire surface of the intestine between the intestinal villi. The surface of both the crypts and villi are covered by an epithelium that contains two types of cells—goblet cells that secrete mucus (lubricates and protects the intestinal surface) and enterocytes present in the crypts secrete large amount of water and electrolytes. Those enterocytes on the surface of the adjacent villi reabsorb the water and electrolytes along with the end products of digestion. This secretion is known as succus entericus.
Volume of secretion: 1800 ml/day
pH: Alkaline (7.5 to 8.0).

Mechanism of Secretion

1. Active secretion of chloride ions into the crypt.
2. Active secretion of HCO_3^- ions.
3. Secretion of both these ions causes electrical drag of positively charged sodium ions through the membrane.
4. All these ions together cause osmotic movement of water into the lumen.

Digestive Enzymes in Small Intestinal Secretions

1. Peptidases which split small peptides to amino acids.
2. *Disaccharidases:* Sucrase, maltase, isomaltase, which split disaccharides to monosaccharides.
3. *Intestinal lipase:* Splits neutral fats into glycerol and fatty acids.

Regulation of small intestine secretion: By local enteric nervous reflexes.

Large Intestine: Secretion

Mucus secretion: The mucus of the large intestine has many crypts of Liberkuhn. There are no villi. The epithelial cells contain no enzymes, instead they have mucus cells that secrete only mucus. In addition, small amount of bicarbonate ions are secreted by non-mucus secreting epithelial cells.

Factors that Influence Secretion

Pelvic nerves that carry parasympathetic innervation cause marked increase in mucus secretion. Extreme parasympathetic stimulation during emotional disturbances causes large amount of mucus secretion which increases the bowel movement.

Mucus in the large intestine protects the intestinal wall. In addition, it also provides an adherent medium for holding faecal matter together. It also protects the intestinal wall from the bacterial activity taking place in the feces. The alkalinity of the mucus provides a barrier to keep acid formed in the feces from attacking the intestinal wall.

22. MOVEMENTS OF GASTROINTESTINAL TRACT OR GI MOTILITY

Structure of the esophagus. It is a narrow, tubular structure, 1.5 cm in diameter and 25 cm long, extending from the lower end of the pharynx to the cardiac orifice of the stomach. It is covered by an outer fibrous coat under which is the muscular layer made up of outer longitudinal and inner circular muscle.

The upper 1/3 is composed of striated muscle and the lower 1/3 smooth muscle and a mixture of both in the middle third. The submucosa has many mucus secreting glands. The mucous membrane is lined by stratified epithelium.

The mucus secretion protects the mucosa, also lubricates it and facilitates the smooth passage of food. The esophagus is innervated by vagus and sympathetic nerves (Fig. 5.10).

MASTICATION

Mastication is a process of chewing of food whereby the large food particles are broken down into smaller size and thoroughly mixed with the saliva.

This aids in the swallowing and digestion of food. The number of chews ranges from 20 to 25 for each bolus of food. Chewing results in reflex salivation.

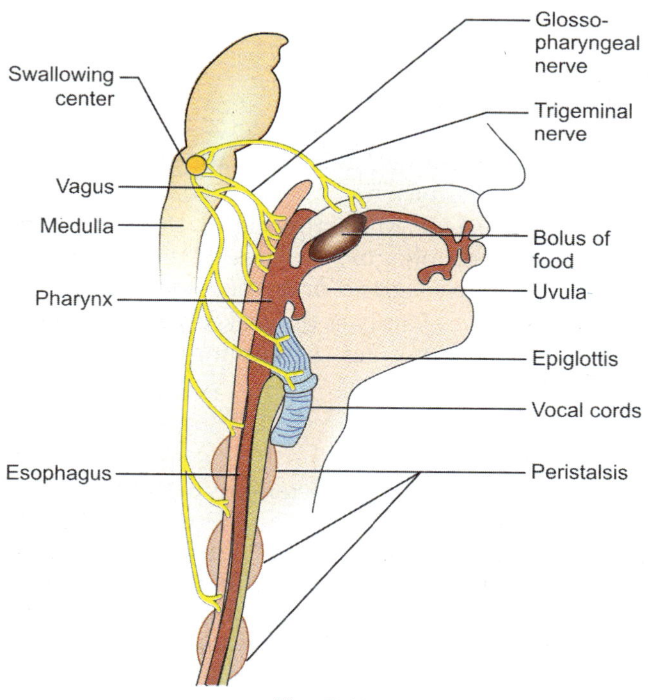

Fig. 5.10

As the food moves in the mouth, the taste buds are stimulated.

The muscles of mastication are the masseter, temporalis, internal, external pterygoids and the buccinator. All these muscles except the buccinators are innervated by the mandibular division of the trigeminal nerve. The facial nerve supplies the buccinator. Though mastication is a voluntary act and forms a part of the conscious activity of the person, it tends to become an automatic reflex activity.

Reflex mastication is carried by the combined action of the muscles of the jaw, lips, cheek and tongue in addition to the muscles of mastication. These are co-ordinated by impulses which travel via the V, VII, IX, X, XI, XII cranial nerves.

5

DEGLUTITION (SWALLOWING)

Deglutition is a process by which the masticated bolus of food passes from the mouth into the stomach. It is a reflex response that is triggered by afferent impulses in the trigeminal, glossopharyngeal and vagus nerves. The entire process takes a few seconds and is divided into three stages:

1. Oral or buccal stage
2. Pharyngeal stage
3. Esophageal stage.

Oral or Buccal Stage

The oral stage consists of passage of food from the oral cavity into the oropharynx. The first stage of swallowing is initiated voluntary but like mastication tends to become a reflex action largely under-conscious control. The bolus is maneuvered to a constant position on the surface of the tongue called the preparatory position.

The mouth is then closed. The whole of the anterior part of the tongue is pressed against the palate, thus forcing the palate posteriorly. This is followed by the sudden backward elevation of the posterior part of the tongue, due to the contraction of the mylohyoid, styloglossus and hyoglossus muscles, resulting in the passage of the bolus through the isthmus of the fauces into the oropharynx. The sequence of events takes place within 0.3 seconds. The first stage is preceeded by a short inspiration of swallowing.

Pharyngeal Stage

In this stage, the food passes through the pharynx into the esophagus. The food in the oropharynx has four outlets:

i. *Into the mouth:* Which is prevented by continued opposition of the tongue against the roof of the mouth and the approximation of the pillars of the fauces.

ii. *Into the nasopharynx:* Which is prevented by the elevation of the soft palate which closes the posterior nares.

iii. *Into the larynx:* Prevented by
   a. Reflex inhibition of respiration (deglutition apnea) which lasts throughout the second stage.
   b. Closure of the glottis by approximation of the vocal cord.
   c. Movements of the larynx upwards and forwards which brings it under the epiglottis and base of the tongue.

iv. It can move down to the esophagus. Since all the other openings are closed, the only avenue for the passage of the bolus is the esophagus.

Involuntary contraction of the pharyngeal constrictor muscles propel the food into the esophagus.

5

Esophageal Stage

The food in the esophagus is transmitted to the stomach by peristaltic waves. They are of three types:

1. *Primary peristalsis:* Which is a continuation of the wave of contraction associated with pharyngeal stage of swallowing. It moves at a rate of 2 to 4 cm per second. The transit time for the food in the esophagus is 6 to 12 seconds.
2. *Secondary peristaltic wave:* It is due to the local stimulation or distension of the esophagus by food retained in the esophagus. It helps to transport the food left behind due to ineffective primary peristalsis. It is not as strong as the primary wave.
3. *Tertiary peristaltic wave:* It is seen occasionally. They are neither peristaltic or propulsive and occur simultaneously in different parts of the esophagus. Swallowing occurs not only when food and fluids are taken but also at other times when awake and during sleep.

A person swallows about 200 times while eating and drinking and about 400 times during the rest of the time which includes 50 swallows during sleep.

Deglutition Reflex

It is a nervous mechanism. The first stage is under voluntary control but is affected without conscious effort. The second and third stages are involuntary and reflex. Contact of food with the mucosa of the fauces and pharynx stimulates the touch receptors located here. The impulses travel up to the deglutition center via the afferent nerve fibers in the branches of the V, IX and X cranial nerves.

Deglutition center is located in the floor of the fourth ventricle in the medulla near the dorsal nucleus of the vagus. It lies close to but separate from the respiratory center and this enables the respiration to be inhibited during the second stage of swallowing.

The efferent fibers pass:

1. Via the V cranial nerve to the mylohyoid muscle.
2. Via the IX and X cranial nerves to the muscles of the pharynx and the esophagus.
3. Via the XII cranial nerve to the muscles to the tongue.

The esophagus is normally relaxed with the upper and lower esophageal sphincter remaining contracted and closed except during swallowing. The closure of the upper esophageal sphincter helps to prevent the entry of air during inspiration and also prevents the reflux of material from the esophagus into the hypopharynx from where it may be aspirated into the respiratory tract.

Applied

1. *Dysphagia*

Difficulty in swallowing. May be for solids alone or for both. Cause may be:

1. *Mechanical:* Due to narrowing of the lumen like stricture of esophagus, tumors or external compression by thyroid gland or aortic aneurysm.
2. *Neuromuscular:* Paralysis or weakness of pharyngeal or esophageal muscles as in motor neuron disease, myasthenia gravis.

2. *Achalasia Cardia*

The lower esophageal sphincter is hypertonic and fails to relax during swallowing. There is loss of co-ordinated peristalsis in the esophagus. The esophagus becomes greatly dilated and the food accumulates in it, trickling very slowly into the stomach. There may be dysphagia. There is degeneration of myenteric plexus in the esophagus due to reduced release of VIP at the nerve endings. Treatment includes:

a. Forcible distension of the lower esophageal sphincter using a balloon or a bag.
b. Muscle in the region can be surgically split without damaging the mucosa.
c. *Calcium channel blockers:* Nifedipine can also be given.

3. Gastroesophageal Reflux

Occurs due to incompetence of the lower esophageal sphincter. Regurgitation of the gastric contents can result in heart burn. Over a longer period, it causes the inflammation of the esophagus (esophagitis), which can later cause ulcer formation.

Treatment

H2 receptor blockers (cimetidine).

4. Hiatus Hernia

It is a herniation of the stomach through the diaphragmatic hiatus. May be associated with reflux esophagitis.

GASTRIC MOTILITY

Hunger Contractions

The contractions which occur when the stomach is empty or near empty are called hunger contractions. They begin three hours after a meal. The duration of the contractions is about 20 seconds.

Initially they are mild peristaltic contractions, but gradually increase in intensity, becoming forceful contractions over the stomach with no intervening pause.

There are three types of contractions:

1. *Type I:* Where the tone is low and there is interval between contractions.
2. *Type II:* The tone is high, amplitude is large with no intervening pause.
3. *Type III:* Tone is very high, duration is long and there is a incomplete tetanus.

Hunger contractions associated with discomfort or pain is known as hunger pangs. As the food enters the stomach, the smooth muscles in the wall especially in the fundus and the body of the stomach relax. This is called receptive relaxation.

It is a reflex initiated by the process of swallowing and begins even before the food enters the stomach. This prepares the stomach to receive the food and enables it to accommodate large volume without much increase in the intragastric pressure. Vagotomy abolishes the receptive relaxation that accompanies swallowing indicating that is neurally mediated.

Gastric peristalsis (mixing and propulsive movements): Peristaltic movements of the stomach help to mix the food thoroughly with the gastric juice and macerate the food which is softened by the digestive juices. It also propels the food through the pylorus into the intestine. The food after being mixed with the digestive juices form a homogeneous semifluid mass called chyme.

The peristaltic waves begins in the middle of the stomach as a weak ring of contraction and passes downwards towards to the pylorus, becoming more powerful and rapid. The pyloric part is more actively motile and its activity increases as the digestive process progresses (digestive peristalsis).

The peristaltic wave reaches the antrum, the pylorus narrows and only a small quantity of about 5 ml of chyme is pushed into the duodenum. The rest of the chyme is pushed back into the stomach.

This antral mechanism permits the discharge of semifluid chyme but retains the solid unmacerated food in the stomach. The duration of the contraction lasts for about 10 seconds and this contractions are known as antral systole.

Gastric Emptying

The pyloric antrum, sphincter and the duodenal bulb contract as one unit, with the contractions of the antrum, sphincter and duodenum occurring one after the other. The pyloric sphincter is relaxed most of the time and closes only when a peristaltic wave passes over it.

Functions

1. Regulates and limits the rate of flow into the duodenum.
2. Increases the effectiveness of antral mixing and churning by closing as the wave passes over it.
3. Prevents reflux of duodenal contents into the stomach as the sphincter remains constricted slightly longer than the duodenum.

Fluids leave the stomach almost immediately after entering the stomach. Solids take longer time. Carbohydrates empty earlier than proteins and fats are emptied last. It takes 3 to 4 ½ hours for the stomach to empty a mixed meal.

Regulation

Both the nervous and humoral mechanisms regulate the gastric motility. The nervous regulation is mediated by the vagus and the local reflex mechanism. Humoral mechanism are by the GI hormones. Factors influencing the gastric emptying:

1. *Gastric Factors*
   a. Gastric distension due to increase in the gastric volume, reflexly increases the gastric peristalsis via the vagovagal reflexes. Vagotomy slows the gastric emptying. It may be increased to 12 hours causing gastric atony and distension.
   b. *Gastrin:* Released due to distension also increases gastric peristalsis.

2. *Duodenal Factors*

They reduce gastric motility and emptying:

a. Duodenal distension or irritation of upper small intestine
b. Fats and fatty acids
c. Acids
d. Products of protein digestion
e. Hypertonic solution.

All these act via enterogastric reflex which is a vagovagal reflex and inhibit gastric motility.

Hormones which inhibit gastric motility and emptying are:

1. CCK-PZ
2. VIP
3. GIP

Hormones which increase gastric motility: Motilin. Some emotions like fear prolong gastric emptying while excitement hastens gastric emptying.

Applied Aspects

Vomiting

Vomiting or emesis is the abnormal emptying of the stomach and upper small intestine through the esophagus and mouth. It is a complex reflex act, which is co-ordinated by the vomiting center (Fig. 5.11).

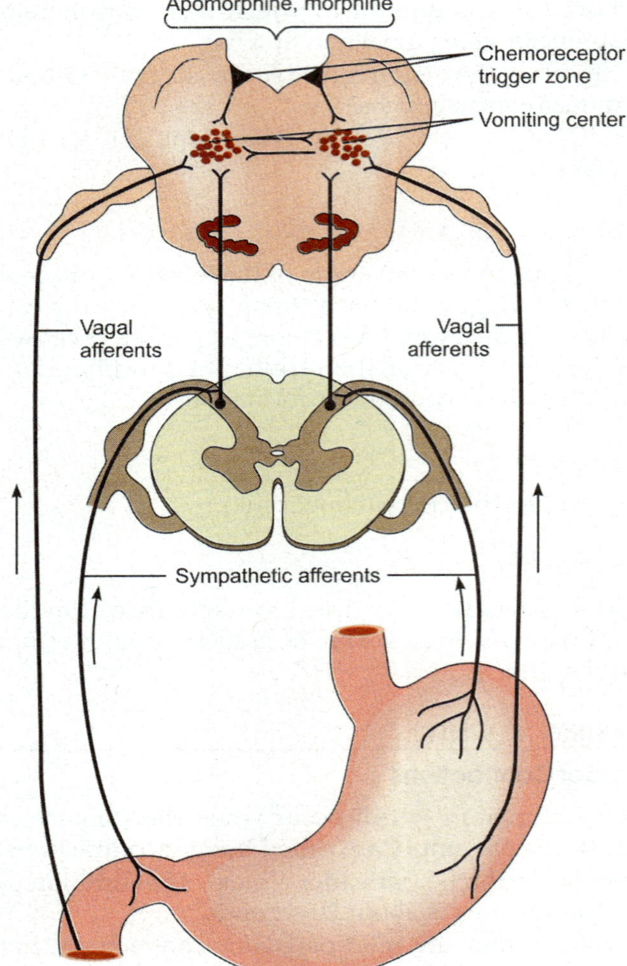

Fig. 5.11

Causes

1. Irritants in the GIT
2. Nauseating sight or odor
3. Drugs like chemotherapeutic agents
4. Central nervous disorders which increase intracranial pressure
5. Metabolic: Uremia
6. Severe pain: Myocardial infarction
7. Pregnancy
8. Psychogenic

Nausea: Unpleasant sensation that induces urge to vomit. It precedes vomiting

Retching: It is a strong involuntary movement that intensifies the feeling of vomiting.

The afferent impulses that mediate vomiting reflex arise from the receptors in the irritated gastrointestinal mucosa.

It travels:

a. Via the sympathetic and vagal afferents
b. Also from pain receptors in the periphery
c. From the vestibular apparatus (motion sickness)
d. From various parts of the brain including the limbic system and the hypothalamus.
e. 5-HT receptor in the small intestine and 5-HT release from the ECL cells initiate impulses in the afferents that trigger vomiting.

Vomiting Center

It is a group of neurons located in the reticular formation of the medulla, near the vagus nucleus. Circulating chemical substances do not act directly on the medullary vomiting center instead at the chemoreceptor trigger zone (CTZ) located on the medullary surface, near the area postrema.

The efferent pathway is the motor impulses from the vomiting center transmitted through V, VII, IX, X and XII cranial nerves and spinal nerves to upper GIT, diaphragm and abdominal muscles.

Emetics are substances that induce vomiting, e.g. apomorphine. Antiemetics prevent or inhibits vomiting, e.g. chlorpromazine, haloperidol, phenothiazines, benzodiazepam. Prolonged vomiting leads to dehydration, hypokalemia and alkalosis.

Vomiting in comatose patients leads to aspiration into the respiratory tract resulting in aspiration pneumonia.

Movements of Small Intestine

Functions

1. Mix the food thoroughly with the digestive enzymes.
2. To bring it into intimate contact with absorptive surface.
3. Propel the contents slowly down the alimentary canal.

Types of Movements

1. Segmental contraction
2. Tonic contraction
3. Peristalsis
4. Pendular movements.

Segmental Contraction

Movements of intestine (Fig. 5.12) mainly due to contraction of circular muscle layer. Longitudinal muscles contract over short distance prior to circular muscle contraction during peristaltic movements. In segmental contractions they are:

1. Rhythmic
2. Occur at regular intervals
3. Intervals are divided into segments of varying length by contraction of the circular muscle.

Segmental contractions of the intestine. Arrows indicate how areas of relaxation become areas of contraction and vice versa. At the end of 1 to 3 seconds, these segments relax and the adjacent segments contracts. This process is repeated by alternate contraction and relaxation of same area of the intestine.

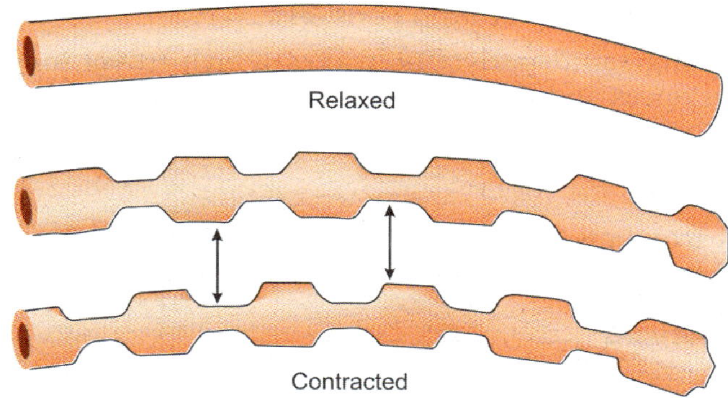

Fig. 5.12

Functions

1. Mixing the chyme with digestive juice
2. Bringing it in contact with absorptive surface.

Tonic Contractions

Prolonged sustained contractions of segments of intestine, which isolates one segment from another.

Peristalsis

Reflex mechanism; distension causes contraction behind the stimulus and relaxation in front of the stimulus and this travels as (Fig. 5.13):

Velocity of peristaltic wave: 1 to 3 cm/sec.

Movement of chyme: 1 cm/min.

Intestinal peristalsis infrequent during fasting and begins when food is eaten and occurs at regular intervals when food enters the intestine.

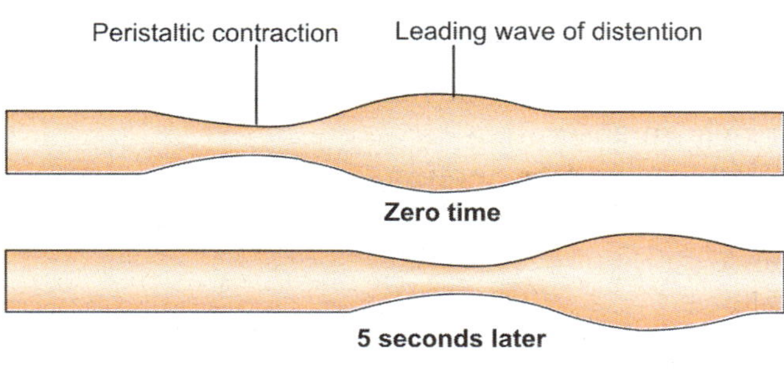

Fig. 5.13

Peristaltic Rush or Rush Peristalsis

Strong rapid peristaltic waves which travel long distances and quickly sweep the intestinal contents into the colon.

Cause

1. Irritation (cathartics)
2. Increased distension.

Functions

Peristaltic waves propel food in the intestine.
Transit time in intestine: 3 to 5 hours.
Peristalsis occurs from oral to aboral end.

If the intestine is cut and resutured in reverse direction, peristaltic waves stop at the site of anastomosis. This is because the excitability, rhythmicity, tone and force of contraction decrease from duodenum to terminal ileum.

Law of Gut (or) Intestine

This was first observed by Bayliss and Starling who called it the law of gut.

Pendular Movements

Not seen in man, seen in rabbits. Simple constrictions of intestinal wall which move up and down for short distances and cause to and fro movement of chyme in the lumen and aid in mixing and exposure of contents to absorptive surface.

Movements of Intestinal Villi

At rest: They lie on the surface of mucosa. Stimulus to movements can be chemical, mechanical, nervous (parasympathetics: increase the movements, sympathetics: decrease the movements and blood supply and hence villi appears pale). Movement types:
1. Lashing
2. Swaying
3. Up and down: Elongation and shortening.

Functions

1. Cause stirring of the fluid bathing surface of villi
2. Help in absorption
3. Movements of lymph in lacteals.

Factors Regulating Intestinal Motility

1. Local
2. Neural
3. Hormonal

Myogenic: Segmental and pendular.

Peristaltic waves are also myogenic but is dependent on the integrity of the Auerbach's and Meissner's plexus. Peristalsis is intrinsic neural reflex elicited by mechanical or chemical excitation of the gut wall.

Distension or stretch stimulates mucosal receptors which send impulses via neurons of submucosal plexus to transmit effect of stretching of myenteric plexus. Here it activates the motor neurons and this causes smooth muscle to contract initiating peristaltic reflex arc which has one cholinergic synapse since ganglion blocking drugs inhibit this reflex. Local anesthetics also block reflex. Acetylcholine and substance P cause constriction behind stimulus, VIP and NO: relaxation in front.

Food in stomach initiates gastroenteric reflex, which is transmitted through myenteric plexus along the wall from the stomach to intestine.

Extrinsic Nerves

Vagus (ACh-parasympathetics) increases tone and intestinal motility. Noradrenaline (sympathetics) decrease motility.

Humoral Factors

1. Serotonin: Secreted by enterochromaffin cells increase peristalsis.
2. Motilin, CCK, gastrin: Causes intestinal contraction and movements.
3. Secretin and glucagon inhibit movements.
4. Histamine acts directly on smooth muscle and causes contraction.

Movements of Large Intestine

Food enters the cecum 4 hours after a meal and is mixed and propelled slowly along the colon. The colonic transit time is as follows:
1. *Ileum:* 8 hours after a meal
2. *Cecum and ascending colon:* 13 to 17 hours
3. *Sigmoid colon:* 18 hours
4. *Rectum:* 24 hours which is followed by defecation.

The colon shows a basic electrical rhythm, the pacemaker cells being located in the submucosal border of the circular muscle layer.

The frequency of the waves increases from 2 per minute in the ileocecal valve to 6 per minute in the sigmoidal colon.

Types of Colonic Movements

1. *Segmentation contractions:* Seen more in the ascending and transverse colon.
2. *Haustral contractions or churning:* In which the colonic walls roll back and forth over the contents.
3. *Kneading movements:* In which large segments contract while adjacent segments relax, followed by contraction and relaxation in the opposite phase.
4. *Pendular type of movements:* (Peristalsis cum antiperistalsis) seen in short segments of the colon. These movements help in the rolling of the colonic contents, mixing them and exposing them to the mucosal surface and not with propulsion of the intestinal contents.
5. There is peristalsis similar to that seen in the small intestine but its frequency is slower.
6. *Mass peristalsis:* Occurs infrequently about 1 to 3 or 4 times per day.

They are forceful contractions which simultaneously involve the contractions of the large segments of the colon and show peak pressures up to 100 mm Hg. These movements help to empty the proximal regions and propel the contents into the distal colon. They may be vigorous enough to push the contents into the rectum and induce the desire or sensation for defecation. Mass peristalsis occur when the colon is irritated or overdistended.

It can occur even after meals: Due to the distension of the stomach and the duodenum-gastrocolic and duodenocolic reflex mediated by the extrinsic ANS.

Defecation

The distension of the rectum with feces initiates the reflex contraction of its musculature and the desire to defecate.

The sympathetic nerve to the internal anal sphincter is excitatory while the parasympathetic nerve is inhibitory. The desire to defecate arises when a pressure of 20 to 25 cm of water is present in the rectum. When the pressure reaches 70 to 80 cm of water, defecation occurs.

Anorectal Motor Mechanism

There are two anal sphincter:

1. External anal sphincter
2. Internal anal sphincter.

The internal anal sphincter is formed by the thickening of the terminal part of the circular muscle layer of the rectum. It precedes the parasympathetic nerve through the pelvic nerves (which is inhibitory) and sympathetic supply via the hypogastric (which causes contraction of the sphincter).

The external anal sphincter consists of three distinct bundles of striated muscle, which forms a collar around the anal canal and keeps it in a tonic contracted state.

The external sphincter has somatic innervation through the pudendal nerve and is under voluntary and reflex control.

Unique features of external sphincter is:

1. Denervation does not cause degeneration of the muscle fiber and they still respond to electrical stimuli, which is of significance. In paraplegia, where electrical stimulus can be used to reduce fecal incontinence.
2. It continues its activity even during sleep, maintained by a spinal reflex originating in the muscle itself.
3. Voluntary control of the external sphincter however strong can only be maintained for a brief period of less than a minute.

Mechanism of Defecation or Defecation Reflex

Defecation is initiated by defecation reflexes. It is intrinsic reflex mediated by the local ENS in the rectal wall (Fig. 5.14).

The fecal matter on entering the rectum, distenses the rectal wall, which initiates afferent signals that spread along the myenteric plexus to initiate peri-

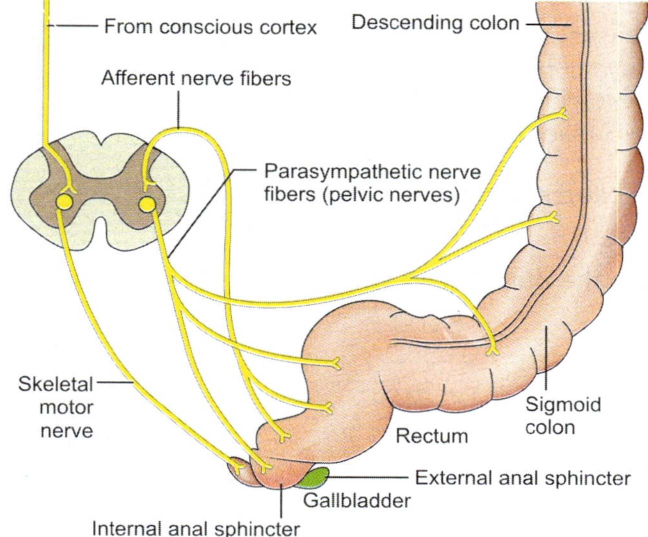

Fig. 5.14

5

staltic waves in the descending colon, sigmoid and rectum, which forces the fecal matter towards the anus.

As the wave of peristalsis reaches the anus, the internal anal sphincter is relaxed by inhibitory signals from the myenteric plexus. If the external anal sphincter is also relaxed at the same time, defecation occurs. The intrinsic ENS—myenteric defecation reflex is normally weak.

To cause effective defecation, it is attenuated by another defecation reflex called the parasympathetic defecation reflex, which involves the sacral segments of the spinal cord.

When the rectal nerve endings are stimulated, signals are transmitted first to the spinal cord and then reflexly back to the descending colon, sigmoid, rectum and anus by pelvic nerves of the parasympathetic system. These parasympathetic signals greatly increase the peristaltic waves along with relaxation of internal anal sphincter. This converts the myenteric defecation reflex into a powerful defecation process which is even effective in emptying the large bowel all the way from the splenic flexure of the colon to the anus.

Signals of defecation initiate other effects

a. Taking a deep breath
b. Closure of glottis
c. Abdominal wall muscle contraction to force the fecal contents downwards and also causing the relaxation of pelvic floor to evacuate the feces.

If it is convenient for the person to defecate, the defecation reflex is activated by deep breath, thus forcing fecal matter into the rectum causing new reflexes.

Defecation reflex causing automatic emptying due to relaxation of external anal sphincter:

1. Newborns
2. Transection of spinal cord.

Applied Aspects

Constipation

It is the difficulty in defecation.

Cause

Anxiety, change of bowel habits. Symptoms are abdominal discomfort and distension.

Treatment

Dietary fiber, laxatives.

Dietary Fiber

In humans, the ingested cellulose escape digestion and absorption (due to absence of microorganisms that break them). The increased bulk of this undigested residue stimulates intestinal peristalsis, which in turn increases the bulk of feces. Thus, high fiber diet plays an important role in prevention and treatment of constipation. Other roles of dietary fiber:

a. It reduces the sudden increase in blood glucose after meal (postprandial hyperglycemia), which helps in prevention and treatment of diabetes mellitus.
b. It reduces the blood cholesterol level by binding with the bile salts. So, useful in obesity, atherosclerosis, hypercholesterolemia.
c. It decreases the incidence of carcinoma of colon by binding and diluting the carcinogens.

Diarrhea

Increase in the frequency of passage of stools.

Cause

Infection (bacterial, viral, protozoal), gastroenteritis (food poisoning), ulcerative colitis.

Hirschsprung's Disease or Aganglionic Megacolon

Due to congenital absence of the ganglionic cells in both the plexus (myenteric and submucous) or degeneration of myenteric plexus. Children defecate only once in 3 weeks. Treated by surgery. There is loss of electrolytes and water in the diarrheal stools which when severe lead to dehydration, electrolyte imbalance, shock, collapse and even death.

23. EXPERIMENTAL EVIDENCES IN GASTROINTESTINAL TRACT

SALIVARY GLANDS

1. Cannulation of salivary ducts has been the classical method used to obtain pure, uncontaminated salivary secretions, from submandibular and parotid gland since these glands open by a single duct.

   Difficulties

   1. Effects of anesthesia
   2. Surgical procedure, so cannot be easily obtained.
2. Pavlov to study conditioned reflexes in dog exteriorized the parotid duct of dog.
3. In human experiments, a cannula is introduced into the opening of parotid or submandibular duct and uncontaminated saliva can be obtained. Radiographs obtained after introduction of radiopaque substances through the cannula will delineate and outline the duct system. This technique is known as sialography, which is detecting and locating calculi in ducts.
4. Carlson and Crittenden in 1915, devised a special collecting vessel held by suction inside of the cheek opposite the opening of the parotid duct.

Daily secretory volume of saliva: 1000 to 1500 milliliter

Resting secretory rate is 0.25 ml/minute
Submandibular gland contributes: 70%
Parotid gland: 20%
Sublingual gland: 5%
Lingual and buccal gland: 5%
Specific gravity of saliva: 1.002 to 1.012.

STOMACH

Methods of Study

In the 18th century Reaumur (1752), a French scientist and later Spallanzani, an Italian priest and scientist, tried to examine the nature of gastric digestive mechanism.

After making animals swallow small perforated wooden and metal tubes containing food, they recovered these containers intact from the feces to find the food inside digested, substantiating the chemical nature of the process.

Spallanzani himself swallowed a small linen bag containing bread and examined it.

Dr. William Beaumont, an US Army surgeon had the unique opportunity to make systemic study of human gastric physiology. He made several observations on his patients.

Alexis St. Martin, a French Canadian, who received a gunshot wound which did not heal completely and left an opening between the stomach and abdominal wall (gastric fistula). He made several observations on various aspects of human gastric physiology including effects of emotions.

Later extensive studies were done on patients with gastric fistula following esophageal burns.

EXPERIMENTAL PROCEDURES IN ANIMALS

Sham Feeding (False Feeding)

Pavlov made animal preparation (in dogs) to study the cephalic phase of gastric secretion. The esophagus was cut in the neck and the two ends were made to open separately on the surface (esophagostomy). Gastric juice was collected from an opening made through the abdominal wall into the stomach.

When the animal was fed, it enjoyed the food and experienced all the sensations associated with eating, but on swallowing the food did not enter the stomach but it came out of the esophageal fistula.

The cephalic phase of gastric secretion was studied this way. The effects of sight and smell of food was also studied.

In humans, the cephalic phase of gastric secretion was studied by collecting the juice through gastric fistula. The patient was made to spit out the food after chewing, so it did not enter the stomach.

DENERVATED AND INNERVATED GASTRIC POUCH

Heidenhain Pouch

It is a vagally denervated pouch with intact blood supply. The gastric glands are distributed throughout the mucosa and have no single duct. Hence, collection of uncontaminated gastric juice secreted in response to food, is not possible in the intact stomach. This basic problem has been circumvented in experimental animals, by surgical procedures which have been devised to collect pure gastric secretions.

The pioneer in this field was Heidenhain, who removed a small portion of the greater curvature of the stomach and formed a pouch with only blood supply intact.

The pouch drains its secretions to the outside through a fistulous opening. During the procedure, the vagal nerve supply is severed. Hence, Heidenhain pouch is a vagally denervated pouch.

24. PANCREAS

5

PHYSIOANATOMY OF THE PANCREAS

The pancreas is both an exocrine and endocrine organ.

It consists of three parts: the head, body and tail. The head lies in the concavity of the duodenum and continues as the body which forms the major part of the gland. It ends in a pointed tongue-like tail which lies in close contact with the spleen.

The portion of the pancreas that subserves the exocrine function is made up of compound alveolar tissue. It is made up of numerous secretory units or acini which form the parenchyma of the gland. The acini empty through the duct systems which coalesce to form the main duct of the pancreas—the duct of Wirsung. The main pancreatic duct joins with the common bile duct to form a dilatation called the ampulla of Vater and opens into the duodenum through the duodenum papilla. The opening is guarded by a smooth muscle sphincter called the sphincter of Oddi. The duct of Santorini is the accessory pancreatic duct which also opens into the duodenum.

The pancreas receives parasympathetic nerve supply through the vagus. The postganglionic fibers innervate both the acinar cells and smooth muscles of the duct. The sympathetic fibers supply the blood vessels and is vasomotor in function. Pain fibers travel in the sympathetic afferents.

Composition of Pancreatic Juice

Volume: 1000 to 1500 ml/day
Specific gravity: 1.010 to 1.018
pH: 7.8 to 8.4
Water: 98.5%
Solids: 1.5%
Electrolytes: Cations: Na^+, K^+, Ca^{++}, Mg^{++}, Zn^{++}
Anions: HCO_3^-, Cl^- , and traces of SO_4^{--},HPO_4^-.

Enzymes

1. Pancreatic α-amylase
2. Pancreatic lipase
3. Pancreatic phospholipase A
4. Pancreatic cholesterol hydrolase
5. Pancreatic colipase
6. Pancreatic proteolytic enzymes: These are powerful protein splitting enzymes that are secreted as inactive proenzymes:
   i. Trypsinogen
   ii. Chymotrypsinogen
   iii. Procarboxypeptidase A and B
   iv. Ribonuclease
   v. Deoxyribonuclease
   vi. Proelastase

The pancreatic enzymes can act only in an alkaline medium. The high bicarbonate content of the pancreatic juice (>100 mEq/L) neutralizes the acid chyme which enters the duodenum, raising the pH to 6 to 7, which ensures the alkalinity in the intestines.

Activation of the Proenzyme

Trypsinogen is converted into the active form trypsin by the enteropeptidase or enterokinase secreted in the small intestine. Trypsin thus formed autocatalyzes the process of activation of trypsinogen. Trypsin then converts the other proenzymes to their active forms:

- Chymotrypsinogen to chymotrypsin
- Proelastase to elastase
- Procarboxypeptidase to carboxypeptidase
- Colipase to active colipase
- Phospholipase A to active phospholipase A

The pancreatic acinar cells contain a trypsin inhibitor which prevents the autodigestion of the pancreas by the activated trypsin.

Action of Pancreatic Enzymes

1. *Pancreatic a-amylase:* Acts on starch and converts it to maltose, maltotriose and α-limit dextrins. It acts on uncooked starch.
2. *Pancreatic lipase:* Hydrolysis the neutral and long chain fats (triglycerides) to mono-and diglycerides, fatty acids and glycerol. Pancreatic lipase is water soluble and acts in the presence of colipase at the lipid water interphase. This lipid water interphase is provided by the emulsifying action of the bile salts.
3. *Pancreatic cholesterol hydrolase:* Hydrolysis cholesterol esters to form cholesterol.
4. *Pancreatic colipase:* Enables pancreatic lipase to act on emulsified fat by binding to the carboxy terminal of lipase, opens the lid which covers the active site of action.

5. *Trypsin and chymotrypsin:* Acts on proteoses, peptones and peptides and converts them to polypeptides. Some amino acids are also formed. Both the enzymes are endopeptidases and act on the interior peptide bonds at the carboxyl side. Chymotrypsin coagulates milk.
6. *Carboxypeptidases A and B* are exopeptidases that act on the C-terminal of peptides.Type A acts on aromatic amino acids while type B acts on basic chains (arginine, lysine).
7. *Ribonuclease and deoxyribonuclease:* Act on RNA and DNA respectively to form nucleotides.
8. *Elastase:* Digest the elastin fibers in meat. It is an endopeptidase.

Formation of Pancreatic Juice

There are three steps in the formation:

i. Synthesis of the enzyme in the granular endoplasmic reticulum of the acinar cells.
ii. Storage of the enzyme in zymogen granules in Golgi apparatus.
iii. Discharge of the granules by exocytosis.

Bicarbonates and other electrolytes are secreted by the centroacinar cells, and cells lining intercalated ducts. When the secretion passes through the larger ducts the bicarbonate is absorbed in exchange for chloride. Hence, when the rate of secretion is low, more bicarbonate gets absorbed and so its content in the excreted juice is less.

Regulation of Secretion

i. Nervous regulation
ii. Humoral regulation

Nervous Regulation

Stimulation of vagus causes the secretion of pancreatic juice rich in enzymes mediated via acetylcholine.

Hormonal Regulation

Two GI hormones secretin and cholecystokinin-pancreozymin (CCK-PZ) stimulate the secretion of pancreas.

Secretin causes the secretion of pancreatic juice which is watery and alkaline, rich in bicarbonates. It acts on the pancreatic ducts where bicarbonates are absorbed in exchange for chlorides. CCK-PZ causes the secretion of thick viscous juice small in volume but rich in enzymes. It acts on the acinar cells and causes the release of zymogen granules.

Phases of Pancreatic Secretion

i. *Cephalic phase:* Forms about 15 to 20% of the total secretion. The sight smell and thought of food causes the secretion of enzyme rich pancreatic juice.
ii. *Gastric phase:* Forms 5 to 10% of the secretion. Presence of food in the stomach causes distension, leading to the secretion of small volume of pancreatic juice rich in enzymes. This is mediated via the gastropancreatic reflex through the vagus.
iii. *Intestinal phase:* Contributes to 75% of the total secretion. Entry of food into the duodenum causes the secretion of the hormones secretin and CCK-PZ which is responsible for this phase of the secretion.

Pancreatic Function Tests

1. *Estimation of serum amylase:* Normal: 50 to 120 units/L. Increased in acute pancreatitis.
2. *Fecal fat excretion test:* Fat is split mainly by the pancreatic lipase. Therefore, in the pancreatic insufficiency, the fat content of stools markedly increases. Normal fat excretion: 5 to 6 gm/day. In pancreatic insufficiency, it is increased to 40 to 50 gm/day.
3. *Lundh test:* This assesses the function of trypsin in the pancreatic juice. Pancreatic juice is obtained by duodenal intubation following a meal. The average trypsin activity of less than 6 IU/L indicates pancreatic insufficiency.
4. *Secretin and CCK-PZ stimulation test:* This is done by aspirating the duodenal contents following the injection of secretin intravenously followed by CCK-PZ. The total volume of the juice aspirated, the pH, HCO_3^- and enzyme concentration is measured and analyzed.
5. *Cytological examination:* Fresh uncontaminated duodenal aspirate is collected and cytological analysis done for cancer cells.

Applied Aspects

Acute Pancreatitis

Here there is activation of the pancreatic enzymes within the gland resulting in autodigestion and chemical inflammation of the gland. There is marked elevation of amylase and other enzymes along with impairment of the endocrine functions of the gland.

Hypofunction of the gland can occur following surgical resection of the pancreas, chronic pancreatitis, neoplastic tumors of the pancreas and fibrocystic disease of the pancreas.

Decreased secretion of pancreatic enzymes results in steatorrhea (excessive excretion of fat in the feces) characterized by bulky, frothy , foul-smelling stools.

Fibrocystic disease of the pancreas is a rare condition which occurs in childhood. It affects other glands like the sweat glands and shows changes in the electrolyte composition of sweat.

Carcinoma of the head of the pancreas can obstruct the bile duct resulting in obstructive jaundice.

25. LIVER

5

PHYSIOANATOMY OF THE LIVER

The liver is the largest organ in the body. It weighs 1.5 kg in the adult. It is reddish brown in color, located in the right hypochondrium, extending into the epigastrium and left hypochondrium. It is enclosed in a fbrous capsule and divided into right and left lobes.

Histology

It contains both parenchymal and connective tissue. The functional unit of the liver is the liver lobule which are made up of cyclindrical column of hepatic cells, forming the syncytium around the central vein (Fig. 5.15).

The portal vein divides into branches—interlobular veins which surround the lobules. From these veins, the blood passes between the hepatic cells in sinusoids to reach the center of the lobule, i.e. the central vein which drains into the hepatic vein via the intralobular branches and from there into the inferior vena cava. The hepatic artery also divides into branches which accompany the branches of the portal vein between the lobules. The hepatic arterial blood also enters the sinusoids where it mixes with the blood from the portal vein.

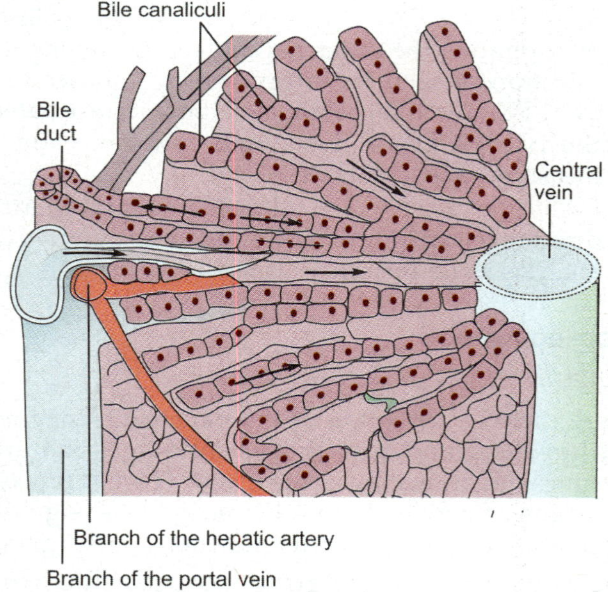

Fig. 5.15

The portal triad is formed by the portal vein, hepatic artery and the bile duct. It is enclosed in a fibrous tissue and is located in the periphery of the lobule to form the portal tract.

The sinusoids lie between the hepatocytes, lined by endothelial cells, phagocytic macrophages called Kupffer cells. The sinusoidal spaces are filled with blood from the portal vein and the hepatic artery. It is highly permeable and has fat storage cells.

The spaces of Disse is the space between the sinusoids and hepatocytes. It contains fluid that drain into lymphatic vessels. The plasma proteins diffuse freely into these spaces.

Blood Supply

Mainly through the portal vein and hepatic artery. The hepatic artery is a branch of celiac artery. It drains into the sinusoids along with the branches of the portal vein.

The portal vein supplies 1000 to 1100 ml/minute while the hepatic artery supplies 300 to 400 ml/min.

Venous Drainage

The portal vein is formed by the union of the superior mesenteric vein, splenic vein and inferior mesenteric vein. The entire blood draining from the GIT, pancreas and spleen enter the liver via the portal vein. The portal vein divides into branches within portal tract and form sinusoids which empty into the central vein of each lobule. These joins together to form the sublobular vein which inturn gives rise to hepatic vein which drains into the inferior vena cava.

Nerve Supply

It receives parasympathetic supply through the vagus nerve and sympathetic supply via celiac ganglion.

The main function of the ANS is the regulation of blood flow through the intrahepatic vessels.

The sensory fibers pass through the right phrenic nerve.

Functions of the Liver

1. Metabolic Functions

a. *Carbohydrate metabolism*
   1. Liver stores large amount of glycogen: Formed from glucose (glycogenesis).
   2. The stored glycogen is broken down to glucose (glycogenolysis)
   3. It forms glucose from noncarbohydrate sources like amino acids, glycerol and triglycerides (gluconeogenesis).
   4. It helps in the regulation of blood glucose level (glucose buffer function).

b. *Protein metabolism*

   It synthesizes all the plasma proteins except part of gammaglobulins. It also synthesizes blood clotting factors, enzymes, urea and lipoproteins from amino acids.

c. *Fat metabolism*

   It helps in the beta oxidation of fatty acid to form active acetate (acetoacetic acid). Nonesterified fatty acids are esterified to form triglycerides in the liver. It helps in the synthesis of lipoproteins HDL, VLDL, LDL, chylomicrons. It helps in the synthesis of saturated fatty acids from the active acetates via Kreb's cycle. It helps in the synthesis of cholesterol and phospholipids (lecithin, sphingomyelin, cephalin) for the cell membrane.

2. Bile Secretion

Liver synthesizes bile salts and bile acids from the cholesterol which helps in the activation of lipase and in the emulsification of fats. It conjugates free bilirubin by bile pigments with uridine diphosphates glucuronic acid (UDPGA) in the presence of glucuronyl transferase to form water soluble bilirubin glucuronides.

3. Synthesis

Liver synthesizes plasma proteins, especially albumin but does not synthesize immunoglobulins. Clotting I, II, V, VII, IX, X are synthesized in the liver. It is site of formation and destruction of RBC. The following enzymes are synthesized in the liver: alkaline phosphatase, serum glutamatic-oxaloacetic transaminase (SGOT), serum glutamatic pyruvic transaminase (SGPT), serum isocitrate dehydrogenase (SICD). It synthesizes urea from ammonia.

4. Storage Functions

a. *Storage of vitamins:* Vitamin A, B_{12} and D are stored in the liver.

b. *Iron storage:* Hepatic cells contain apoferritin. When iron concentration in the blood increases, it combines with apoferritin to form ferritin and gets stored in the liver.

5

5. Detoxicating and Protecting Function

It causes complete destruction of drugs like nicotine and short-acting barbiturates. Kupffer cells form part of the reticuloendothelial system and helps in immune mechanism. By conjugating with sulphates, glycine, glucuronic acid, acetic acid, it helps in the excretion of several substances in the urine.

6. Hormone Inactivation

Liver inactivates many hormones like cortisol, aldosterone, insulin, glucagon, testosterone and thyroxine.

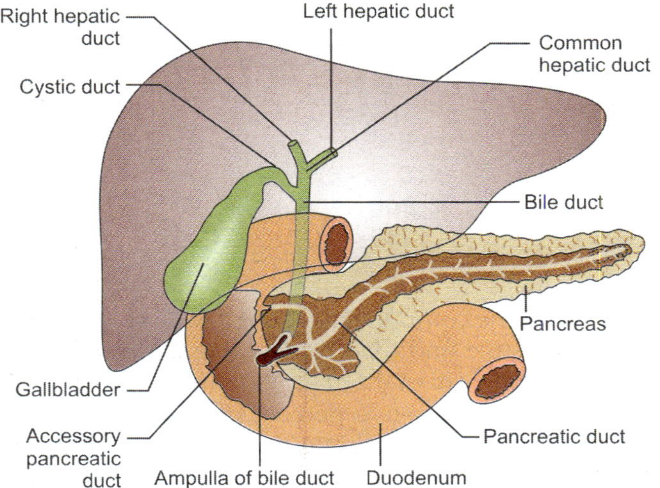

Fig. 5.16

BILE

Bile is secreted by the hepatic cells into the bile capillaries, from where is collected by the hepatic ducts which joins with the cystic duct to form the common bile duct (Fig. 5.16).

Bile is made up of bile salts, bile pigments and other substances dissolved in an alkaline electrolyzed solution (resembling pancreatic juice).

Composition of Bile

Daily secretion	500 to 1000 ml per day
Color	Golden yellow
pH	7.8 to 8.6
Water	97%
Bile salts	0.7% (sodium and potassium salts of bile acids)
Bile pigments	0.2% (biliverdin and bilirubin)
Fats	0.1%
Enzymes	Alkaline phosphatase—helps in converting organic phosphate to free phosphate
Electrolytes	
1. Cations: Na^+, K^+, Ca^{++}	
2. Anions: Cl^-, HCO_3^-	

5

Composition of Hepatic and Gallbladder Bile

	Hepatic bile (mmol/l)	*Gallbladder bile (mmol/l)*
Water	97%	86%
Solids	3%	14%
Bile salts	26	145
Bile pigments	0.7	5.1
Lecithin	0.5	3.9
Fatty acid	3.6	29
Cholesterol	2 to 6	16
HCO_3	28	10
pH	8.6	Neutral
Ca	5	23
Cl	100	25
Na	145	130
K	5	12

Some of the components of the bile are reabsorbed in the intestine and then excreted again by the liver (enterohepatic circulation) as shown in Fig. 5.17.

Ninety to ninety-five percent of the bile salts are absorbed from the small intestine. Some are absorbed by nonionic diffusion, but most are absorbed from the terminal ileum by an efficient Na^+, bile salt cotransport system powered by basolateral Na^+ K^+ ATPase.

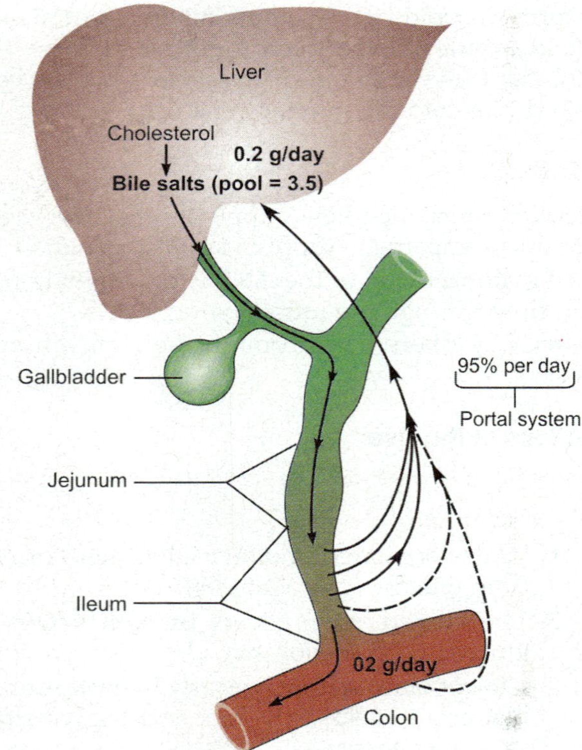

Fig. 5.17: Enterohepatic circulation

The remaining 5–10% of the bile salts enter the colon and are converted to the salts of deoxycholic acid and lithocholic acid.

The absorbed bile salts are transported back to the liver in the portal vein and re-excreted in the bile which is called enterohepatic circulation.

The total bile salt pool of 3.5 gm recycles via the enterohepatic circulation The entire pool recycles twice per meal and six to eight times per day.

Severe malabsorption of fat soluble vitamin results when bile is excluded from the intestine and up to 50% of ingested fat appears in the feces. Enterohepatic circulation is impaired:

1. Resection of the terminal ileum
2. Disease in this portion of the small intestine.

In this condition, bile salt reabsorption is impaired, so the amount of fat in stools is increased.

Production of bile is increased by vagal nerve stimulation and hormone secretin which increases the water and HCO_3^- content of bile.

Functions of Gallbladder

1. Bile is concentrated by absorption of water (liver bile is 97% water, gallbladder bile is 89%)
2. Acidification of bile.

Cholagogues: Substances that cause contraction of the gallbladder.

Cholerectics: Substances that increase bile secretion

Cholelithiasis: Presence of gallstones.

Two types:

1. Calcium bilirubinate stones
2. Cholesterol stones

Factors involved in the formation of gallstones:

1. Bile stasis: Stone formed in bile is sequestrated in the gallbladder.
2. Supersaturation of the bile with cholesterol.
3. Nucleation factors.

Liver Function Tests

Liver function tests measure the concentrations of various different proteins and enzymes in blood that are either produced by liver cells or released when liver cells are damaged.

Liver function tests are done in people suspected with liver disease.

a. *Tests of liver's biosynthetic capacity:* Serum proteins, serum ceruloplasmin, procollagen, prealbumin, prothrombin time.
b. *Tests that detect injury to hepatocytes (serum enzyme tests):* Alanine aminotransferases, alkaline phosphatases, gamma glutamyl transpeptidases, 5-nucleotidases.
c. *Tests to assess metabolic functions of the liver*
d. *Tests to assess bile secretory capacity:* Serum bilurubin, urine bilurubin, urobilinogen and stercobilinogen-
e. *Tests to assess detoxicating power of liver:* Hippuric acid excretion test. Bromsulphalein excretion test (BSP).
f. *Other tests:* Isotope scan, ultrasound scan, CT, liver biopsy.

Tests of Liver's Biosynthetic Capacity

In hepatic cell damage, serum albumin (A) decreases and globulin (G) increases leading to reversal of A/G ratio.

1. *Albumin*

- Albumin is the major protein present within the blood.
- It is synthesized by the liver.
- It is a major synthetic protein and a marker for the ability of the liver to synthesize proteins.

2. *Prothrombin Time (PT)*

It is a measure of hepatic synthetic function.

Prothrombin time is affected by proteins synthesized in the liver. Particularly, these proteins are associated with the incorporation of vitamin K metabolites into a protein. This allows normal coagulation (clotting of blood).

In patients with prolonged prothrombin times, liver disease may be present.

3. *There is a Increase in Blood and Urine Ammonia*

Tests that Detect Injury to Hepatocytes (Serum Enzyme Tests)

1. *Alanine Aminotransferase (ALT)*

- ALT is the enzyme produced within the cells of the liver.
- ALT is increased in conditions of inflamed liver or cell death.
- As the cells are damaged, the ALT leaks into the bloodstream leading to a rise in the serum levels.
- ALT is the most sensitive marker for liver cell damage.

Increased levels of ALT

- Chronic hepatitis C
- Chronic hepatitis B
- Acute viral hepatitis (A to E, EBV, CMV)
- Steatosis/Steatohepatitis
- Hemochromatosis
- Medications/Toxins
- Autoimmune hepatitis
- 1-antitrypsin deficiency
- Wilson's disease

2. *Aspartate Aminotransferase (AST)*

This enzyme also reflects damage to the hepatic cell. It is less specific for liver disease. It may also be elevated in conditions like myocardial infarction (heart attack).

Increased levels of AST

- Hepatic
  - Alcohol-related liver injury
  - Steatosis/Steatohepatitis
  - Cirrhosis
- Nonhepatic
  - Hemolysis
  - Myopathy

- Thyroid disease
- Strenous exercise

3. Alkaline Phosphatase

Alkaline phosphatase is an enzyme associated with the biliary tract. It is also found in bone and placenta, renal or intestinal damage

If the alkaline phosphatase is elevated, biliary tract damage and inflammation should be considered.

4. Gammaglutamyl Transpeptidase (GGT)

This is most commonly due to alcohol abuse or enzyme inducing drugs.

5. Lactate Dehydrogenase (LDH)

5

Lactate dehydrogenase is an enzyme found in many body tissues, including the liver. Elevated levels of LDH may indicate liver damage

6. 5-Nucleotidase (5-NTD)

5-nucleotidase is another test specific for cholestasis or damage to the intra or extrahepatic biliary system. It is used as a substitute for GGT for ascertaining whether an elevated ALP is of biliary or extrabiliary origin.

Tests to Assess Metabolic Functions of the Liver

1. For Carbohydrate Metabolism

a. Galactose tolerance test
b. Serum glucose estimation

The liver's ability to produce glucose gluconeogenesis) is lost in liver failure.

2. For Protein Metabolism

a. Estimation of blood amino acid
b. Urine amino acid estimation.

3. For Fat Metabolism

Estimation of serum cholesterol, triglycerides, phospholipids, total lipids and ketone bodies.

Tests of Liver's Biosynthetic Capacity

Total serum bilirubin increases in liver insufficiency. There is bilirubinuria (urine bilirubin: normally absent).

BILIRUBIN

Bilirubin is derived from the breakdown of haem in the red blood cells within the reticuloendothelial system.

- The unconjugated bilirubin then binds albumin and is taken up by the liver.
- In the liver it is conjugated which then makes it water soluble and thus allows it to be excreted into the urine (Fig. 5.18).
- Normally, total serum bilirubin is measured, however, the unconjugated and conjugated portions can be determined by measures of the fractions of indirect bilirubin and direct bilirubin respectively.

Metabolism of Bilirubin (Fig. 5.19)

Determination of bilirubin concentration. Van den Bergh reaction (aqueous).

- Conjugated bilirubin reacts readily—direct reaction
- Unconjugated, hydrophobic, reacts slowly
- Both conjugated and unconjugated react same in methanol—gives total bilirubin value
- Subtraction of direct from total gives indirect.

Normal	*Basis of abnormality*	*Associated liver disease*	*Extrahepatic sources*
Bilirubin 0–1 mg/dl	Decreased hepatic clearance	Jaundice hyperbilirubinemia	Hemolysis, ineffective erythropoeisis
Amino-transferases ALT = 10–55 U/l AST = 10–40 U/l	Leakage from damaged tissues	Hepatitis	ALT-hepatocytic necrosis
Alkaline phosphatases 45–115 U/l	Overproduction and leakage in blood	Granulomatous hepatitis	Bone diseases, placenta, tumor
Gamma-glutamyl transpeptidases 0–30 U/l	Overproduction and leakage in blood	Alcohol and drug abuse	Kidney, spleen, heart, pancreas
Prothrombin time 10–14 sec	Decreased synthetic capacity	Biliary obstruction, vit K related liver disease	Vitamin K deficiency
Serum albumin 3.5–5.5 g/l	Decreased synthesis	Chronic liver disease, cirrhosis	Nephrotic syndrome, malignancy

Applied Aspects

Jaundice and Cholestasis

- Jaundice is the yellow discoloration of the skin, the mucous membranes, or the eyes. The yellow

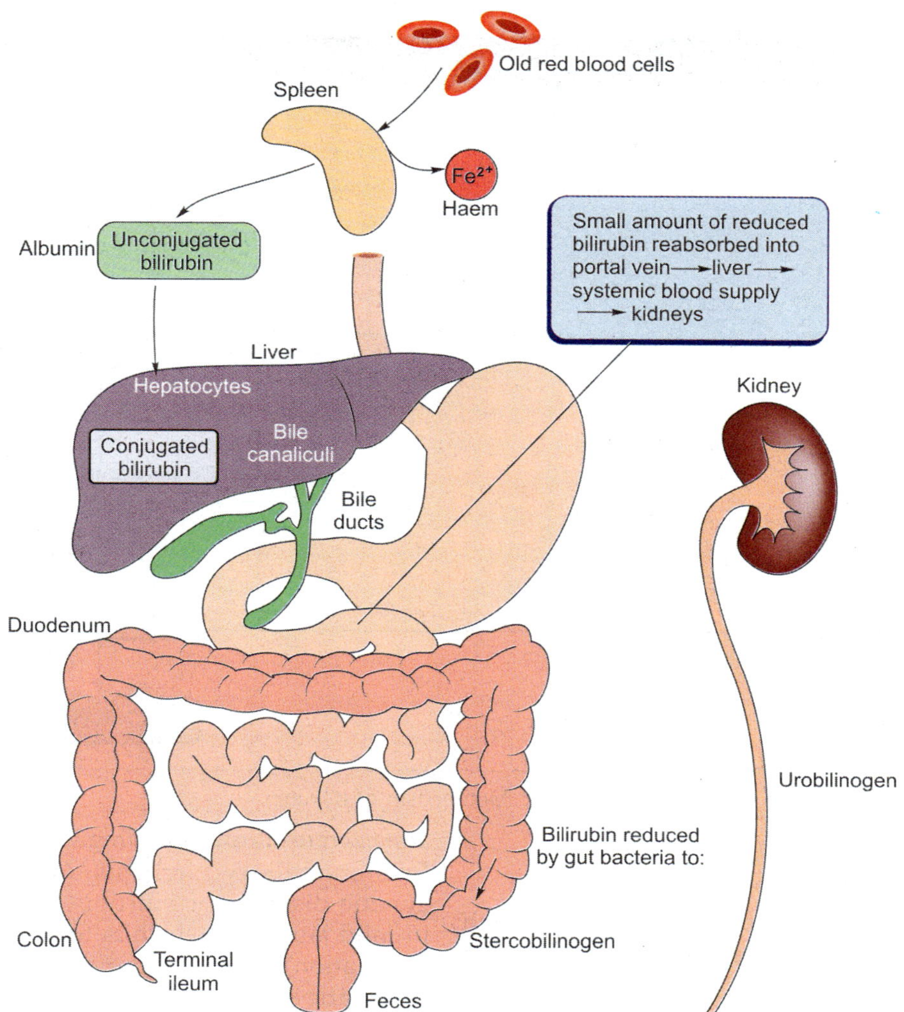

Fig. 5.18

pigment is from bilirubin, a byproduct of old red blood cells.

- Jaundice is detected clinically when plasma bilirubin exceeds 3 mg/dl.

Causes of Jaundice

- Unconjugated hyperbilirubinemia
- Excess production of bilirubin
- Hemolytic anemias
- Resorption of blood from internal hemorrhage
- Ineffective erythropoiesis syndromes (e.g. pernicious anemia, thalassemia)
- Reduced hepatic uptake
- Drug interference with membrane carrier systems
- Some cases of Gilbert syndrome
- Impaired bilirubin conjugation
- Physiologic jaundice of the newborn (decreased UGT1A1 activity, decreased excretion)
- Genetic deficiency of UGT1A1 activity (Crigler-Najjar syndrome types I and II) Gilbert syndrome (mixed etiologies) diffuse hepatocellular disease (e.g. viral or drug-induced hepatitis, cirrhosis)
- Conjugated hyperbilirubinemia
- Deficiency of canalicular membrane transport
- Impaired bile flow.

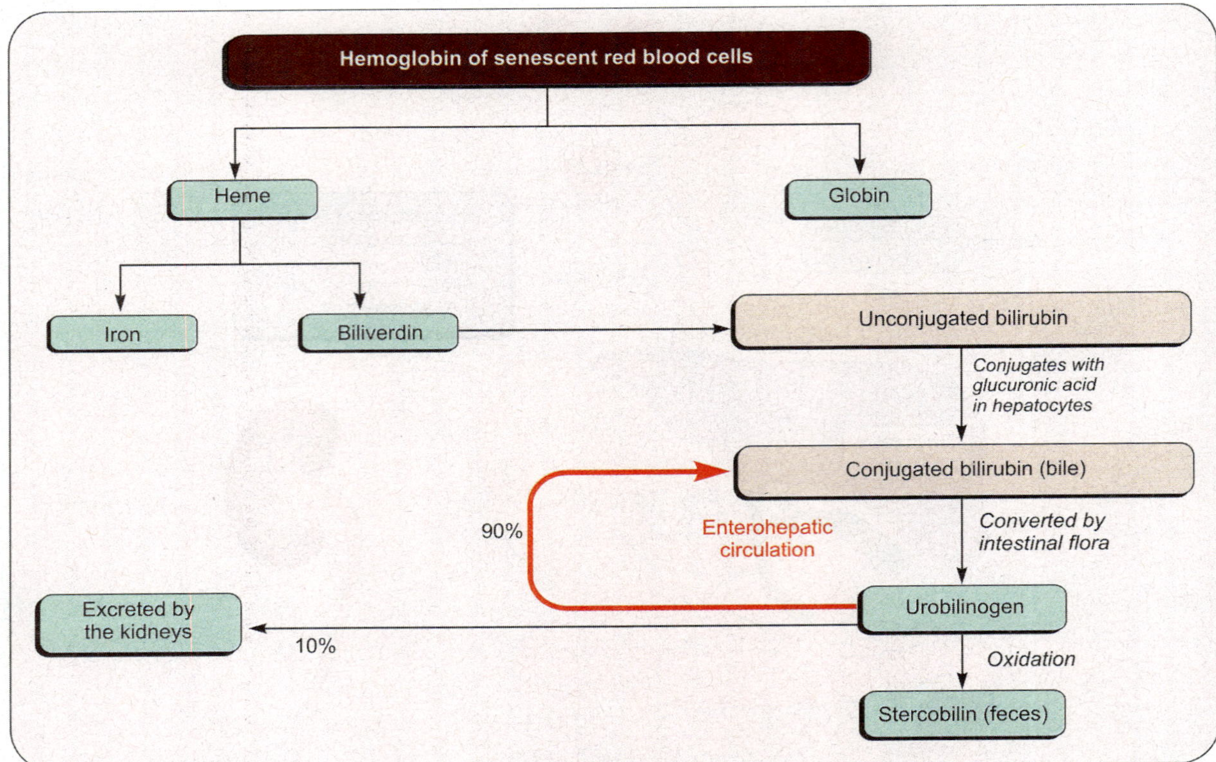

Fig. 5.19: Metabolism of bilirubin

5

Types of Jaundice

1. *Prehepatic Jaundice*

Prehepatic jaundice is caused by anything which causes an increased rate of hemolysis (breakdown of red blood cells).

Sickle cell anemia, spherocytosis, glucose-6-phosphate dehydrogenase deficiency, blood trasfusion reactions can lead to increased red cell lysis and therefore hemolytic jaundice.

Diseases of the kidney, such as hemolytic uremic syndrome, defects in bilirubin metabolism also present as jaundice. Rat fever (leptospirosis) can also cause jaundice.

Laboratory findings

- *Urine:* No bilirubin present, urobilirubin >2 units (except in infants where gut flora has not developed).
- *Serum:* Increased unconjugated bilirubin.

Hepatic Jaundice

Causes

Acute hepatitis, hepatotoxicity and alcoholic liver disease. These reduce the liver's ability to metabolize and excrete bilirubin leading to a build up in the blood. Primary biliary cirrhosis, Gilbert's syndrome (a genetic disorder of bilirubin metabolism can result in mild jaundice, which is found in about 5% of the population). Neonatal jaundice is common, occurring as hepatic and the machinery for the conjugation and excretion of bilirubin does not fully mature until approximately two weeks of age.

Laboratory findings include:

Urine: Conjugated bilirubin present, urobilirubin >2 units but variable (except in children)

2. *Posthepatic Jaundice*

- Posthepatic or obstructive jaundice, is caused by an interruption to the drainage of bile in the biliary system.
- Common causes are gallstones in the common bile duct, and pancreatic cancer in the head of the pancreas.
- Also, a group of parasites known as "liver flukes" live in the common bile duct, causing obstructive jaundice.
- Biliary atresia, ductal carcinoma, pancreatitis and pancreatic pseudocysts.

Cholestatic Jaundice

Etiology and pathogenesis

- Conjugated bilirubin is unable to enter the bile canaliculi and passes back into blood.
- Failure of clearance of unconjugated bilirubin arriving at the liver cells.

Causes

Failure of hepatocytes to generate bile flow. Obstruction to the bile flow in bile ducts in the portal tracts.

Obstruction to bile flow in the extrahepatic bile ducts between porta-hepatis and papillae of Vater.

Symptoms

- Discoloration
- Itching, which can be intense
- Nausea
- Vomiting
- Headache
- Fever
- Dark-colored urine
- Abdominal pain, loss of appetite, abdominal swelling, and light-colored stools.

Diagnosis

- The diagnosis is made by recognition of the patient's appearance and accompanying symptoms.
- A blood test will confirm the raised bilirubin level and other tests such as those for hepatitis and hemolysis are also done on the blood.
- Ultrasound is a good way to inspect the liver and bile ducts for signs of obstruction, and often can give useful information onto the pancreatic gland.
- CT scanning also helps to diagnose obstructive jaundice accurately.

Treatment

- Treatment depends on the underlying cause, and may involve removal of the offending agent.
- Administration of antibiotic, antiviral, antifungal, or antiparasitic drugs; surgery to correct blockage.
- The use of chemotherapy, anti-inflammatory, or steroid medications, dietary changes.

26. DIGESTION AND ABSORPTION

DIGESTION

It is the process by which complex food substances (carbohydrates: CHO, proteins and fats) are broken down into absorbable units.

ABSORPTION

It is the products of digestion and vitamins, minerals and water which cross the mucosa and enter the lymph or blood.

Mucosal Cells of Intestine

1. Called as enterocytes
2. Towards the luminal side, they have a brush border made up of numerous microvilli lining the apical surface.
3. This border is rich in enzymes.
4. Luminal border is lined by a layer rich in neutral and amino sugar called glycocalyx.
5. Membranes of mucosal cells contain glycoproteolytic enzymes which hydrolyse CHO and peptides.
6. Below the glycocalyx and brush border is an unstirred layer similar to the layer beneath other biological membrane.
7. Solutes diffuse through this layer to reach the mucosal cells.
8. The mucous coat overlying the cells also forms a significant barrier to diffusion.
9. Substances pass from intestinal lumen into enterocyte and from enterocyte to interstitial fluid.
10. The process of diffusion across the luminal membrane is different from that of the basal and lateral cell membrane.

Carbohydrate Digestion

Dietary CHO are polysaccharides: Starch, glycogen.

- Disaccharides
- Monosaccharides
- Polysaccharides

In glycogen

1. Glucose molecules are long chains with 1:4 α-linkage.
2. Branching of chain produced by 1: 6 α-linkages.

Glycogen present in animal food. Amylase and amylopectin are present in plant food.

Disaccharides: Lactose and sucrose.

Monosaccharides: Fructose and glucose.

Enzymes of Carbohydrate Digestion (Fig. 5.20)

Salivary α-Amylase

1. Optimal pH: 6.7
2. Action inhibited by acid gastric juice
3. Action stops in stomach but continues in small intestine along with pancreatic α-amylase and hydrolyses 1:4 α-linkages.
4. Both α-amylase convert polysaccharides into:
   a. Oligosaccharides
   b. Disaccharides: Maltose
   c. Trisaccharides: Maltotriose
   d. α Dextrins: Which contain eight or more glucose molecules with 1:6 α-linkages.
5. α-Amylases do not act upon the 1:6 α branching linkage and terminal 1:4 α-linkages.

Enzymes acting at brush border (outer portion) present at the microvilli are:

1. *α Dextrins:* Also called isomaltose. Hydrolyses 1: 6 α-linkages. Along with maltase and sucrase, it breaks down dextrin, maltotriose and maltose.
   It is synthesized along with sucrase as a single glycoptic chains which is inserted into the brush border membrane.
   Then, hydrolyzed by pancreatic proteases into sucrase and a dextrinase.
2. *Lactase:* Hydrolyses lactose to glucose and galactose
3. *Sucrase:* Hydrolyses sucrose to glucose and fructose
4. *Trehalase:* Hydrolyses trehalose to two glucose molecules.

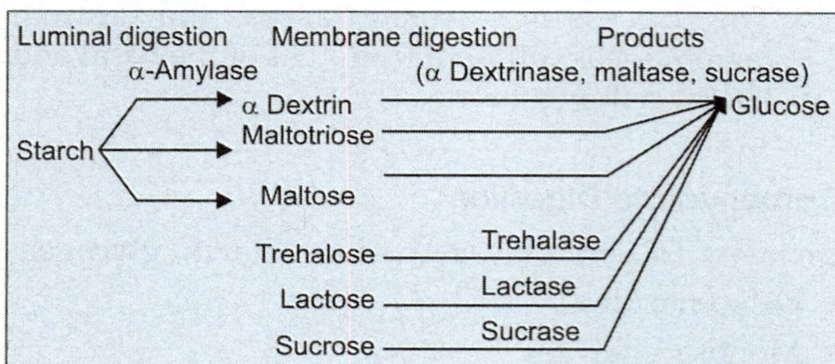

Fig. 5.20

Deficiency of brush border enzymes causes:

1. *Diarrhea:* Increased number of osmotically active oligosaccharide molecules in internal lumen.
2. *Bloating and flatulence:* Due to production of CO_2 and H_2 from disaccharide residues in lower small intestine and colon.

Lactose Intolerance

1. Children by low lactase level with intolerance to milk.
2. Lactase level is high at birth and decline to low levels during childhood and adulthood.
3. Lactose intolerance more commonly seen in blacks, Orientals, Americans, Indians and Mediterran.
4. Yogurt is better tolerated by these people because it contains bacterial lactase.
5. Commercial lactase preparation available are expensive.

Carbohydrate Absorption

1. Absorption of hexoses completed before food reaches terminal part of ileum.
2. Hexoses pass from mucosal cells 'capillary blood' draining into portal vein.
3. Absorption of carbohydrates at luminal side by Na^+ dependent glucose transporter cotransporter or symport since Na^+ and glucose are in high concentration in the internal lumen.
4. Na^+ glucose transporter belong to SGLT-1 and SGLT-2 family and are responsible for facilitated diffusion.
5. SGLT crosses the cell membrane twelve times and have their –COOH and NH_2 terminals at the cytoplasmic side of the membrane.
6. After entering the enterocyte, Na^+ concentration is low inside the cell and moves along the concentration gradient. Glucose moves in along with sodium and once inside the cytoplasm they separate.
7. Na^+ passes through the lateral intercellular spaces into the lumen.
8. Glucose is transported by GLUT-2 into the interstitium 'blood capillaries'.
9. Glucose is transported by secondary active transport.
10. Energy for transport of glucose is obtained indirectly from the transport of Na^+ actively out of the cell.

11. This maintains the concentration gradient across the luminal border and facilitates further transport of glucose.

Applied Aspects

Glucose Galactose Malabsorption

Due to congenital defect in Na^+ glucose co-transporter.

Symptoms

Severe diarrhea: Unless glucose and galactose removed from diet, may be fatal.

Galacotse absorption: Same as glucose.

Fructose: By facilitated diffusion from the intestinal lumen into the enterocytes by GLUT-5 and out of the enterocytes into interstitium by GLUT-2.

Some fructose gets converted to glucose

Pentoses: Absorbed by simple diffusion. Insulin has little effects on intestinal absorption of sugars.

Absorption resembles that of glucose absorption in proximal convoluted tubule of kidneys.

Absorption of glucose depressed by drug phlorhizin.

Maximal rate of glucose absorption from the intestine is 120 gm/hour.

Glucose transporters: Secondary active transport (Na^+ glucose cotransport).

SGLT-1: Present in small intestine and renal tubules.

SGLT-2: Renal tubules.

Facilitated Diffusion (GLUT-1 to 7)

Transporter	*Mechanism*	*Site*
GLUT-1	Basal glucose uptake	Placenta, brain and kidney
GLUT-2	B cell glucose sensor Transport out of internal and renal epithelial cells	B cells of islets, liver, epithelial cells of intestine, kidneys
GLUT-5	Fructose transport	Jejunum, sperm

Digestion of Proteins and Nucleic Acids

Protein digestion starts in the stomach. Pepsin is secreted as its precursor proenzyme pepsinogen and activated by gastric HCl. Pepsin has two immunohistochemically distinct groups:

1. *Pepsinogen I:* Found in acid secreting region. Maximal acid secretion correlates with its level.
2. *Pepsinogen II:* Found in pyloric region.

Pepsin hydrolyses the bonds between aromatic amino acids (e.g. phenyl alanine and tyrosine) and another amino acid and produces polypeptides of various sizes.

Optimum pH for pepsin action: 1.6 to 3.2.

Pepsin acts until food mixes with alkaline pancreatic juice when pH at duodenal cap is 2 to 4.0 but ceases in the intestine where pH is 6.5. Stomach also secretes gelatinase, which liquefies gelatin.

Chymosin (Rennin) is a milk clotting gastric enzyme found in animals.

In the intestine: Pancreatic enzymes:

1. Endopeptidases
2. Exopeptidases

Endopeptidases

1. Trypsin
2. Chymotrypsin act on interior peptide bonds
3. Elastase

They are secreted in proenzyme form.

Exopeptidases

1. Carboxypeptidases: Hydrolyse amino acid at the carboxyl and amino end of polypeptide
2. Aminopeptidase

Some di-and tripeptides are actively transported into the cells of intestine and hydrolyzed by intracellular peptidases and amino acid enter the blood stream.

Therefore, digestion of proteins to amino acids occurs in three locations:

1. Internal lumen
2. The brush border
3. Cytoplasm of enterocytes.

ABSORPTION

Seven different transport systems transport amino acids into enterocytes.

Five require Na^+ to cotransport amino acids in a fashion similar to cotransport of Na^+ and glucose.

Among the five, two require Cl^- in addition to Na^+. Two systems transport amino acid independent of Na^+, di- and tripeptides are transported into enterocytes by a system which requires H^+ instead of Na^+.

Within the enterocytes, amino acids are released into cytoplasm and transported out of the basolateral membrane by five transport systems.

Two of these sytems depend of Na^+ and three do not. Amino acids then enter the portal blood.

Absorption of amino acids are maximum in duodenum and jejunum and minimum in the ileum.

50% of digested protein → food

25% of digested protein → digestive juices

25% of digested protein → desquamated mucous cells

2–5% escape digestion, but some may be digested by intestinal bacteria in the colon.

Hartnup Disease

Cogenital defect in the transport of neutral amino acid in the intestine and renal tubule.

Cystinuria

Congenital defect in the transport of basic amino acid.

5

Passive Immunity througth Colostrum in Neonates

Protein antibody in maternal colostrum are largely secretory.

Ig (IgA) the production of which is increased in late pregnancy.

It crosses mammary epithelium by transcytosis and enter the circulation of infant from the intestine, providing passive immunity against infections.

Absorption is by endocytosis and subsequent exocytosis.

Protein absorption decreases with age. Foreign proteins that enter the circulation provoke formation of amino acids.

These antibodies enter the circulation and then are deposited in Peyer's patches where they can produce allergic reaction on second exposure to same antigen.

Absorption of protein antigens especially bacterial and viral antigens takes place in large microfold cells or M cells which overlie aggregates of lymphoid tissue (Peyer's patches).

These cells pass the antigens to the lymphoid cells and lymphocytes are activated. The activated lymphoblast later return to intestinal mucosa and secrete IgA.

Secretory immunity is an important defence mechanism. Food allergy occurs in 8% of children to sea food.

Nucleic Acids

Nucleic acids → Nucleotides
(Pancreatic nucleases)

Nucelotides → Nucleoside + phosphoric acid
(by enzymes in luminal surface of enterocyte)

Nucleoside → ribose (or) deoxyribose (sugar) + purine (or) pyrimidine (base)

Bases are absorbed by active transport.

Lipid Digestion

Lipid digestion starts in the mouth.

Ebner's glands on the dorsal surface of the tongue secretes lingual lipase.

Gastric lipase is also present but only of significance in pancreatic insufficiency.

Lingual lipase is active in stomach and digests up to 30% of dietary triglycerides, in the duodenum.

Pancreatic Lipase

It is the important enzyme which hydrolyses the 1:3 bonds of triglycerides and the products are fatty acids and 2 monoglycerides.

Pancreatic lipase acts on emulsified fats.

Colipase

It is a protein with molecular weight 11,000, and is also secreted in pancreatic juice. When it binds to the –COOH terminal domain of the pancreatic lipase, it causes opening of the amphipathic helix that covers the active site of pancreatic lipase, like a lid and activates it.

Colipase is secreted in inactive form and is activated in the internal lumen by trypsin.

Bile salt activated lipase is the second enzyme present in the pancreas, which has a molecular weight of 100,000 kDa. Activated by bile salts. Represents about 4% of the total protein in pancreatic juice.

It catalysis the hydrolyses of cholesterol esters, esters of fat soluble vitamins and phospholipids and triglycerides. Pancreatic lipase I is 10 to 60 times more active than bile salt activated lipase.

Cholesteryl Ester Hydrolase

It hydrolyses dietary cholesteryl esters in the internal lumen. Fats being insoluble cannot cross the unstirred border and enter the mucosal cells by themselves.

They are emulsified by the detergent action of bile salts, lecithin and monoglycerides. Bile salts and lipids interact spontaneously to form micelles.

Micelles

Take up lipids at various concentration and contain fatty acids, monoglycerides and cholesterol in their hydrophobic centers.

The micelles move down the concentration gradient and pass through the unstirred layer and enter the brush border of the mucosal cells.

The lipids diffuse out of the micelles and a saturated aqueous solution of lipids is maintained in contact with the brush border.

Applied Aspects

Steatorrhea

Destruction of exocrine portion of pancreas causes pancreatic lipase deficiency which leads to steatorrhea.

There is fatty, bulky, clay colored stools due to impaired digestion and absorption of fat.

Steatorrhea can also occur in:

1. Increased secretion of gastric acid
2. Defective absorption of bile salts in distal ileum.

Fat Absorption

Initially thought that absorption of fat is by passive diffusion.

Now evident that carriers are involved. Inside the cells, lipids are rapidly esterified, thus maintaining concentration gradient.

Uptake of bile salts in jejunum is low and so formation of new micelles is high.

Fat of fatty acids inside enterocyte depend on size. Fatty acids containing <10 to 12 carbon atoms are water soluble and actively transported to portal blood where they circulate as free fatty acids (FFAs).

Fatty acids with >10 to 12 carbon atoms are re-esterified to triglycerides, some cholesterol is also esterified.

The triglycerides and cholesteryl esters are then coated with a layer of protein, cholesterol and phospholipid to form chylomicrons.

By exocytosis, they leave the cell and enter the lymphatics.

From 2-monoglycerides by acylation → triglycerides → occurs in smooth endoplasmic reticulum.

Glucose 'glycerophosphate', glycerophospholipids, chylomicrons occurs in rough endoplasmic reticulum.

Carbohydrates is added to protein in Golgi apparatus and finished chylomicrons extruded by exocytosis from the basal or lateral aspects of the cell

95% of ingested fat is absorbed in upper part of small intestine.

Short Chain Fatty Acids (SCFAs) in Colon

SCFAs are 2 to 5 carbon weak fatty acids. They have a normal concentration of 80 mmol/liter in lumen

60%: As actetate
25%: Propionate
15%: Butyrate

SCFAs are formed by action of colonic bacteria on complex CHO, resistant starch and other components of dietary fiber which escape digestion in upper GIT.

Absorbed SCFAs are metabolized and make a significant contribution to the total caloric intake. They exert:

1. Atrophic effect on the colonic epithelial cells
2. Combat inflammation
3. Are absorbed in exchange for hydrogen
4. Thus maintain acid base balance
5. Promote absorption of sodium.

Cholesterol Absorption

Cholesterol is readily absorbed from small intestine, if bile, fatty acids and pancreatic juice are present. Absorbed cholesterol is incoporated into chylomicrons and enter circulation through lymphatics. Plant sterols are poorly absorbed.

Plant sterols acts as competitive inhibitor for cholesterol absorption competing with cholesterol for esterification with fatty acids.

Water Absorption

Daily water turnover in GIT.

Water (H_2O) ingested	*Volume* 2000 ml
Secretions	
1. Salivary glands	1500 ml
2. Stomach	2500 ml
3. Bile	500 ml
4. Pancreas	1500 ml
5. Intestine	1000 ml
Total secretions	7000 ml
Total input	(H_2O ingested + total secretions): 9000 ml
Reabsorbed	
1. Jejunum	5000 ml
2. Ileum	2000 ml
3. Colon	1300 ml
Total absorbed	8300 ml
Excreted in stools	(Total input – total absorbed) 9000 ml – 8300 ml = 700 ml

5

Only small amounts of water move across the gastric mucosa. In small and large intestine, because of the osmotic gradient, large amount of water moves in both direction.

Sodium

Sodium diffused in or out of small intestine depending on the concentration gradient. The basolateral membrane contains Na^+K^+ATPase, the luminal membrane of both small and large intestine are permeable to Na^+ and so Na^+ is actively absorbed throughout the intestines.

In small intestine, Na^+ acts as a cotransporter for glucose and amino acid absorption by secondary active transport. So, glucose increase Na^+ absorption.

Hence, in treatment of diarrhea—solution containing NaCl (sodium chloride) and glucose are given to prevent Na^+ and H_2O loss. Cereals containing CHO are also useful. This is the treatment of cholera.

Chlorides

Chlorides enter enterocytes from the interstitial fluid via $Na^+K^+2Cl^-$ cotransporters in basolateral membrane.

Cl^- is secreted into the intestinal lumen via channels regulated by protein kinases, e.g. protein kinase A activated by cAMP. cAMP concentration is increased in cholera.

Cholera bacillus stays in the lumen but it produces a toxin which binds to GM I ganglioside receptors and this permits part of the 'A' subunit of the toxin to enter the cell.

The 'A' peptide binds adenosine diphosphate ribose to the α subunit of G2 inhibiting its GTPase activity. Therefore, the constitutively activated G protein produces prolonged stimulation of adenyl cyclase and a marked increase in cAMP concentration.

This causes increased secretion of Cl^- into the lumen. Also function of mucosal carrier for Na^+ is reduced and this reduces Na^+ reabsorption. The resultant increase in H_2O and electrolyte contents in intestine causes diarrhea. The Na^+K^+ATPase and Na^+ glucose cotransporters are unaffected and so coupled reabsorption of glucose and Na^+ bypasses the defect.

Water

Movement of H_2O occurs to and fro until osmotic pressure of intestinal contents equals plasma. In duodenum, the contents may be hypertonic or hypotonic. But in the jejunum, osmolality is close to plasma and is maintained throughout the rest of the intestine.

Osmotically active particles produced by digestion causes H_2O to move out along the osmotic gradient.

In the colon, Na^+ is pumped out and water moves passively out along the osmotic gradient. Saline cathartics such as $MgSO_4$ are poorly absorbed and retain their osmotic equivalent of H_2O in intestine, thus increasing internal volume content and exerting a laxative effect.

Potassium

K^+ is secreted into the lumen as a component of mucus K^+ channels are present in the luminal wall and basolateral membrane of colon. So, potassium is secreted in the colon.

K^+ also moves passively down the electrochemical gradient. The accumulation of K^+ in the colon is partially offset by H^+ K^+ ATPase in the luminal membrane of cells in distal colon with resulting active transport of K^+ into the cells. But loss of ileal and colonic fluids in chronic diarrhea can cause severe hyperkalemia. When dietary intake of K^+ is high for a long time, aldosterone secretion is increased and more K^+ enters colon.

Aldosterone increases Na^+K^+ ATPase pumps in basolateral membrane of colon and therefore increased intracellular K^+ and K^+ diffusion across the luminal membrane of the cells.

Vitamins

Fat soluble vitamins are absorbed along with fat and so decrease in bile and pancreatic enzyme decreases its absorption. Most vitamins are absorbed in upper small intestine. Vitamin B_{12} absorbed in ileum.

It binds with intrinsic factor in stomach and the complex is absorbed in ileal mucosa. Vit B_{12} and folate absorption are Na^+ independent. But, all the other H_2O soluble vitamins are absorbed by carriers that are Na^+ cotransporters.

27. GASTROINTESTINAL HORMONES

Gastrointestinal hormones play an important role in the regulation of gastrointestinal secretions and motility. They are biologically active peptides secreted by nerve cells and gland cells in the mucosa. They act in a paracrine fashion, but they also enter the circulation.

They are classified into two families:

I. The gastrin family
  i. Gastrin
  ii. Cholecystokinin (CCK)

II. The secretin family
  i. Secretin
  ii. Glucagon
  iii. Glicentin (GLI)
  iv. Vasoactive intestinal polypeptide (VIP)
  v. Gastric inhibitory polypeptide (GIP)

Gastrin

It is secreted by the G cells or gastrin cells which are located in the deeper portion of the antral glands in the gastric mucosa.

The G cells are flask shaped cells containing gastrin granules in the lower part of the cell. The G cells are amine precursors uptake and decarboxylation (APUD) cells. They are of neural origin and are also found in the pituitary gland, hypothalamus, medulla oblongata, vagus and sciatic nerves.

Gastrin is secreted in its inactive form (progastrin) and is converted into gastrin by the action of hydrochloric acid and the products of digestion.

There are three isoforms of gastrin: G34, G17 and G14. The gastrin present in the GIT is mostly of G17 isoform. It has a half life of 2 to 3 minutes. It is inactivated in the kidneys and in the small intestine.

Functions

1. It increases the secretion of gastric acid as well as pepsin.
2. It has a trophic action on the gastric mucosa.
3. It increases the intestinal motility, and also causes the contraction of the lower esophageal sphincter.
4. It causes feeble contraction of the gallbladder.
5. After a protein meal it stimulates the secretion of insulin and glucagon.

Factors influencing gastrin secretion

- Gastrin secretion increased by:
  i. Luminal factors
    a. Distension of the pyloric antrum
    b. Products of protein digestion.
  ii. Neural factors
    Increased vagal discharge acts through GRP to increase gastrin secretion.
  iii. Chemical factors
    Calcium and epinephrine.
- Gastrin secretion is decreased by:
  i. Luminal factors
  Acid in the pyloric antrum acts directly on the G cells and inhibits secretion by a negative feedback mechanism.
  Increased gastric secretion → increase acid secretion
  ↑ ↓.
  ← ← Inhibit ← ← ↓
  ii. Chemical factors

Hormones of secretin family
- Glucagon
- Calcitonin

Cholecystokinin–Pancreozymin (CCK–PZ)

Earlier it was thought that a hormone called cholecystokinin caused contraction of the gallbladder and a separate hormone caused secretion of pancreatic juice rich in enzymes. Now, it is known that both the functions are carried out by the same hormone, and hence it came to be called cholecystokinin-pancreozymin (CCK-PZ).

It is secreted by the cells in mucosa of the upper part of the small intestine. It exhibits heterogeneity: The large fragment containing 58 amino acid, and others containing 39 AA, 33 AA and 12 AA. It has a half life of 5 minutes.

Functions

- It causes the contraction of the gallbladder to release bile.
- It acts on the pancreatic acinar cells and causes the release of pancreatic juice rich in enzymes.
- It has a trophic effect on the pancreas.
- It inhibits gastric emptying.

- It increases the secretion of enterokinase from the duodenum.
- It increases the motility of the small and large intestine.
- It also stimulates the secretion of glucagon.

Factors that increase CCK-PZ secretion:
Presence of products of digestion of carbohydrates, proteins and fats in the small intestine increases CCK-PZ secretion. Acid in the duodenum is a weak stimulation for secretion.

Secretin

It was the first hormone to be discovered (in 1902 by Bayliss and Starling). It is secreted by the S cells located deep in the mucosa of the upper portion of the small intestine. There is only one form of the hormone. It contains 27 amino acids and has a structure similar to that of glucagon, GLI, VIP, and GIP. Its half life is about 5 minutes.

Functions

- It causes an increase in pancreatic secretion rich in water and bicarbonates.
- It stimulates the secretion of bile.
- It augments the action of CCK-PZ on the pancreas.
- It decreases the secretion of HCl.

Along with CCK-PZ it causes the contraction of the pyloric sphincter.

Factors that increase secretion:
i. Presence of acid in the intestine
ii. Products of protein digestion.

Feedback control of secretin secretion:

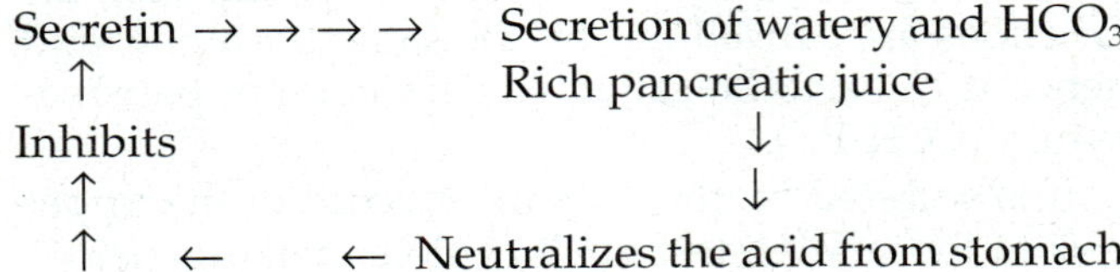

Gastric Inhibitory Polypeptide (GIP)

GIP contains 42 amino acids. It is secreted by the K cells present in the mucosa of the duodenum and jejunum.

Function

It stimulates the secretion of insulin. Therefore, it is called glucose dependent insulotrophic polypeptide In high doses it decreases gastric secretion and motility. Hence, called gastric inhibitory polypeptide.

Factors increasing GIP secretion
Glucose and fat in the duodenum.

Vasoactive Intestinal Peptide (VIP)

- It contains 28 amino acids.
- It is found in the nerves of GIT and also in the blood brain and autonomic nerves.
- It has a half life of 2 minutes in the blood.

Functions

- It greatly enhances intestinal secretion of electrolytes and water.
- It causes relaxation of intestinal smooth muscle including sphincters.
- Dilation of peripheral blood vessels.
- Inhibits gastric acid secretion.
- Increases the action of acetylcholine on the salivary glands.

Glucagon

- It is secreted by the cells of the stomach and duodenum and by the α-cells in the pancreatic islets
- It plays an important role in hyperglycemia of diabetes.

Peptide YY

- It is secreted in the small intestine and colon
- It inhibits gastric acid secretion and motility
- Its level is low in obese individuals.

On infusion, it reduces appetite in normal and obese individuals.

Ghrelin

- It is a 22 amino acid polypeptide
- It is one of the endogenous ligands for the growth hormone secretogogue receptors in the anterior pituitary gland.
- Its name is derived from the Proto-Indian European word 'ghre' which means growth. Its main source is the stomach. The levels of ghrelin are reduced when food is eaten and increased during fasting. Ghrelin increases food intake by acting on the arcuated nucleus.

Motilin

- It is a polypeptide containing 22 amino acid.
- It is secreted by the enterochromaffin cells and Mo cells in the stomach, small intestine and colon.

Functions

- It causes the contraction of the smooth muscle of the stomach and small intestine.
- It is a major regulator of migrating motor complexes that control gastrointestinal motility in between meals.

Somatostatin

- It is the growth hormone inhibiting hormone.
- It is secreted by the D cells in the pancreatic islets.
- It exists in 2 isoforms: Somatostatin 14 and Somatostatin 28.

Functions

- It inhibits the secretion of gastrin, VIP, GIP, secretin and motilin.
- Inhibits gastric acid secretion and motility causing dyspepsia.
- Inhibits gallbladder contraction and precipitates formation of gallstones.
- It inhibits the absorption of glucose, amino acids and triglycerides.

Factors that increase secretion

- Acid in the stomach
- Factors that increase insulin secretion.

Neurotensin

It is a 13 amino acid polypeptide:

- Produced by neurons and cells in the mucosa of the ileum
- It inhibits gastrointestinal motility
- It increases ileal blood flow
- Fatty acids stimulate its release.

Substance P

- It is found in the endocrine and nerve cells in the gastrointestinal tract
- It increases the motility of the small intestine.

Gastrin Releasing Peptide (GRP)

- It is present in the vagal nerve endings that terminate on G cells
- It acts as a neurotransmitter at vagal nerve endings to cause increase in gastrin secretion.

Guanylin

It is made up of 15 amino acid residues secreted by the cells of the intestinal mucosa from the pylorus to the rectum.

It binds to guanylyl cyclase and increases the concentration of intracellular cGMP. This in turn increases the activity of cystic fibrosis regulated Cl^- channels and increases the release of chloride ions into the intestinal lumen. Most of the guanylin acts in a paracrine fashion, but guanylin receptors are also found in the kidneys, female reproductive tract and liver where it may act in a endocrine fashion to regulate fluid movement in these tissues.

Heat stable enterotoxin of diarrhea producing strains of *E. coli* has a structure similar to guanylin and activates guanylin receptors in the intestine.

Applied Aspects

Cells that secrete gastrointestinal polypeptides can form tumours. 50% are gastrinomas, 25% are glucagonomas. Others like VIPomas, neurotensinomas also occur rarely.

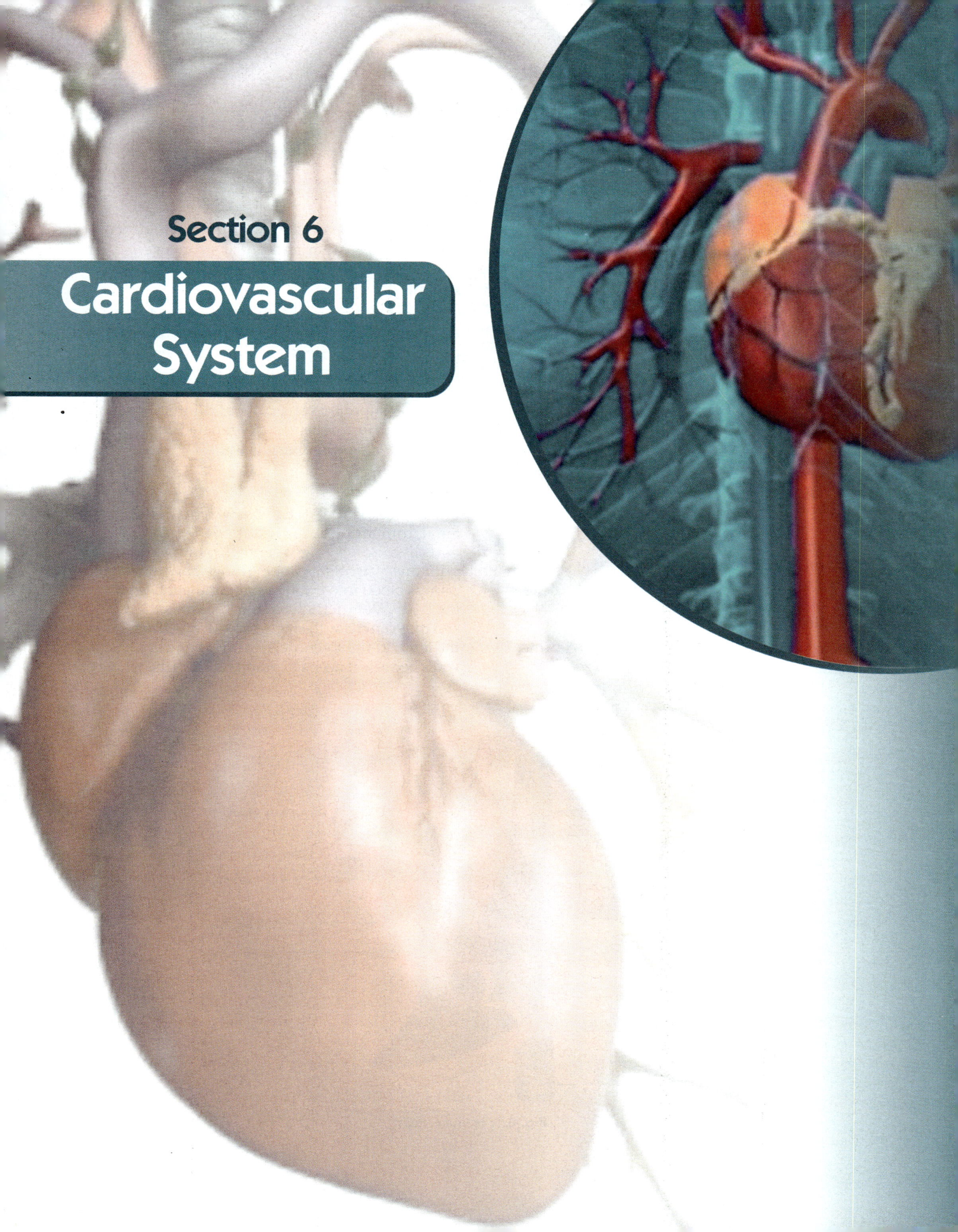

Section 6

Cardiovascular System

28. CARDIOVASCULAR SYSTEM

Cardiovascular system is the system of heart and blood vessels that circulates blood throughout the body. The heart is the life-giving, ever-beating muscle in our chest. From inside the womb until death, the thump goes on. Within weeks of conception the heart starts its mission of supplying the body with nutrients. The primary function of the heart is to pump blood through the arteries, capillaries, and veins. Blood transports oxygen, carbon dioxide, nutrients, hormones and has other important functions as well.

THE HEART

The heart is a hollow, muscular organ about the size of a fist. It is responsible for pumping blood through the blood vessels by repeated, and rhythmic contractions. The term "cardiac" means "related to the heart" and comes from the Greek word kardia, for "heart". It is a four-chambered, double pump and is located in the thoracic cavity between the lungs (Fig. 6.1).

Heart Chambers

The heart has four chambers, two atria and two ventricles.

The atria are smaller with thin walls, while the ventricles are larger and much stronger.

Atrium

There are two atria on either side of the heart. On the right side is the atrium that contains blood which is poor in oxygen. The left atrium contains blood which has been oxygenated and is ready to be sent to the body. The right atrium receives deoxygenated blood from the superior vena cava and inferior vena cava. The left atrium receives oxygenated blood from the left and right pulmonary veins.

Ventricles

The ventricle is a heart chamber which collects blood from an atrium and pumps it out of the heart. There are two ventricles: the right ventricle pumps blood into the pulmonary circulation for the lungs, and the left ventricle pumps blood into the systemic circulation for the rest of the body. Ventricles have thicker walls than the atria, and thus can create the higher blood pressure. Comparing the left and right ventricle, the left ventricle has thicker walls because it needs to pump blood to the whole body.

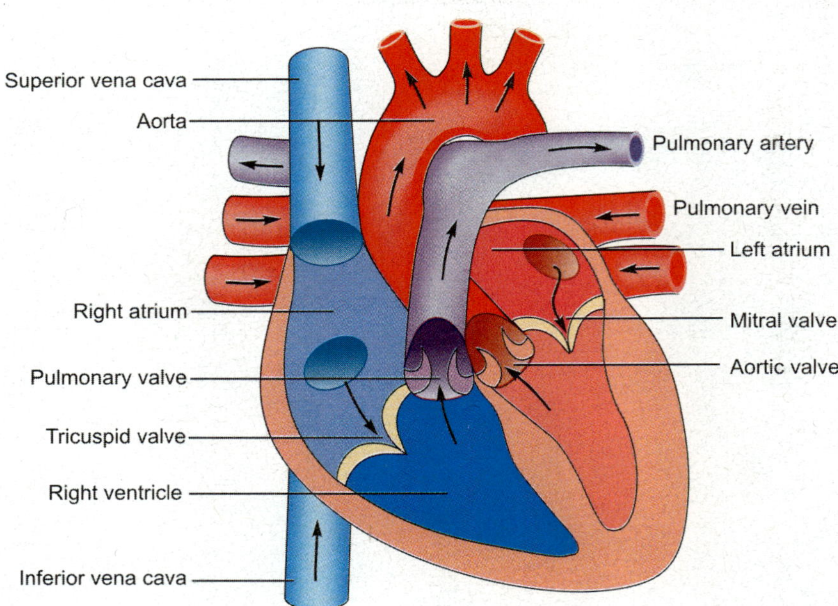

Fig. 6.1: Human heart

Layers of the Heart

Endocardium

Smooth endothelial lining of the heart and entire cardiovascular system. This helps to reduce friction of blood flow and prevent clotting.

Myocardium

The myocardium is the muscular tissue of the heart. The myocardium is composed of specialized cardiac muscle cells with an ability not possessed by muscle tissue elsewhere in the body. Cardiac muscle, like other muscles, can contract, but it can also conduct electricity, like nerves. The blood to the myocardium is supplied by the coronary arteries.

Pericardium

Surrounding the heart is a sac known as the pericardium, which consists of two membranes. The outer layer being the fibrous parietal pericardium and the inner layer being the serous visceral pericardium. It is the serous visceral pericardium that secretes the pericardial fluid into the pericardial cavity (the space between the two pericardial layers). The pericardial fluid reduces friction within the pericardium by lubricating the epicardial surface allowing the membranes to glide over each other with each heart beat.

Septum

The interventricular septum is the thick wall separating the lower chambers (the ventricles) of the heart from one another. The greater portion of it is thick and muscular and constitutes the muscular ventricular septum. Its upper and posterior part, which separates the aortic vestibule from the lower part of the right atrium and upper part of the right ventricle, is thin and fibrous, and is termed the membranous ventricular septum. The interatrial septum separates right and left atrium.

Valves

The two atrioventricular (AV) valves are one-way valves that ensure that blood flows from the atria to the ventricles, and not the other way. The right AV valve is also called the tricuspid valve because it has three flaps. It is located between the right atrium and the right ventricle. The tricuspid valve allows blood to flow from the right atrium into the right ventricle. The left AV valve is also called the bicuspid valve because it has two flaps. It is also known as the mitral valve due to the resemblance to a bishop's mitre (liturgical headdress). This valve prevents blood in the left ventricle from flowing into the left atrium.

The two semilunar (SL) valves are present in the arteries leaving the heart; they prevent blood from flowing back into the ventricles. They have flaps that resemble half moons. The pulmonary semilunar valve lies between the right ventricle and the pulmonary trunk. The aortic semilunar valve is located between the ventricle and the aorta.

The sound heard in a heartbeat is due to the closure of the heart valves.

Subvalvular Apparatus

The chordae tendinae are attached to papillary muscles that cause tension to better hold the valve. Together, the papillary muscles and the chordae tendinae are known as the subvalvular apparatus. The function of the subvalvular apparatus is to keep the valves from prolapsing into the atria when they close. The subvalvular apparatus have no effect on the opening and closing of the valves. This is caused entirely by the pressure gradient across the valve.

THE CIRCULATORY SYSTEM (Fig. 6.2)

The double circulatory system of blood flow refers to the separate systems of pulmonary circulation and the systemic circulation.

Pulmonary Circuit

In the pulmonary circuit, blood is pumped to the lungs from the right ventricle of the heart. It is carried to the lungs via pulmonary arteries. At lungs, oxygen in the alveoli diffuses to the capillaries surrounding the alveoli and carbon dioxide in the blood diffuses to the alveoli. As a result, blood is oxygenated which is then carried to the left atrium via pulmonary veins. Oxygen rich blood is prepared for the whole organs and tissues of the body. This is important because mitochondria inside the cells should use oxygen to produce energy from the organic compounds.

The Systemic Circuit

The systemic circuit supplies oxygenated blood to the organ system. Oxygenated blood from the lungs is returned to the left atrium, then the ventricle contracts and pumps blood into the aorta. Systemic arteries split from the aorta and direct blood into the capillaries.

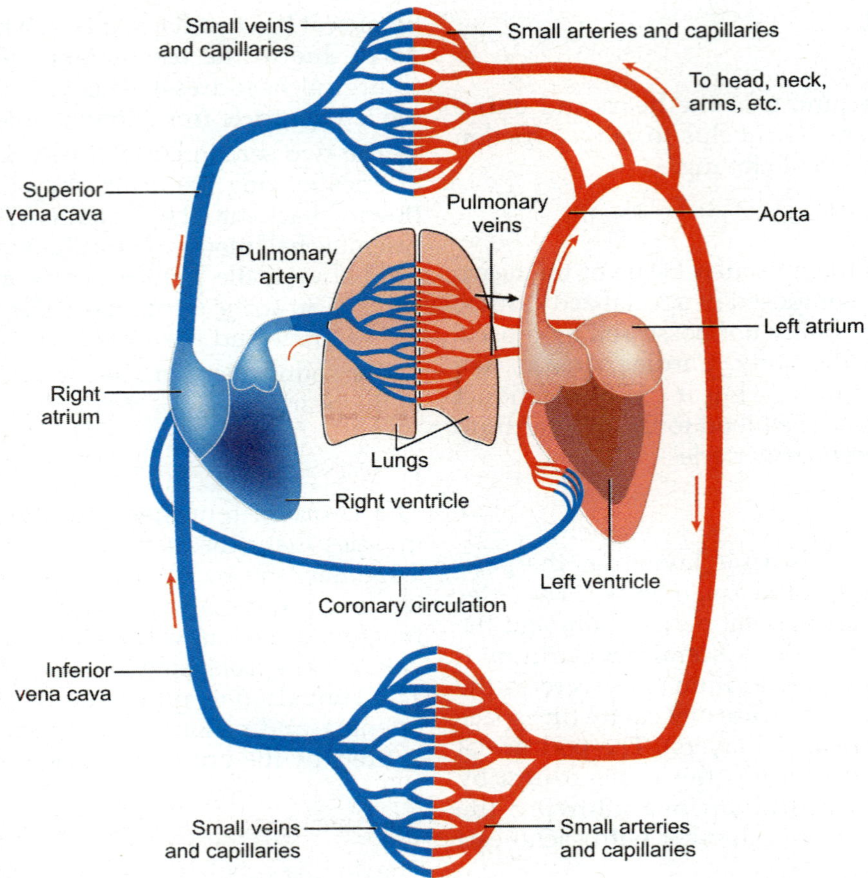

Fig. 6.2: Cardiovascular system

Cells consume the oxygen and nutrients and add carbon dioxide, wastes, enzymes and hormones. The veins drain the deoxygenated blood from the capillaries and return the blood to the right atrium.

29. STRUCTURE OF CARDIAC MUSCLE

Cardiac muscle is a type of involuntary striated muscle found in the walls of the heart, specifically the myocardium. Cardiac muscle is one of three major types of muscle, the others being skeletal and smooth muscle. The cells that comprise cardiac muscle are seen as intermediate between these two other types in terms of appearance, structure, metabolism, excitation-coupling and mechanism of contraction. Cardiac muscle shares similarities with skeletal muscle with regard to its striated appearance and contraction, with both differing significantly from smooth muscle cells.

The cardiac muscle fibers are of three types:

1. Contractile or working muscle fibers which form the bulk of atria and ventricles.
2. Nodal tissues are in the sinoatrial node and atrioventricular node.
3. Conducting tissues are the bundle of His, Purkinje fibers, and atrial internodal fibers.

Appearance

Cardiac muscle cells, also called cardiocytes or cardiac myocytes, are relatively small, averaging 10–20 μm in diameter and 50–100 μm in length. A typical cardiac muscle cell has a single, centrally placed nucleus, although a few may have two or more (Fig. 6.3).

Striations

Cardiac muscle exhibits cross striations formed by alternating segments of thick and thin protein filaments. Like skeletal muscle, the primary structural proteins of cardiac muscle are actin and myosin. The actin filaments are thin causing the lighter appearance of the I bands in striated muscle, while the myosin filament is thicker lending a darker appearance to the alternating A bands as observed with electron microscopy. However, in contrast to skeletal muscle, cardiac muscle cells may be branched instead of linear and longitudinal.

T-Tubules

Another histological difference between cardiac muscle and skeletal muscle is that the T-tubules in cardiac muscle are shorter, broader and run along the Z-discs. There are fewer T-tubules in comparison with skeletal muscle. Additionally, cardiac muscle forms dyads instead of the triads formed between the T-tubules and the sarcoplasmic reticulum in skeletal muscle. T-tubules play critical role in excitation-contraction coupling (ECC).

Intercalated Discs

Each cardiac muscle cell contacts several others at specialized sites known as intercalated discs. Intercalated discs play a vital role in the function of cardiac muscle. At an intercalated disc, the cell membranes of two adjacent cardiac muscle cells are extensively intertwined and bound together by gap junctions and desmosomes. These connections help stabilize the relative positions of adjacent cells and maintain the three-dimensional structure of the tissue. The gap junctions allow ions and small molecules to move from one cell to another. This arrangement creates a direct electrical connection between the two muscle cells. An action potential can travel across an intercalated disc, moving quickly from one cardiac muscle cell to another.

6

Syncytium

Myofibrils in the two interlocking muscle cells are firmly anchored to the membrane at the intercalated disc. Because their myofibrils are essentially locked together, the two muscle cells can "pull together" with maximum efficiency. Because the cardiac muscle cells are mechanically, chemically, and electrically connected to one another, the entire tissue resembles a single, enormous muscle cell. For this reason, cardiac muscle has been called a functional syncytium. The heart has two syncytia (pleural of syncytium), the atrial myocardium is one, the ventricular myocardium is the other. They are separated from one another by a fibrous septum. An impulse cannot pass from one to another directly, but must travel through the heart's conduction system.

Metabolism

Cardiac muscle is adapted to be highly resistant to fatigue: it has a large number of mitochondria, enabling continuous aerobic respiration via oxidative phosphorylation, numerous myoglobins (oxygen-storing pigment) and a good blood supply, which provides nutrients and oxygen. The heart is so tuned

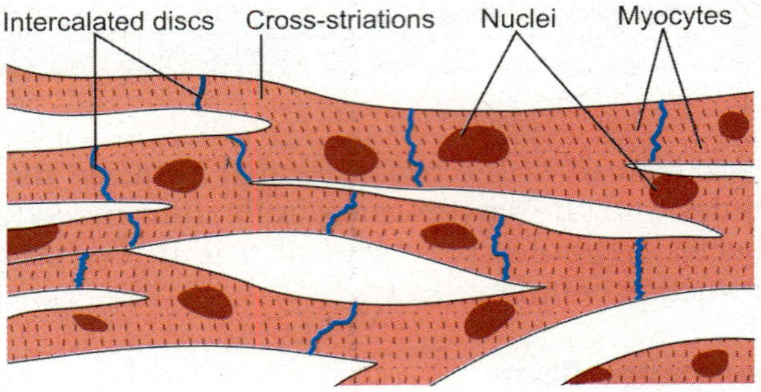

Fig. 6.3: Cardiac muscle

to aerobic metabolism that it is unable to pump sufficiently in ischaemic conditions. At basal metabolic rates, about 1% of energy is derived from anaerobic metabolism. This can increase to 10% under moderately hypoxic conditions, but, under more severe hypoxic conditions, not enough energy can be liberated by lactate production to sustain ventricular contractions.

Under basal aerobic conditions, 60% of energy comes from fat (free fatty acids and triglycerides), 35% from carbohydrates, and 5% from amino acids and ketone bodies. However, these proportions vary widely according to nutritional state.

30. PROPERTIES OF THE CARDIAC MUSCLE AND CONDUCTING SYSTEM OF HEART

The physiological properties of the cardiac muscle are:

1. Rhythmicity
2. Excitability
3. Contractility
4. Conductivity

I. RHYTHMICITY/AUTOMATICITY/CHRONOTROPISM

In the myocardium, automaticity is the ability of the cardiac muscles to depolarize spontaneously, without external electrical stimulation from the nervous system.

Primary Pacemaker

The sinoatrial node (SA node) is a group of cells positioned on the wall of the right atrium, near the entrance of the superior vena cava. These cells are modified cardiac myocytes. They possess some contractile filaments, though they only contract relatively weakly.

Cells in the SA node spontaneously depolarize, resulting in contraction, approximately 100 times per minute. This native rate is constantly modified by the activity of sympathetic and parasympathetic nerve fibers, so that the average resting cardiac rate in adult humans is about 70 beats per minute. Because the sinoatrial node is responsible for the rest of the heart's electrical activity, it is sometimes called the primary pacemaker.

Secondary Pacemaker

If the SA node does not function, a group of cells further down the heart will become the heart's pacemaker, this is known as an ectopic pacemaker. These cells form the atrioventricular node (AV node), which is situated beneath the endocardium at the lower right posterior portion of the interatrial septum near the opening of the coronary sinus above the tricuspid valve.

The cells of the AV node normally discharge at about 40–60 beats per minute, and are called the secondary pacemaker.

Tertiary Pacemaker

Further down the electrical conducting system of the heart is the bundle of His. The left and right branches of this bundle, and the Purkinje fibers, will also produce a spontaneous action potential at a rate of 30–40 beats per minute, if the SA and AV node both do not function. The reason the SA node controls the whole heart is that its action potentials are released most often to the heart's muscle cells; this will produce contraction. The action potential generated by the SA node passes down the cardiac conduction system, and arrives before the other cells have had a chance to generate their own spontaneous action potential. This is the normal conduction of electrical activity within the heart.

Generation of Action Potentials

There are three main stages in the generation of an action potential in a pacemaker cell.

Pacemaker Potential

The key to the rhythmic firing of pacemaker cells is that, unlike muscle and neurons, these cells will slowly depolarize by themselves.

The resting potential of a pacemaker cell (–55 mV to –60 mV) is caused by a continuous outflow or "leak" of potassium ions through ion channels in the membrane. This potassium permeability decreases as time goes on, partly causing the slow depolarization. As well as this, there is a slow inward flow of sodium, called the funny current, as well as an inward flow of calcium, through transient Ca^{2+} channel (T-channel). This all serves to make the cell more positive.

This relatively slow depolarization continues until the threshold potential is reached. Threshold is between –40 mV and –50 mV. When threshold is reached, the cells enter phase of depolarization (Fig. 6.4).

Depolarization

Though much faster than the depolarization caused by the funny current and decrease in potassium permeability above, the upstroke in a pacemaker cell is slow compared to that in an axon.

The SA and AV node do not have fast sodium channels like neurons, and the depolarization is mainly caused by a slow influx of calcium ions. (The funny current also increases). The calcium is let into the cell by voltage-sensitive calcium channels (long lasting or L-type channel) that open when the threshold is reached.

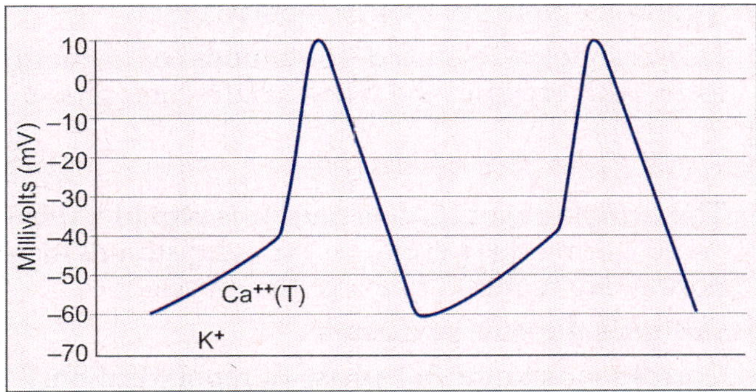

Fig. 6.4: Pacemaker action potential

Repolarization

The calcium channels are rapidly inactivated, soon after they open. Sodium permeability is also decreased. Potassium permeability is increased, and the efflux of potassium (loss of positive ions) slowly repolarises the cell.

Factors Affecting Myocardial Rhythmicity (Fig. 6.5)

1. *Cardiac Innervation*

a. *Sympathetic stimuli*

It releases noradrenaline, which acts on the beta1 receptors causing rapid opening of Ca channels, accelerating the rate of depolarisation. As a result, the slope of depolarization increases, causing increased rate of SA node firing and increased heart rate.

Parasympathetic stimuli (vagus)

It releases acetylcholine which acts on the muscarinic receptors, causing opening of K^+ channels, increases SA node membrane permeability to K^+ results in more K^+ efflux and decreased membrane permeability to Ca^{2+} results in less Ca^{2+} influx. As a result, the pre-potential slope decreases, causing decreased rate of SA node firing and decreased heart rate.

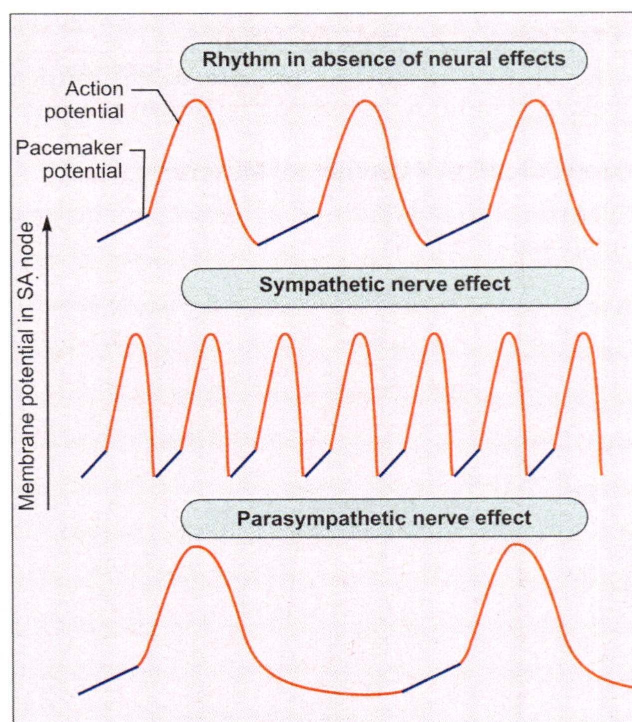

Fig. 6.5: Myocardial rhythmicity

6

2. *Effect of Ion Concentrations in ECF*

a. *K^+ Ions*

Decreased K^+ increases rhythmicity. Increased K^+ decreases rhythmicity (stops heart in diastole).

b. Na^+ Ions

If increased, initiate rhythmicity, but cannot maintain it.

3. *Physical Factors*

a. *Warming:* Increases rhythmicity
b. *Cooling:* Decreases rhythmicity.
c. *Exercise:* Increases heart rate as a result of increased sympathetic nerve stimulation and decreased vagal inhibition to SA node.
d. *Endurance-trained athletes:* Resting bradycardia due to high vagal activity.

4. *Chemical Factors (Drugs)*

a. *Thyroid hormones and catecholamines:* Increases rhythmicity.
b. Acetylcholine decreases rhythmicity.
c. *Hypoxia:* Decreases rhythmicity.

6

II. EXCITABILITY (BATHMOTROPISM)

Is the ability of cardiac muscle to respond to adequate stimuli by generating an action potential.

Action Potential of Ventricular Muscle (Fig. 6.6)

- Ventricular muscle has a resting membrane potential of –90 mV.

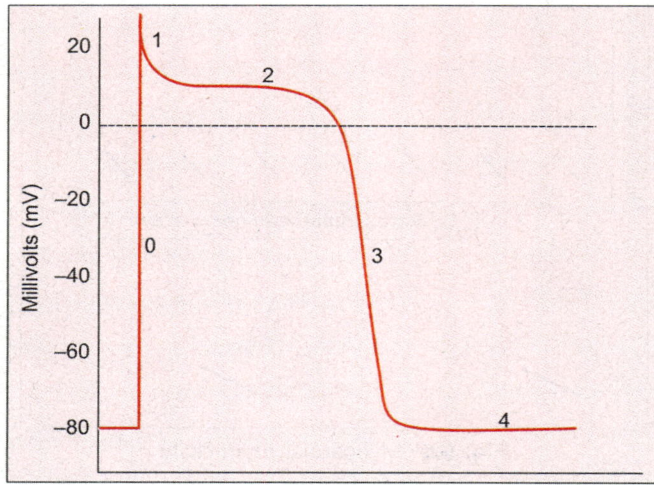

Fig. 6.6

- The transmembranous action potential overshoots to a potential of +20 mV.
- Transmembranous action potential of ventricular muscle is characterized by presence of 5 phases.
  Phase 0 = Rapid depolarization.
- Opening of fast Na^+ channels increased Na^+ influx.
  Phase 1 = Rapid repolarization/1st rapid repolarization.
- Closure of Na^+ channels, decreased K^+ permeability, and Cl^- influx.
  Phase 2 = A plateau.
- Opening of slow Ca^{2+} channels (slow Ca^{2+} Na^+ channels) increased Ca^{2+} influx, with slow opening of K^+ channels.
  Phase 3 = Slow repolarization/2nd rapid repolarization.
- Closure of slow Ca^{2+} channels, with increased K^+ permeability increased K^+ efflux.
  Phase 4 = Complete repolarization.
- Active Na^+ K^+ pump $2K^+$ in/$3Na^+$ out.

Excitability changes during the action potential
Passes through 2 periods:
1. Absolute refractory period (ARP)
2. Relative refractory period (RRP).

Refractory Periods

Absolute Refractory Period (ARP) (Fig. 6.7)

- The excitability of cardiac muscle is completely lost during this period, i.e. does not respond to 2nd stimulus however strong it may be.
- The duration is very long that occupies the whole period of systole.
- Corresponds to the period of depolarization (phase 0), and the first 2 phases of repolarization.
- Heart cannot be tetanized (continuous contraction), as its ARP occupies the whole contraction phase.

Relative Refractory Period (RRP)

- The excitability of cardiac muscle is partially recovered during this period, i.e. stronger stimuli than normal are required to excite the muscle.
- Occupies the time of diastole.
- Corresponds to the 3rd phase of repolarization.
- Can be affected by the heart rate, temperature, vagal stimulation, sympathetic stimulation and drugs.

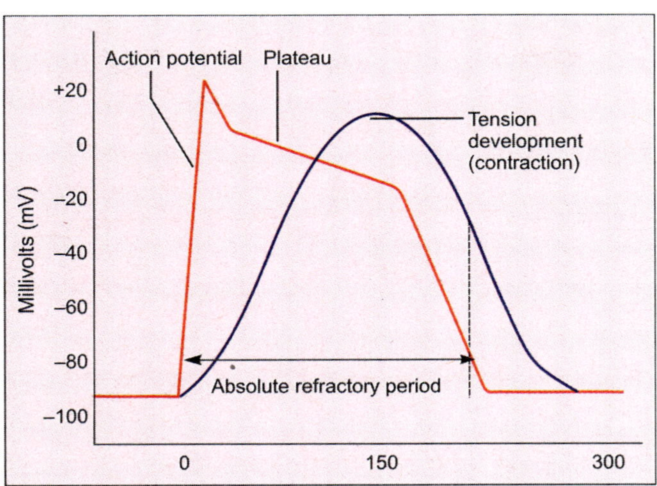

Fig. 6.7

Extrasystole and Compensatory Pause

The refractory periods can be demonstrated in the beating heart of frog. If an stimulus is applied during systole, there is no response. If stimulus is applied during diastole, there is a contraction called extrasystole, which is of higher amplitude due to beneficial effect. The extrasystole is followed by a compensatory pause. This pause occurs because when the next normal impulse from the sinus arrives, the heart is in absolute refractory period of extrasystole. Therefore, it has to wait for the next normal impulse to arrive. The interval between the contractions preceding and following the extrasystole is equal to the length of 2 cardiac cycles.

Postextrasystolic Potentiation

Ventricular extrasystole increases myocardial contractility so that the contraction following the extrasystole is stronger than the contraction preceding it. This is mainly due to greater availability of Ca^{++} ions resulting from previous contraction. This is called as postextrasystolic potentiation.

Factors Affecting Myocardial Excitability

1. *Cardiac Innervation*
   - Sympathetic nerve stimulation increases excitability.
   - Parasympathetic nerve stimulation (vagus) decreases excitability.
2. *Effect of Ions Concentration in ECF*
   - Increased Ca^{2+} and increased Na^{+} → increases excitability.
   - Increased K^{+} → increases excitability.
3. *Physical Factors*
   - Rise in temperature increases excitability.
   - Decrease in temperature decreases excitability.
4. *Blood Flow*
   - Insufficient blood flow to cardiac muscle decreases excitability and myocardial metabolism for three reasons:
     1. Lack of O_2
     2. Excess accumulation of CO_2
     3. Lack of sufficient food nutrients.
5. *Chemical Factors (Drugs)*

   Digitalis increases excitability.

Relation between the Action Potential and the Mechanical Response (Fig. 6.8)

- The mechanical response consists of contraction (systole) and relaxation (diastole).
- Cardiac muscle begins to contract a few milliseconds after the action potential begins, and continues to contract until a few milliseconds after the action potential ends.
- Duration of contraction: 0.2 sec in atrial muscle, and 0.3 sec in ventricular muscle.
- Diastole begins at the end of the plateau.
  2nd rapid repolarization is completed at about the middle of diastole.

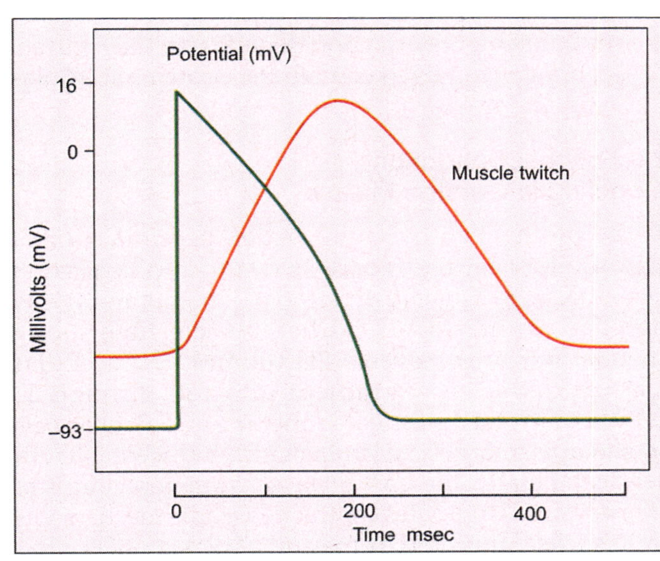

Fig. 6.8

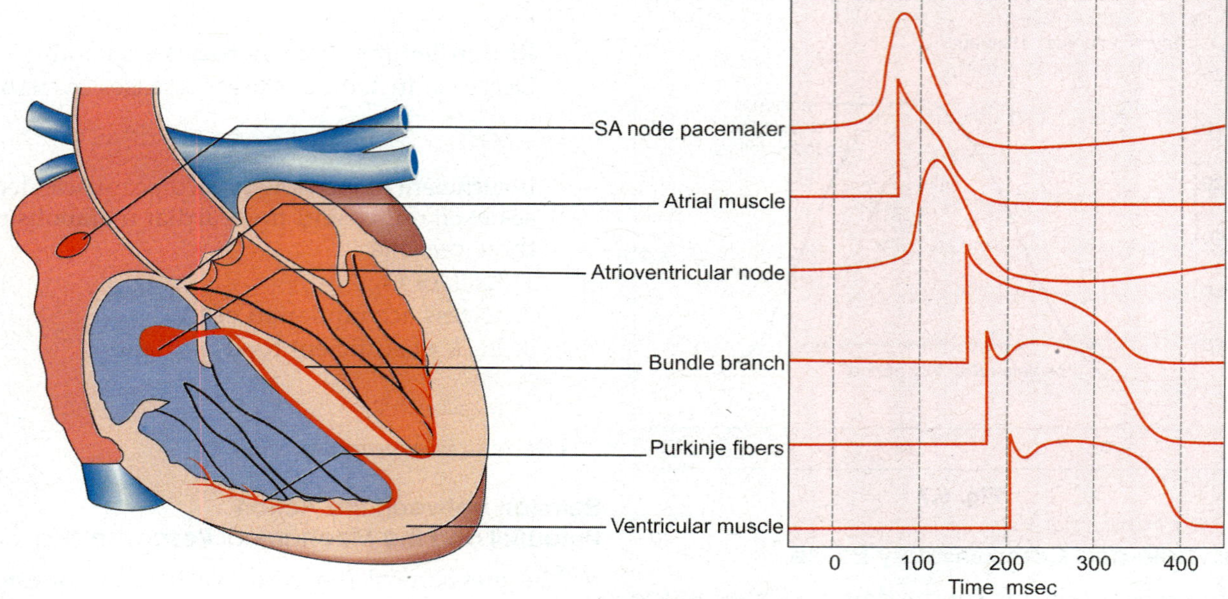

Fig. 6.9

6

Action potential of different types of cardiac muscle is shown in Fig. 6.9.

III. CONTRACTILITY/INOTROPISM

Is the ability of the cardiac muscle to convert electrical energy into mechanical work.

Myocardial fibers have 'functional syncytium' and not 'anatomical syncytium', because they present in contact but not in continuity.

- Strength of myocardial contraction determines the heart pumping power.
- Mechanism of contraction depends on the contractile filaments, which contain the protein molecules (actin and myosin).

Excitation-Contraction Coupling in Cardiac Muscle

Is the mechanism by which action potential causes myofibrils of cardiac muscle to contract. When action potential passes over cardiac muscle membrane, it also spreads to interior of cardiac muscle fiber along membranes of transverse (T) tubules. Extracellular Ca^{2+} diffuses down gradient into cell through T-tubules. This Ca^{2+} stimulates opening of Ca^{2+} channels in sarcoplasmic reticulum (calcium induced calcium release). Finally, the Ca^{2+} released from here, binds to troponin and stimulates contraction (same mechanisms as in skeletal muscle). At the end of plateau of cardiac action potential, i.e. during repolarization, Ca^{2+} in sarcoplasm is rapidly and actively transported and pumped out of the cell via a Na^{+}- Ca^{2+}- exchanger, back into both sarcoplasmic reticulum and T-tubules resulting in cessation of the contraction until new action potential occurs.

Factors affecting Myocardial Contractility

1. *Cardiac Innervation*
   - Sympathetic nerve stimulation increased force of contraction.
   - Parasympathetic nerve stimulation (vagus) decreased atrial force of contraction with no significant effect on ventricular muscle.
2. *Oxygen Supply*

   Hypoxia decreases contractility.
3. *Calcium and Potassium Ions Concentration in ECF*
   - Increase in Ca^{2+} increases contractility.
   - Increase in K^{+} increases contractility.
4. *Physical Factors*
   - Warming increases contractility.
   - Cooling decreases contractility.
5. *Hormonal and Chemical Factors (Drugs)*
   - Positive inotropics: (Adrenaline, noradrenaline, alkalosis, digitalis, Ca^{2+}, caffeine).

- Negative inotropics: [Acetylcholine, acidosis, ether, chloroform, some bacterial toxins (e.g. diphtheria toxins), K^+].

Characteristics of Contractility

a. Cardiac muscle obeys 'all-or-none law'. A single subminimal stimulus does not evoke any response, but minimal or threshold stimuli lead to maximal cardiac contraction, and further increase in stimulus strength does not increase the contraction.
b. Cardiac muscle cannot be stimulated while it is contracted, because its excitability during contraction is zero due to long absolute refractory period, so it cannot be tetanized.
c. Cardiac muscle can perform both isometric and isotonic types of contractions.
d. Starling's law of the heart "Length–tension relation-ship". Within physiological limits, the greater the initial length of the fiber, the stronger will be the force of its contraction; however, overstretching the fiber as in heart failure its power of contractility decreases.
e. Staircase phenomenon/Treppe: If several adequate stimuli of same strength are applied in quick succession, the first few contractions show a progressive increase in amplitude, after that it becomes standstill. The initial increase is due to increase of temperature, H^+ ion and Ca^{++} ion concentrations resulting from previous contractions. This is referred to as staircase phenomenon.
f. Summation of subminimal stimuli. A single subminimal stimulus is ineffective. But if two or more such stimuli are applied in quick succession, there is a response. This is due to summation of all the local excitatory states caused by each sub-minimal stimulus.

IV. CONDUCTIVITY (DROMOTROPISM)

Is the ability of cardiac muscle fibers to conduct the cardiac impulses that are initiated in the SA node (the pacemaker of the heart) (Fig. 6.10).

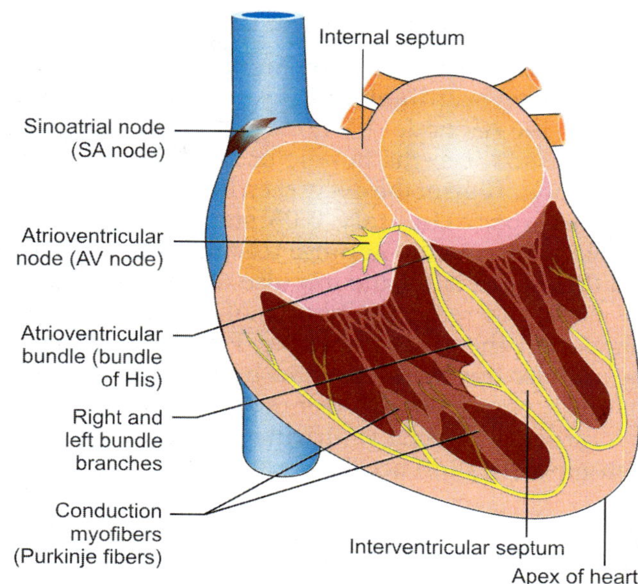

Fig. 6.10

SA Node

Under normal conditions, electrical activity is spontaneously generated by the SA node, the physiological pacemaker. This electrical impulse is propagated throughout the right atrium, and through Bachmann's bundle to the left atrium, stimulating the myocardium of both atria to contract. As the electrical activity is spreading throughout the atria, it travels via specialized pathways, known as internodal tracts, from the SA node to the AV node.

Internodal Tracts

They comprise of three namely, anterior bundle of Bachmann, middle-Wenkebach, and posterior bundle of Thorel.

AV Node

The AV node functions as a critical delay in the conduction system. Without this delay, the atria and ventricles would contract at the same time, and blood would not flow effectively from the atria to the ventricles.

Bundle of His

The distal portion of the AV node is known as the bundle of His. The bundle of His splits into two branches in the interventricular septum, the left bundle branch and the right bundle branch. The left bundle branch activates the left ventricle, while the right bundle branch activates the right ventricle. The left bundle branch is short, splitting into the left anterior fascicle and the left posterior fascicle.

Purkinje Fibers/Ventricular Myocardium

The two bundle branches taper out to produce numerous Purkinje fibers, which stimulate individual groups of myocardial cells to contract.

Sequence of Events in Cardiac Conduction

SA node depolarizes and the impulse spreads across the atrial myocardium and through the internodal fibers to the AV node. AV node picks up the impulse and transfers it to the bundle of His. This produces the major portion of the delay seen in the cardiac cycle. It takes approximately 0.03 sec from SA node depolarization to the impulse reaching the AV node, and 0.13 seconds for the impulse to get through the AV node and reach the bundle of His. Also during this period the atria repolarize. From the AV node the impulse travels through the bundle branches and through the Purkinje fibers to the ventricular myocardium, causing ventricular depolarization and then repolarization occurs.

The Direction of the Impulse (Fig. 6.11)

1st → Atrial spread from SA node conductive tissue to ventricles

2nd → Ventricular spread from apex of the heart to base, via Purkinje fibers to the endocardial surface of ventricles.

6

Note: Left bundle branch starts before right bundle branch, as left ventricular wall is thicker so the impulse needs more enough time to reach. Accordingly both ventricles will contract together.

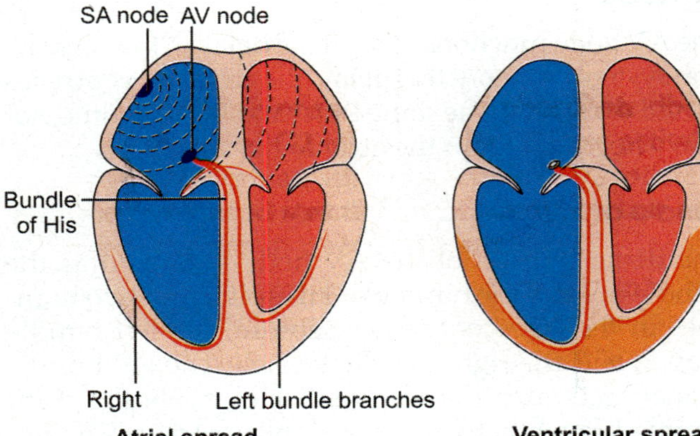

Fig. 6.11

The Conduction Velocities of the Impulse

SA node	0.05 m/sec
AV node	0.01 m/sec (slowest)
Bundle of His	1.00 m/sec
Purkinje fibers	4.00 m/sec (fastest)
Atrial and ventricular muscles	0.3 to 0.4 m/sec

The slowest conduction velocity in AV node: Because it has few number of intercalated discs.

Importance: To allow sufficient time for ventricles to be filled with blood before they contract.

The fastest conduction velocity in Purkinje fibers

Importance: To allow the 2 ventricles to contract at the same time simultaneously.

Factors affecting Myocardial Conductivity

1. *Cardiac Innervation*
   - *Sympathetic nerve stimulation: Increases conductivity.*
   - *Parasympathetic nerve stimulation (vagus): Decreases conductivity.*

2. *Effect of Ions Concentration in ECF*
   - Increase in Ca^{2+} → Increases conductivity.
   - Increase in K^+ → Increases conductivity.

3. *Physical Factors*
   - Rise of temperature increases conductivity.
   - Decreases temperature decreases conductivity.

4. *Blood Flow*

Insufficient blood flow to cardiac muscle decreases conductivity and myocardial metabolism for three reasons:

1. Lack of O_2
2. Excess accumulation of CO_2
3. Lack of sufficient food nutrients.

5. *Chemical Factors (Drugs)*

Digitalis → Increases conductivity.

31. CARDIAC CYCLE

Cardiac cycle is the term referring to all of the events that occurs from the beginning of one heartbeat to the beginning of the next. The frequency of the cardiac cycle is the heart rate (*see* Fig. 6.16).

Duration: The time taken to complete one cardiac cycle is 0.8 sec and is called as cardiac cycle time.

It can be subdivided into two major phases, the systolic (contraction) phase and the diastolic (relaxation) phase.

EVENTS OF CARDIAC CYCLE

1. Mechanical changes
2. Pressure changes
3. Volume changes
4. Electrical changes
5. Phonocardiogram

Mechanical Changes

Atrial Events

- Atrial systole (0.1s)
- Atrial diastole (0.7s)

Atrial systole initiates the cycle, because of presence of pacemaker SA node and is followed by atrial diastole. At the end of diastole, the atrial systole returns, and the cycle goes on.

Ventricular Events

Ventricular Systole (0.3s)

- Isovolumetric contraction phase
- Rapid ejection
- Reduced ejection

Ventricular Diastole (0.5s)

- Protodiastole
- Isovolumetric relaxation
- First rapid filling
- Diastasis
- Second rapid filling

At the end of atrial systole, ventricular systole (0.3s) starts. This is followed by ventricular diastole (0.5s). At the end of diastole, the ventricular systole repeats, and the cycle goes on like this.

Description

Cardiac cycle begins with the atrial systole. During this period, the atria contract and expel their contents into the ventricles. The LA being away from the SA node, contract a little after the RA. But practically their contractions are simultaneous.

After atrial systole, comes atrial diastole. During this period, the atria relax and receive blood from the great veins. RA from vena cavae, and LA from pulmonary veins.

Ventricular systole commences at the end of atrial systole. This is because the impulse originating in the SA node after passing through the atria, will travel down the junctional tissues and enter the ventricles resulting in contraction. Systoles of atria and ventricles will never overlap.

At the end of ventricular systole, the first heart sound occurs. It is caused by sudden closure of AV valves due to sharp rise in intraventricular pressure. The semilunar valves open a little later, because, until the intraventricular pressure goes above that in the aorta and pulmonary artery, SL valves will not open. Thus, at the beginning of ventricular systole, there is a brief period during which both the valves are closed and the ventricles are contracting as closed cavities. No blood passes out and hence, no shortening of the muscle will occur. This period is called isovolumetric contraction phase (0.05s).

At the end of this period, SL valves open and ejection phase starts (0.25s). During this phase, blood is expelled from the ventricles, from LV to systemic aorta and from RV to pulmonary artery. In the first part of this period (0.11s), the outflow is very rapid. Hence, this is known as rapid ejection phase. In the last part, (0.14s) the rate of outflow slows down. Hence, this is called reduced ejection phase. Here, the ventricular systole ends and the diastole starts.

As soon as the ventricles relax, the intraventricular pressure starts falling.The blood column in the aorta and pulmonary trunk try to roll back towards ventricles, but are stopped by the sharp closure of SL valves.This produces the second heart sound. The second sound occurs at the end of ventricular systole. But this statement is not exact, because, till the falling of intraventricular pressure goes below the intra-aortic pressure, the SL valves will not close.

Consequently, there will be short interval between the onset of diastole and the closure of SL valves. This is called protodiastolic phase (0.04s).

Although the SL valves have closed, yet the AV valves are still not open. Because the falling intraventricular pressure takes a little time to go below that of atria, so that the AV valves may open. So, there will be a brief interval during which both the valves remain closed and ventricles are relaxing as closed cavities. Since no blood enters the ventricles there will be no lengthening of cardiac muscle fibers. This phase is called as isovolumetric relaxation phase (0.05s).

At the end of isometric relaxation phase, the AV valves open. Blood rushes into the ventricles and ventricular filling begins. The first part of this phase is known as the first rapid filling phase (0.11s). Because, as soon as the AV valves open, blood accumulating so long in the atria rushes into the ventricles. The steep fall of the intraventricular pressure during the isometric relaxation phase, makes the inflow all the more intense. Although the duration is less, yet the largest part of ventricular filling takes place during it. The rapid rush of blood produces a third heart sound.

In the next phase, the rate of filling slows down. The ventricles are already full to a large extent and ventricular pressure slowly rises. Consequently, the rate of inflow from the atria will be gradually slower. This phase is called diastasis or slow filling phase (0.16s). Although this is the longest phase of ventricular diastole, the amount of filling during this phase is minimum.

Then comes the last phase of ventricular diastole which corresponds to atrial systole. Due to atrial contraction, blood rushes into the ventricles rapidly and this is called second rapid filling phase (0.1s). The rapid rush of blood produces a fourth heart sound. Here the ventricular diastole ends. Again the ventricular systole starts and the cycle repeats.

Characteristics

Quiescent period: Period when all chambers are at rest and filling. 70% of ventricular filling occurs during this period. The AV valves are open, the semilunar valves are closed.

Atrial systole: Pushes the last 30% of blood into the ventricle.

Pressure Changes

Atrial Pressure Changes

During atrial systole, atrial pressure rises ('a' wave). During atrial diastole, since the AV valves bulge into the atrial cavity in isometric contraction period of ventricle, intra-atrial pressure rises ('c' wave).

Then pressure falls during rapid ejection period of ventricles due to three reasons:

a. Atrial relaxation continues
b. As the ventricular muscle shortens, the AV ring is pulled down, so that atrial cavity enlarges
c. Due to reduction of ventricular volume, mediastinal pressure falls. Owing to this negative pressure, the thin walled atria dilate and atrial pressure falls.

In the later part of ventricular systole, intra-atrial pressure slowly rises ('v' wave) due to accumulation of blood in the atria as a result of venous filling, and AV valves remaining closed. This rise slowly continues until AV valves open.

During isovolumetric relaxation phase, AV ring rises up and is an additional cause for pressure rising.

As soon as the AV valves open, atrial blood rushes into the ventricles, so that intra-atrial pressure decreases. This fall continues till about middle of ventricular diastole.

As the ventricles fill up during diastasis, intra-atrial pressure slowly rises. After this atrial pressure comes down again.

Ventricular Pressure Changes

a. During Ventricular Systole

1. *In the isometric contraction phase:* Intraventricular pressure rises.
2. *In the rapid ejection phase:* For a short period, force of contraction is more than the rate of outflow intraventricular pressure rises. Then, gradually equalize: horizontal plateau at the summit.
3. *In the reduced ejection phase:* Force of contraction is less than the rate of outflow: intraventricular pressure decreases.

b. During Ventricular Diastole

4. *In the protodiastolic phase:* Intraventricular pressure decreases.
5. *In the isovolumetric relaxation phase:* Ventricles are relaxing as closed cavities—intraventricular pressure decreases.

6. *In the first rapid filling phase:* Rate of relaxation is more than filling intraventricular pressure decreases slowly to some extent.
7. *In diastasis:* Ventricles are no more relaxing, blood accumulates in it intraventricular pressure rises slowly.
8. *In second rapid filling phase:* Intraventricular pressure rises.

Aortic Pressure Changes (Fig. 6.12)

During isovolumetric contraction phase of ventricles, a slight rise of aortic pressure is due to bulging of SL valves into the aorta.

With the opening of SL valves, blood enters the aorta and aortic pressure smoothly rises and falls running parallel to intraventricular pressure.

The fall of aortic pressure in reduced ejection phase is due to two causes:

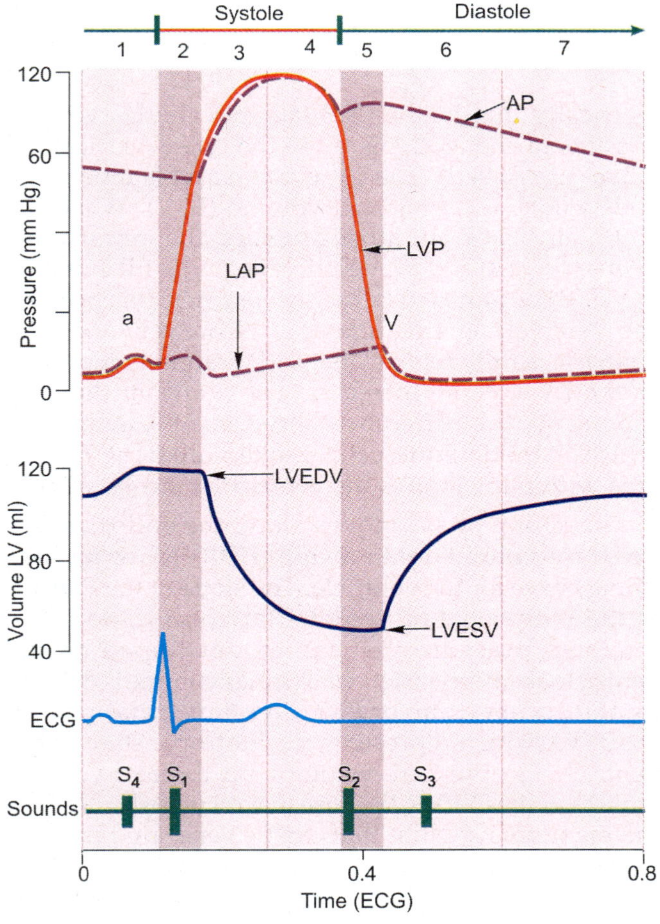

Fig. 6.12

a. Ventricle is contracting less forcibly than before, so that a comparatively less amount blood is entering the aorta now.
b. More blood is running out into the periphery than is entering the aorta from the ventricles.

With the onset of diastole, ventricular pressure sharply falls causing a backward flow of the aortic blood towards ventricles. Owing to this, aortic pressure drops causing the 'incisura'. The blood column is reflected back by the sudden closure of SL valves, thus causing a sharp rise in the aortic pressure. The aortic pressure then slowly falls due to continuous passage of blood to periphery. The fall continues till ventricles contract again.

Volume Changes

Ventricular Volume Changes

The volume changes of ventricles are to some extent the reverse of its pressure changes.

1. During atrial systole, ventricular volume rises due to rapid filling. This rise is maintained during isovolumetric contraction phase of ventricles, because no blood is going out.
2. During ejection phase, ventricular volume smoothly and continuously falls up to the end of systole.
3. In isovolumetric relaxation phase, volume remains same, because no blood is entering.
4. During first rapid filling phase, volume rises.
5. During diastasis, ventricular volume very slowly increases.

The stroke volume is the volume of blood, in milliliters (ml), pumped out of the heart with each beat, 70 ml/beat.

The output per minute is also called as minute volume. End-diastolic volume (EDV) is the amount of blood in the ventricle at the end of diastole. Normal value is about 120 ml.

Ejection fraction (EF) is the portion of end diastolic volume that is pumped out during one systole. EF = SV/EDV = 70/120 x 100 = 60%

End-systolic volume (EDV) is the amount of blood in the ventricle at the end of systole. Normal value is about 50 ml.

Ventricular Pressure-Volume Relationship

Left ventricular pressure-volume (PV) loops are derived from pressure and volume information found

6

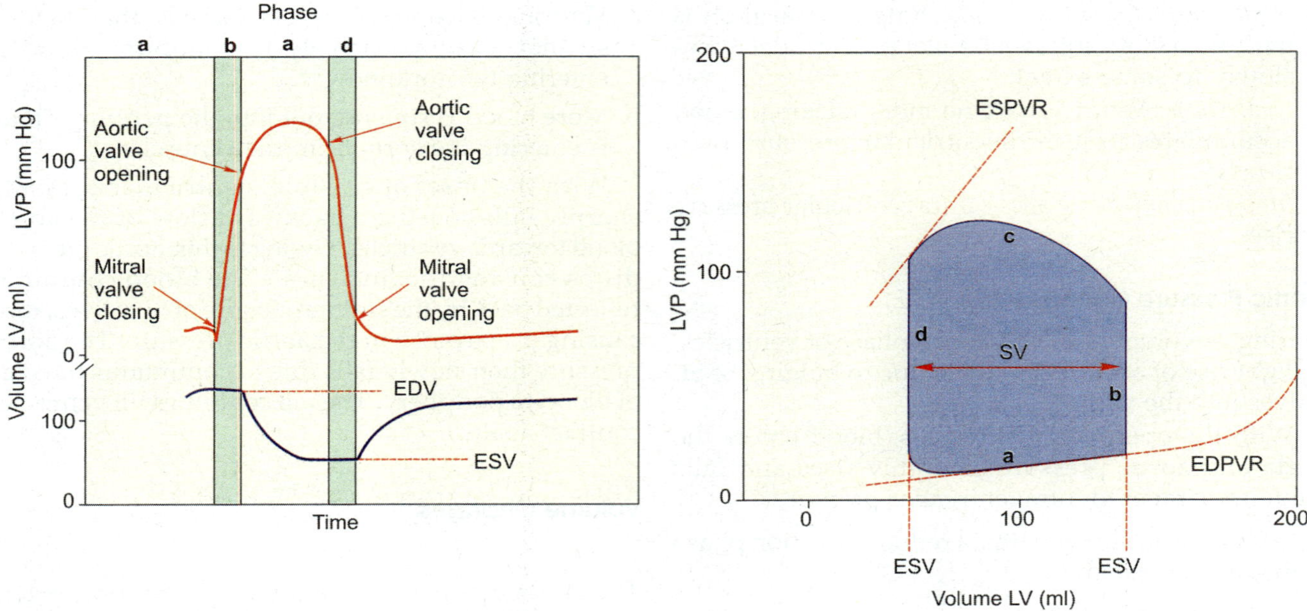

Fig. 6.13

in the cardiac cycle diagram (*see* left panel of Fig. 6.13). To generate a PV loop for the left ventricle, the left ventricular pressure (LVP) is plotted against left ventricular (LV) volume at multiple time points during a complete cardiac cycle. When this is done, a PV loop is generated (right panel of Fig. 6.13).

To illustrate the pressure-volume relationship for a single cardiac cycle. The cycle can be divided into four basic phases:

- Ventricular filling (phase A, diastole)
- Isovolumetric contraction (phase B)
- Ejection (phase C)
- Isovolumetric relaxation (phase D).

Point 1 on the PV loop is the pressure and volume at the end of ventricular filling (diastole), and therefore, represents the end-diastolic pressure and end-diastolic volume (EDV) for the ventricle. As the ventricle begins to contract isovolumetrically (phase B), the LVP increases but the LV volume remains the same, therefore, resulting in a vertical line (all valves are closed). Once LVP exceeds aortic diastolic pressure, the aortic valve opens (point 2) and ejection (phase C) begins. During this phase the LV volume decreases as LVP increases to a peak value (peak systolic pressure) and then decreases as the ventricle begins to relax. When the aortic valve closes (point 3), ejection ceases and the ventricle relaxes isovolumetrically that is, the LVP falls but the LV volume remains unchanged, therefore the line is vertical (all valves are closed). The LV volume at this time is the end-systolic (i.e. residual) volume (ESV). When the LVP falls below left atrial pressure, the mitral valve opens (point 4) and the ventricle begins to fill. Initially, the LVP continues to fall as the ventricle fills because the ventricle is still relaxing. However, once the ventricle is fully relaxed, the LVP gradually increases as the LV volume increases. The width of the loop represents the difference between EDV and ESV, which is by definition the stroke volume (SV). The area within the loop is the ventricular stroke work.

The filling phase moves along the end-diastolic pressure-volume relationship (EDPVR), or passive filling curve for the ventricle. The slope of the EDPVR is the reciprocal of ventricular compliance. The maximal pressure that can be developed by the ventricle at any given left ventricular volume is defined by the end-systolic pressure-volume relationship (ESPVR), which represents the inotropic state of the ventricle. The pressure-volume loop, therefore, cannot cross over the ESPVR, because that relationship defines the maximal pressure that can be generated under a given inotropic state. The end-diastolic and end-systolic pressure-volume relationships are analogous to the passive and total tension curves used to analyze muscle function.

Electrical Changes

Electrocardiogram

ECG stands for *electrocardiogram* and represents the electrophysiology of the heart. Cardiac electrophysiology is the science of the mechanisms, functions, and performance of the electrical activities of specific regions of the heart. The ECG is the recording of the heart's electrical activity as a graph. The graph can show the heart's rate and rhythm, it can detect enlargement of the heart, decreased blood flow, or the presence of current or past heart attacks (Fig. 6.14).

- The P is the atrial depolarization.
- QRS is the ventricular depolarization, as well as atrial repolarization.
- T is the ventricular repolarization.

Apical Impulse

During ventricular systole, all the diameters of the heart are reduced, and the base of the heart is pulled down towards the apex. On account of the spiral arrangement of the cardiac muscle fibers, the apex of the heart is rotated anteriorly and to the right, bringing most of the left ventricle to the front. Due to this movement, as well as the hardening of the ventricular wall during contraction, there is a forward thrust of the apical region against the chest wall. This causes an impulse which is visible and palpable on the chest wall during each contraction and is called the apical impulse. This is felt on the left 5th intercostal space, 1/2 an inch internal to the midclavicular line. Palpation of the apical impulse gives useful clinical information.

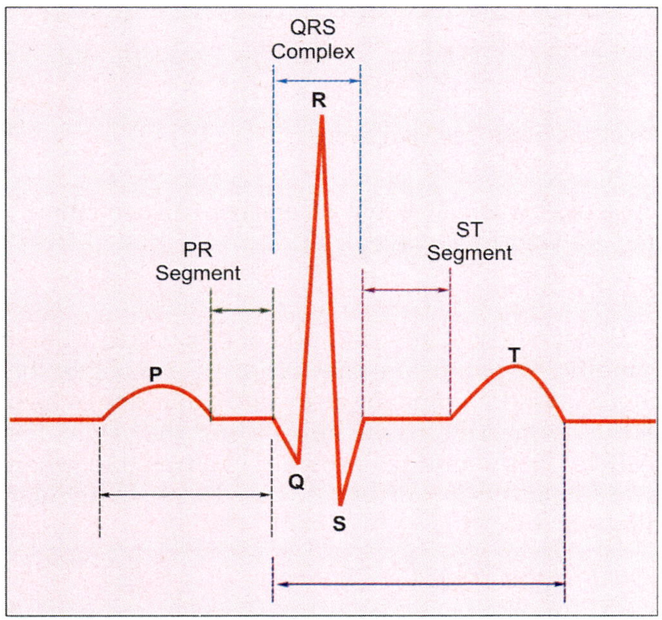

Fig. 6.14: Electrocardiogram

Phonocardiogram

In healthy adults, there are two normal heart sounds often described as a *lub and a dub (or dup)*, that occur in sequence with each heart beat. These are the first heart sound (S1) and second heart sound (S2). In addition to these normal sounds, other sounds may be present including gallop rhythms S3, S4 and heart murmurs (Fig. 6.15).

In cardiac auscultation, an examiner uses a stethoscope to listen for these sounds, which provide important information about the condition of the heart.

The aortic area, pulmonary area, tricuspid area and mitral area are areas on the surface of the chest where the heart is auscultated.

Pulmonary area	Second intercostal space	Left upper sternal border
Aortic area	Second intercostal space	Right upper sternal border
Mitral area	Fifth intercostal space	Medial to left midclavicular line
Tricuspid area	Fourth intercostal space	Lower left sternal border

First Heart Sound

S1 is a soft, low pitched sound of long duration 0.1–0.17s and frequency of 25–45 Hz. Best heard at the apex.

Causes

1. Sudden closure of AV valves
2. Vibrations set up by the turbulence of blood due to accelerations and decelerations caused by ventricular contractions
3. Vibrations set up in the ventricular muscle fibers as it begins contracting.

S1 is normally slightly split (~0.04 sec) because mitral valve closure precedes tricuspid valve closure. however, this very short time interval cannot normally be heard with a stethoscope so only a single sound is perceived. It coincides with the spike of the QRS complex of the ECG and just precedes the C wave of the atrial pressure curve.

6

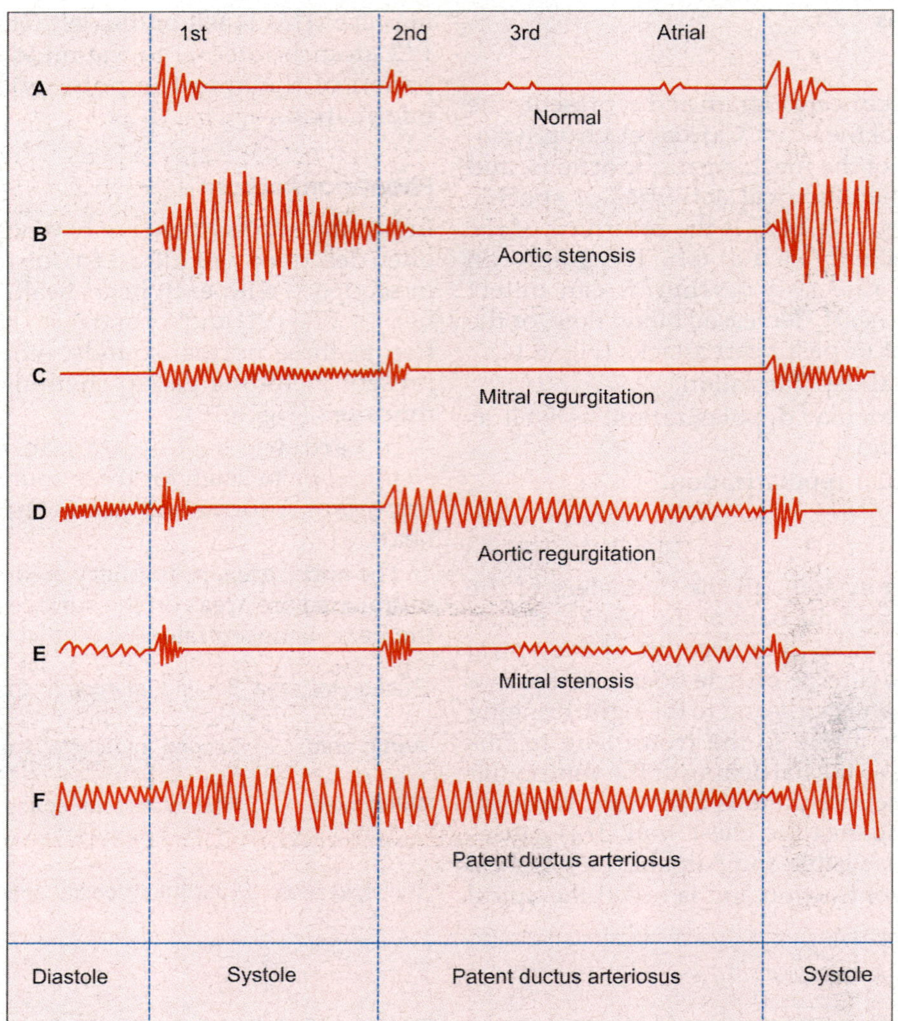

Fig. 6.15: Phonocardiograms from normal and abnormal heart sounds

Second Heart Sound

S2 is shorter, sharper and of slightly higher pitch, best heard at the base, having a duration of 0.1–0.14s and a frequency of 50 Hz.

Causes

1. Sudden closure of SL valves
2. Vibrations set up in the blood columns and in the walls of aorta and pulmonary artery.

S2 is physiologically split because aortic valve closure normally precedes pulmonary valve closure. This splitting is not of fixed duration. S2 splitting changes depending on respiration, body posture and certain pathological conditions. It coincides with the upstroke of the V wave of atrial pressure curve , and the end of T wave of ECG.

Third Heart Sound

S3 is low pitched, and duration of 0.1s occurs in first rapid filling phase, and may represent tensing of the chordae tendinae and the atrioventricular ring, which is the connective tissue supporting the AV valve leaflets. This sound is normal in children, but when heard in adults it is often associated with ventricular dilation.

Fourth Heart Sound

Is normally not heard, but only seen in phonocardiogram recording. It has a low frequency of 20 Hz and is

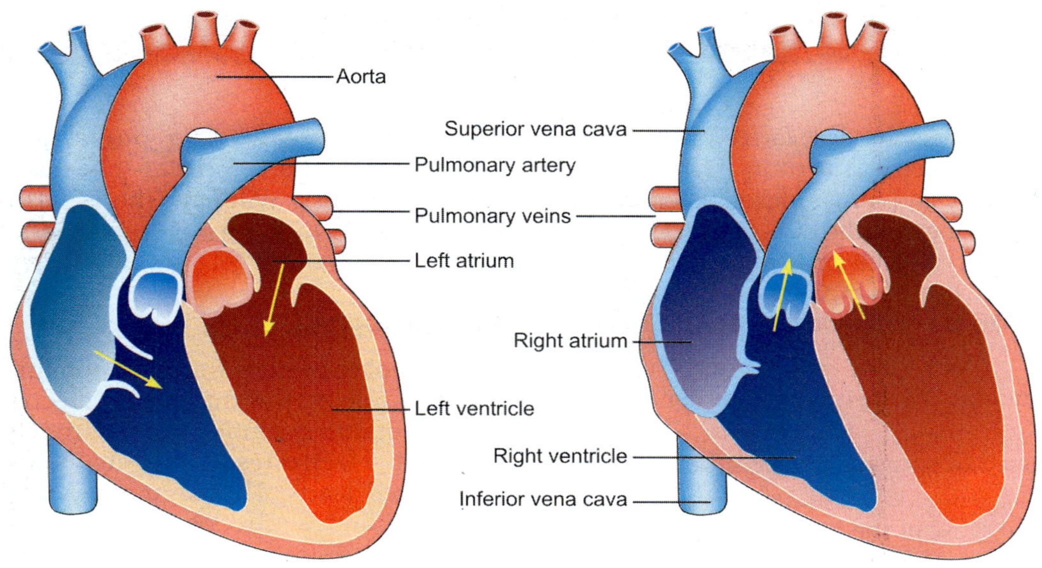

Fig. 6.16: Cardiac cycle

caused by vibration of the ventricular wall during atrial contraction. This sound is usually associated with a stiffened ventricle (low ventricular compliance), and therefore is heard in patients with ventricular hypertrophy, myocardial ischemia, or in older adults.

Heart Murmurs

Heart murmurs are generated by turbulent flow of blood, which may occur inside or outside the heart. Murmurs may be physiological (benign) or pathological (abnormal).

Physiologic Murmurs

Physiologic murmurs also called functional murmurs can occur in the absence of valvular pathology. Very high flow velocities in the aorta can lead to turbulent flow which will result in murmurs during the ejection phase of the cardiac cycle. Examples of this include high cardiac outputs in trained athletes and high output states during anemia. Another example is pregnancy where the increase in cardiac output especially when coupled with anemia can result in physiologic ejection murmurs.

Abnormal Murmurs

Abnormal murmurs can be caused by stenosis restricting the opening of a heart valve, resulting in turbulence as blood flows through it. Abnormal murmurs may also occur with valvular insufficiency (or regurgitation), which allows backflow of blood when the incompetent valve closes with only partial effectiveness. Different murmurs are audible in different parts of the cardiac cycle, depending on the cause of the murmur.

32. ELECTROCARDIOGRAM (ECG)

At every beat, the heart is depolarized to trigger its contraction. This electrical activity is transmitted throughout the body and can be picked up on the skin. This is the principle behind the ECG. An ECG machine records this activity via electrodes on the skin and displays it graphically. An ECG involves attaching 10 electrical cables to the body. One to each limb and six across the chest.

ECG terminology has two meanings for the word "lead".

- The cable used to connect an electrode to the ECG recorder.
- The electrical view of the heart obtained from any one combination of electrodes.

The standard ECG uses 10 cables to obtain 12 electrical views of the heart. The different views reflect the angles at which electrodes "look" at the heart and the direction of the heart's electrical depolarization.

6

Limb Leads

Three bipolar leads and three unipolar leads are obtained from three electrodes attached to the left arm, the right arm, and the left leg, respectively. (An electrode is also attached to the right leg, but this is an earth electrode.) The bipolar limb leads reflect the potential difference between two of the three limb electrodes.

- The limb leads form the points of Einthoven's triangle (an equilateral triangle used as a model of the standard limb leads used in electrocardiography).
- Einthoven's law: The potential differences between the bipolar leads measured simultaneously will have the values II = I + III.
- Lead I = LA ↔ RA, Lead II = LL ↔ RA, Lead III = LL ↔ LA (Fig. 6.17).

Augmented Limb Leads

The unipolar leads reflect the potential difference between one of the three limb electrodes and an estimate of zero potential: derived from the remaining two limb electrodes. These leads are known as augmented leads. The augmented leads and their respective limb electrodes are (Fig. 6.18).

- aVR lead: Right arm
- aVL lead: Left arm
- aVF lead: Left leg

Chest Leads

Another six electrodes, placed in standard positions on the chest wall, give rise to a further six unipolar leads: the chest leads (also known as precordial leads), V_1–V_6. The potential difference of a chest lead is recorded between the relevant chest electrode and an estimate of zero potential—derived from the average potential recorded from the three limb leads (Fig. 6.19).

PLACEMENT OF ELECTRODES

Electrode label	Electrode placement
RA	On the right arm, avoiding bony prominences
LA	In the same location that RA was placed, but on the left arm this time

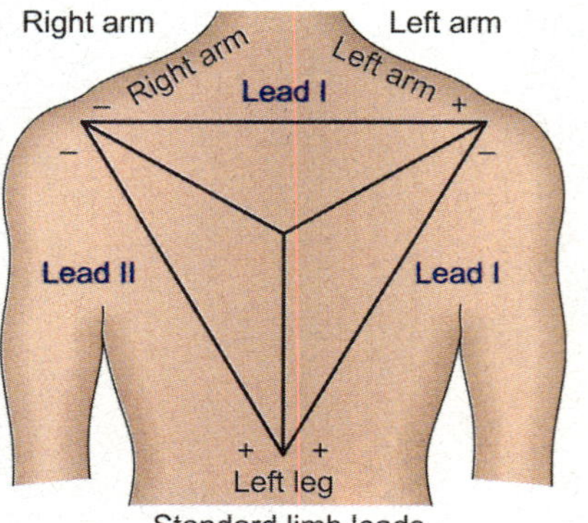

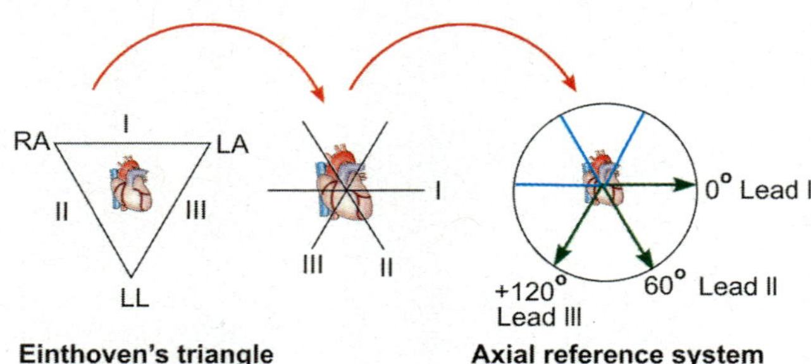

Fig. 6.17: ECG leads

RL	On the right leg, avoiding bony prominences
LL	In the same location that RL was placed, but on the left leg this time
V_1	In the fourth intercostal space (between ribs 4 and 5) just to the right of the sternum
V_2	In the fourth intercostal space (between ribs 4 and 5) just to the left of the sternum
V_3	Between leads V_2 and V_4
V_4	In the fifth intercostal space (between ribs 5 and 6) in the midclavicular line
V_5	Horizontally even with V_4, but in the anterior axillary line
V_6	Horizontally even with V_4 and V_5 in the midaxillary line

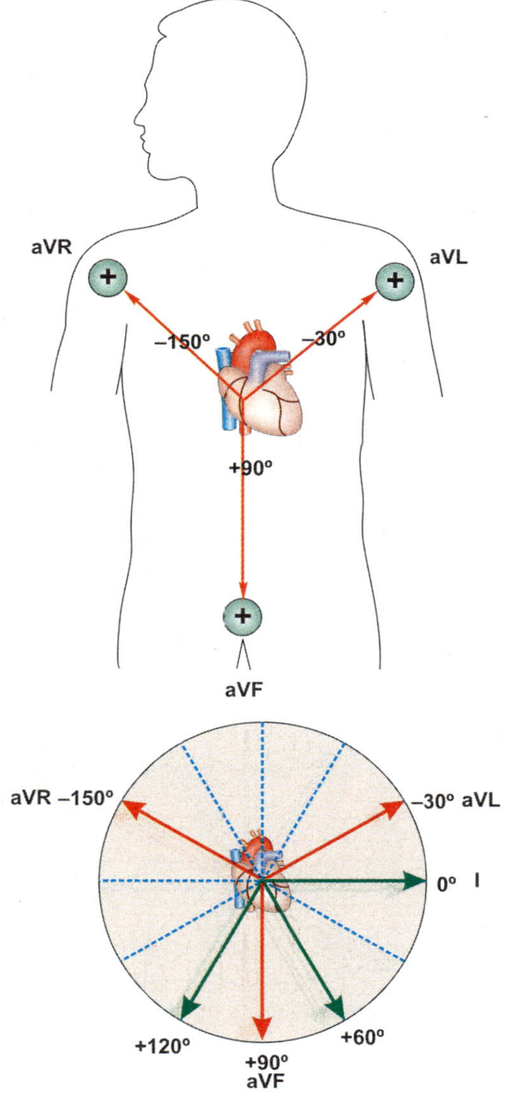

Fig. 6.18: Augmented limb leads

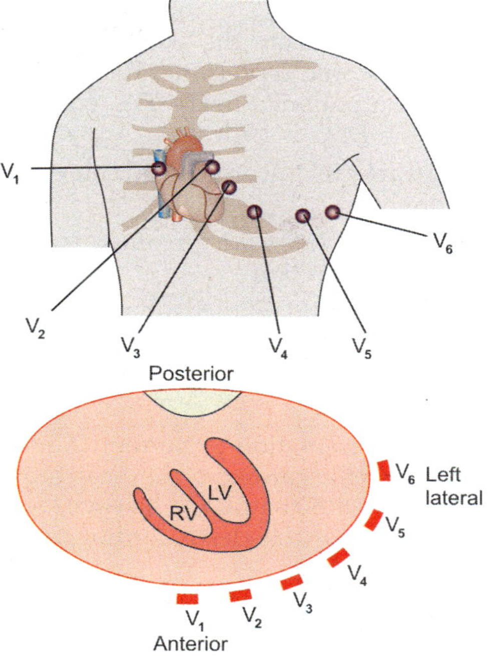

Fig. 6.19: Chest leads

Planes of View

The limb leads looking at the heart in a vertical plane, whereas the chest leads look at the heart in a horizontal plane. In this way, a three-dimensional electrical picture of the heart is built up (Fig. 6.20).

ECG leads and their respective views of the heart.

View	Lead
Inferior	II, III, aVF
Anterior	I, aVL, V_1–V_3
Septal	V_3, V_4
Lateral	V_4–V_6

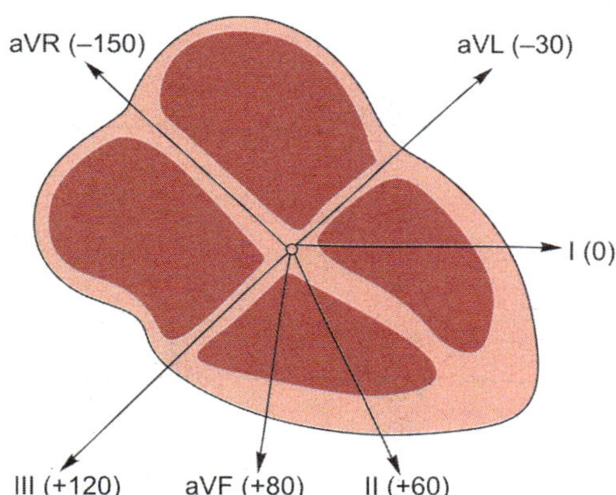

Fig. 6.20

The ECG trace: The ECG machine processes the signals picked up from the skin by electrodes and produces a graphic representation of the electrical activity of the patient's heart (Fig. 6.21). The basic pattern of the ECG is logical:

- Electrical activity towards a lead causes an upward deflection
- Electrical activity away from a lead causes a downward deflection
- Depolarization and repolarization deflections occur in opposite directions.

Normal Results

Schematic representation of normal ECG. A typical ECG tracing of the cardiac cycle (heartbeat) consists of a P wave, a QRS complex, a T wave, and aU. The baseline voltage of the electrocardiogram is known as the isoelectric line.

Waves and Intervals

P Wave

It is due to atrial depolarization. Its duration is 0.1 sec and just precedes the atrial systole. Its amplitude is about 0.1–0.3 mV. The cardiac impulse reaches the AV node at the summit of P wave.

QRS Complex

The QRS complex reflects the rapid depolarization of the right and left ventricles. They have a large muscle mass compared to the atria and so the QRS complex usually has a much larger amplitude than the P wave. Q wave is a small downward deflection which represents septal depolarization. R is a prominent positive wave and S is a small negative wave. Both R and S are due to depolarization of ventricular muscle. Duration of QRS complex is 0.08 sec and its amplitude is about 1 mV (Fig. 6.22).

T Wave

It is due to the ventricular repolarization. It is a broad wave of variable duration and of low amplitude. Its duration is 0.27 sec and amplitude is about 0.15–0.5 mV.

U Wave

U Wave is rarely seen, and thought to possibly be the repolarization of the papillary muscles.

PR Interval

PR interval is measured from the beginning of the P wave to the beginning of the QRS complex. The PR

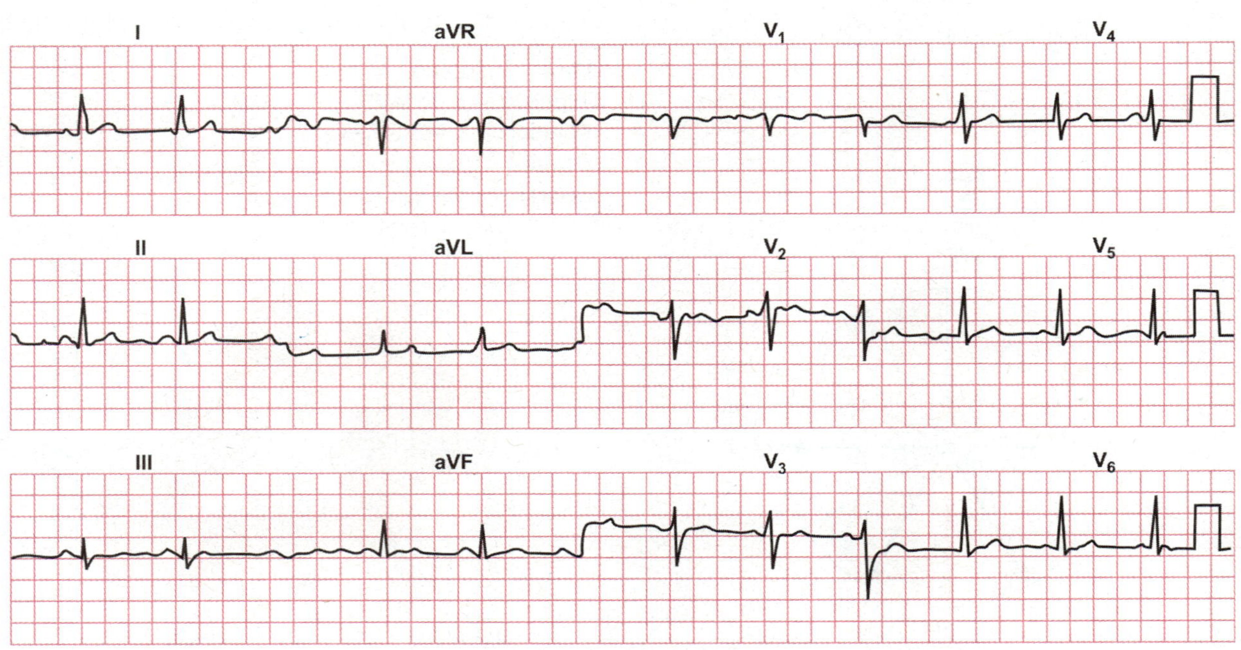

Fig. 6.21: ECG

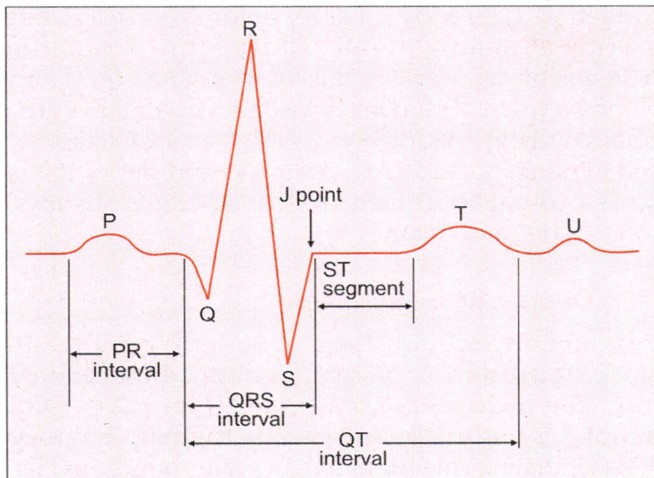

Fig. 6.22: Schematic representation of normal ECG

interval reflects the time the electrical impulse takes to travel from the sinus node through the AV node and entering the ventricles. The PR interval is therefore a good estimate of AV node function. The normal duration is 0.12–0.16 sec and does not exceed 0.2 sec. If it is more than 0.2 sec, it indicates conduction delay. PR interval corresponds to the A–C interval of the jugular pulse tracing.

QT Interval

This is measured from the beginning of the QRS complex to the end of the T wave. The average duration is 0.4 sec. A prolonged QT interval is a risk factor for ventricular tachyarrhythmias and sudden death.

ST Interval

The ST interval is measured from the J point to the end of the T wave. The average duration is 0.32 sec.

J Point

The point at which the QRS complex finishes and the ST segment begins. Used to measure the degree of ST elevation or depression present.

ST Segment

The ST segment connects the QRS complex and the T wave and it is isoelectric. Its duration is 0.05 sec.

Electrical Axis

The heart's electrical axis refers to the general direction of the heart's depolarization wavefront (or mean electrical vector) in the frontal plane. With a healthy conducting system the cardiac axis is related to where the major muscle bulk of the heart lies. Normally this is the left ventricle with some contribution from the right ventricle. It is usually oriented in a right shoulder to left leg direction, which corresponds to the left inferior quadrant of the hexaxial reference system, although –30° to +90° is considered to be normal. If the left ventricle increases its activity or bulk then there is said to be "left axis deviation" as the axis swings round to the left beyond –30°, alternatively in conditions where the right ventricle is strained or hypertrophied then the axis swings round beyond +90° and "right axis deviation" is said to exist. Disorders of the conduction system of the heart can disturb the electrical axis without necessarily reflecting changes in muscle bulk.

Normal	–30° to 90°		
Left axis deviation	–30° to –90°	May indicate left anterior fascicular block or Q waves from inferior myocardial infarction	Left axis deviation considered normal in pregnant women and those with emphysema
Right axis deviation	+90° to +180°	May indicate left posterior fascicular block, Q waves from high lateral myocardial infarction, or a right ventricular strain pattern	Right deviation is considered normal in children and is a standard effect of dextrocardia

Specific Arrhythmias

- *Sinus bradycardia:* Low sinus rate less than 60 beats/min.
- *Sinus tachycardia:* High sinus rate of 100–180 beats/min as occurs during exercise or other conditions that lead to increased SA nodal firing rate.
- *Sick sinus syndrome:* A disturbance of SA nodal function that results in a markedly variable rhythm (cycles of bradycardia and tachycardia).
- *Atrial tachycardia:* A series of 3 or more consecutive atrial premature beats occurring at a frequency more than 100/min usually due to abnormal focus within the atria and paroxysmal in nature, therefore appearance of P wave is altered in different ECG leads. This type of rhythm includes paroxysmal atrial tachycardia (PAT).
- *Atrial flutter:* Sinus rate of 250–350 beats/min.
- *Atrial fibrillation:* Uncoordinated atrial depolarizations.

- *Junctional escape rhythm:* SA node suppression can result in AV node-generated rhythm of 40–60 beats/min (not preceded by P wave).
- *AV nodal blocks:* A conduction block within the AV node (or occasionally in the bundle of His) that impairs impulse conduction from the atria to the ventricles.

First-Degree AV Nodal Block

The conduction velocity is slowed so that the P–R interval is increased to greater than 0.2 seconds (Fig. 6.23). Can be caused by enhanced vagal tone, digitalis, beta-blockers, calcium channel blockers, or ischemic damage.

Second-Degree AV Nodal Block

The conduction velocity is slowed to the point where some impulses from the atria cannot pass through the AV node (Fig. 6.24). This can result in P waves that are not followed by QRS complexes. For example, 1 (as shown below) or 2 P waves may occur alone before one is followed by a QRS. When the QRS follows the P wave, the PR interval is increased. In this type of block, the ventricular rhythm will be less than the sinus rhythm.

There are two subtypes of second-degree AV blocks: *Mobitz I* and *Mobitz II.*

In *Mobitz I* (Wenkebach block), the PR interval gradually increases over several beats until it is sufficiently prolonged (that is, AV conduction is sufficiently impaired) that the impulse fails to pass into the ventricles (i.e. a P wave will not be followed by a QRS).

Mobitz II occurs when the PR interval is fixed in duration, but some P waves are not followed by a QRS (as illustrated). If complete heart block develops suddenly, there occurs a delay before ventricles start beating at their own rate. During this period the systemic blood pressure falls to a very low level and blood supply to brain becomes inadequate. If ventricular standstill lasts for few seconds, it causes dizziness, and fainting, called Stokes-Adams syndrome, or if it is more prolonged, it leads to loss of consciousness, convulsions and death.

Third-Degree AV Nodal Block

Conduction through the AV node is completely blocked so that no impulses are able to be transmitted from the atria to the ventricles (Fig. 6.25). QRS complexes will still occur (escape rhythm), but they will originate from within the AV node, bundle of His, or other ventricular regions. Therefore, QRS complexes will not be preceded by P waves. Furthermore, there will be complete asynchrony between the P wave and QRS complexes. Atrial rhythm may be completely normal, but ventricular rhythm will be greatly reduced depending upon the location of the site generating the ventricular impulse. Ventricular rate typically range from 30 to 40 beats/min.

- *Supraventricular tachycardia (SVT):* Usually caused by re-entry currents within the atria or between ventricles and atria producing high heart rates of 140–250, the QRS complex is usually normal width, unless there are also intraventricular conduction blocks (e.g. bundle branch block).
- *Ventricular premature beats (VPBs):* Caused by ectopic ventricular foci; characterized by widened QRS, often referred to as a premature ventricular complex, or PVC.
- *Ventricular tachycardia (VT):* High ventricular rate caused by aberrant ventricular automaticity (ventricular foci) or by intraventricular re-entry can be

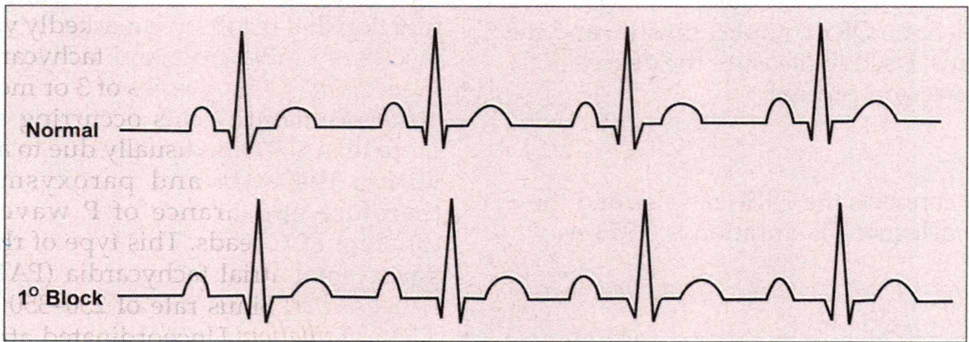

Fig. 6.23: First-degree AV nodal block

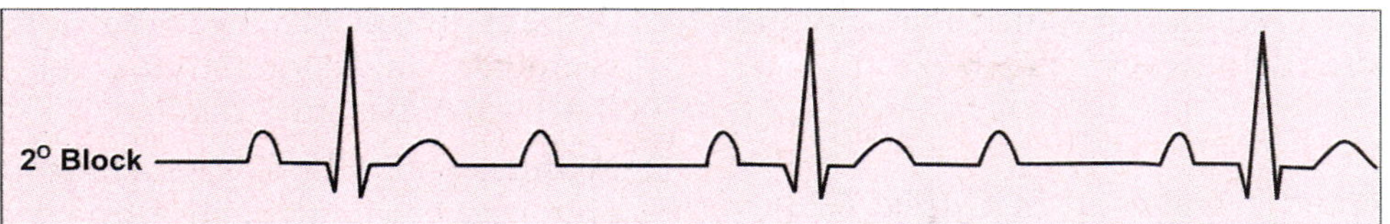

Fig. 6.24: Second-degree AV nodal block

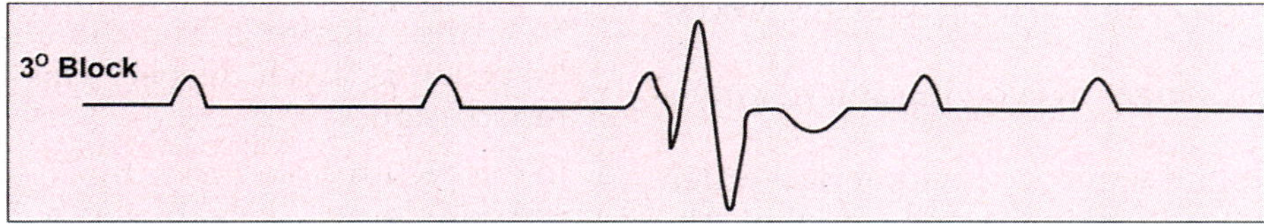

Fig. 6.25: Third-degree AV nodal block

sustained or nonsustained (paroxysmal) usually characterized by widened QRS (>0.14 sec) rates of 100 to 280 beats/min, life-threatening.

- *Ventricular flutter:* Very rapid ventricular depolarizations >250/min, since wave appearance; leads to fibrillation.
- *Ventricular fibrillation:* Uncoordinated ventricular depolarizations; leads to death if not quickly converted to a normal rhythm or at least a rhythm compatible with life.

Bundle Branch Block (BBB)

A problem in the bundle of His presents in an identical fashion to a combined block of both bundles, i.e. complete heart block. However, a more common occurrence is an isolated left or right bundle branch block. The patterns of the ECG are characteristic, but highly variable; the hallmark is a wide QRS complex. In left bundle branch block (LBBB), the pattern is best detected in V_6 where there is an "M" pattern, while in V_1 there is a "W" pattern.

In right bundle branch block (RBBB), the pattern is best detected in V_1 where there is an RSR complex, while in V_6 there is a QRS complex (Fig. 6.26).

Ventricular Pre-excitation

Wolff-Parkinson-White syndrome (WPW syndrome) Pre-excitation is defined as an early depolarization of the ventricular myocardium that occurs prior to any conduction through the AV node. The most common condition in which this is seen is WPW syndrome, where there is an accessory AV pathway called the bundle of Kent. The anomalous conducting system can be located anywhere around the mitral or tricuspid rings. Conduction through the accessory connection is faster and is independent of the heart rate. Consequently, the ventricular myocardium is activated from two directions: through the normal system and through the accessory pathway. The resulting QRS complex is a product of fusion of the two distinct activation wavefronts. Since conduction over the accessory pathway is faster, the initial part

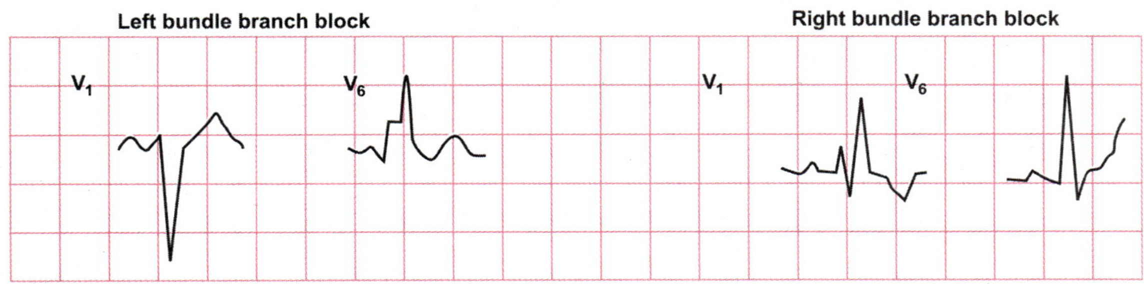

Fig. 6.26

of the QRS complex represents ventricular activation through this route (delta wave—Fig. 6.27).

Hyperkalemia

Note the tall, tented T waves in ECG (Fig. 6.28).

Sequence of Changes in Myocardial Infarction

The ECG sequence shown in Fig. 6.29 gives you an idea as to how ST elevation would develop with this process of necrosis.

Image: Sequence of changes in evolving anterior myocardial infarction.

Let's work through the sequence in numerical order:

1. This picture shows a normal sinus complex. The ST segment is on the isoelectric line. At the onset of pain the ECG would be normal but the ST segment would soon start to change. In this picture, the T wave has grown taller.
2. Within an hour the ST segment would be noticeably elevated, indicating the onset on myocardial necrosis (tissue death).
3. If thrombolysis is administered, we would be looking for specific changes on the ECG. In this picture, the ST elevation has reduced by more than 50% from picture 2. You can also see the T wave invertion is much deeper. This is a good sign of reperfusion.
4. In this picture you can see the ST segment is back on the isoelectric line but the T wave remains inverted.

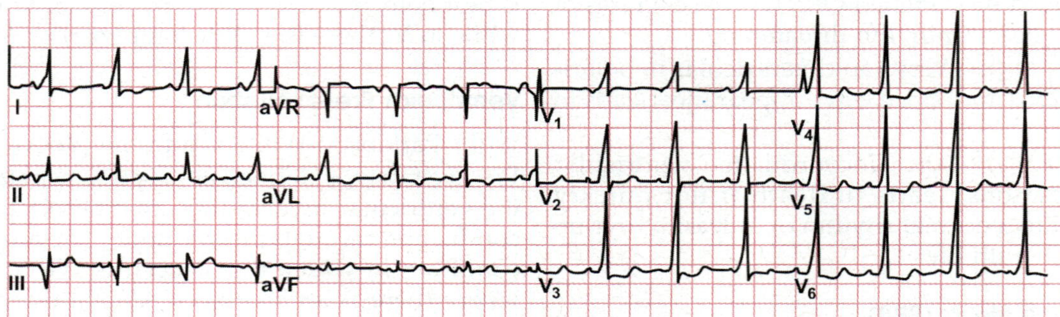

Fig. 6.27

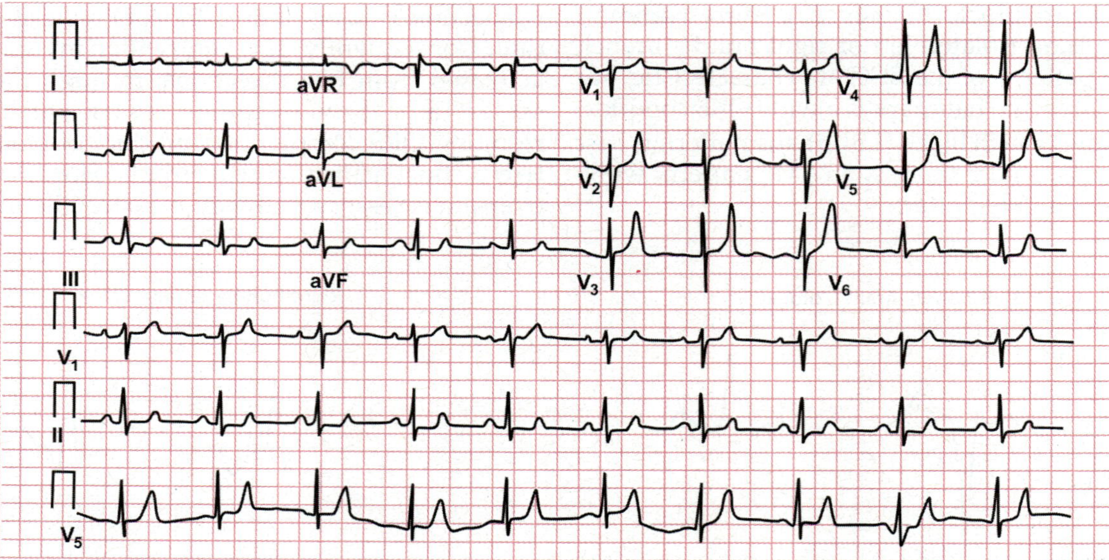

Fig. 6.28

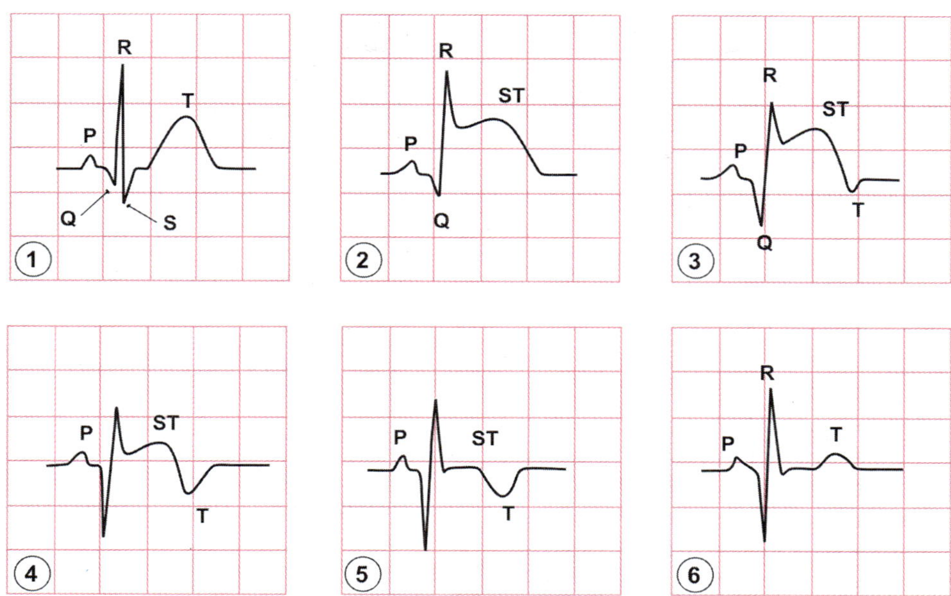

Fig. 6.29: Sequence of ECG changes in myocardial infarction

5. Six, in some cases, after a few months the ECG looks relatively normal. Compare picture 6 with picture 1. They look much the same but for the deep Q wave in picture 6. A deep Q wave is an indicator myocardial tissue death and will remain on the ECG.

6

33. CARDIAC OUTPUT

CARDIAC OUTPUT

It is the volume of blood pumped by the heart per minute. Cardiac output is a function of heart rate and stroke volume.

The heart rate is simply the number of heartbeats per minute, 70 beats/minute.

The stroke volume is the volume of blood, in milliliters (ml), pumped out of the heart with each beat, 70 ml/beat.

Increasing either heart rate or stroke volume increases cardiac output.

Cardiac output = Heart rate × Stroke volume
in ml/min (beats/min) (ml/beat)

Cardiac output = 70 (beats/min) × 70 (ml/beat)
= 4900 ml/minute.

The total volume of blood in the circulatory system of an average person is about 5 liters (5000 ml). According to our calculations, the entire volume of blood within the circulatory system is pumped by the heart each minute (at rest).

The output per minute is also called as minute volume.

End-diastolic volume (EDV) is the amount of blood in the ventricle at the end of diastole. Normal value is about 120 ml.

Ejection fraction (EF) is the portion of end-diastolic volume that is pumped out during one systole, EF = SV/EDV.

Cardiac Index

It is defined as cardiac output divided by body surface area. An average surface area is 1.73 square meters (m^2). Therefore, a person with an average cardiac output of 5 liter/min would have a cardiac index of: 5 liter/min ÷ 1.73 m^2 = 2.89 l/min/m^2. The normal range for cardiac index is approximately 2.6–4.2. A cardiac index less than 2.5 may indicate mild left heart failure. Shock is suggested by a cardiac index less than 1.8.

Stroke volume index is stroke volume divided by body surface area.

Cardiac Reserve

It is the maximum percentage increase in cardiac output above normal that can be achieved. During vigorous exercise, the cardiac output can increase up to 20–25 liter/min (300–400%) while a trained athlete can increase up to 30–35 liters/min (500–600%).

Alterations in Cardiac Output in Health and Disease

Physiological

1. *Exercise*

Increased skeletal muscle metabolism increases the total O_2 demands. Increased blood flow to muscle decreases peripheral resistance to flow. This along with the muscle pumping action and respiratory pump action, increases venous return and cardiac output. Cardiac output can increase 4 to 6-fold in exercise.

In spite of the reduced peripheral resistance, arterial pressure does not decrease in exercise because of the baroreceptor reflex.

6

2. *Emotional States*

In anxiety and fear cardiac output is increased.

3. *Posture*

Standing, after sitting or lying, decreases cardiac output by as much as 20% due to pooling of blood in the veins of the legs with a resultant reduction of venous return.

4. *Pregnancy*

Cardiac output increases by as much as 10% during pregnancy, partially due to the increased body mass and blood volume, but also due to the low resistance of the placental and uterine vasculature producing a shunt of blood from arterial to venous sides. Cardiac output is reflexly increased to maintain arterial pressure.

5. *Digestion*

About 1–3 hrs after a meal, cardiac output is increased.

6. *Temperature*

Cardiac output is increased in high environmental temperature.

Pathological

Anemia

Two factors increase cardiac output. Anemia lowers blood viscosity which marginally reduces resistance to blood flow. More importantly, anemia reduces O_2 content of blood. Delivering more blood per minute to transport the same quantity of O_2 must compensate this.

Hemorrhage

Decrease blood volume (decreased circulatory filling pressure) reduces venous return.

Metabolic

Hyperthyroidism, like fever and exercise, increases tissue metabolic activity and O_2 demand.

Cardiac Failure

Includes syndromes in which myocardial cells fail to contract normally.

Factors Determining Cardiac Output

The cardiac output is affected by four important factors:
- Venous return
- Force of contraction
- Heart rate
- Preipheral resistance.

Venous Return

Venous return is the amount of blood entering the right atrium via the veins in one minute. Over a period of time, the cardiac output is equal to the venous return. The resting venous return is 5 liter/min, but increases up to 35 liter/min during exercise. The venous return is extremely important as it determines the cardiac output and also the filling of the heart, the end diastolic volume, the preload, and the fiber length.

Determinants of Venous Return

1. *Respiratory Pump*

During inspiration the intrathoracic pressure becomes more negative and increases the intrathoracic volume, which by distending the thoracic veins increases the return of blood to the heart. Also the descent of diaphragm during inspiration increases the intra-abdominal pressure and squeezes the blood out of the splanchnic veins into the thorax. The effect of negative intrathoracic pressure is referred to as 'vis a fronte' which means force from the front.

If the intrathoracic pressure becomes positive, venous return decreases (positive pressure breathing or valsalva maneuver).

2. *Muscle Pump*

When skeletal muscle contract, they squeeze the veins in the muscles and drive the blood towards the heart and increases the venous return.

3. *Venous Tone*

The pressure in the veins helps to propel blood towards the heart. Increase in venous tone and vasoconstriction increases intrathoracic blood volume and in turn venous return. This is called 'vis a tergo' means force from behind. Distension of the veins has the opposite effect.

4. *Gravity*

In the erect posture, as there is pooling of blood in the dependent parts, venous return decreases.

5. *Blood Volume*

Blood volume and venous return are directly proportional to each other.

Force of Contraction

Increase in force of contraction increases stroke volume and cardiac output. The force of contraction depends upon the following factors:

1. Initial length of cardiac muscle fiber
2. Autonomic nerve activity
3. Ions.

1. *Initial Length of Cardiac Muscle Fiber*

The initial length of the cardiac muscle fiber is determined by the EDV which is the preload. The greater is the initial length of the cardiac muscle fiber, the greater is the force of contraction within physiological limits. This is known as the Frank-Starling's law of the heart.

If the venous return increases, the diastolic filling increases and thus EDV (preload). This stretches the cardiac muscle and increases the muscle length and force of contraction. The regulation of cardiac force by alteration in the length of muscle fiber is called as heterometric regulation (Fig. 6.30).

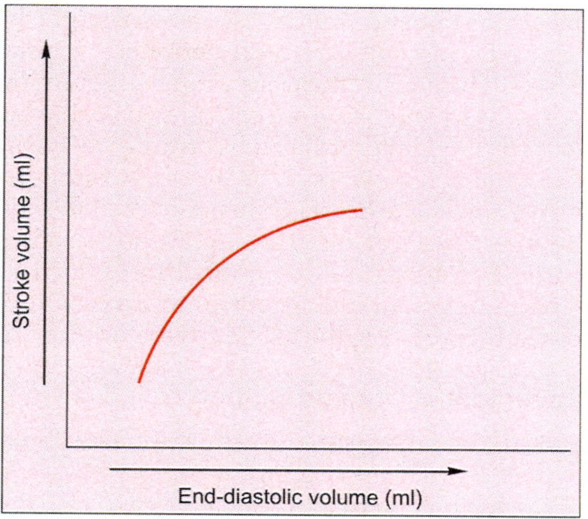

Fig. 6.30

2. *Autonomic Nerve Activity*

The sympathetic stimulation increases and parasympathetic stimulation decreases the force of contraction. This neural regulation without change in fiber length is referred to as homometric regulation.

3. *Ions*

Optimal ionic concentrations are essential for heart's action. Na is necessary for excitability and Ca for contraction while K favours diastole.

Heart Rate

Increase in heart rate increases cardiac output, if venous filling is maintained or is not much reduced. In rapidly beating heart, the diastolic phase is much reduced and hence initial fiber length is smaller, and thus stroke volume and cardiac output are reduced. If the heart is beating slowly, the diastolic phase is longer, and hence venous filling and end-diastolic volume are increased and thus stroke volume and cardiac output are increased. In muscular exercise however, a great increase in heart rate is associated with moderate increase in stroke volume as well so that the cardiac output is considerably increased.

Peripheral Resistance (Afterload)

If the resistance to flow against which the ventricle has to pump is increased, the amount of blood pumped out by the ventricle is reduced. Aortic pressure (and/or aortic valve diameter) is the major determinant of afterload on the left heart.

The effects of venous return, distension of the heart and cardiac muscle length, and peripheral resistance have been studied in the heart, lung preparation in dogs. The heart and lungs are cannulated so that blood flows from the aorta to the right atrium via a system of tubes and reservoir, back to the aorta through the heart and lungs. The heart is functioning but the nerves of the heart are not functioning. Venous return is increased by raising the reservoir thereby increasing the venous pressure. The peripheral resistance is increased by reducing the caliber of the outflow tube.

Measurement of Cardiac Output

Determination of cardiac output is based on two principles:
1. Fick principle
2. Indicator dilution technique.

The Fick Principle

6

The Fick principle relies on the observation that the total uptake of (or release of) a substance by the peripheral tissues is equal to the product of the blood flow to the peripheral tissues and the arterial-venous concentration difference (gradient) of the substance.

The essence of the Fick principle is that blood flow to an organ can be calculated using a marker substance if the following information is known:
- Amount of marker substance taken up by the organ per unit time.
- Concentration of marker substance in arterial blood supplying the organ.
- Concentration of marker substance in venous blood leaving the organ.

Direct Fick Principle

In the determination of cardiac output, the substance most commonly measured is the oxygen content of blood, and the flow calculated is the flow across the pulmonary system. This gives a simple way to calculate the cardiac output. The O_2 uptake can be measured by rebreathing through a spirometer filled with O_2 and by analyzing the spirometer gas samples before and after rebreathing. Arterial and venous O_2 concentrations can be measured by withdrawing and analyzing blood from both vessels. Arterial O_2 content is measured from femoral or brachial artery. Venous blood from pulmonary artery, i.e. by cardiac catheterization. Therefore:

$$\text{Cardiac output} = \frac{\text{Oxygen consumption}}{\text{Arterial} - \text{venous oxygen gradient}} \times 100$$

If the minute O_2 consumption is 250 ml and O_2 content of 1 liter of arterial and venous blood are 190 and 140 ml respectively, then

Cardiac output = 250 ÷ (190–140) = 5 liter/min.

Indirect Fick Method

Here arterial and venous CO_2 concentrations were calculated from the analysis of an alveolar air before and after breathing gas in mixtures containing different CO_2 %. This method is not in use nowadays.

Indicator Dilution Technique

A known quantity of a dye is injected into the right atrium via catheter. Small amounts of blood are continuously withdrawn from the arterial system with an indwelling catheter and passed through a photosensitive device that measures dye concentration. The concentration of the dye rises rapidly, reaches peak and then declines, but again rises due to recirculation. The downslope is extrapolated to time scale, and this gives the time taken for the first passage of the dye through the circulation. The area under the dye-dilution curve can be calculated and approximates the average concentration of dye over time. Knowing the quantity of dye injected, the cardiac output can be determined by:

$$\text{Cardiac output} = \text{Quantity of dye injected} \div \text{Area under the curve}$$

It is critical that the dye must be well mixed in the blood, should not be lost from the circulation, must not be toxic, or have any cardiac effects of its own.

Another variation on this theme is the thermodilution technique in which a bolus of cold dextrose solution substitutes for the dye. The procedure is the same, but blood temperature is measured instead of dye color. The thermodilution technique uses a special thermistor-tipped catheter (Swan-Ganz catheter) that is inserted from a peripheral vein into the pulmonary artery. A cold saline solution of known temperature and volume is injected into the right atrium from a proximal catheter port. The injectate mixes with the blood as it passes through the ventricle and into the pulmonary artery, thus cooling the blood. The blood temperature is measured by a thermistor at the catheter tip, which lies within the pulmonary artery, and a computer is used to acquire the thermodilution profile, that is, the computer quantifies the change in blood temperature as it flows over the thermistor surface. The computer then calculates flow (cardiac output from the right ventricle) using the blood temperature information, and the temperature and volume of the injectate.

Indicator injected (I)	5.0 mg
Mean dye conc. (C)	1.6 mg/l
Duration of 1st circulation (T)	39 sec

CO = I ÷ (C × T) = 5.0 mg ÷ (1.6 mg/I × 39/80)

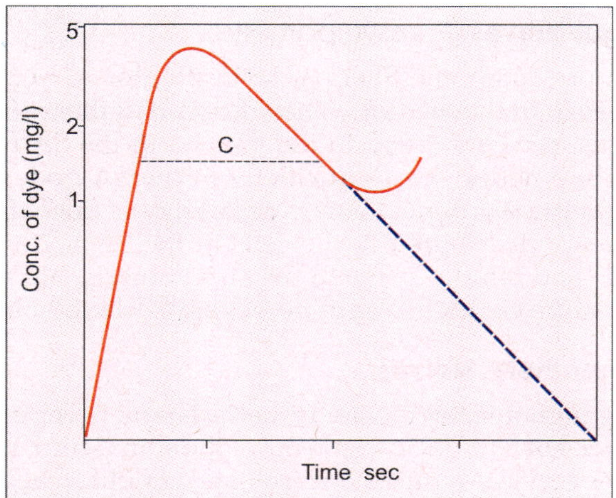

Fig. 6.31: Cardiac output determined by indicator dilution

Echocardiographic techniques and radionuclide imaging techniques can be used to estimate real-time changes in ventricular dimensions, thus computing stroke volume, which when multiplied by heart rate, gives cardiac output (Fig. 6.31).

BALLISTOCARDIOGRAPHY

It is based on Newton's Third Law, that every action has equal and opposite reaction. Thus the forward thrust of the heart during systole is balanced by the recoil of the body. By measuring the small thrust and the recoil and applying the formula developed, the stroke volume was calculated. This is an old age method and is not in use nowadays.

Distribution of Cardiac Output

Liver (splanchnic)	1400 ml/min
Kidney	100 ml/min
Skeletal muscle	800 ml/min
Brain	750 ml/min
Heart	250 ml/min
Skin	300 ml/min
Others	600 ml/min

Liver is the organ which receives highest amount of blood flow per minute (1400 ml/min).

Kidney is the organ which receives highest amount of blood flow per 100 gm of tissue per minute (350–400 ml/100 gm/min).

6

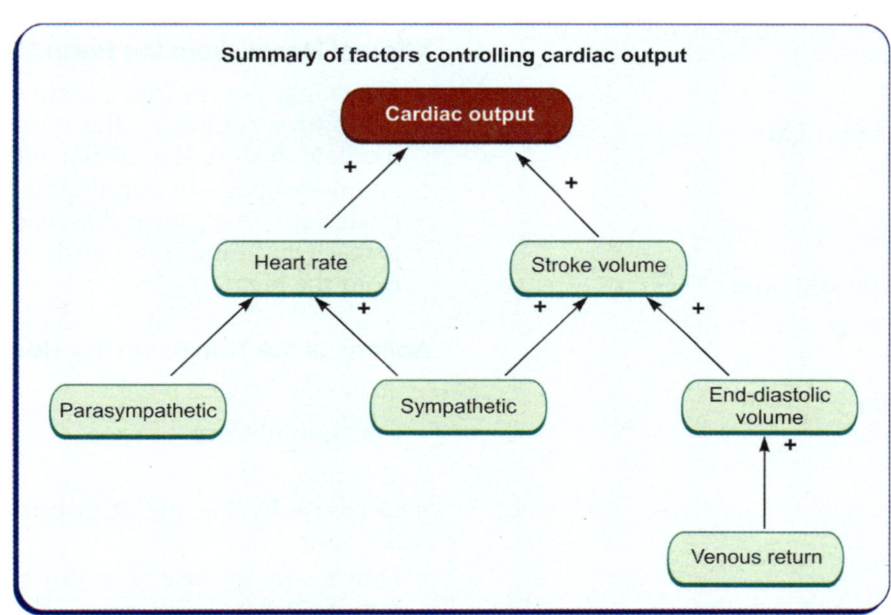

34. HEART RATE

HEART RATE

It is the number of heart beats per minute. The resting heart rate is about 72/minute (60–80/minute).

Intrinsic Heart Rate

Heart rate is normally determined by the pacemaker activity of the sinoatrial node (SA node) located in the posterior wall of the right atrium. The SA node exhibits automaticity that is determined by spontaneous changes in Ca^{++}, Na^{+}, and K^{+} conductances. This intrinsic automaticity, if left unmodified by neurohumoral factors, exhibits a spontaneous firing rate of 100–115 beats/min. This intrinsic firing rate decreases with age.

Tachycardia

Increase in heart rate >100/min.

6

Physiological

1. Newborn 120–150/min
2. Comparatively high in females, and in pregnancy
3. Emotional excitement
4. Exercise
5. Diurnal variation: High in evening.

Pathological

1. Fever (for 1 degree rise, there is increase of 10–14 beats/min)
2. Thyrotoxicosis
3. Atrial flutter and fibrillation
4. Circulatory shock

Bradycardia

Decrease in heart rate <60/min

Physiological

1. Athletes
2. Sleep

Pathological

1. Myxedema
2. Heart block
3. General weakness and debility

Innervation of the Heart

Heart is innervated by fibers from autonomic nervous system which contain both afferent and efferent fibers (Fig. 6.32).

Vagus Nerves (Parasympathetic)

The preganglionic fibers arise in the dorsal nucleus of vagus in the medulla. They descend in the trunk of vagus nerve, and end in the ganglia in the SA node and AV nodes, the right chiefly in the SA node and left in the AV node. Short postganglionic fibers from here are distributed to the cells in the SA node, AV node and bundle, some to the atrial muscle, but very few to the ventricle. Vagus nerves are cardioinhibitory.

Sympathetic Nerves

Preganglionic fibers arise from the lateral horns of the upper 4 or 5 thoracic segments of the spinal cord, relay in the cervical sympathetic (stellate) ganglia, reach the heart and innervate the SA and AV nodes, bundle of His and branches and atrial and ventricular muscles. Vagal and sympathetic fibers mingle in the superficial and deep cardiac plexus. Sympathetic fibers cause acceleration and augmentation of the heart.

Atrial and ventricular muscles have much sympathetic innervations but vagal innervation is sparse, especially to the ventricular muscle.

Afferent Nerves from the Heart Travel Via

- The vagal nerves into the medulla to the cardioinhibitory region of the vasomotor area. They mediate most of the cardiac reflexes.
- Along sympathetic nerves enter the spinal cord via posterior nerve root and ascend up the spinal cord to reach the brain. They mostly convey pain impulses from the heart.

Actions of the Nerves on the Heart

I. *Actions of Vagus*

Cardioinhibitory

Weak stimulation causes

- Decrease in the rate of impulse formation in the SA node
- Diminishes the rate of conduction in the AV node, bundle and its branches

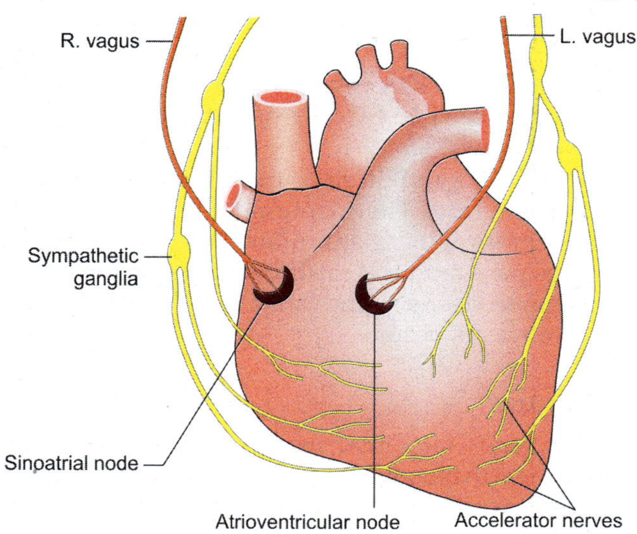

Fig. 6.32

- Diminishes the force of atrial contraction
- There is no direct action on the ventricles. The ventricular slowing is the effect of:
  - Decreased impulse formation in the SA node.

Strong stimulation causes

- Stoppage of impulse formation in the SA node
- Stoppage of impulse transmission through the AV junction.

With strong stimulation, initially both atria and ventricles stop beating completely, but after a varying interval, the ventricles begin to beat on their own, but at a much smaller rate (20–40/min). This phenomenon is called vagal escape. It is the ventricles that escape from the effect of vagus.

Right vagal stimulation predominantly reduces impulse formation in the SA node, whereas the left vagal stimulation predominantly reduces AV conduction.

Mode of Action of Vagus Nerve

Vagus acts by release of Acetylcholine at its post-ganglionic terminals. The acetylcholine increases K^+ permeability and K^+ efflux resulting in hyper-polarization of the membrane and the tissue becomes less excitable.

Vagal Tone

Impulses from cardioinhibitory region of the medulla are continually passing down the vagus nerves to the heart and keep the heart rate slower. This is called vagal tone. Vagal tone is minimal in the newborn and is well-developed in athletes.

II. Actions of Sympathetic Nerves

Acceleration and augmentation

- Increases the rate of impulse formation in the SA node (positive chronotropism)
- Increases the conductivity (positive dromotropism)
- Increases the force of contraction (positive inotropism).

Mode of Action of Sympathetic

It acts by releasing noradrenaline at the postganglionic terminals. Noradrenaline increases heart rate by acting on SA nodal cells causing reduction in K^+ efflux, followed by opening of transient Ca^{++} channels. Adrenaline also has a similar action.

Sympathetic Tone

It is due to impulses from the medulla and hypothalamus.

Homometric Regulation

Nervous control of force of contraction without change in muscle fiber length is called as homometric regulation.

Medullary Centers Controlling Heart Rate

The vasomotor center is located bilaterally in the reticular formation of the medulla oblongata and contains the following areas:

Vasoconstrictor Area (Cardioaccelerator Area)

It is located in the upper anterolateral region of the medulla. The fibers from here pass down the spinal cord to connect with the cells of origin of the sympathetic nerves which innervate both blood vessels and heart.

Vasodilator Area (Cardioinhibitory Area)

It is more medially placed close to the dorsal motor nucleus of vagus and the nucleus ambiguous which send impulses via the vagus nerves.

Sensory Area

It is located in the upper posterolateral region of the medulla in the nucleus tractus solitarius. This area receives afferents from the baroreceptors and other receptors mainly via the vagus and glossopharyngeal nerves which in turn conveys impulses to the vasomotor areas.

Regulation of Heart Rate

There are two different factors involved in heart rate management:

1. Intrinsic
2. Extrinsic.

Intrinsic regulation of heart rate is the result of the unique nature of cardiac tissue. It is self-regulating and maintains its own rhythm without direction.

Extrinsic controls are those that come from both hormonal responses as well as the commands from the nervous system: The central nervous system and the autonomic nervous system. Extrinsic regulation can cause the heart rate to change rapidly because of chemicals that circulate in the blood or by direct action of nerves that go to the heart.

Hormonal Control

The sympathetic components increase heart rate by releasing the neural hormone catecholamines: epinephrine and norepinephrine.

The parasympathetic components decrease heart rate. These neurons release the neurohormone acetylcholine, which inhibits heart rate.

Nervous Control

Higher brain (hypothalamus): Stimulates the center in response to exercise, emotions, "fight or flight", and temperature.

Reflex Control

Sinoaortic Baroreceptor Reflex

Baroreceptors present are

- Carotid sinus which is a dilatation at the commencement of the internal carotid artery
- The arch of aorta.

They are branched and coiled myelinated nerve endings which respond to changes in blood pressure. Even though both rapid and sustained change stimulates baroreceptors, the effects are greater for the former. The impulses from the carotid sinus are carried by the carotid sinus nerve, a branch of glossopharyngeal nerve and from the aortic arch by the vagus. The impulses are sent up to the nucleus tractus solitarius and then to the vasomotor centers. The nerves are together called as sinoaortic nerves and are referred to as buffer nerves, since they buffer blood pressure changes.

Normally there is low frequency impulse discharge in these nerves, which are responsible for vagal tone. When blood pressure rises, the rate of discharge is increased, and when BP decreases, the discharge rate is slowed down.

When the arterial BP rises, there is a reflex slowing of the heart rate. The increased BP stimulates the baroreceptors, which stimulates NTS, from where impulses pass onto the cardioinhibitory region, then via vagus to decrease the heart rate. When BP falls, opposite effects occur.

Marey's Law

Marey's Law states that the heart rate is inversely proportional to blood pressure. This is due to sinoaortic baroreceptor reflex. There are two exceptions, they are exercise and sleep.

Reflexes from Sinoaortic Chemoreceptors

Chemoreceptors are present in the carotid and aortic bodies. These are stimulated by hypoxia, hypercapnea and H^+. Chemoreceptor stimulation increases heart rate, but is of minor importance.

Bainbridge Reflex

The venous engorgement of the right side of the heart (atria and great veins) causes tachycardia, and is brought about by stimulation of stretch receptors. The vagus is the afferent pathway and the efferents are both vagus and sympathetic nerves. A part of this reflex may be mechanical, resulting from stretching of SA node when right atrium is distended (to prevent accumulation of blood in the atria and the great veins).

Bezold-Jarish Reflex (Coronary Chemoreflex)

Injection of substances like phenyl diguanidine, serotonin, veratridine into the left ventricle via coronary artery supplying the left ventricle in experimental animals causes reflex slowing of the heart, hypotension, apnea followed by rapid shallow breathing. This is called as Bezold-Jarish reflex. The receptors are unmyelinated C fiber endings.

Pulmonary Chemoreflex

Injection of substances like phenyl diguanidine, serotonin, veratridine into the pulmonary vascular bed produces bradycardia, hypotension, apnea followed by rapid shallow breathing. This is called as pulmonary chemoreflex. The receptors are unmyelinated C fiber endings located close to the pulmonary capillaries, the juxtacapillary J receptors of Paintal.

Respiratory Sinus Arrhythmia (RSA)

It is a naturally occurring variation in heart rate that occurs during a breathing cycle. Heart rate increases during inspiration and decreases during expiration. It may be:

- Reflexly produced by afferent impulses from stretch receptors in the lungs. When the lungs inflate during inspiration, the impulse discharge along the vagus increases and on deflation, the impulse discharge decreases.
- Irradiation of impulses from the respiratory center to the cardioinhibitory areas.

Oculocardiac Reflex

Pressure on the eyeball causes reflex slowing of the heart, by increasing the vagal tone. The afferent impulses pass via the trigeminal nerve. Most painful stimuli also increase heart rate.

Cerebral ischemia due to raised intracranial pressure causes bradycardia by indirect effect due to rise of BP.

35. HEMODYNAMICS (PRESSURE, FLOW AND RESISTANCE)

Hemodynamics can be defined as the physical factors that govern blood flow. These are the same physical factors that govern the flow of any fluid, and are based on Ohm's Law.

$$F = \frac{\Delta P}{R} = \frac{(P_A - P_V)}{R}$$

For the flow F of blood in a blood vessel, the ΔP is the pressure difference between any two points along a given length of the vessel and R is the resistance to flow.

The above relationship also indicates that there is a linear and proportionate relationship between flow and perfusion pressure. This linear relationship, is not followed when pathological conditions lead to turbulent flow, because turbulence, increases resistance to flow.

Resistance to Blood Flow

Resistance to blood flow is determined by:

1. The size of vessels (length and diameter).
2. The organization of the vascular network (series and parallel arrangements).
3. Physical characteristics of the blood (viscosity, laminar flow versus turbulent flow).
4. Extravascular mechanical forces acting upon the vasculature.

Of the above factors, changes in vessel diameter are most important quantitatively for regulating blood flow within an organ, as well as for regulating arterial pressure. Changes in vessel diameter, particularly in small arteries and arterioles, enable organs to adjust their own blood flow to meet the metabolic requirements of the tissue. Therefore, if an organ needs to adjust its blood flow (and therefore, oxygen delivery), cells surrounding these blood vessels release vasoactive substances that can either constrict or dilate the resistance vessels.

Regulation of Blood Flow

The ability of an organ to regulate its own blood flow is termed local regulation of blood flow and is mediated by vasoconstrictor and vasodilator substances released by the tissue surrounding blood vessels (vasoactive metabolites) and by the vascular endothelium. There is also a mechanism intrinsic to the vascular smooth muscle (myogenic mechanism) that is involved in local blood flow regulation.

In organs such as the heart and skeletal muscle, mechanical activity (contraction and relaxation) produces compressive forces that can effectively decrease vessel diameters and increase resistance to flow during muscle contraction.

Besides local regulatory mechanisms, there are extrinsic mechanisms acting on the vasculature to regulate vessel diameter. One important extrinsic mechanism regulating vascular diameter operates through the autonomic innervation of blood vessels. In general, sympathetic adrenergic influences acting through vascular alpha-adrenoceptors cause resistance vessels as well as veins to be partially constricted under basal conditions. This is termed "sympathetic vascular tone." Therefore, removal of sympathetic adrenergic influences (for example, by administration of an alpha-adrenoceptor antagonist or by sympathectomy) leads to vasodilation and an increase in organ blood flow. A second type of extrinsic influence on the vasculature is circulating vasoactive hormones such as angiotensin II, epinephrine and norepinephrine, vasopressin (antidiuretic hormone, ADH), atrial natriuretic peptide (ANP), and endothelin. Both the neural and humoral factors, while affecting organ blood flow, primarily serve the function of regulating arterial pressure by altering systemic vascular resistance.

Determinants of Resistance to Flow (Poiseuille's Equation)

There are three primary factors that determine the resistance to blood flow within a single vessel: vessel diameter (or radius), vessel length, and viscosity of the blood.

6

Vessel resistance (R) is directly proportional to the length (L) of the vessel and the viscosity (η) of the blood, and inversely proportional to the radius to the fourth power (r^4).

$$R \propto \frac{n.L}{r^4}$$

If the above expression for resistance is combined with the equation describing the relationship between flow, pressure and resistance ($F = \Delta P/R$), then

$$F \propto \frac{\Delta P.r^4}{n.L}$$

This relationship (Poiseuille's equation) was first described by the 19th century French physician Poiseuille. It is a description of how flow is related to perfusion pressure, radius, length, and viscosity.

Viscosity of Blood

The viscosity of whole blood is strongly influenced by four factors: hematocrit, temperature, flow and vessel diameter as described below.

1. *Hematocrit* is an important determinant of the viscosity of blood. As hematocrit increases, there is a disproportionate increase in viscosity. 50% increase in hematocrit from a normal value increases blood viscosity by about 100%.
2. Temperature also has a significant effect on viscosity. As temperature decreases, viscosity increases.
3. The flow rate of blood also affects viscosity. At very low flow states in the microcirculation, the blood viscosity can increase significantly.
4. At small vessel diameters, (e.g. in arterioles less than 300 microns), there is a paradoxical decrease in blood viscosity (Fahraeus-Lindqvist effect). This occurs because the hematocrit decreases in small vessels relative to the hematocrit of large feed arteries.

Laminar Flow

Laminar flow is the normal condition for blood flow throughout most of the circulatory system. It is characterized by concentric layers of blood moving in parallel down the length of a blood vessel. The highest velocity (V_{max}) is found in the center of the vessel. The lowest velocity ($V = 0$) is found along the vessel wall. The flow profile is parabolic once laminar flow is fully developed. This occurs in long, straight blood vessels, under steady flow conditions (Fig. 6.33).

One practical implication of parabolic, laminar flow is that when flow velocity is measured using a Doppler flowmeter, the velocity value represents the average velocity of a cross-section of the vessel, not the maximal velocity found in the center of the flow stream.

The orderly movement of adjacent layers of blood flow through a vessel helps to reduce energy losses in the flowing blood by minimizing viscous interactions between the adjacent layers of blood and the wall of the blood vessel. Disruption of laminar flow leads to turbulence and increased energy losses.

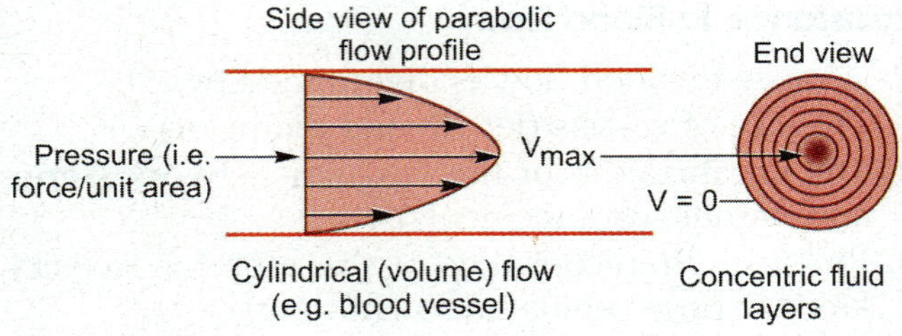

Fig. 6.33: Laminar flow

Turbulent Flow

Generally in the body, blood flow is laminar.

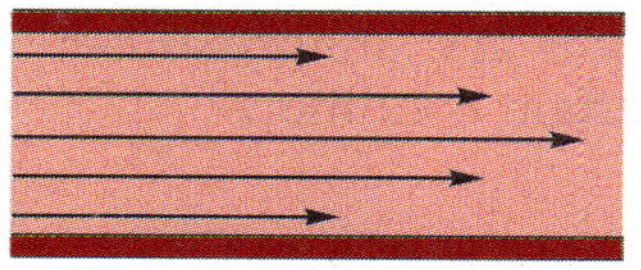

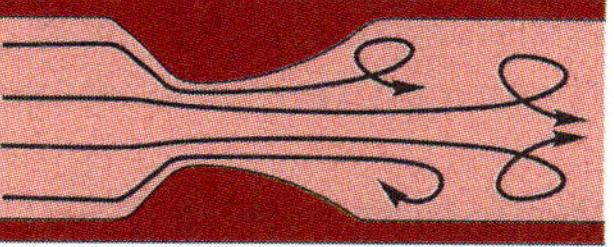

Fig. 6.34

Turbulence (Fig. 6.34) occurs when a critical Reynolds number (Re) is exceeded. The equation for Reynolds number is:

$$Re = \frac{(\bar{v}.D.\rho)}{\eta}$$

Where v = mean velocity, D = vessel diameter, ρ = blood density, and η = blood viscosity.

Bernoulli's principle is a physical phenomenon that was named after the Swiss scientist Daniel Bernoulli who lived during the eighteenth century. Bernoulli studied the relationship of the speed of a fluid and pressure.

The principle states that "the pressure of a fluid (liquid or gas) decreases as the speed of the fluid increases." Within the same fluid (air in the example of aircraft moving through air), high-speed flow is associated with low pressure, and low-speed flow is associated with high pressure.

The continuity equation relates the speed of a fluid moving through a pipe to the cross-sectional area of the pipe. It says that as the radius of the pipe decreases the speed of fluid flow must increase and vice versa.

Distensibility of a blood vessel is the fraction of increase of the initial volume for each mm Hg.

Compliance or Capacitance is the volume change per unit pressure change.

Elastance is the reciprocal of compliance.

Critical closing pressure: The pressure at which the blood flow ceases in a small blood vessel is called as critical closing pressure.

36. ARTERIAL PULSE AND VENOUS PULSE

ARTERIAL PULSE

It is the regular, recurrent expansion and contraction of an artery, produced by waves of pressure caused by the ejection of blood from the left ventricle of the heart as it contracts. The pulse is easily detected on superficial arteries, such as the radial and carotid arteries, and corresponds to each beat of the heart.

Arterial Pulse Tracing

The arterial pulse wave can be measured by a sphygmograph. The resulting tracing shows ascending and descending limbs.

The ascending limb is steep and is called anacrotic limb or the percussion wave. It is due to expansion of the artery resulting from rapid ejection phase of ventricular systole.

The descending limb is called the catacrotic limb. Here, the dicrotic notch and dicrotic wave is present. Sometimes, a small tidal wave is present soon after the percussion wave.

Dicrotic notch: When the pressure in the ventricle falls below that in aorta at the end of systole, the aorta recoils now, causing the blood column to sweep back toward the heart resulting in dicrotic notch.

Dicrotic wave: The reverse flow of blood closes the aortic valve and the blood column rebounds from the closed aortic valve resulting in dicrotic wave.

Abnormal Pulses

a. Water-Hammer: Large amplitude, rapidly rising
   - Hypertrophic cardiomyopathy
   - Aortic regurgitation
   - Mitral regurgitation (severe)
   - Patent ductus arteriosus
b. Pulses parvus et tardus (small amplitude, slow rising)
   - Aortic stenosis
   - Diminished cardiac output
c. Pulsus alternans (alternating strong and weak pulse)
   - Left ventricular systolic dysfunction
d. Pulsus paradoxus (diminished pulse on inspiration)
   - Cardiac tamponade
   - Congestive heart failure (severe)

- Chronic obstructive pulmonary disease (severe)
- Asthma
- Constrictive pericarditis

e. Pulsus bisferiens (double-peak pulse)
- Aortic regurgitation
- Hypertrophic cardiomyopathy.

VENOUS PULSE (Fig. 6.35)

Description

The jugular venous pressure (JVP) provides an indirect measure of central venous pressure. The internal jugular vein connects to the right atrium without any intervening valves—thus acting as a column for the blood in the right atrium. The JVP consists of certain waveforms and abnormalities of these can help diagnose certain conditions.

Waveforms of the JVP

a: Presystolic; produced by right atrial contraction.
c: Bulging of tricuspid valve into the right atrium during ventricular systole (isovolumic phase).
v: Occurs in late systole; increased blood in right atrium from venous return.

Descents

x: Combination of atrial relaxation, downward movement of the tricuspid valve and ventricular systole.
y: Tricuspid valve opens and blood flows into the right ventricle.

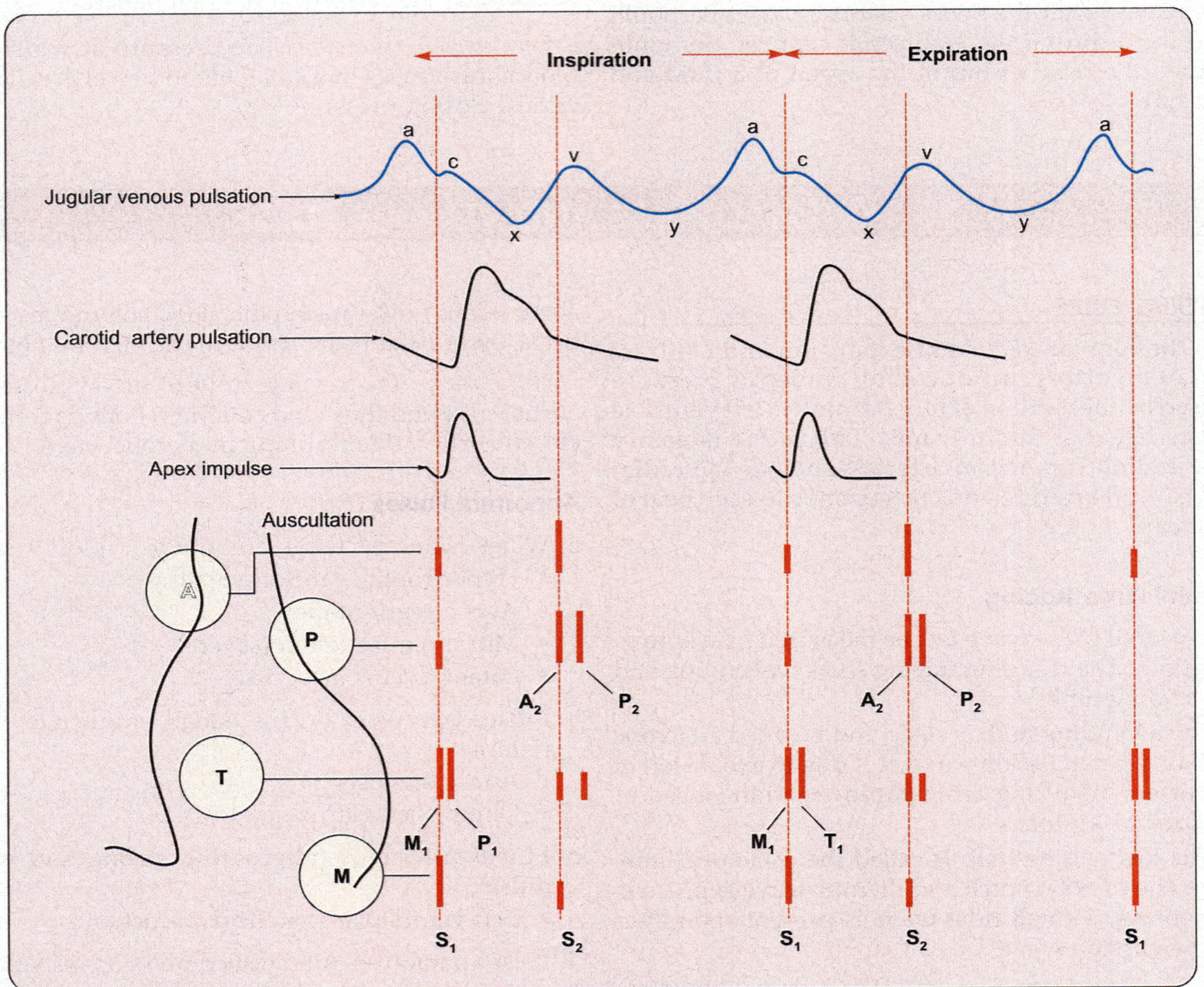

Fig. 6.35

Causes of a Raised JVP

- Heart failure
- Constrictive pericarditis (JVP increases on inspiration called Kussmaul's sign)
- Cardiac tamponade
- Fluid overload, e.g. renal disease
- Superior vena cava obstruction (no pulsation).

Abnormalities of the JVP

Abnormalities of the a Wave

- Disappears in atrial fibrillation
- Large a waves occur in any cause of right ventricular hypertrophy (pulmonary hypertension and pulmonary stenosis) and tricuspid stenosis
- Extra large a waves (called cannon waves) in complete heart block and ventricular tachycardia.

Prominent v Waves

Tricuspid regurgitation is called cv or v waves and occur at the same time as systole (combination of v wave and loss of × descent); there may be ear lobe movement.

Slow y Descent

- Tricuspid stenosis
- Right atrial myxoma

Steep y Descent

- Right ventricular failure
- Constrictive pericarditis
- Tricuspid regurgitation

(The last two conditions have a rapid rise and fall of the JVP called Friedreich's sign).

Central Venous Pressure

Central venous pressure (CVP) describes the pressure of blood in the thoracic vena cava, near the right atrium of the heart. CVP reflects the amount of blood returning to the heart and the ability of the heart to pump the blood into the arterial system.

It is a good approximation of right atrial pressure, which is a major determinant of right ventricular end-diastolic volume.

Measurement

CVP can be measured by connecting the patient's central venous catheter to a special infusion set which is connected to a small diameter water column. If the water column is calibrated properly the height of the column indicates the CVP.

Normal values are 2–8 mm Hg.

Factors Affecting CVP

a. *Factors that increase CVP*

1. Hypervolemia
2. Forced exhalation
3. Tension pneumothorax
4. Heart failure
5. Pleural effusion
6. Decreased cardiac output
7. Cardiac tamponade

b. *Factors that decrease CVP*

1. Hypovolemia
2. Deep inhalation
3. Distributive shock

6

37. BLOOD PRESSURE

BLOOD PRESSURE (BP)

It is the lateral pressure exerted by the blood on the walls of the blood vessels. Pressure in the arterial system fluctuates with the cardiac cycle. Blood pressure reaches a peak in systole and is lowest in diastole.

Systolic pressure is the maximum pressure in the arteries during systole (120 mm Hg).

Diastolic pressure is the minimum pressure in the arteries during diastole (80 mm Hg).

Pulse pressure is the difference between the systolic and diastolic pressures.

Pulse pressure = systolic pressure – diastolic pressure (40 mm Hg).

Mean arterial pressure represents the average pressure in the arterial system. This value is important because it is the difference between MAP and the venous pressure that drives blood through the capillaries of the organs. Because more time is spent in diastole than in systole, MAP is not simply the average of the systolic and diastolic pressures. A simple formula for calculation of MAP is:

MAP = Diastolic pressure + 1/3 pulse pressure (94 mm Hg).

Measurement of Blood Pressure

Palpation Method

A more accurate value of systolic BP can be obtained with a sphygmomanometer and palpating for when a radial pulse returns. The diastolic blood pressure can not be estimated by this method. Palpation is used to get an estimate before using the auscultatory method.

Auscultatory Method

The auscultatory method (from the Latin word for listening) uses a stethoscope and a sphygmomanometer. This comprises an inflatable (Riva-Rocci) cuff placed around the upper arm at roughly the same vertical height as the heart, attached to a mercury manometer. The mercury manometer, considered the gold standard, measures the height of a column of mercury, giving an absolute result. A cuff of appropriate size is fitted smoothly and snugly, then inflated manually by repeatedly squeezing a rubber bulb until the artery is completely occluded. Listening with the stethoscope to the brachial artery at the elbow, the examiner slowly releases the pressure in the cuff. When blood just starts to flow in the artery, the turbulent flow creates a "whooshing" or pounding (first Korotkoff sound). The pressure at which this sound is first heard is the systolic BP. The cuff pressure is further released until no sound can be heard (fifth Korotkoff sound), at the diastolic arterial pressure.

The auscultatory method has been predominant since the beginning of BP measurements.

Oscillometric Method

The Oscillometric method was first demonstrated in 1876 and involves the observation of oscillations in the sphygmomanometer cuff pressure which are caused by the oscillations of blood flow. The electronic version of this method is sometimes used in long-term measurements. It uses a sphygmomanometer cuff like the auscultatory method, but with an electronic pressure sensor (transducer) to observe cuff pressure oscillations, electronics to automatically interpret them, and automatic inflation and deflation of the cuff. The pressure sensor should be calibrated periodically to maintain accuracy.

According to Bernoulli, in a tube or a blood vessel, the sum of kinetic energy of flow and pressure energy is constant. When the end pressure is measured, the flow of blood is interrupted, and all the kinetic energy is converted into pressure energy. But, when side pressure is measured, there is no interruption of flow and so the side pressure is lower by the kinetic energy of flow.

Physiological Variations

1. *Age*

In children, the normal ranges are lower than for adults. As adults age, systolic pressure tends to rise and diastolic tends to fall. In the elderly, BP tends to be above the normal adult range, largely because of reduced flexibility of the arteries.

2. *Sex*

In adult females, both systolic and diastolic pressures are slightly lower.

3. *Exercise*

Systolic BP increases due to increase in stroke volume. The change in diastolic pressures depends on the degree of peripheral vascular resistance.

4. *Emotional Reactions and Stress*

Systolic BP increases.

5. *Posture*

Diastolic pressure is higher in the standing than in sitting position and is lowest in the lying posture. When posture is changed from lying to standing, blood accumulates in the dependent parts and the pressure falls in the upper parts of the body. This stimulates the sinoaortic baroreceptors and rise in pressure.

6. *Digestion*

Slight rise of systolic pressure after a meal and slight fall of diastolic pressure due to dilatation of vessels of digestive tract.

7. *Sleep*

Systolic pressure is reduced.

Classification of Blood Pressure for Adults

Category	*Systolic (mm Hg)*	*Diastolic (mm Hg)*
Hypotension	<90	<60
Normal	90–120	and 60–80
Pre-hypertension	120–139	or 81–89
Stage 1 Hypertension	140–159	or 90–99
Stage 2 Hypertension	≥160	or ≥100

Factors Affecting Blood Pressure

1. Cardiac output = Stroke volume × heart rate
2. *Starling effect:* Increased stretching of heart muscle leads to increased contraction.
3. *Sympathetic stimulation:* Causes an increase in heart rate, and in force of contraction.
4. *Parasympathetic stimulation:* Mainly decreases the heart rate and slight decrease in force.
5. *Peripheral resistance:* Particularly of the arterioles. Sympathetic nerves are extremely important in regulating blood pressure and thus blood flow. If these arteriole vessels constrict, then the outflow to the veins is temporarily reduced and thus MAP is increased, whilst if vessels dilate, MAP is decreased. Variations in the diameter of the arterioles of the abdominal (splanchnic) region are more effective than other areas in causing changes in MAP. The splanchnic vessels when fully dilated have an immense capacity to hold blood volume. Sudden strong emotion may cause their dilation, and thus a fall in MAP and may lead to fainting.
6. *Blood volume:* A sufficient amount is required to overfill the arterial system. Hemorrhage causes a decrease in blood volume and thus MAP falls. Atrial natriuretic peptide (ANP or ANF), released from the atria due to stretching of atria, can decrease blood volume in minutes, by action on the kidney to increase water loss, decrease sodium reabsorption, and also decrease release of ADH and renin/aldosterone. It also causes vasodilation of arteries and veins. Blood volume can be increased by the hormones renin, angiotensin II, aldosterone and ADH, which can thus raise blood pressure.
7. *Viscosity:* Blood is 5 times more viscous than water. Thus increased viscosity causes an increase in resistance to blood flow and thus increased work for the heart.
8. *Elasticity of the arterial walls:* Elasticity (and thus the recoil of the vessel walls) and the peripheral resistance (to prevent escape of too much blood to the venous system) are essential for the development of the diastolic pressure.

Vasomotor Center

The vasomotor center in the medulla of the brain is responsible for the overall control of blood distribution and pressure throughout the body.

Impulses from the vasomotor center are mostly in the sympathetic nervous system (exception—those to the genitalia) and mostly cause vasoconstriction (exception—the skeletal muscles and coronary arteries which are vasodilated).

Inputs to the vasomotor center are similar to those innervating the cardiac center—baroreceptors located throughout the body and the hypothalamus.

1. The baroreceptors allow maintenance of normal blood pressure.
2. The hypothalamus stimulates responses associated with exercise, emotions, "Fight or Flight", and thermoregulation.

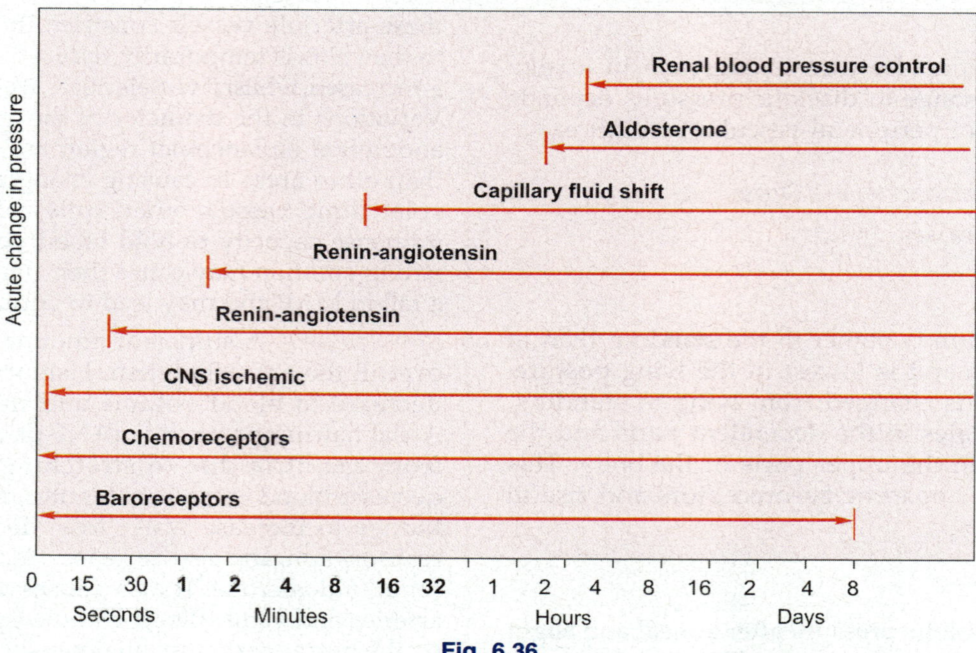

Fig. 6.36

6

Neurohumoral Mechanism Maintaining Blood Pressure (Fig. 6.36)

1. Rapidly acting pressure control mechanisms to return blood pressure to physiological levels. All are nervous mechanisms: Within seconds or minutes:
   a. Baroreceptor
   b. Chemoreceptor
   c. CNS ischemic response.
2. Intermediate mechanisms that acts in minutes or hours:
   a. Stress relaxation of vasculature
   b. Renin angiotensin vasoconstrictor mechanism
   c. Capillary fluid shift mechanism.
3. Long-term mechanisms for arterial pressure regulation; to return blood volume to normal levels. Essentially involves kidney control via several hormonal mechanisms: in takes days, months and years.
   a. Renal blood volume pressure control mechanism
   b. Aldosterone.

SHORT-TERM REGULATION OF MEAN ARTERIAL BLOOD PRESSURE

Baroreceptor Reflexes

Anatomy

1. Baroreceptors are especially abundant in the:
   a. Carotid sinuses (located in wall of ICA just above carotid bifurcation)
   b. Walls of the aortic arch
2. Impulses are transmitted from
   a. Carotid sinus via the glossopharyngeal nerve (CN-IX) to the medulla
   b. Aortic arch via the vagal nerve (CN-X) to the medulla.

Responses of Baroreceptors to Pressure (Fig. 6.37)

- <60 mm Hg see no stimulation of baroreceptors
- 60–160 mm Hg see maximum stimulation.
- See maximum $\frac{\Delta I}{\Delta P}$ at normal pressures (I = impulses)
- The baroreceptors respond much more to a rapidly changing pressure than to a stationary pressure.
- They adapt in 1–2 days to whatever pressure they are exposed to have no long-term effect in BP regulation.

Baroreceptor Reflex

1. Stimulated baroreceptors inhibit vasoconstrictor center of medulla:
   a. Vasodilation of peripheral vasculature.
   b. Decreased HR and contractility → reduced BP (low BP has an opposite effect).

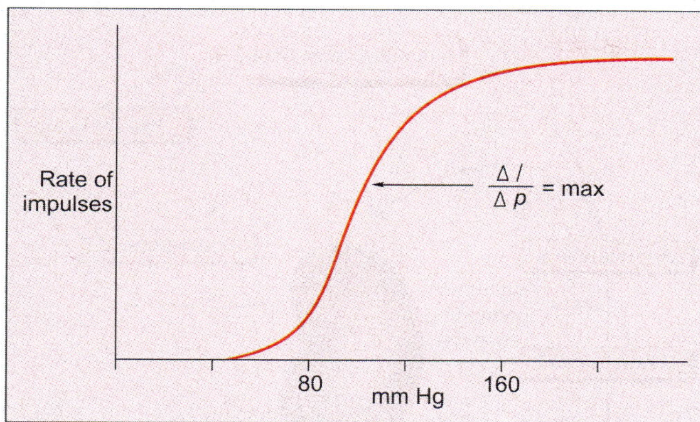

Fig. 6.37: Response of baroreceptors at different BP

2. Baroreceptors play a major role in maintaining BP during postural changes (Fig. 6.38).

Chemoreceptor Reflexes

Anatomy

1. Chemoreceptors are located in the:
   a. Carotid bodies (located in the carotid bifurcation)
   b. Aortic bodies in walls of the aortic arch.
2. Impulses are transmitted via the vagus (along with nerve fibers from baroreceptors) into the vasomotor center.
3. Each body has its own blood supply → each body is in close contact with arterial blood.

Chemoreceptor Reflex

- Primary reduced arterial BP → reduced O_2 increased CO_2 and H^+ → stimulate chemoreceptors → excite vasomotor center → increase BP (and increased respiratory stimulation).
- Primary reduced O_2; increased CO_2 and H^+ → stimulate chemoreceptors → excite vasomotor center → increase BP.
- Only works strongly with BP <80 mm Hg.

Atrial and Pulmonary Artery Reflexes

Anatomy

- Both the atria and pulmonary arteries have stretch receptors in their walls-low pressure receptors.
- Pulmonary artery receptors are similar to baroreceptors in operation. Atrial receptors operate as follows:

Atrial Reflexes

1. Stretched atria:
   a. Reflex dilatation of afferent arterioles of kidney because of release of ANP → increased urine production.
   b. Increased HR (Bainbridge reflex) → offload fluid from heart.

CNS Ischemic Response

- Reduced blood flow to vasomotor center in brainstem → ischemia of medulla → increased local (CO_2) → excite vasomotor center → increased BP
- It has a tremendous magnitude in increasing BP: It is one of the most powerful activators of the sympathetic vasoconstrictor system
- Only becomes active at arterial BP <50 mm Hg: 'last ditch stand'

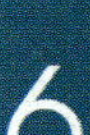

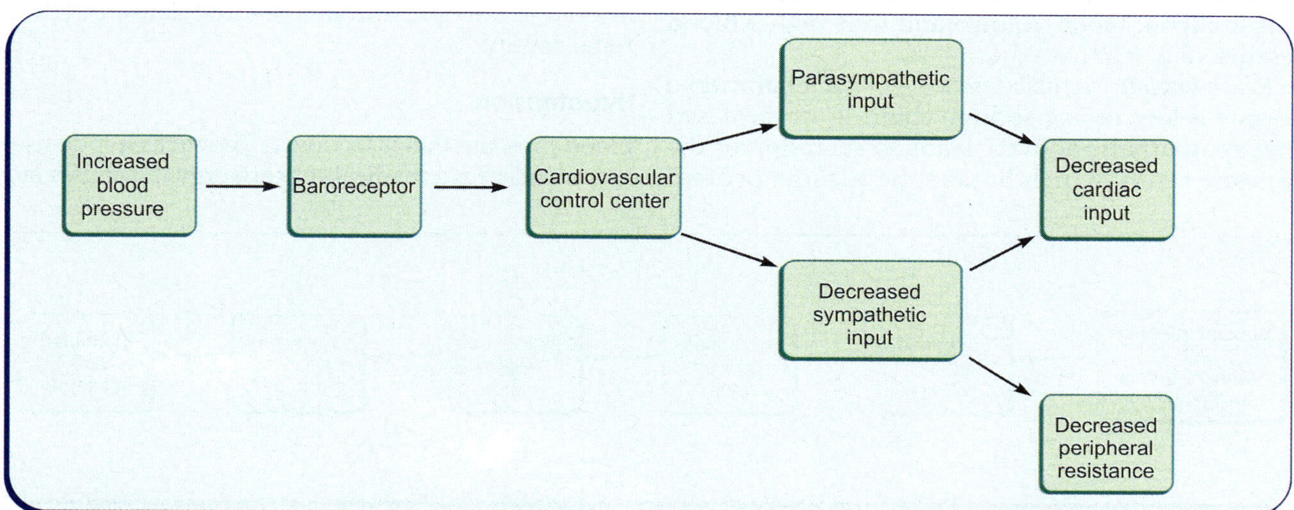

Fig. 6.38

- Cushing reaction: Increased intracranial pressure → compression of arteries in brain → CNS ischemic response → increased BP.

Intermediate Mechanism

i. *Stress relaxation of vasculature:* When the pressure in the blood vessels is too high, they become stretched and keep on stretching more and more results in decrease of pressure to normal. The continued stretch of the vessel causes stress relaxation of the vasculature.
ii. *Renin angiotensin vasoconstrictor mechanism:* At least 20 minutes are required before this system can become fully active.
iii. *Capillary fluid shift mechanism:* When the capillary pressure decreases, fluid is absorbed by osmosis from tissues to circulation. Conversely, when the capillary pressure increases, fluid escapes into the tissues from circulation.

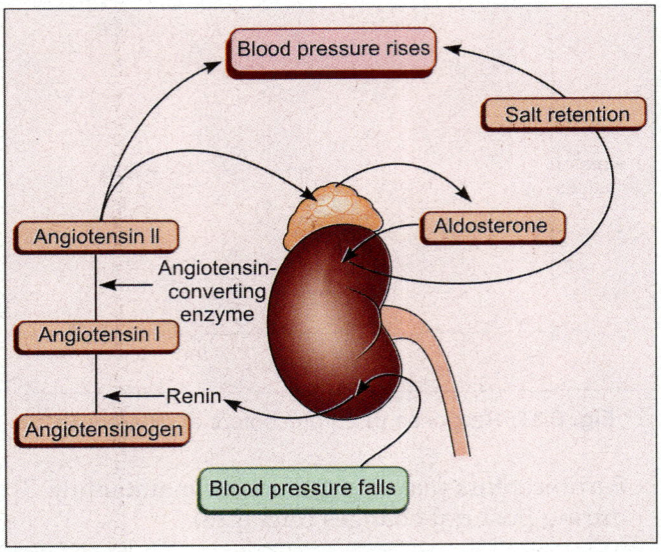

Fig. 6.40

Long-term Control

Blood volume is directly related to blood pressure. If the blood volume is increased then venous return of blood to the heart will increase, thus stroke volume will increase, thus cardiac output will increase and the blood pressure will rise. Therefore, blood pressure can be controlled by controlling blood volume.

Plasma, the liquid portion of blood, is part of the extracellular fluid (ECF). If the kidneys retain water, then the volume of the ECF rises and blood volume rises. If the kidneys retain salt (NaCl), then the ECF becomes saltier and thus capable of retaining more water (water follows solute). Higher ECF volume leads to higher blood volume and thus higher blood pressure (Fig. 6.39).

"*Renin-angiotensin-aldosterone system:* If renal arterial pressure is low, or low sodium chloride, or increased renal sympathetic activity leads to secretion of the hormone renin, which breaks the plasma protein angiotensinogen into angiotensin I and then angiotensin II. The latter is a powerful vasoconstrictor (half-life 30s), and also increases sodium reabsorption by proximal tubule, and stimulates the release of aldosterone (and cortisol) from adrenal cortex, which reabsorbs sodium and also stimulates ADH release (Fig. 6.40)".

Hypertension

Hypertension or high blood pressure is a medical condition wherein the blood pressure is chronically elevated. Persistent hypertension is one of the risk factors for strokes, heart attacks, heart failure and arterial aneurysm, and is a leading cause of chronic renal failure.

Hypotension

Blood pressure that is too low is known as hypotension. Hypotension is a medical concern only if it causes signs

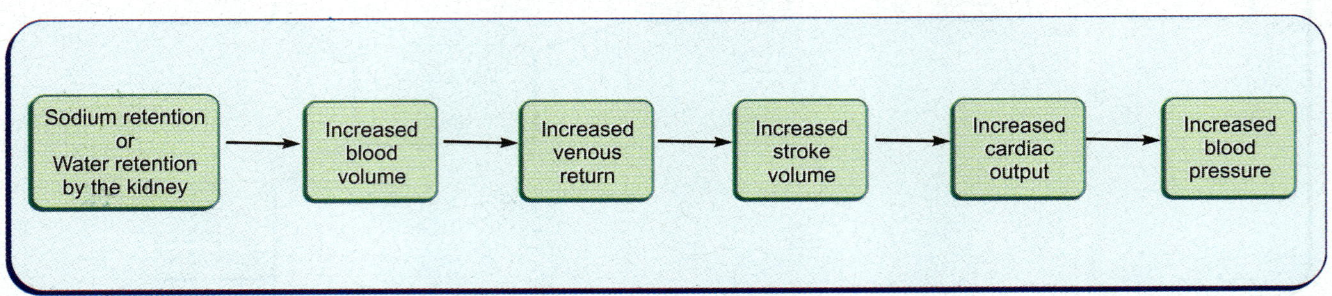

Fig. 6.39

or symptoms, such as dizziness, fainting, or in extreme cases, shock. When arterial pressure and blood flow decrease beyond a certain point, the perfusion of the brain becomes critically decreased (i.e. the blood supply is not sufficient), causing lightheadedness, dizziness, weakness or fainting.

Sometimes the arterial pressure drops significantly when a patient stands up from sitting. This is known as orthostatic hypotension (postural hypotension); gravity reduces the rate of blood return from the body veins below the heart back to the heart, thus reducing stroke volume and cardiac output.

When people are healthy, the veins below their heart quickly constrict and the heart rate increases to minimize and compensate for the gravity effect. This is carried out involuntarily by the autonomic nervous system. The system usually requires a few seconds to fully adjust and if the compensations are too slow or inadequate, the individual will suffer reduced blood flow to the brain, dizziness and potential blackout. Increases in G-loading, such as routinely experienced by aerobatic or combat pilots 'pulling Gs', greatly increases this effect. Repositioning the body perpendicular to gravity largely eliminates the problem.

Other causes of low arterial pressure include:
- Sepsis
- Hemorrhage: Blood loss
- Toxins including toxic doses of BP medicine
- Hormonal abnormalities, such as Addison's disease.

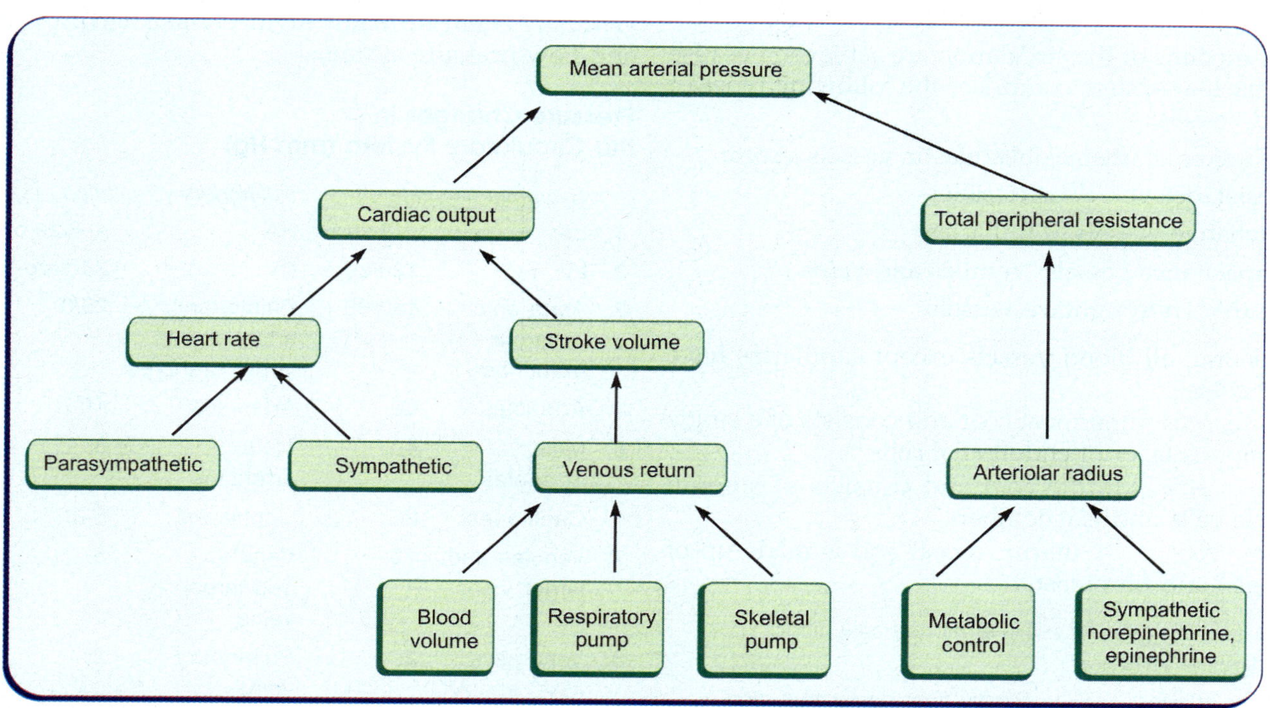

Fig. 6.41: Factors that affect mean arterial pressure

6

38. CIRCULATORY SYSTEM

Functions of the Circulation

1. To supply the tissues of the various organs with nutrient substances, hormones and immunological agents.
2. To remove waste products of tissue metabolism
3. Controls blood flow to the skin and limbs to regulate heat loss to environment.
4. Aids in body's defence mechanisms by delivering antibodies, platelets and leukocytes to affected areas of the body.

Organization of the Circulatory System

The functions of the circulation are achieved because the vascular system comprises the following types of blood vessels:

a. Windkessel/distensible/elastic vessels: Aorta
b. Resistance vessels: Arterioles
c. Exchange vessels: Capillaries
d. Capacitance vessels: Venules and veins
e. Shunt/Thoroughfare vessels.

In general, all blood vessels except capillaries have three coats:
Tunica intima: Innermost coat and consists of a single continuous layer of endothelial cells.
Tunica media: Middle coat and consists of smooth muscle cells and elastic fibers.
Tunica adventitia: Outermost coat and is made up of collagen and fibroblasts.

Aorta and big arteries (windkessel vessels)	Have more elastic fiber
Smaller arteries	Elastic fiber decreases, and smooth muscle increases
Arterioles (muscular arteries)	No elastic fibers, only smooth muscle
Capillaries	Single layer of endothelium and no media and adventitia
Veins	Thinner than arteries

Elastic property is low and also low smooth muscle content. Heart provides the pressure for the circulation, how? Blood flows from the heart to the periphery and then via the veins back to the heart only because of pressure gradient.

Pressure Changes in the Circulatory System

Blood enters the left atrium or right atrium at a pressure near 'zero' which rises to 7–8 mm Hg in left atrium and 4–6 mm Hg in right atrium during systole. Pressure changes in the arterial system (ventricles, aorta, pulmonary artery and their large branches) is pulsatile in nature, i.e. pressure rises to a peak value during systole and decreases to minimum during diastole. But, the pressure in the periphery is steady. This is due to the elastic recoil of the arterial system and resistance to blood flow offered by the arterioles.

Based on the pressure changes, the whole of the vascular system is broadly divided into: High pressure and Low pressure system.

Pressure Changes in the Circulatory System (mm Hg)

Systemic circulation		*Pulmonary circulation*	
1. LA	7–8/zero	RA	4–6/zero
2. LV	120/zero	RV	25/zero
3. Aorta and its larger branches	120/80	Pulmonary artery and its larger branches	25/8
4. Arterioles	60	Arterioles	10
5. Meta arterioles	40	Meta arterioles	8
6. Capillaries	25	Capillaries	6–8
7. Venules and larger veins	10	Venules and larger veins	5
8. Vena cava (SVC and IVC)	2	Pulmonary veins	2
High pressure		Low pressure	
High resistance		Low resistance	
Responsible for control of: • Systems arterial BP • Distribution of blood flow		Responsible for control of: • Blood volume • Venous return	

Aorta

The aorta is the largest of the arteries in the systemic circuit. The blood is pumped from the left ventricle into the aorta and from there it branches to all parts of the body. The aorta is an elastic artery, and as such is able to distend. When the left ventricle contracts to force blood into the aorta, the aorta expands (windkessel effect). This stretching gives the potential energy that will help maintain blood pressure during diastole, as during this time the aorta contracts passively.

Arteries

Arteries are muscular blood vessels that carry blood away from the heart. The pulmonary arteries will carry deoxygenated blood to the lungs and the systemic arteries will carry oxygenated blood to the rest of the body.

Arterioles

An arteriole is a small artery that extends and leads to capillaries.

Capillaries

Capillaries are the smallest of a body's vessels; they connect arteries and veins, and most closely interact with tissues.

Venules

A venule is a small vein that allows deoxygenated blood to return from the capillary beds to the larger blood veins, except in the pulmonary circuit where the blood is oxygenated.

Veins

Veins carry blood to the heart. The pulmonary veins will carry oxygenated blood to the heart while the systemic veins will carry deoxygenated to the heart. Most of the blood volume is found in the venous system. Most veins have one-way valves called venous valves to prevent backflow caused by gravity. They also have a thick collagen outer layer, which helps maintain blood pressure and stop blood pooling. If a person is standing still for long periods or is bedridden, blood can accumulates in veins and can cause varicose veins. Veins are used medically as points of access to the bloodstream, permitting the withdrawal of blood specimens (venipuncture) for testing purposes, and enabling the infusion of fluid, electrolytes, nutrition, and medications (intravenous delivery).

Superior Vena Cava

The superior vena cava (SVC) is a large but short vein that carries deoxygenated blood from the upper half of the body to the heart's right atrium.

Inferior Vena Cava

The inferior vena cava (IVC) is a large vein that carries deoxygenated blood from the lower half of the body into the heart.

Distribution of blood volume in the vascular system.

At rest, 64% of the circulating blood volume is in systemic veins.

7%	:	Heart
13%	:	Arteries
7%	:	Arterioles and capillaries
9%	:	Pulmonary circulation

39. THE BLOOD CIRCULATION

CORONARY CIRCULATION

Introduction

Coronary circulation is the circulation of blood in the blood vessels of the heart muscle (myocardium).

Normal coronary blood flow at rest is about 60–80 ml/100 gm/min (or) 250 ml/min blood supply.

In general there are two main coronary arteries, the left and right (Fig. 6.42):

- Right coronary artery
- Left coronary artery.

Both of these arteries originate from the beginning (root) of the aorta, immediately above the aortic valve. The left coronary artery originates from the left aortic sinus, while the right coronary artery originates from the right aortic sinus.

The right coronary artery branches to smaller arteries including the marginal, which leads down the margin or edge of the right ventricle. The main portion of the right coronary artery proceeds to the back of the heart becoming the posterior interventricular.

The left coronary artery divides to form the circumflex which curves to the back of the heart, and the anterior interventricular which descends between the two ventricles. The arteries anastomose to provide collateral circulation to the ventricular myocardium.

In 20% individuals	Myocardium is predominantly supply by LCA
50% supplied by	RCA
30% supplied by	Both equally

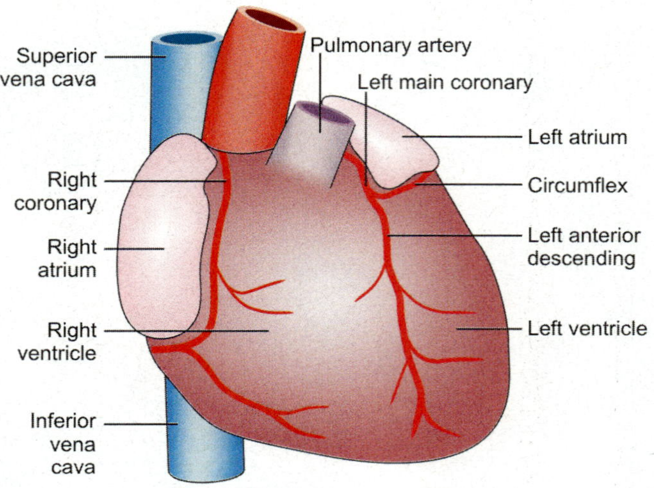

Fig. 6.42: Coronary arteries

Coronary veins drain the myocardium from the anterior interventricular area through the great cardiac (or coronary) vein, from the right atrial area through the small cardiac vein, and from the posterior interventricular area through the middle cardiac vein. All of these come together to form the coronary sinus which drains directly into the right atrium, the only systemic venous drainage not through the vena cavae. There are also anterior cardiac veins and thebesian veins drain directly into the cardiac chambers.

The left and right coronary arteries and their branches lie on the surface of the heart, and therefore, are sometimes referred to as the epicardial coronary vessels. These vessels distribute blood flow to different regions of the heart muscle. The arterioles branch into numerous capillaries that lie adjacent to the cardiac myocytes. A high capillary-to-cardiomyocyte ratio and short diffusion distances ensure adequate oxygen delivery to the myocytes and removal of metabolic waste products from the cells (e.g. CO_2 and H^+).

Measurements of Coronary Blood Flow

1. *Kety Method*

This method is based on Fick's principle.

Fick's principle: It states that the amount of a substance taken up by an organ (or by the whole body) per unit of time is equal to the arterial level of the substance minus the venous level (A–V difference) times the blood flow.

Amount of substance taken/min = (A–V difference) × blood flow/min

$$\text{Blood flow/min} = \frac{\text{Amt. of substance taken/min}}{\text{(A – V) difference of the substance}}$$

The subject inhales a mixture of air and an inert gas till the gas has distributed itself in tissues in accordance to partition coefficient. Arterial blood sample can be collected from any peripheral artery. Venous blood sample can be collected from any coronary sinus. Coronary blood flow is calculated as the ratio of the amount of the inert gas passing through the coronary arteries in unit time to the time—integrated average (A–V) gas con. difference. Inert gases suitable are N_2O radionucleotide, hydrogen and helium.

2. *Radionuclide Utilization Technique*

Radioactive tracers that can be detected with scintillation cameras over the chest have been used to study regional blood flow in the heart and to detect areas of ischemia and myocardial infarction.

A suitable radionuclide such as radioactive thallium (^{201}Th) is injected. Gamma cameras are placed in front of the (heart) chest for monitoring ^{201}Th uptake by the heart. The uptake proportional to blood flow. So areas of ischemia can be detected by their low uptake.

Conversely, radiopharmaceuticals, e.g. technitium 99m stannous pyrophosphate (^{99m}Tc-PYP) are selectively taken up by infarct tissue and make infarcts stand at as Hot Spots on scintiscans of the chest.

3. *Coronary Angiography*

This can be combined measurement of ^{133}Xe washout to provide detailed analysis of coronary blood flow. Radiopaque contrast medium is first injected into the coronary arteries, X-rays being used to outline their distribution. The angiographic camera is thus replaced with a multiple-crystal scintillation camera and ^{133}Xe wash out is measured.

4. *Direct Measurement*

Flow can be measured directly by placing an electromagnetic flow meter around a coronary artery. This method can be used in man only during open heart surgery.

Coronary Flow

The following summarizes important features of coronary blood flow:

- Flow is tightly coupled to oxygen demand. This is necessary because the heart has a very high basal oxygen consumption (8–10 ml O_2/min/100 g) and the highest A–VO_2 difference of a major organ (10–13 ml/100 ml). In nondiseased coronary vessels, whenever cardiac activity and oxygen consumption increases, there is an increase in coronary blood flow (active hyperemia) that is nearly proportionate to the increase in oxygen consumption.
- Good autoregulation between 60 and 200 mm Hg perfusion pressure helps to maintain normal coronary blood flow whenever coronary perfusion pressure changes due to changes in aortic pressure.
- Adenosine is an important mediator of active hyperemia and autoregulation. It serves as a metabolic coupler between oxygen consumption and coronary blood flow. Nitric oxide is also an important regulator of coronary blood flow.
- Activation of sympathetic nerves innervating the coronary vasculature causes only transient vasoconstriction mediated by α_1-adrenoceptors. This brief (and small) vasoconstrictor response is followed by vasodilation caused by enhanced production of vasodilator metabolites (active hyperemia) due to increased mechanical and metabolic activity of the heart resulting from β_1-adrenoceptor activation of the myocardium. Therefore, sympathetic activation to the heart results in coronary vasodilation and increased coronary flow due to increased metabolic activity (increased heart rate, contractility) despite direct vasoconstrictor effects of sympathetic activation on the coronaries. This is termed "functional sympatholysis."
- Parasympathetic stimulation of the heart, (i.e. vagal nerve activation) elicits modest coronary vasodilation (due to the direct effects of released acetylcholine on the coronaries). However, if parasympathetic activation of the heart results in a significant decrease in myocardial oxygen demand due to a reduction in heart rate, then intrinsic metabolic mechanisms will increase coronary vascular resistance by constricting the vessels.
- Progressive ischemic coronary artery disease results in the growth of new vessels (termed angiogenesis) and collateralization within the myocardium. Collateralization increases myocardial blood supply by increasing the number of parallel vessels, thereby reducing vascular resistance within the myocardium.

During contraction of the ventricular myocardium (systole), the subendocardial coronary vessels (the vessels that enter the myocardium) are compressed due to the high intraventricular pressures. However, the epicardial coronary vessels (the vessels that run along the outer surface of the heart) remain patent. Because of this, blood flow in the subendocardium stops. As a result most myocardial perfusion occurs during heart relaxation (diastole) when the subendocardial coronary vessels are patent and under low pressure (Fig. 6.43).

In the presence of coronary artery disease, coronary blood flow may be reduced. This will increase oxygen extraction from the coronary blood and decrease the venous oxygen content. This leads to tissue hypoxia and angina which is intense chest pain. Severe ischemia can cause the heart muscle to die from hypoxia, such as during a myocardial infarction.

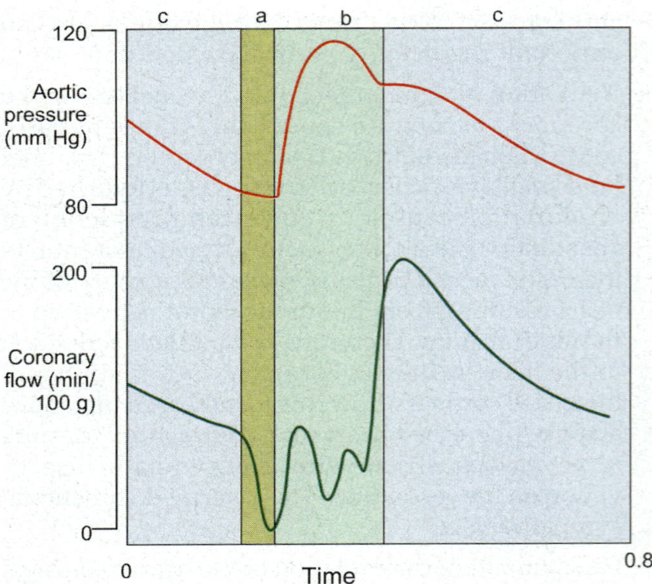

Fig. 6.43: Pulsatile nature of left coronary artery blood flow. Flow is lower during phases of isovolumetric contraction (a) and ejection (b) than during diastolic (c)

6

If the lack of blood flow is due to a fixed stenotic lesion in the coronary artery (because of atherosclerosis), blood flow can be improved within that vessel by:

1. Placing a stent within the vessel to expand the lumen
2. Using an intracoronary angioplasty balloon to stretch the vessel open
3. Bypassing the diseased vessel with a vascular graft. If the insufficient blood flow is caused by a blood clot (thrombosis), a thrombolytic drug that dissolves clots may be administered. Anti-platelet drugs and aspirin are commonly used to prevent the recurrence of clots.

If the reduced flow is due to coronary vasospasm, then coronary vasodilators can be given (e.g. nitrodilators, calcium channel blockers) to reverse and prevent vasospasm.

CEREBRAL CIRCULATION

Introduction

The brain, though representing 2% of the total body weight, it receives one-fifth of the resting cardiac output. The amount of blood that the cerebral circulation carries is known as cerebral blood flow.

Blood Supply

This blood supply is carried by the two internal carotid arteries (ICA) and the two vertebral arteries that anastomose at the base of the brain to form the circle of Willis.

Carotid arteries and their branches (referred to as the anterior circulation) supply the anterior portion of the brain while the vertebrobasilar system (referred to as posterior circulation) supplies the posterior portion of the brain.

Venous Drainage

Venous blood flows peripherally via superficial cerebral veins and centrally via the deep cerebral veins into the venous sinuses which drain into the internal jugular vein. The cerebral veins are thin-walled and have no valves. There are numerous venous connections between cerebral veins and dural sinuses and venous systems of the meninges, skull, scalp and nasal sinuses so facilitating propagation of thrombus or spread of infection between these vessels.

General Features

1. Adult brain weighs 1400 gm (2% of body weight), 60% is composed of white matter, 40% is composed of grey matter.
2. Cerebral blood flow is 750 ml/min or 50–60 ml/min/100 gm.
3. Cerebral O_2 consumption is 3.3 ml/min/100 g. Since grey matter consists of cell bodies, O_2 consumption is more here, i.e. 3 ml/min/100 gm white matter consists of only axons and so O_2 consumption is less, about 0.3 ml/min/100 gm.
4. Total O_2 consumption is 42–49 ml/min, which is nearly 17–20% of the total O_2 consumption of the body (250 ml).
5. Brain tissue is highly susceptible to O_2 lack. Sudden cessation of O_2 supply or blood flow to the brain results in loss of consciousness within 10 sec and deprivation of O_2 for 3–4 min results in irreversible brain damage. Minimum level of blood flow is essential for maintaining brain function. Critical blood flow level is approximately 18 ml/min/100 gm, i.e. flow less than this level causes unconsciousness.
6. Glucose is the chief source of energy for the brain. Hence, hypoglycemia also leads to damage of the brain tissue.
7. Cranium contains the brain (1400 gm), blood (75 ml) and CSF (75 ml). All these three are incompressible because of rigid cranium. Hence, the contents of the cranial cavity remains constant. This is known as Monro-Kellie doctrine.

Regulation of Cerebral Blood Flow

CBF is tightly regulated to meet the brain's metabolic demands. Too much blood (a condition known as hyperemia) can raise intracranial pressure (ICP), which can compress and damage delicate brain tissue. Too little blood flow (ischemia) results if blood flow to the brain is below 18 to 20 ml per 100 g per minute, and tissue death occurs if flow dips below 8 to 10 ml per 100 g per minute.

CBF is equal to the cerebral perfusion pressure (CPP) divided by the cerebrovascular resistance (CVR): CBF = CPP/CVR.

Control of CBF is considered in terms of the factors affecting CPP and the factors affecting CVR.

1. *Cerebral Perfusion Pressure or CPP*

CPP is the net pressure gradient causing blood flow to the brain (brain perfusion). It is defined as the difference between mean arterial and intracranial pressures.

$$CPP = MAP - ICP$$

Under normal circumstances cerebral blood flow is relatively constant due to protective autoregulation. (MAP between 60 to 150 mm Hg and ICP about 10 mm Hg).

Outside of the limits of autoregulation, raising MAP raises CPP and raising ICP lowers it (this is one reason that increasing ICP in traumatic brain injury is potentially deadly). CPP is normally between 70 and 90 mm Hg in an adult human, and cannot go below 70 mm Hg for a sustained period without causing ischemic brain damage.

2. *Cerebrovascular Resistance*

Cerebrovascular resistance can be modulated by local-chemical and endothelial factors, by autacoids, and by release of transmitters from perivascular nerves.

a. *Local-chemical* factors such as H^+, K^+, CO_2, adenosine, and osmolarity are involved in the regulation of cerebrovascular resistance during cortical activation and under pathological conditions such as hypoxia or ischemia. They cause vasodilation of cerebral vessels.

b. *Endothelial factors* such as thromboxane A2, endothelin (ET), endothelium derived constrictor factor and endothelium derived relaxing [EDRF, identified as nitric oxide (NO)] or hyperpolarizing (EDHF) factor, and prostacyclin (PGI_2), can be released by physical stimuli such as shear stress or hemorrhage, by autacoids, by neurotransmitters, and by cytokines. Several of these factors (NO, PGI_2, ET) can also be released from neurons and astrocytes thus enabling a coupling between parenchymal function and flow.

c. Autacoids like histamine, bradykinin, eicosanoids, and free radicals influence cerebrovascular resistance, capacitance vessels and the permeability of the blood-brain barrier under pathological conditions. They are released by trauma, ischemia, seizures and inflammation and causes vasodilation.

d. *Neural control:* Cerebral arteries are innervated by several systems. The sympathetic-noradrenergic fibers originate from the superior cervical ganglion. By releasing the constricting transmitters norepinephrine and neuropeptide Y, this system extends the range of autoregulation. The parasympathetic cholinergic system with the dilating transmitters acetylcholine and vasoactive intestinal polypeptide may prevent ischemia.

Measurement

1945 Kety and Schmidt described a method of quantifying cerebral blood flow in humans, based on the Fick principle, that utilized nitrous oxide, a metabolically inert and highly lipid-soluble gas, as the tracer of blood flow.

A major advance toward the broad clinical application of cerebral blood flow measurement came with the substitution of radiolabeled ^{85}Kr for nitrous oxide and scintillation counting as the direct measure of tracer movement within the tissue. The latter measure being substituted for the difference of the arterial and venous concentrations of the tracer. This approach provided a regionality of blood flow determination that was lacking in the global blood flow measures provided by nitrous oxide.

In recent years most centers have turned to intravenous bolus introduction of ^{133}Xe as a simpler means of delivering the tracer.

Single photon emission computed tomography (SPECT) imaging system for ^{133}Xe. SPECT CBF derived with radiolabeled isotopes today provide relatively high-resolution three-dimensional qualitative CBF imaging.

Diffusion imaging with magnetic resonance imaging provides information concerning the presence or absence of blood movement.

Direct monitoring of cortical blood flow is available today utilizing either thermal dilution or laser Doppler technologies.

MICROCIRCULATION

Structure

The microcirculation is a term used to describe the small vessels in the vasculature which are embedded within organs and are responsible for the distribution of blood within tissues.

The vessels on the arterial side of the microcirculation are called the arterioles. Arterioles carry the blood to the capillaries. Blood flows out of the capillaries into the venules. The blood flows from venules into the veins. In addition to these blood vessels, the microcirculation also includes lymphatic capillaries and collecting ducts.

Arterioles

- Small precapillary resistance vessels (10–50 μ) composed of an endothelium surrounded by one or more layers of smooth muscle cells.
- The endothelium provides a smooth surface for the flow of blood and regulates the movement of water and dissolved materials in the plasma between the blood and the tissues.
- The endothelium also produce molecules that discourage the blood from clotting unless there is a leak.
- The smooth muscle cells can contract and decrease the size of the arterioles and thereby regulate blood flow and blood pressure.
- Richly innervated by sympathetic adrenergic fibers and highly responsive to sympathetic vasoconstriction via both α_1 and α_2 postjunctional receptors.
- Represent a major site for regulating systemic vascular resistance.
- Primary function within an organ is flow regulation, thereby determining oxygen delivery and the washout of metabolic byproducts.
- Regulate, in part, capillary hydrostatic pressure and therefore influence capillary fluid exchange.

Capillaries

- Small exchange vessels (6–10 μ) composed of highly attenuated (very thin) endothelial cells surrounded by basement membrane. There is no smooth muscle.
- This layer is so thin that molecules such as oxygen, water and lipids can pass through them by diffusion and enter the tissues. Waste products such as carbon dioxide and urea can diffuse back into the blood to be carried away for removal from the body.
- They are very prevalent in the body; total surface area is about 6,300 square meters. Because of this, no cell is very far from a capillary, no more than 50 micrometers away.
- The "capillary bed" is the network of capillaries present throughout the body. These beds are able to be "opened" and "closed" at any given time, according to need. This process is called autoregulation and capillary beds usually carry no more than 25% of the amount of blood it could hold at any time. The more metabolically active the cells, the more capillaries it will require to supply nutrients.

Three structural classifications (Fig. 6.44).

Continuous (Nonfenestrated)

- Found in muscle, skin, lung, central nervous system
- Basement membrane is continuous and intercellular clefts are tight (i.e. have tight junctions); these capillaries have the lowest permeability.

Fenestrated

- Found in exocrine glands, renal glomeruli, intestinal mucosa.
- Perforations (fenestrae) in endothelium result in relatively high permeability.

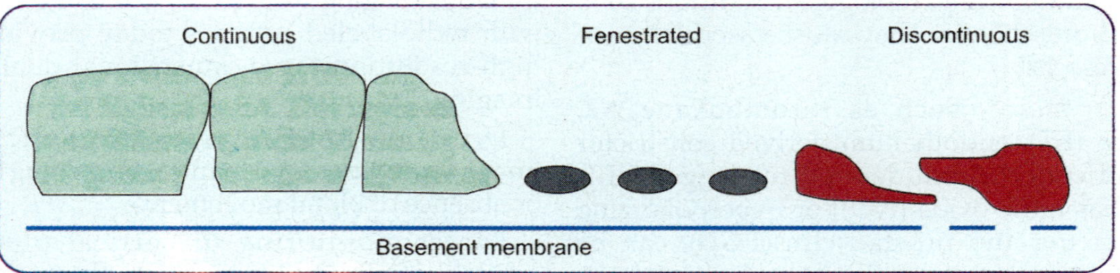

Fig. 6.44: Three structural classifications

Sinusoidal (Discontinuous)

- Found in liver, spleen, bone marrow
- Large intercellular gaps and gaps in basement membrane result in extremely high permeability.

Venules (Fig. 6.45)

- Small vessels (10–50 μ) composed of endothelial cells surrounded by basement membrane (smallest postcapillary venules) and smooth muscle (larger venules).
- Fluid and macromolecular exchange occur most prominently at venular junctions.
- Sympathetic innervation of larger venules can alter venular tone which plays role in regulating capillary hydrostatic pressure.

Terminal Lymphatics

- Composed of endothelium with intercellular gaps surrounded by highly permeable basement membrane and are similar in size to venules: terminal lymphatics end as blind sacs.
- Larger lymphatics also have smooth muscle cells.
- Spontaneous and stretch-activated vasomotion is present which serves to "pump" lymph.
- Sympathetic nerves can modulate vasomotion and cause contraction.
- One-way valves direct lymph away from the tissue and eventually back into the systemic circulation via the thoracic duct and subclavian veins (2–4 liters/day returned).

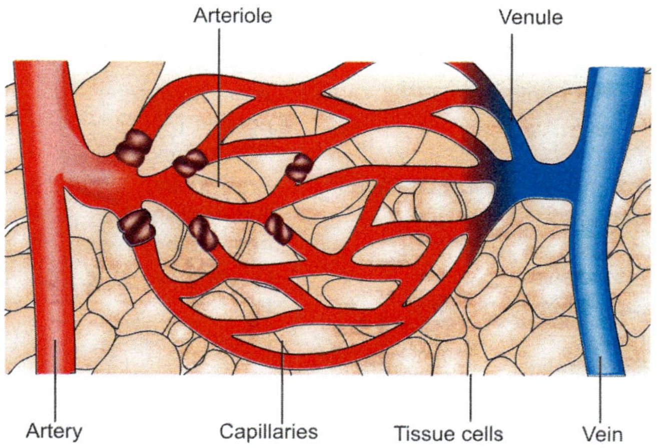

Fig. 6.45: Capillaries, arterioles and venules

Functions

The main functions of the microcirculation include the:

1. Regulation of blood flow and tissue perfusion. Flow is determined by the diameter and the length of the vessels of the microcirculation. The Hagen-Poiseuille equation predicts the flow of blood through the vessels.
2. Regulation of blood pressure, by capillary fluid shift mechanism.
3. Regulation of tissue fluid (swelling or edema), by capillary exchange of water. The starling equation is an equation that describes the roles of hydrostatic and oncotic forces (the so-called Starling forces) in the movement of fluid across capillary endothelium.
4. Delivery of oxygen and other nutrients and removal of CO_2 and other metabolic waste products, by capillary exchange of solutes. Small solutes move across the endothelium by passing through the spaces formed by the tight junctions formed where the edges of adjacent endothelial cells abut.
5. Regulation of body temperature. Triple response (of Lewis): It is a physiological reaction of the skin to stroking with a blunt instrument: first a red line develops at the site of stroking, due to capillary dilatation because of release of histamine or a histamine-like substance, then a flare develops, i.e. redness in the surrounding area due to arteriolar dilatation mediated by axon reflex, and lastly a wheal is formed as a result of exudation of fluid from capillaries and venules.

PULMONARY CIRCULATION

Physiologic Anatomy of the Pulmonary Circulatory System

The quantity of blood flowing through the lungs is essentially equal to that flowing through the systemic circulation.

Pulmonary Vessels

The pulmonary trunk extends only 5 cm beyond the apex of the right ventricle and then divides into the right and left main branches, which supply blood to the two respective lungs. The pulmonary artery is also thin with a wall thickness one-third that of the aorta. The pulmonary arterial branches are all very short. However, all the pulmonary arteries, smaller arteries and arterioles have larger diameter than their counterpart systemic arteries. Pulmonary arterioles subdivide to form network of pulmonary capillaries which surrounds the alveoli and are sandwiched between their walls. Alveoli are kept in a basket of capillaries.

Effective wall surface area at rest is 60 m^2 and transit time across the capillaries is 0.8 sec. During heavy exercise, it increases to 90 m^2. Pulmonary venules and veins receive oxygenated blood from the capillaries; they join to form 4 main veins which finally open into the left atrium.

The pulmonary veins like the pulmonary arteries are short but their distensibility characteristics are similar to those of the veins in the systemic circulation.

Bronchial Vessels

Blood also flows to the lungs through several bronchial arteries, amounting to about 1–2% of cardiac output. This bronchial arterial blood is oxygenated blood. It supplies the supporting tissues of the lungs, including the connective tissue, septa and large and small bronchi. From this, deoxygenated blood enters into the pulmonary veins and enters the left atrium, rather than passing back to the right atrium.

Therefore, the flow into the left atrium and left ventricular output are about 1–2% greater than the right ventricular output.

6

Lymphatics

Lymphatics extend from all the supportive tissue of the lung, beginning in the connective tissue spaces that surrounded the terminal bronchioles and coursing to the hilum of the lung and hence mainly into the right lymphatic duct. Particulate matter entering the alveoli is partly removed by way of these channels, and plasma protein leaking from the lung capillaries is also removed from the lung tissue, thereby helping to prevent edema.

Pressures in the Pulmonary System

Right ventricle	25/0 mm Hg
Pulmonary artery	25/8 mm Hg
Pulmonary capillary	7 mm Hg
Left atrium	1–5 mm Hg

Blood Volume of the Lungs

The blood volume of the lungs is about 450 ml (9% of cardiac output)

70 ml	Capillaries
190 ml	Arteries
190 ml	Veins

Lungs acts as a blood reservoir. During emergency, there is shift of blood from lungs into systemic vessels.

Blood Flow through the Lungs and its Distribution

Factors Affecting Pulmonary Circulation

1. The blood flow through the lungs is equal to cardiac output.
2. Therefore, the factors that control cardiac output, mainly peripheral factors also control pulmonary blood flow.
3. Under most conditions, the pulmonary vessels act as passive, distensible tubes that enlarge with increase in pressure and narrow with decrease in pressure.
4. For adequate aeration of the blood, it is important for the blood to be distributed to those segments of the lungs where the alveoli are best oxygenated. Hypoxia causes vasoconstriction. So, there is shift of blood flow to better aerated area of the lungs which provides automatic control system for distributing blood flow to the different pulmonary areas in proportion to their degree of ventilation.
5. Autonomic nervous control of blood flow in the lungs.

   Stimulation of sympathetic nerves: Slight increase in pulmonary vascular resistance. Stimulation of vagus: Slight decrease in pulmonary vascular resistance.

   Stimulation of sympathetic nerves causes constriction of large pulmonary capacitance vessel (veins) which causes displacement of blood from lungs to other segments where it is needed to combat low pressure.
6. Chemicals

Constrictors	Dilators
Hypoxia	Adenosine
Hypercapnia	Atrial natriuretic peptide (ANP)
TXA_2	ACh (acetylcholine)
Adrenergic catecholamines	Bradykinin
Histamine	Beta-adrenergic catecholamines
Angiotensin	Dopamine
Serotonin	PGI
PGE_2	NO
Endothelin	
Vasopressin	

7. *Effect of exercise:* During heavy exercise, the blood flow through the lungs increases 4 to 7 fold.

This extra flow is accommodated in the lungs in three ways:

1. By increasing the number of open capillaries: recruitment
2. By distending all the capillaries—distension
3. By increasing pulmonary arterial pressure.

In the normal person, the first 2 changes together decrease the pulmonary vascular resistance so much that the pulmonary arterial pressure rises very little even during maximum exercise.

Blood Flow

Blood flow through the lungs depends upon the relationship between the pulmonary arterial pressure, pulmonary venous pressure and alveolar pressure.

The difference between the pulmonary arterial and pulmonary venous pressure is the driving pressure (force).

Secondly, pulmonary capillary pressure must be above the alveolar pressure for the blood flow to continue.

Gravity affect the regional distribution of blood flow through the lungs by altering the pulmonary vascular pressure.

Regional Blood Flow: Zone 1, 2 and 3 of Pulmonary Blood Flow

The capillaries in the alveolar walls are distended by the pressure inside them, but simultaneously, they are compressed by the alveolar pressure on their outside. Under different normal and pathological lung conditions, one may find any one of three possible zones of pulmonary blood flow as follows:

Zone 1: No blood flow during any part of the cardiac cycle because local capillary pressure in that area of the lung never rises higher than the alveolar pressure during any part of the cardiac cycle.

Zone 2: Intermittent blood flow only during the pulmonary arterial pressure peaks because the systolic pressure is greater than the alveolar pressure but the diastolic pressure is less than alveolar pressure.

Zone 3: Continuous blood flow: because the capillary pressure remains greater than alveolar pressure during the entire cardiac cycle.

Normally, the lungs have only Zone 2 (apex) and Zone 3 (base) blood flow.

When a person is in upright position, the pulmonary arterial pressure at the lung apex is about 15 mm Hg less than the pressure at heart level. Therefore, apical systole pressure is only 10 mm Hg, i.e. 25 mm Hg at heart level – 15 mm Hg pressure difference.

This is more than zero alveolar pressure so that blood flows through the pulmonary apical blood vessels during systole.

On the other hand, during diastole, pulmonary arterial pressure is 8 mm Hg – 15 mm Hg = 7 mm Hg. So, no blood flow during diastole. Zone 2 extends from the level of lungs which is 10 cm above the level of the heart to the top.

In the lower regions of the lungs, from about 10 cm above the level of the heart to the bottom, the pulmonary arterial pressure during both systole and diastole remain more than zero alveolar pressure. Therefore, there is continuous flow. Also, when a person is in a lying position, no part of the lung is more than a few cm above the level of the heart. Blood flow then in a normal person is entirely Zone 3 in lying position.

Zone 1 blood flow occurs only under abnormal conditions, i.e. when alveolar pressure is too high or capillary pressure is too low. For example (Fig. 6.46):

1. If an upright person is breathing against a positive air pressure so that intra-alveolar pressure is atleast 10 mm Hg more than normal, but the pulmonary capillary pressure is normal—zone 1 blood flow.
2. In hypovolemic states, pulmonary capillary pressure is too low—zone 1 blood flow.

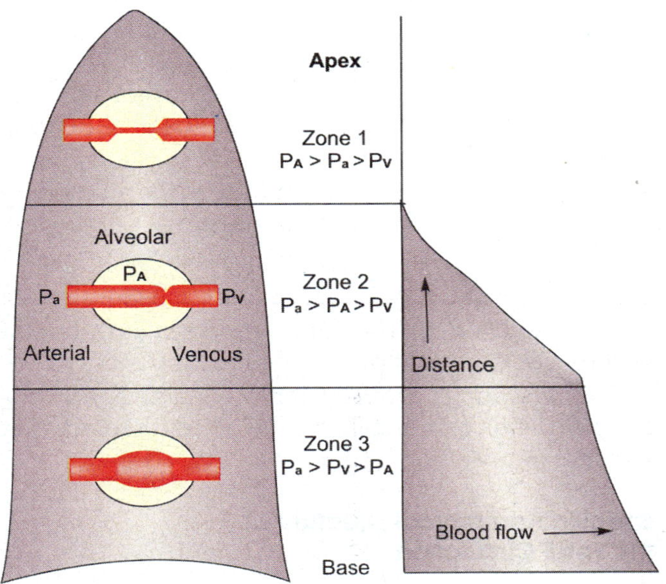

Fig. 6.46

6

Measurement

Regional blood flow through the lungs has been assessed by using radioactive gases. In one method, a person take a single breath of 15 CO_2, and holds the breath for 15 secs. Scintillation counters are placed in pairs at the front and back of the chest. The initial rise in radioactivity is due to the distribution of gas by ventilation (the greater the rise, better the ventilation in the region). The latter fall in radioactivity is due to removal of the gas by blood. Faster the fall in a region of the lung, higher the blood flow through the region.

Alternatively, radioactive xenon (^{133}Xe) may be dissolved in saline and injected into the superior vena cava. It soon travels to the pulmonary blood vessels. If counters are placed around the chest the relative distribution of radioactivity in different regions of the chest can be assessed. Greater the concentration of radioactivity in a region, higher the blood flow through the region. Both the radioactive CO_2 and ^{133}Xe methods have shown the blood flow to be higher at the base than at the apical region of the lungs.

6

Pulmonary Vascular Reflexes

1. Stimulation of baroreceptor causes reflex dilatation of pulmonary vessels. While stimulation of chemoreceptor causes reflex pulmonary vasoconstriction.
2. In pulmonary trunk and its main branches, vagal mechanoreceptors are present. Therefore, increase in pulmonary arterial pressure leads to bradycardia and hypotension.
3. Stimulation of vagal mechanoreceptors at the junction of pulmonary vein with left atrium produces tachycardia and diuresis which helps in regulating blood volume.
4. Stimulation of vagal nerve endings in the pulmonary small vessels produces tachypnea.

FETAL CIRCULATION

The circulation of the fetus shows a number of differences from that of the postnatal infant.

The fetal lungs are functionally inactive, and the fetus depends completely on the placenta for O_2 and nutrient supply.

Specific Anatomical Structure of the Fetal Circulation

Oxygenated blood from the placenta passes through the umbilical vein to the liver. A minor fraction passes through the liver and a major fraction bypasses the liver to the inferior vena cava through the ductus venous. In the inferior vena cava, blood from the ductus venosus joins blood returning from the lower trunk and extremities; this combined stream is in turn joined by blood from the liver through the hepatic veins. The streams of blood maintain their identity in the inferior vena cava and are divided into 2 streams of unequal size by the edge of the interatrial septum.

The larger stream, which is mainly blood from the umbilical vein, is shunted to LA through foramen ovale.

The other stream passes into right atrium, where it is joined by superior vena caval blood returning from the upper parts of the body and by blood from myocardium.

In contrast to the adult, in whom the right and left ventricles pump in series; in fetus the ventricles operate in parallel.

Because of the large pulmonary resistance, less than 1/3rd of right ventricle output goes through the lungs. The remainder passes through the ductus arteriosus from the pulmonary artery to the aorta at a point distal to the origin of the arteries to the head and upper extremities. Flow from pulmonary artery to aorta occurs because pulmonary arterial pressure is 5 mm Hg higher than that of aorta.

The large volume of blood coming through foramen ovale into left atrium is joined by blood returning from the lungs and is pumped out by left ventricle into the aorta.

About 1/3rd of aortic blood goes to the head, upper thorax and arms; remaining 2/3rds go to the rest of the body and the placenta (via 2 umbilical arteries).

- Fetal blood leaving the placenta is 80% saturated, but the saturation of the blood passing through the foramen ovale is reduced to 67% by mixing with desaturated blood returning from the lower part of the body and the liver. Addition of the desatura-ted blood from the lungs reduces the O_2 saturation of left ventricular blood to 62%, which is the level of saturation of the blood reaching the head and upper extremities.

The blood in the right ventricle, a mixture of desaturated superior vena caval blood, coronary venous blood, and inferior vena caval blood, is only 52% saturated with O_2. when the major portion of the blood traverses the ductus arteriosus and joins that pumped by the left ventricle, the resultant O_2 saturation of blood traveling to the lower part of the body and back to the placenta is 58% saturated.

Thus, it is apparent that the tissue receiving blood of the highest O_2 saturation are the liver, heart and upper parts of the body, including the head.

At the placenta, the chorionic villi dip into the maternal sinuses, and O_2, CO_2, nutrients, and metabolic waste products exchange across the membranes. The barrier to exchange is quite large, and the equilibrium of O_2 tension between the two circulations is not reached at normal rate of blood flow. Therefore, the O_2 tension of the fetal blood leaving the placenta is very low.

Since, the fetal hemoglobin has higher O_2 affinity, oxygen dissociation curve is shifted to the left.

Changer in the Fetal Circulation at Birth

1. Primary changes in pulmonary and systemic vascular resistance at birth
2. Closure of the foramen ovale
3. Closure of the ductus arteriosus
4. Closure of the ductus venosus.

Primary Changes in Pulmonary and Systemic Vascular Resistance

First, loss of the tremendous blood flow through the placenta, approximately doubles the systemic vascular resistance at birth. This increases the aortic pressure as well as the pressure in the left ventricle and left atrium.

Second, the pulmonary vascular resistance greatly decreases as a result of expansion of the lungs. In the unexpanded fetal lungs, the blood vessels had been compressed because of the small volume of the lungs. Immediately on expansion, these vessels are no longer compressed and the resistance to blood flow decreases several fold. Also in fetal life, the hypoxia of the lungs causes considerable tonic vasoconstriction of the lung blood vessels, but vasodilatation takes place when aeration of the lungs eliminates the hypoxia. All these changes together reduce the resistance to blood flow through the lungs as much as five-fold, which reduces the pulmonary arterial pressure, right ventricular and right atrial pressure.

Closure of the Foramen Ovale

The low right atrial pressure and the high left atrial pressure that occur secondarily to the changes in pulmonary and systemic resistances at birth cause blood now to attempt to flow backward through the foramen ovale, i.e. from left atrium into right atrium. Consequently, the small valve that lies over the foramen ovale on the left side of the atrial septum closes over this opening, thereby preventing further flow through the foramen ovale.

In 2/3rds, the valve becomes adherent over the foramen ovale within a few months to a few years and forms a permanent closure. But even if permanent closure does not occur, the left atrial pressure throughout life remains 2–4 mm Hg more than the right atrial pressure and the back pressure keeps the valve closed.

Closure of the Ductus Arteriosus

First, increased systemic resistance elevates aortic pressure; while decreased pulmonary vascular resistance reduces pulmonary arterial pressure.

As a consequence, afterbirth, blood begins to flow backward from the aorta into pulmonary artery through ductus arteriosus. However, after only a few hours the muscle wall of the ductus arteriosus constricts markedly and within 1–8 days, the constriction is usually sufficient to stop all blood flow. This is called functional closure of the ductus arteriosus. Then, during the next 1–4 months the ductus arteriosus ordinarily becomes anatomically occluded by growth of fibrous tissue into its lumen.

The cause of closure is due to increased oxygenation of the blood flowing through the ductus.

In fetal life PO_2	15–20 mm Hg
After birth	100 mm Hg

The degree of contraction of the smooth muscle in the ductus wall is highly related to the availability of O_2.

Bradykinin constrict umbilical vessels and ductus arteriosus while dilating the pulmonary vascular bed. Failure of closure leads to patent ductus arteriosus.

In some instance, cause may be due to the effect of prostaglandins—vasodilatation. The treatment is Indomethacin (prostaglandin inhibitor).

Closure of the Ductus Venosus

In fetal life, the portal blood from the fetus's abdomen joins the blood from the umbilical vein, and then together pass through the ductus venosus directly into the vena cava, thus bypassing the liver. Immediately afterbirth, blood flow through the umbilical vein ceases, but most of the portal blood still flows through the ductus venosus, with only a small amount passing through the channels of the liver. However, within 1–3 hours, the muscle wall of ductus venosus contract strongly and closes this venue of flow. So, portal venous pressure rise from '0' to 6–10 mm Hg, which is enough to force blood flow through the liver sinuses.

Closure of ductus arteriosus before birth causes pulmonary hypertension.

Special Features (Fig. 6.47)

1. All the blood is eventually transferred from the right heart to the aorta, as in the adult. But unlike the adult, it takes three routes to do so. The adult route (via lungs) is taken by only about 13% of right atrial blood. Other 2 unique routes are foramen ovale and ductus arteriosus. They close soon after birth.
2. The aortic flow is distributed to the whole body as in the adult. But a unique artery arising from fetal aorta is umbilical artery which carries blood to placenta. After improving to O_2 content in the placenta, the blood returns to the fetus through the umbilical vein. Thus, the placenta acts like the lungs of the adult. It also acts like the gut and kidneys in the sense that it adds nutrients to and also removes waste products from the fetal blood.

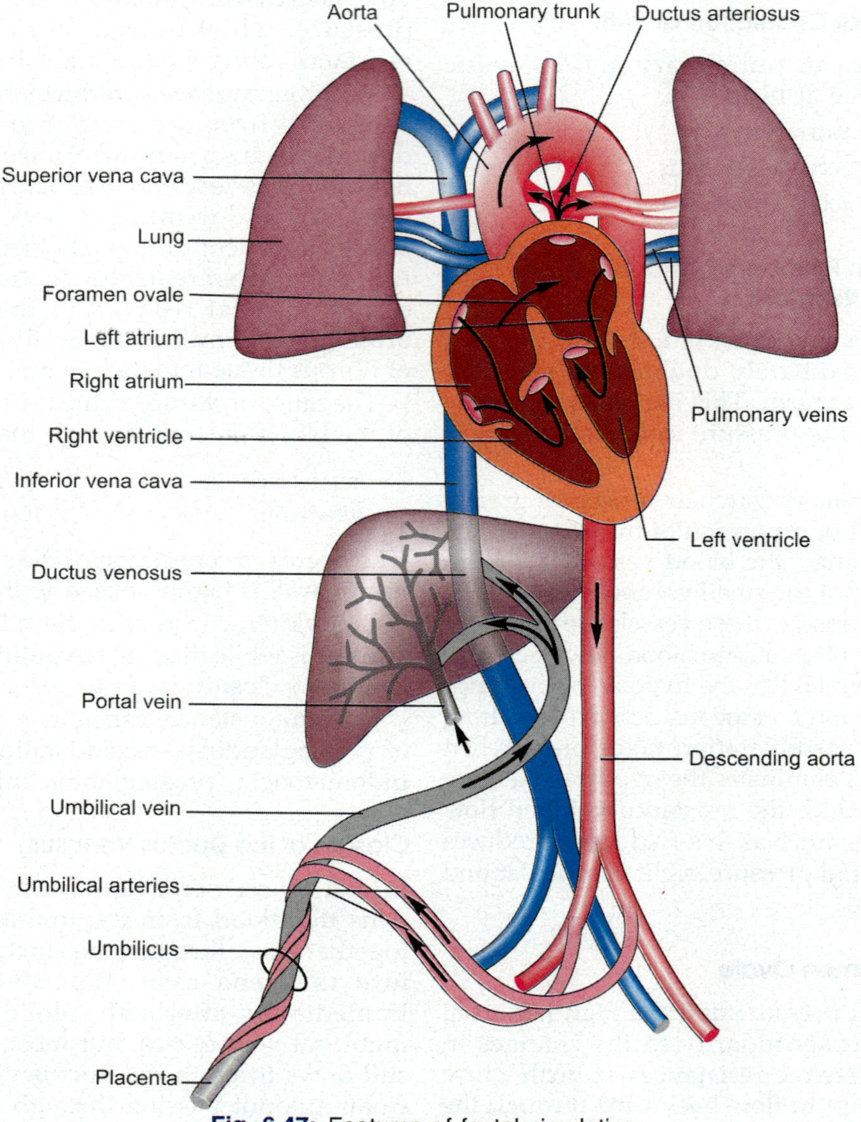

Fig. 6.47: Features of foetal circulation

SPLANCHNIC CIRCULATION

The splanchnic circulation is composed of gastric, small intestinal, colonic, pancreatic, hepatic, and splenic circulations, arranged in parallel with one another. It receives about 1500 ml of blood at rest (30% of cardiac output).

The three major arteries that supply the splanchnic organs are celiac, superior and inferior mesenteric, which give rise to smaller arteries that anastomose extensively:

i. Celiac artery supplies 200 ml to stomach and spleen and 500 ml to liver via hepatic artery.
ii. Superior mesenteric artery supplies 500 ml to pancreas, small intestine and parts of colon.
iii. Inferior mesenteric artery supplies 300 ml to colon.

The Hepatic Vascular System (Fig. 6.48)

The circulatory system of the liver is unlike that seen in any other organ. Of great importance is the fact that a majority of the liver's blood supply is venous blood!

The pattern of blood flow in the liver can be summarized as follows:

1. Roughly 75% of the blood entering the liver is venous blood from the portal vein. Importantly, all of the venous blood returning from the small intestine, stomach, pancreas and spleen converges into the portal vein. One consequence of this is that the liver gets "first pickings" of everything absorbed in the small intestine, which, as we will see, is where virtually all nutrients are absorbed.
2. The remaining 25% of the blood supply to the liver is arterial blood from the hepatic artery.

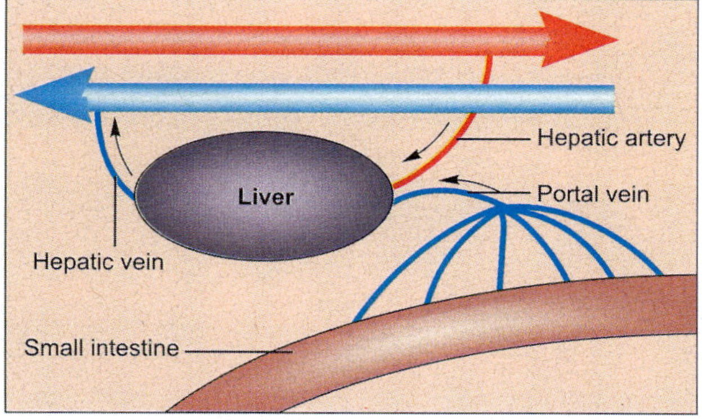

Fig. 6.48: Hepatic vascular system

Terminal branches of the hepatic portal vein and hepatic artery empty together and mix as they enter sinusoids in the liver. Sinusoids are distensible vascular channels lined with highly fenestrated or "holey" endothelial cells and bounded circumferentially by hepatocytes. As blood flows through the sinusoids, a considerable amount of plasma is filtered into the space between endothelium and hepatocytes (the "space of Disse"), providing a major fraction of the body's lymph.

Blood flows through the sinusoids and empties into the central vein of each lobule. Central veins coalesce into hepatic veins, which leave the liver and empty into the vena cava (Fig. 6.49).

Hepatic Blood Volume and Reservoir Function

The liver receives approximately 30% of resting cardiac output and, is therefore, a very vascular organ. The hepatic vascular system is dynamic, meaning that it has considerable ability to both store and release blood—it functions as a reservoir within the general circulation.

In the normal situation, 10–15% of the total blood volume is in the liver, with roughly 60% of that in the sinusoids. When blood is lost, the liver dynamically adjusts its blood volume and can eject enough blood to compensate for a moderate amount of hemorrhage. Conversely, when vascular volume is acutely increased, as when fluids are rapidly infused, the hepatic blood volume expands, providing a buffer against acute increases in systemic blood volume.

Intestinal Circulation

In the intestines the arteries enter the wall and circle round the gut and send branches to the muscular layers, mucosa and the villi. The mucosa receives more blood than other parts. In the villi, the artery and vein are close to and parallel to each other with blood flow in opposite direction (countercurrent). Blood flow responds to changes in metabolic activity.

Skeletal Muscle Blood Flow

Skeletal muscle accounts for about 20% of cardiac output and systemic vascular resistance. During extreme physical exertion, more than 80% of cardiac output can be directed to contracting muscles; therefore, skeletal muscle resistance becomes the primary determinant of systemic vascular resistance during exercise.

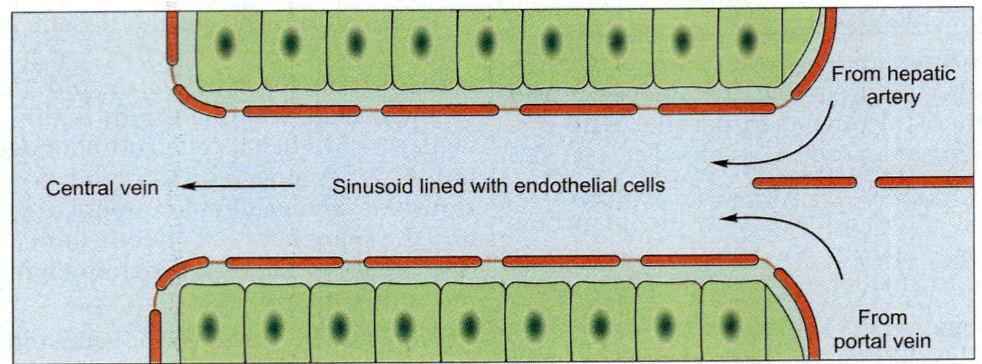

Fig. 6.49

Blood Flow

At rest, skeletal muscle blood flow may be 1–4 ml/min per 100 g. Maximal blood flow may reach 50–100 ml/min per 100 g depending upon the muscle type. Therefore, blood flow can increase 20 to 50-fold with maximal vasodilation or active hyperemia.

Coordinated, rhythmical contractions (e.g. running) enhance blood flow by means of the skeletal muscle pump mechanism.

6

Regulation

1. Sympathetic innervation produces vasoconstriction through α_1 and α_2-adrenoceptors located on the vascular smooth muscle. There is a significant amount of sympathetic tone at rest so that abrupt removal of sympathetic influences (e.g. by using an alpha-adrenoceptor blocker) can increase resting flow 2 to 3-fold. Vascular β_2-adrenoceptors produce vasodilation when stimulated by agonists such as epinephrine. There is evidence for sympathetic cholinergic innervation of skeletal muscle arteries, particularly large arteries. Activation of these autonomic nerves during exercise can cause neural-mediated vasodilation through the release of acetylcholine binding to muscarinic receptors.
2. There is a close coupling between oxygen consumption and blood flow.
3. Blood flow is strongly determined by local regulatory (tissue and endothelial) factors such as tissue hypoxia, adenosine, K^+, CO_2, H^+, and nitric oxide. During exercise, these local regulatory mechanisms override the sympathetic vasoconstrictor influences (termed functional sympatholysis).
4. Skeletal muscle blood flow shows a moderate degree of autoregulation.
5. Like the coronary circulation, muscle blood flow can be significantly compromised by extravascular compression that occurs during strong muscular contractions, especially during sustained tetanic contractions.

40. SHOCK

Definition

Shock is a serious, life-theatening condition characterized by inadequate tissue and oxygen perfusion, which, reduces the delivery of oxygen and other essential nutrients to a level below that required for normal cellular activities. Cellular injury and destruction may occur and tissue and organ functions deteriorate.

Causes

- Cardiogenic: Results from diminished heart pumping ability
- Hypovolemia
  - Hemorrhage
  - Burns
  - Dehydration
- Distributive: Septic shock, anaphylaxis and neurogenic
- Obstructive

Physiology of Shock

Stages of Shock

It has three stages:
1. Nonprogressive
2. Progressive
3. Irreversible

Nonprogressive

1. Loss of effective circulating blood volume initiates reactive changes
2. Redistribution of circulating blood volume occurs
3. Perfusion to coronary and cerebral circulations is maintained by autoregulation
4. Acute hypovolemia results in
   - Reduced central venous pressure
   - Reduced cardiac filling and cardiac output
5. Sympathetic stimulation causes
   - Reduced splanchnic perfusion
   - Cutaneous vasoconstriction
   - Reduced renal perfusion
   - Venous return is increased
   - Increases myocardial contractility
6. Renin-angiotensin system is stimulated
7. Antidiuretic hormone is released
8. Urine output is reduced
9. If compensation is adequate
   - Blood pressure is maintained
   - Oxygen delivery remains adequate.

Progressive

- If compensatory mechanisms are inadequate
- Ischemia and hypoxia occurs
- Anaerobic metabolism results in increased lactate production
- Capillary permeability increases
- Pulmonary edema may occur resulting in ARDS
- Renal hypoperfusion can result in acute tubular necrosis.

Irreversible

- If compensatory mechanisms fail
- Vasodilatation occurs and capillary permeability is increased
- Progressive tissue hypoxia occurs
- When systolic pressure falls below 50–60 mm Hg
  - Reduced coronary circulation results in myocardial ischemia
  - Cerebral ischemia causes vasomotor depression and visceral vasodilatation
- Disseminated intravascular coagulation occurs
- Water and electrolyte disturbances occur.

Physiology of Treatment

- Treat the cause first
- *Replacement therapy:* With blood and plasma transfusion
- Sympathomimetic drugs can be used for treating neurogenic and septic shock

Head down position
- Oxygen therapy
- Glucocorticoids.

6

41. CARDIOVASCULAR RESPONSES TO EXERCISE

Redistribution of Blood Flow

1. Increased blood flow to working skeletal muscle
2. Reduced blood flow to less active organs
   - Liver, kidneys, GI tract
   - Brain BF not affected
3. Changes in muscle and splanchnic blood flow as a function of exercise intensity
4. Increased blood flow to skeletal muscle during exercise
   - Withdrawal of sympathetic vasoconstriction
   - Autoregulation

Changes in CV Parameters with Increasing Exercise Intensity

1. Heart rate increases
2. Stroke volume increases
3. Cardiac output increases
4. Systolic blood pressure increases
5. Diastolic pressure change depends on degree of peripheral resistance.

Changes in CV Parameters with Prolonged Exercise

1. Cardiac output is maintained
2. Gradual decrease in stroke volume
3. Gradual increase in heart rate
4. "Cardiovascular drift"
   - Due to dehydration and increased skin blood flow (rising body temperature).

Cardiovascular Control during Exercise

1. Initial signal to "drive" cardiovascular system comes from higher brain centers
2. Fine-tuned by feedback from:
   - *Chemoreceptors:* In muscle and in carotid bodies, aortic arch
   - *Mechanoreceptors:* In muscle
   - *Baroreceptors:* In carotid sinus.

Effects of Training on CV Parameters

1. Oxygen uptake increases.
2. Increases in maximal exercise capacity with training
3. Factors causing an increase in SV with training:
   - Increased end-diastolic volume ("preload")
   - Increased plasma volume
   - Increased filling time due to lower HR
   - Increased ventricular volume
   - Increased contractility
   - Decreased TPR ("afterload").

6

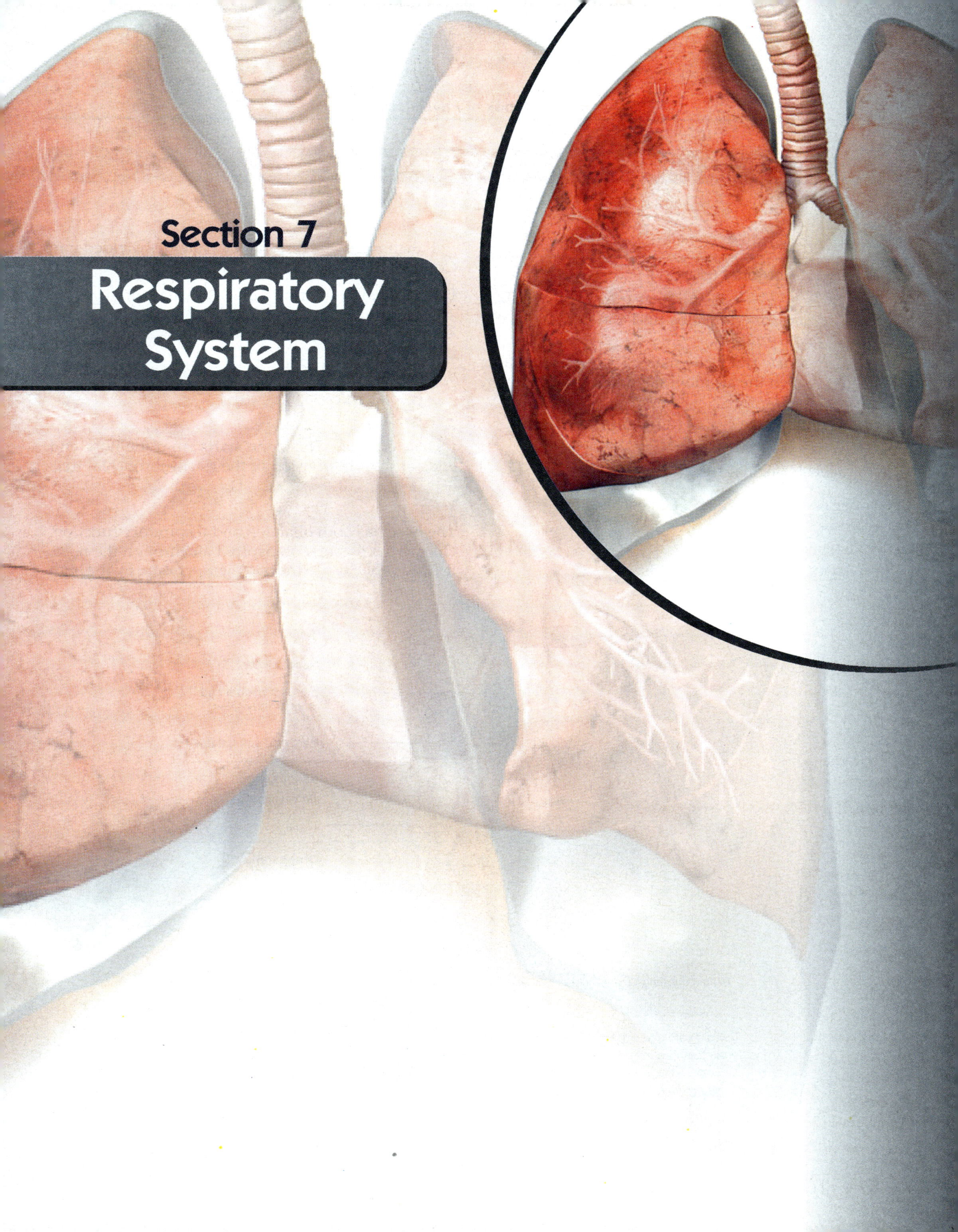

Section 7

Respiratory System

42. RESPIRATORY PHYSIOLOGY

INTRODUCTION

Functional Anatomy (Fig. 7.1)

Organs of respiration: Respiratory tract, lungs, thoracic cage, respiratory muscles and the center for the control of respiration.

Respiratory tract consists of the air passages through which the air moves in and out of the lung.

1. Nose
2. Pharynx
3. Larynx
4. Tracheobronchial tree.

Upper respiratory tract (URT) consists of:

- Nose
- Pharynx
- Larynx up to the vocal cords.

Functionally the respiratory system is divided into Conducting Zone and Respiratory Zone.

Lower respiratory tract (LRT) consists of:

- Trachea
- Bronchi
- Bronchioles
- Terminal bronchioles
- Alveolar duct
- Alveoli

Conducting zone: This zone starts from the nose and ends at the16th division of the tracheobronchial tree.

Nose

The nose has both olfaction and respiratory function. During the passage of inspired air through the nose, it is brought close to the body temperature by the high

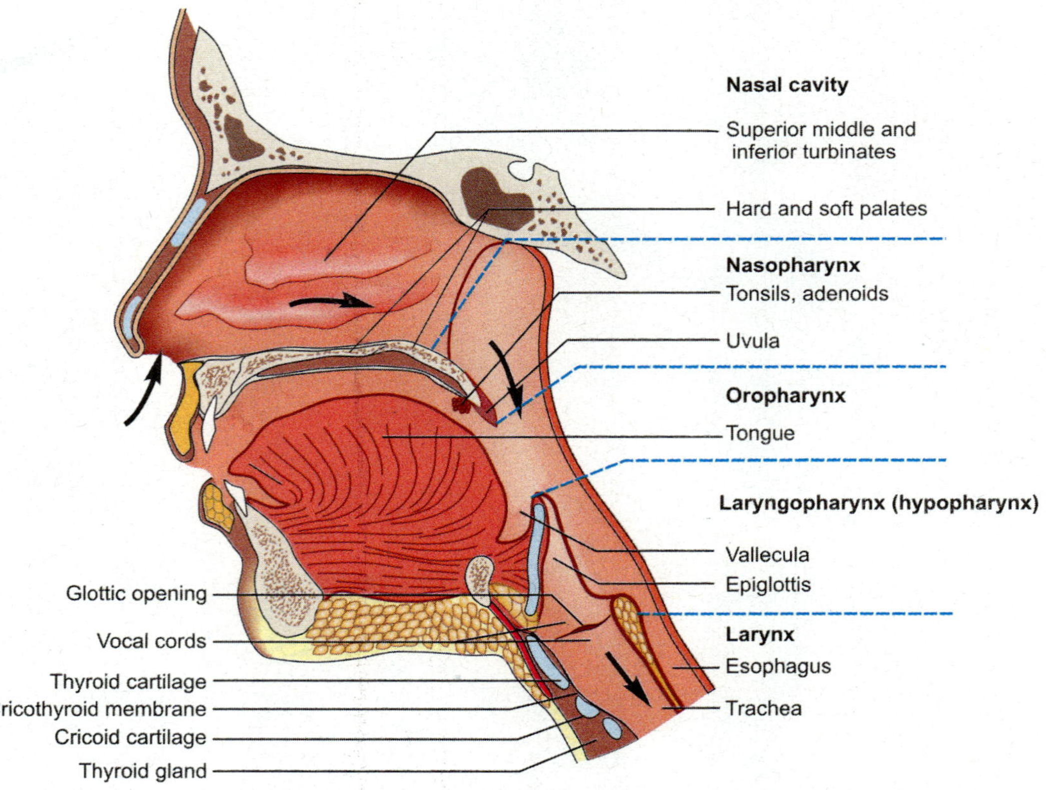

Fig. 7.1: Functional anatomy of upper respiratory tract

vascularity called 'warming'. The nasal mucosal secretion 'humidifies' the air and they have 'bactericidal' properties. Stiff hair of nostrils 'trap' the dust and foreign particles and takes part in 'sneezing reflex'. It acts as a resonator during speech.

Pharynx

The nasal cavities open posteriorly into the nasopharynx. The oral part of pharynx is common pathway of air into larynx and food from the mouth into the esophagus. Swallowing reflex prevent the food from reaching the larynx.

Larynx (Figs 7.2 and 7.3)

They lie in front of lower part of pharynx. It is a cartilaginous box, held together by ligaments. It functions in production of voice, preventing the food entry into trachea during swallowing and vomiting, by causing the closure of the vocal cords.

After passing through the nose, pharynx, larynx the next structure is trachea, which is a tubular structure, the lumen of which is kept patent by a number of C-shaped rings with the posterior gap bridged by the fibroelastic tissue and smooth muscle. The trachea divides into two bronchi which in turn divide 23 times. Bronchioles starts from the 4th division, till the 16th division. It is purely conducting pathway for air and the gas exchange does not occur in these regions. So, till this area it is termed as anatomical dead space.

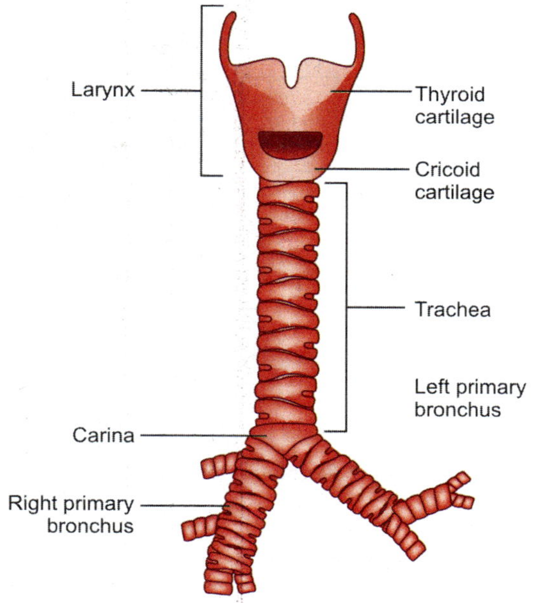

Fig. 7.3: Tracheobronchial tree

Respiratory Zone

From the 17th division, the remaining seven generations forms the transitional and respiratory zone, which are made up of respiratory bronchioles, alveolar ducts and alveoli (Fig. 7.4). These multiple divisions increase the cross-sectional area from 2.5 cm^2 in the trachea to 11, 800 cm^2 in the alveoli.

The alveoli are made up of two types of cells (Fig. 7.24a):

	Name	Division	Diameter (mm)	How many?	Cross-sectional area (cm)
Conducting system	Trachea	0	15–22	1	2.5
	Primary bronchi	1	10–15	2	↓
	Smaller bronchi	2		3	
	↓	3	1–10	↓	
		4			
		5			
		6–11		1×10^4	
	Bronchioles	12–23	0.5–1	2×10^4 ↓ 8×10^4	100 5×10^6
Exchange surface	Alveoli	24	0.3	$3–6 \times 10^4$	$>1 \times 10^6$

Fig. 7.2: Details of lower respiratory tract

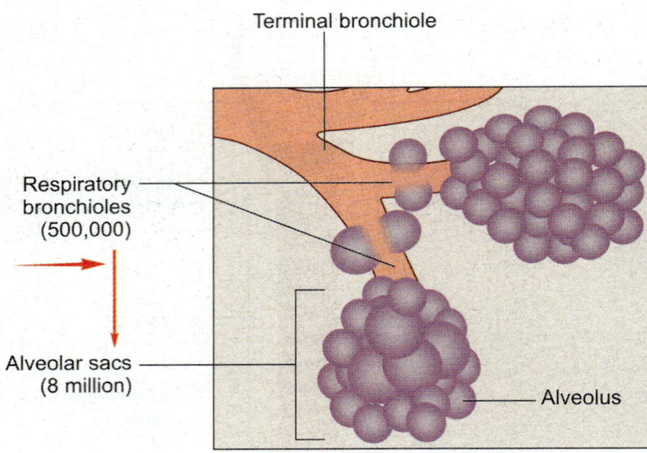

Fig. 7.4: Respiratory zone

i. *Type I:* Primary lining cells with large cytoplasmic extensions.

ii. *Type II:* Granular pneumocytes are thicker and contain numerous inclusion bodies which produce surfactant.

The alveoli are surrounded by pulmonary capillaries and the blood and air are just 0.5 μm apart by the respiratory membrane (alveolar capillary membrane).

Innervations

The walls of the respiratory tract are innervated by

Adrenergic nerves: Bronchodilatation

Cholinergic nerves: Broncoconstriction

Noncholinergic nonadrenergic: Bronchodilatation

Lung

The lungs are large spongy cone shaped structures which occupy most of the thoracic cavity. The substance of the lung is formed by the numerous branches of the respiratory tract with several million air spaces forming the bulk of the lung. Vascular, lymphatic, nervous and the connective tissue forms the rest of the lung. The surface of the lung is lined by a serous membrane, the 'pleura'.

Respiratory Functions

- Supply adequate quantities of oxygen to the tissues
- Elimination of carbon dioxide formed in the tissues during metabolism.

Nonrespiratory Functions

- *Filtration of foreign particle:* The hairs in the nostril filter the particles of size 10 μm which are eliminated by sneezing reflex. Particles of size 2–10 μm are

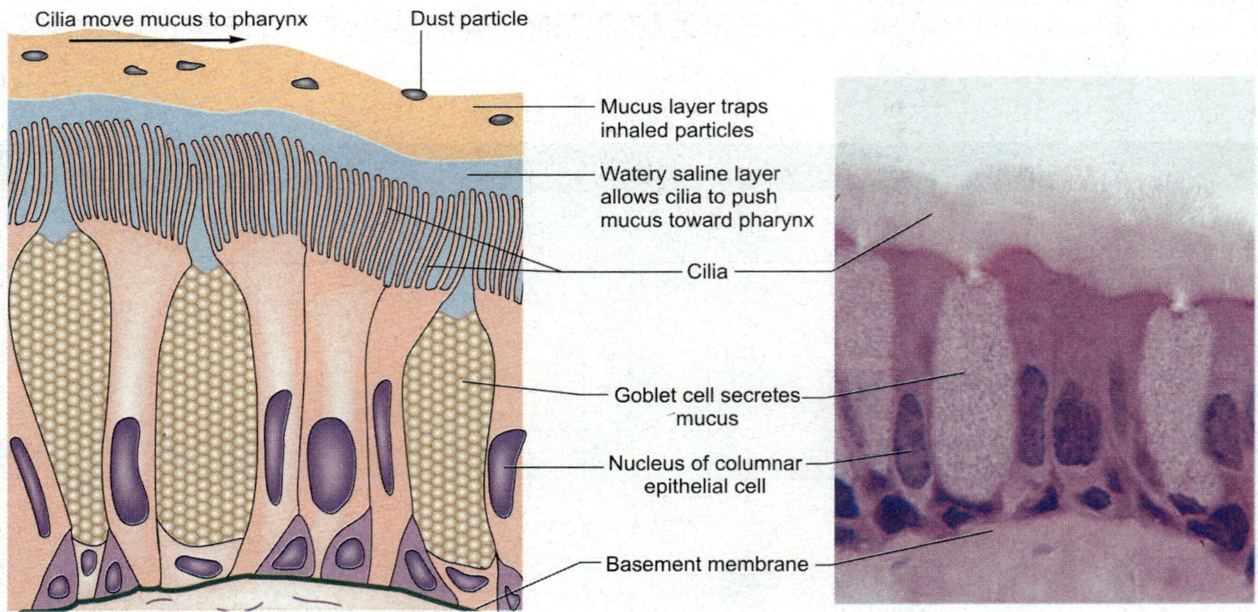

Fig. 7.5: Ciliated epithelium of the trachea

filtered by the cilia lining the bronchi and are escalated towards the upper air way. Particles of size <2 μm reach the alveoli, where they are ingested by macrophages.

- *Defense:* The tonsils and adenoids filter some bacteria. Bronchial secretion contain IgA that deposit in the bronchi. Pulmonary alveolar macrophages (PAM) ingest inhaled bacteria and small particles. Surfactant act as opsonins and promote phagocytosis.
- *Metabolic:* Activate angiotensin I to angiotensin II, remove bradykinin, produce histamine.
- *Synthetic:* Surfactant, serotonin.
- Regulation of body temperature—the circulation.
- Regulation of blood volume and BP-lung can add or remove about 800 ml from the circulation.
- *Storage:* Lungs store blood and puts back into circulation during posture variation and blood volume changes.
- *Fibrinolytic system:* Small clots are lysed by this
- Speech and vocalization.
- *Acid-base balance:* Through carbon dioxide elimination or retention.
- *Olfaction:* Influence the taste through olfaction.
- *Sexual behavior:* Vomeronasal organ in animals helps to detect the pheromones from the opposite sex.

43. PULMONARY CIRCULATION

FUNCTIONAL ANATOMY

Pulmonary Vessels (Fig. 7.6)

The pulmonary artery (PA) extends only 5 cm beyond the apex of the right ventricle and then divides into right and left branches to enter the respective lung. Almost all the blood in the body passes through the pulmonary artery to the capillary bed, where it gets oxygenated and returned to left atrium through the pulmonary veins (PV). The walls of the PA and its larger branches are only about 30% as thick as the systemic vessels and have less smooth muscle. Even the capillaries have some smooth muscles. So, they have larger diameter than the systemic vessels. The walls are thin with an average compliance of about 7 ml/mm Hg, which is equal to the entire systemic compliance. The pulmonary capillaries are large with multiple anastomoses, so that each alveoli sits on a rich capillary basket.

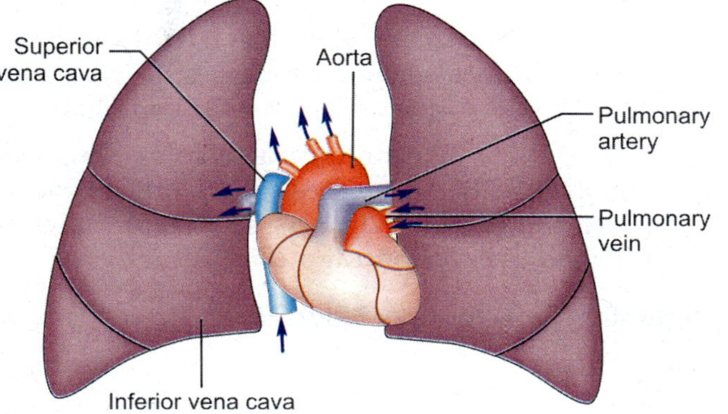

Fig. 7.6: Pulmonary circulation

Bronchial Vessels

The bronchial arteries are three in number, provides oxygenated blood to the lungs amounting to about 1–2% of the cardiac output. It nourishes the walls of the bronchi, bronchioles, blood vessels, nerves connective tissue and the visceral pleura. It does not supply beyond the terminal bronchiole. About 1/3rd returns to right atrium by bronchial vein and the remaining 2/3rds drains into the pulmonary veins, now together called as bronchopulmonary veins into the left atrium causing physiologic shunt.

CHARACTERISTICS OF PULMONARY CIRCULATION

1. The entire pulmonary vascular system is a distensible low pressure system (Fig. 7.7).
2. *Reservoir:* Because of their distensibility, the pulmonary veins act as an important blood reservoir. The volume of blood at any one time in the pulmonary vessels is 1 liter.

   Posture: But, when a person lies down the pulmonary blood volume increases by 400 ml and when the person stands up this blood is discharged into the general circulation. When a person blows air out like blowing a trumpet as much as 250 ml is

7

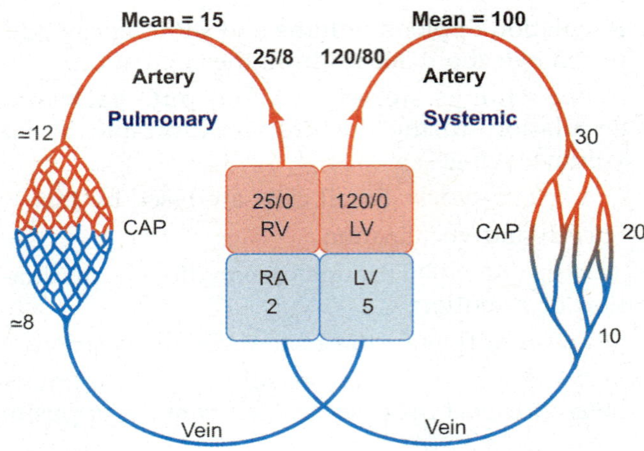

Fig. 7.7: The pulmonary arterial pressure is about 25/8 with a mean pressure of about 15 mm Hg. The left atrtial pressure is about 5–8 so the pressure gradient is about 7 mm Hg compared to 90 mm Hg in the systemic. It is not feasible to measure the left atrial pressure but can often be estimated by pulmonary capillary wedge pressure (PCwP)

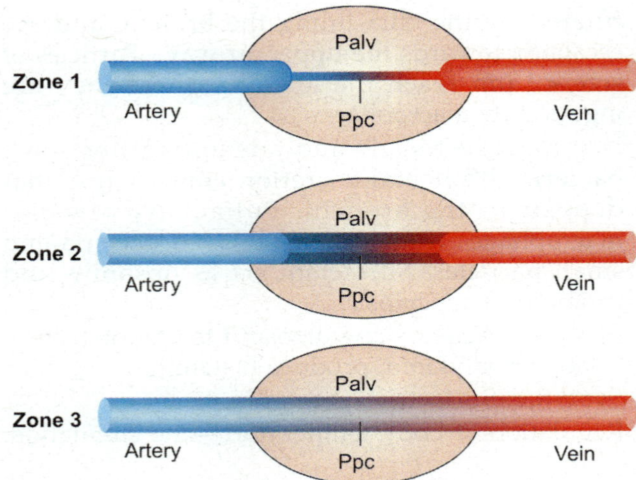

Fig. 7.8: Different zones of respiratory system

expelled into systemic circulation. Loss of blood due to hemorrhage can be met with this automatic shift of blood.

3. *Blood flow:* The pulmonary vessels can be divided into three categories:
   - Alveolar
   - Extra alveolar
   - Microcirculation.

   The extra alveolar vessels are affected by change in lung volume, alveolar vessels caliber depends on the alveolar pressure changes. Microcirculation participates in the liquid and the solute exchange, in the maintenance of fluid balance.

4. *Distribution (effect of gravity):* In the upright position, the upper portion of the lungs is well above the level of the heart, and the bases are below it. Consequently there is marked pressure gradient in the pulmonary arteries from the top to the bottom of the lungs due to the effect of gravity. In a normal upright adult, the lowest point in the lungs is about 30 cm below the highest point. This represents a 23 mm Hg pressure difference, about 15 mm Hg above the heart and 8 below. Such pressure difference has profound effect on the blood flow through different areas of the lungs. To explain such effect the lungs is divided into 3 zones based on the blood flow during the cardiac cycle (Fig. 7.8).

   Zone 1: No blood flow occurs during any phase of the cardiac cycle. because the local alveolar capillary pressure in this area never rises higher than the alveolar air pressure and no blood flows through.

   Zone 2: Intermittent blood flow. Flow occurs only during the systole when the capillary pressure exceeds the alveolar pressure. This is known as 'Water fall effect'.

   Zone 3: Continuous blood flow during the entire cardiac cycle as the capillary pressure remains higher than the alveolar pressure throughout the cycle.

   Normally the lungs have only two zones, 2 intermittent flow in the apices and 3 continuous flow in the lower areas. Zone 1 occurs only under abnormal conditions like positive pressure ventilation artificially and in severe blood loss.

5. *Pulmonary vascular resistance is low:* Low pressure pathway produces less net filtration than produced in the systemic capillaries. It is because of low vascular tone and increased compliance.
6. *Autoregulation:* Pulmonary arterioles constrict when alveolar PO_2 decreases and diverts the blood flow to the ventilated parts so that it matches ventilation/ perfusion ratio (Fig. 7.9).

Regulation of Pulmonary Blood Flow

Active Factors

Autonomic nervous system: Sympathetic reduces the blood flow.

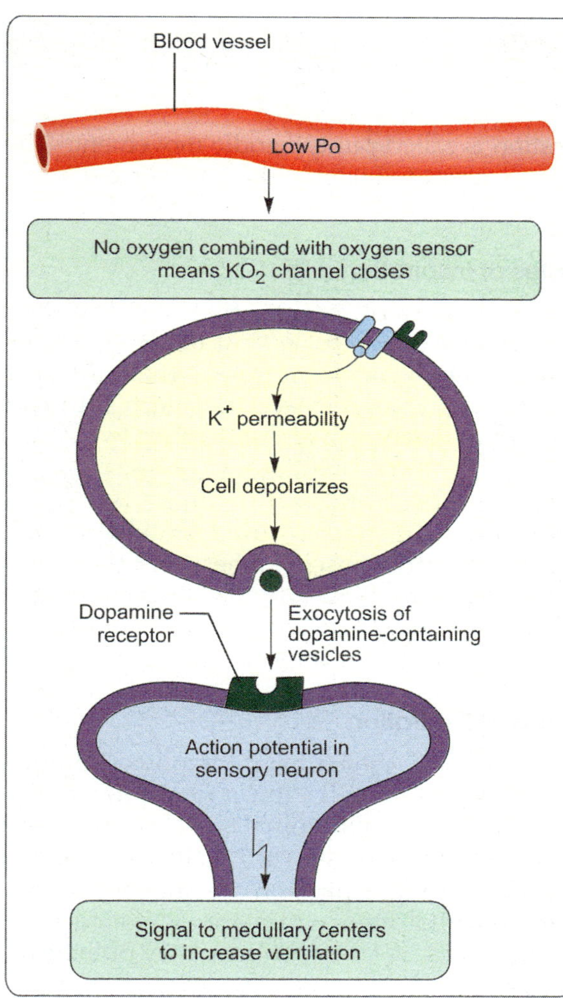

Fig. 7.9

Humoral: Vasoconstriction—angiotensin and thromboxane vasodilatation—bradykinin, vasopressin, ANP and histamine.

Passive factor: Cardiac output, gravity and hypoxia.

PULMONARY CAPILLARY DYNAMICS

The dynamics of fluid exchange across the lung capillary membranes are qualitatively same as in peripheral tissues but differ quantitatively (Fig. 7.10).

- The pulmonary capillary pressure is 7 mm Hg very low when compared to the systemic 17 mm Hg.
- The interstitial fluid pressure is more negative (–8) than peripheral tissues.
- The pulmonary capillaries are leaky to protein molecules, so the interstitial oncotic fluid pressure is 14 mm Hg.

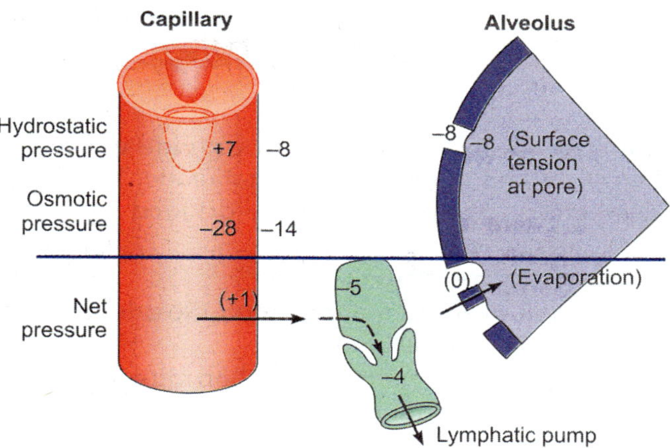

Fig. 7.10: Pressure causing fluid movement

From Fig. 7.10

total outward pressure	= 7 + 14 + 8 = **29**
The total inward force	= **28**
Mean filtration pressure	= 29 – 28 = **1**

This **1** causes flow of fluid from the capillaries in the interstitial space which is taken up by the lymphatic system and the alveoli are kept dry.

PULMONARY EDEMA

Any factor that causes the pulmonary interstitial fluid pressure to rise from negative to positive will result in rapid filling of interstitial space and alveoli with fluid termed as pulmonary edema.

Common Causes

- Left heart failure
- Infections damaging the capillary membranes
- Inhalation of chlorine or sulfur gas
- Lymphatic obstruction.

Safety Factor

Plasma colloid osmotic pressure: As the normal pressure in humans is 28 mm Hg, the pulmonary capillary pressure has to rise from normal 7 mm Hg to this 28 mm Hg in order to cause pulmonary edema. So the acute safety factor is 28 – 7 = 21 mm Hg.

Lymphatics: In chronic conditions the lymph vessels expand greatly and increase their carrying capacity by 10-fold which makes the lung more resistant to edema. When the capillary pressure rises more than 25–30 mm Hg above the safety factor level, death ensues in less than 30 minutes.

44. PULMONARY VENTILATION

The goals of respiration are to provide oxygen to the tissues and to remove carbon dioxide..To achieve these goals, respiration can be divided into four major functions:

1. Pulmonary ventilation
2. Diffusion of oxygen and carbon dioxide between the alveoli and the blood
3. Transport of oxygen and carbon dioxide in the blood and body fluids to and from the body's tissue cells
4. Regulation of ventilation.

This chapter is concerned with the functions of the respiratory system in external respiration, i.e. the processes responsible for the uptake of O_2 and excretion of CO_2 in the lungs.

MECHANICS OF PULMONARY VENTILATION

Muscles that Cause Lung Expansion and Contraction (Fig. 7.11)

7

The lungs can be expanded and contracted in two ways: By downward and upward movement of the diaphragm, to lengthen or shorten the chest cavity. During inspiration, contraction of the diaphragm pulls the lower surfaces of the lungs downward. Then, during expiration, the diaphragm simply relaxes, and the elastic recoil of the lungs, chest wall, and abdominal structures compresses the lungs and expels the air.

The second method for expanding the lungs is to raise the rib cage. When the rib cage is elevated, the ribs project almost directly forward, so that the sternum also moves forward, away from the spine, making the anteroposterior thickness of the chest about 20 percent greater during maximum inspiration than during expiration is called pump handle movement. The rib cage movement to increase the transverse diameter is called Bucket handle movement (Fig. 7.11).

Muscles of Inspiration (Fig. 7.12)

The most important muscles that raise the rib cage are the external intercostals, but others that help are the sternocleidomastoid muscles, which lift upward on the sternum; anterior serrati, which lift many of the ribs and scaleni, which lift the first two ribs.

Movement of the diaphragm accounts for 75% of the change in intrathoracic volume during quiet inspiration. Attached around the bottom of the thoracic cage, this muscle arches over the liver and moves downward like a piston when it contracts. The distance it moves ranges from 1.5 to 7 cm to as much as 7 cm with deep inspiration.

Muscles of Expiration (Fig. 7.12)

Abdominal recti, which have the powerful effect of pulling downward on the lower ribs at the same time that they and other abdominal muscles also compress the abdominal contents upward against the diaphragm.

The ribs during expiration are angled downward, and the external intercostals are elongated forward and downward. As they contract, they pull the upper ribs forward in relation to the lower ribs, and this causes leverage on the ribs to raise them upward, thereby causing inspiration. The internal intercostals function exactly in the opposite manner, functioning as expiratory muscles because they angle between the ribs in the opposite direction and cause opposite leverage.

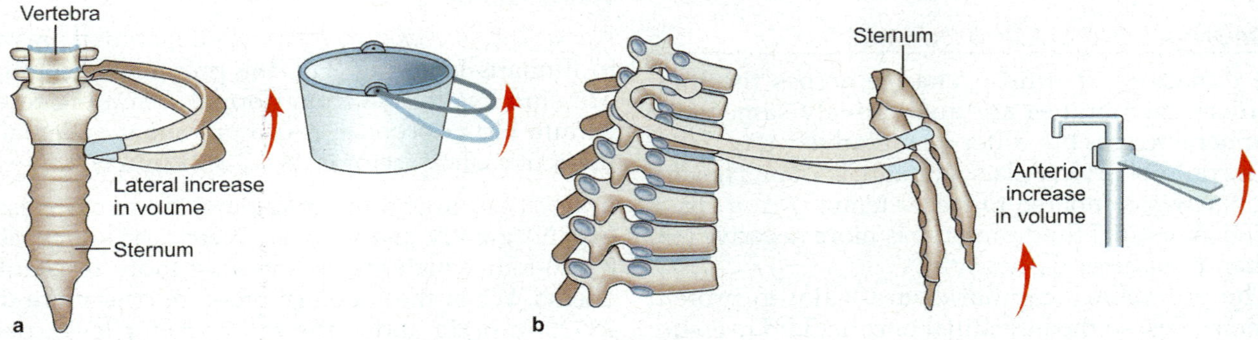

Fig. 7.11

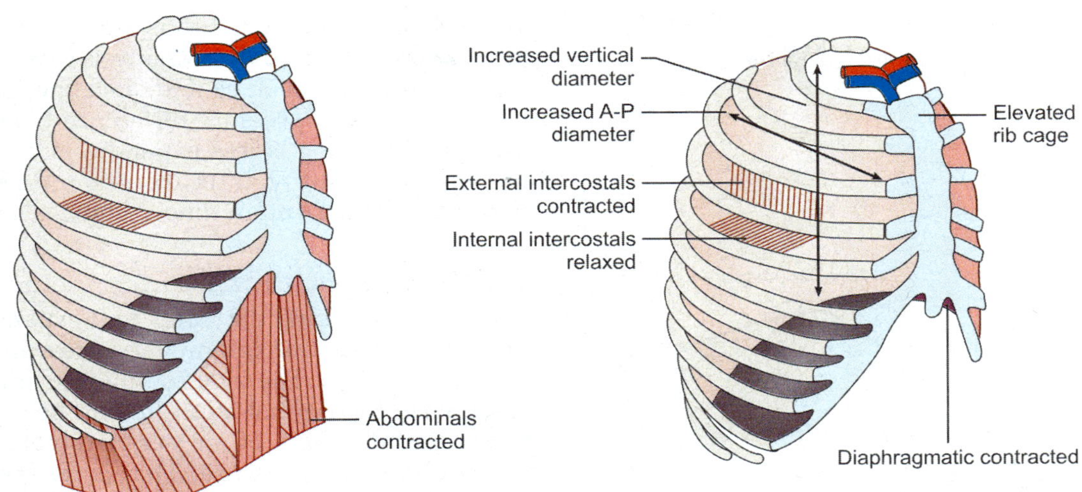

Fig. 7.12: Mechanics of pulmonary ventilation

Glottis

The abductor muscles in the larynx contract early in inspiration, pulling the vocal cords apart and opening the glottis. During swallowing or gagging, there is reflex contraction of the abductor muscles that closes the glottis.

Bronchial Tone

In general, the smooth muscle in the bronchial walls aids respiration the bronchi dilate during inspiration and constrict during expiration. Dilation is produced by sympathetic discharge and constriction by parasympathetic discharge. There is a circadian rhythm in bronchial tone, with maximal constriction at about 6 AM and maximal dilation at about 6 PM.

Movement of Air in and out of the Lungs and the Pressures

The lung "floats" in the thoracic cavity, surrounded by a thin layer of pleural fluid that lubricates movement of the lungs within the cavity. The lungs are held to the thoracic wall as if glued there, except that they are well lubricated and can slide freely as the chest expands and contracts.

Pleural Pressure and its Changes during Respiration (Fig. 7.13)

Pleural pressure is the pressure of the fluid in the thin space between the lung pleura and the chest wall pleura. As this is normally a slight suction, which means a slightly negative pressure, the normal pleural pressure at the beginning of inspiration is about –5 cm of water, which is the amount of suction required to hold the lungs open to their resting level.

Then, during normal inspiration, expansion of the chest cage pulls outward on the lungs with greater force and creates more negative pressure, to an average of about –7.5 cm of water.

Alveolar Pressure

Alveolar pressure is the pressure of the air inside the lung alveoli. When the glottis is open and no air is flowing into or out of the lungs, the pressures in all parts of the respiratory tree, up to the alveoli are equal to atmospheric pressure, which is considered to be zero reference pressure in the airways that is, 0 centimeters water pressure.

To cause inward flow of air into the alveoli during inspiration, the pressure in the alveoli must fall to a value slightly below atmospheric pressure (below 0). During normal inspiration, alveolar pressure decreases to about –1 centimeter of water. This slight negative pressure is enough to pull 0.5 liter of air into the lungs in the 2 seconds required for normal quiet inspiration. During expiration, the alveolar pressure rises to about 1 centimeter of water, and these forces the 0.5 liter of inspired air out of the lungs during the 2 to 3 seconds of expiration.

Transpulmonary Pressure

The difference between the alveolar pressure and the pleural pressure is called the transpulmonary

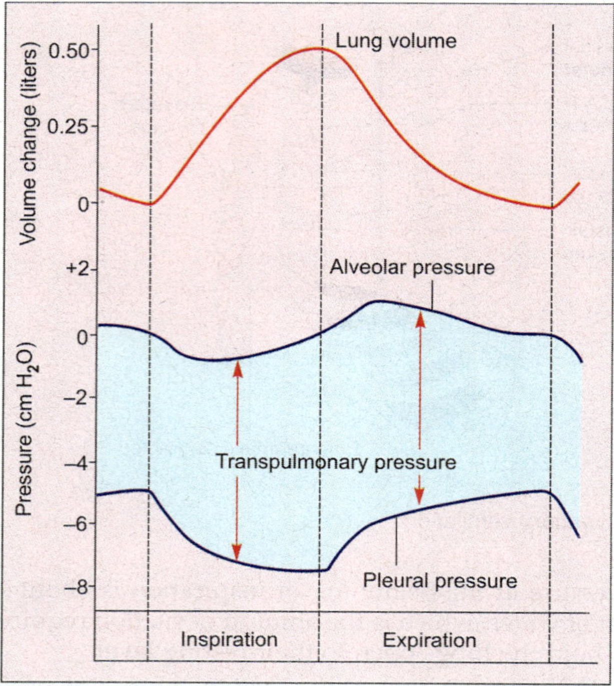

Fig. 7.13: Pleural pressure and its changes during respiration

pressure. It is a measure of the elastic forces in the lungs that tend to collapse the lungs at each instant of respiration called the recoil pressure.

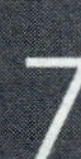

Differences in Ventilation

In the upright position, ventilation per unit lung volume is greater at the base of the lung than at the apex. The reason for this is that at the start of inspiration, intrapleural pressure is less negative at the base than at the apex and since the intrapulmonary-intrapleural pressure difference is less than at the apex, the lung is less expanded. Conversely, at the apex, the lung is more expanded, i.e. the percentage of maximum lung volume is greater.

COMPLIANCE OF THE LUNGS

The extent to which the lungs will expand for each unit increase in transpulmonary pressure is called lung compliance. The total compliance of both lungs together in the normal adult human being averages about 200 milliliters of air per centimeter of water transpulmonary pressure. That is, every time the transpulmonary pressure increases 1 centimeter of water, the lung volume, after 10 to 20 seconds, will expand 200 milliliters.

Note that the relation is different for inspiration and expiration. Each curve is recorded by changing the transpulmonary pressure in small steps and allowing the lung volume to come to a steady level between successive steps. The two curves are called, respectively, the inspiratory compliance curve and the expiratory compliance curve, and the entire diagram is called the compliance diagram of the lungs between successive steps (Fig. 7.14).

The compliance diagrams are determined by the elastic forces of the lungs. These can be divided into two parts:

1. Elastic forces of the lung tissue itself

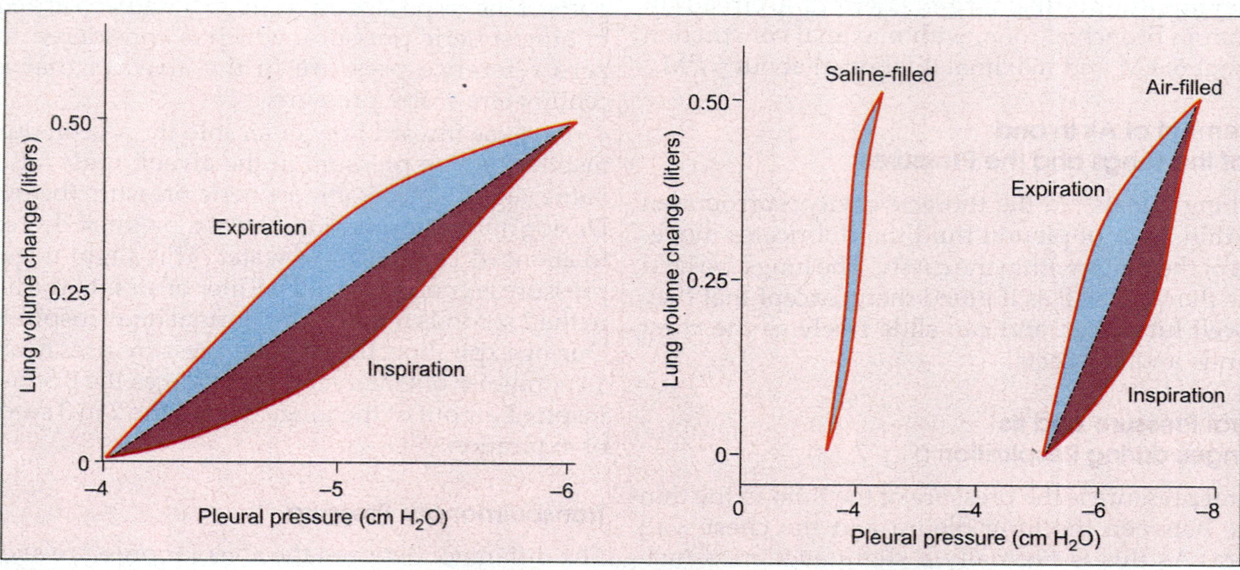

Fig. 7.14: Compliance diagram of the lungs

2. Elastic forces caused by surface tension of the fluid that lines the inside walls of the alveoli and other lung air spaces.

The elastic forces of the lung tissue are determined mainly by elastin and collagen fibers interwoven among the lung parenchyma. In deflated lungs, these fibers are in an elastically contracted and kinked state; then, when the lungs expand, the fibers become stretched and unkinked.

The significance of surface tension is shown in Fig. 3.4, which compares the compliance diagram of the lungs when filled with saline solution and when filled with air. When the lungs are filled with air, there is an interface between the alveolar fluid and the air in the alveoli. In the case of the saline solution-filled lungs, there is no air-fluid interface; therefore, the surface tension effect is not present—only tissue elastic forces are operative in the saline solution-filled lung. Because saline reduces the surface tension to nearly zero, the pressure-volume curve obtained with saline measures only the tissue elasticity, whereas the curve obtained with air measures both tissue elasticity and surface tension. The difference between the two curves, the elasticity due to surface tension, is much smaller at small than at large lung volumes. The surface tension is also much lower than the expected surface tension at a water-air interface of the same dimensions. Thus, one can conclude that the tissue elastic forces tending to cause collapse of the air-filled lung represent only about one-third of the total lung elasticity, whereas the fluid-air surface tension forces in the alveoli represent about two-thirds. The fluid-air surface tension elastic forces of the lungs also increase tremendously when the substance called surfactant is not present in the alveolar fluid.

SURFACTANT, SURFACE TENSION, AND COLLAPSE OF THE ALVEOLI (Fig. 7.15)

The low surface tension when the alveoli are small is due to the presence in the fluid lining the alveoli of surfactant, a lipid surface-tension-lowering agent. Surfactant is a complex mixture of several phospholipids, proteins, and ions. The most important components are the phospholipid dipalmitoyl phosphatidylcholine, surfactant apoproteins, and calcium ions. The dipalmitoylphosphatidylcholine, along with several less important phospholipids. Formation of the phospholipids film is greatly facilitated by the proteins in surfactant. This material contains four unique proteins, SP-A, SP-B, SP-C, and SP-D.

If the surface tension is not kept low when the alveoli become smaller during expiration, they collapse in accordance with the law of Laplace.

Law of Laplace (Fig. 7.16)

In spherical structures like the alveoli, the distending pressure equals 2 times the tension divided by the radius ($P = 2T/r$); if T is not reduced as r is reduced, the tension overcomes the distending pressure.

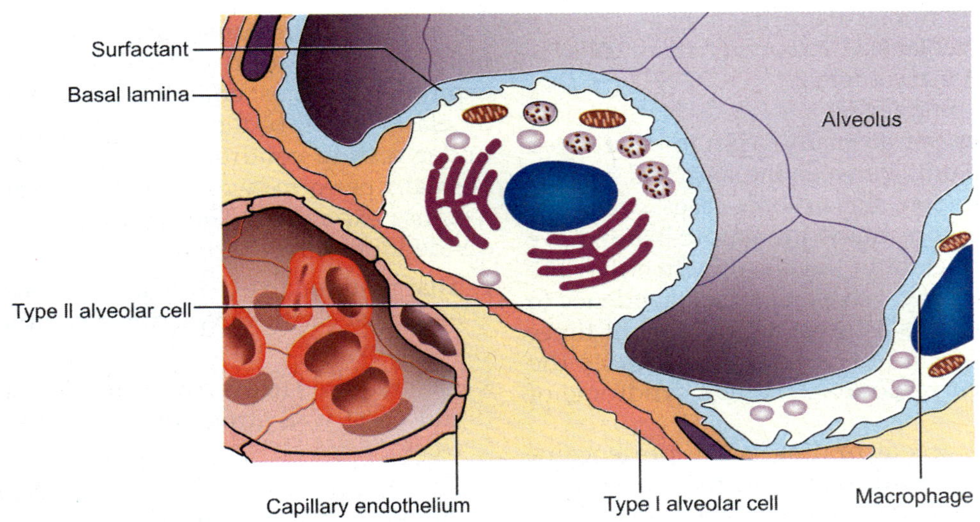

Fig. 7.15: Significance of surface tension

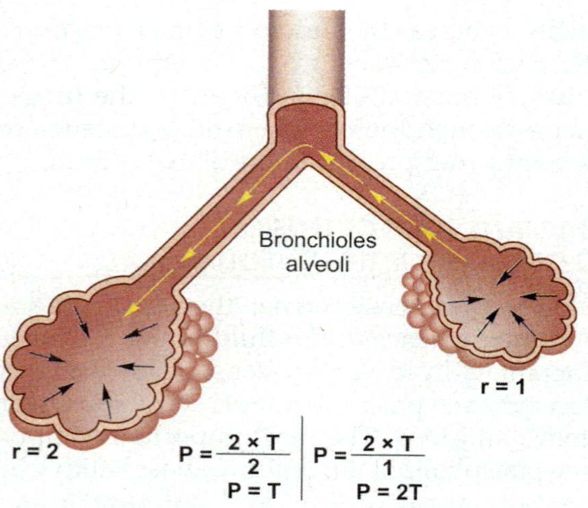

Fig. 7.16: Law of Laplace

Formation

Surfactant is produced by type II alveolar epithelial cells. Typical lamellar bodies, membrane-bound organelles containing whorls of phospholipids, are formed in these cells and secreted into the alveolar lumen by exocytosis. Tubes of lipid called tubular myelin form from the extruded bodies, and the tubular myelin in turn forms the phospholipids film. Some of the protein-lipid complexes in surfactant are taken up by endocytosis in type II alveolar cells and recycled.

7

Functions

1. Reduces alveolar surface tension
2. Reduces the effort required by the respiratory muscles to expand the lungs
3. Reduces the intermolecular attraction
4. Stabilize the alveolar size and prevent their collapse
5. Prevents pulmonary edema
6. Increases the compliance
7. Surfactant does not normally begin to be secreted into the alveoli until between the sixth and seventh months of gestation, and in some cases, even later than that. Therefore, many premature babies have little or no surfactant in the alveoli when they are born, and their lungs have an extreme tendency to collapse, sometimes as great as six to eight times that in a normal adult person. This causes the condition called respiratory distress syndrome of the newborn.
8. An interesting recent finding is the presence of excess surfactant lipids and proteins in mice with the GM-CSF gene knocked out. The role of GM-CSF in hematopoiesis is already known.
9. SP-A and SP-D are members of the collectin family of proteins that are involved in innate immunity.

Applied

1. Surfactant deficiency is an important cause of infant respiratory distress syndrome (IRDS; hyaline membrane disease). Administration of phospholipids alone by inhalation has little value in the treatment of IRDS. However, a synthetic surfactant and a surfactant preparation derived from bovine lungs are available for use by inhalation. Used prophylactically at birth and as replacement therapy.
2. Patchy atelectasis is also associated with surfactant deficiency in patients who have undergone cardiac surgery involving use of a pump oxygenator and interruption of the pulmonary circulation.
3. Surfactant deficiency may play a role in some of the abnormalities that develop following occlusion of a main bronchus, occlusion of one pulmonary artery.
4. There is a decrease in surfactant in the lungs of cigarette smokers.

WORK OF BREATHING

Work is performed by the respiratory muscles in:

- Stretching the elastic tissues of the chest wall and lungs (elastic work)
- Moving inelastic tissues (viscous resistance)
- Moving air through the respiratory passages.

During normal quiet breathing, all respiratory muscle contraction occurs during inspiration; expiration is almost entirely a passive process caused by elastic recoil of the lungs and chest cage. Thus, under resting conditions, the respiratory muscles normally perform "work" to cause inspiration but not to cause expiration. The work of inspiration can be divided into three fractions:

1. That required to expand the lungs against the lung and chest elastic forces, called compliance work or elastic work.
2. That required to overcome the viscosity of the lung and chest wall structures, called tissue resistance work.
3. That required to overcome airway resistance to movement of air into the lungs, called airway resistance work.

Energy Required for Respiration

Estimates of the total work of quiet breathing ranges from 0.3 up to 0.8 kg m/min. The work of breathing is greatly increased in diseases such as emphysema, asthma, and congestive heart failure with dyspnea and orthopnea.

45. PULMONARY VOLUMES AND CAPACITIES

SPIROMETRY—RECORDING CHANGES IN PULMONARY VOLUME

A simple method for studying pulmonary ventilation is to record the volume movement of air into and out of the lungs, a process called spirometry. It consists of a drum inverted over a chamber of water, with the drum counterbalanced by a weight. In the drum is a breathing gas, usually air or oxygen; a tube connects the mouth with the gas chamber. When one breathes into and out of the chamber, the drum rises and falls, and an appropriate recording is made on a moving sheet of paper. For ease in describing the events of pulmonary ventilation, the air in the lungs has been subdivided in this diagram into four volumes and four capacities, which are the average for a young adult.

PULMONARY VOLUMES (Fig. 7.17)

1. The tidal volume is the volume of air inspired or expired with each normal breath; it amounts to about 500 milliliters in the adult male.

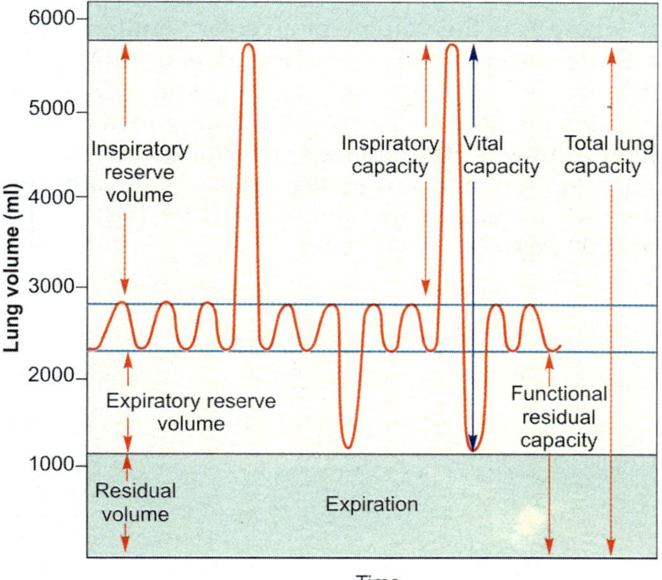

Fig. 7.17: Pulmonary capacities

2. The inspiratory reserve volume is the extra volume of air that can be inspired over and above the normal tidal volume when the person inspires with full force; it is usually equal to about 3000 milliliters.
3. The expiratory reserve volume is the maximum extra volume of air that can be expired by forceful expiration after the end of a normal tidal expiration; this normally amounts to about 1100 milliliters.
4. The residual volume is the volume of air remaining in the lungs after the most forceful expiration; this volume averages about 1200 milliliters.

PULMONARY CAPACITIES

Two or more of the volumes together are called pulmonary capacities.

1. The inspiratory capacity equals the tidal volume plus the inspiratory reserve volume. This is the amount of air (about 3500 milliliters) a person can breathe in, beginning at the normal expiratory level and distending the lungs to the maximum amount.
2. The functional residual capacity equals the expiratory reserve volume plus the residual volume. This is the amount of air that remains in the lungs at the end of normal expiration (about 2300 milliliters).
3. The vital capacity equals the inspiratory reserve volume plus the tidal volume plus the expiratory reserve volume. This is the maximum amount of air a person can expel from the lungs after first filling the lungs to their maximum extent and then expiring to the maximum extent (about 4600 milliliters).
4. The total lung capacity is the maximum volume to which the lungs can be expanded with the greatest possible effort (about 5800 milliliters); it is equal to the vital capacity plus the residual volume. All pulmonary volumes and capacities are about 20 to 25 percent less in women than in men, and they are greater in large and athletic people than in small and asthenic people.

Abbreviations and Symbols Used in Pulmonary Function Studies

A few simple algebraic exercises showing some of the interrelations among the pulmonary volumes and capacities

- VC = IRV + VT + ERV
- VC = IC + ERV
- TLC = VC + RV
- TLC = IC + FRC
- FRC = ERV + RV

Determination of Functional Residual Capacity, Residual Volume, and Total Lung Capacity—Helium Dilution Method

The functional residual capacity (FRC), cannot be measured in a direct way, because the air in the residual volume of the lungs cannot be expired into the spirometer, and this volume constitutes about one half of the functional residual capacity. To measure functional residual capacity, the spirometer must be used in an indirect manner, usually by means of a helium dilution method, as follows:

A spirometer of known volume is filled with air mixed with helium at a known concentration. Before breathing from the spirometer, the person expires normally. At the end of this expiration, the remaining volume in the lungs is equal to the functional residual capacity. At this point, the subject immediately begins to breathe from the spirometer, and the gases of the spirometer mix with the gases of the lungs. As a result, the helium becomes diluted by the functional residual capacity gases, and the volume of the functional residual capacity can be calculated from the degree of dilution of the helium.

Once the FRC has been determined, the residual volume (RV) can be determined by subtracting expiratory reserve volume (ERV), as measured by normal spirometry, from the FRC. Also, the total lung capacity (TLC) can be determined by adding the inspiratory capacity (IC) to the FRC. That is:

RV = FRC – ERV

and

TLC = FRC + IC

Minute Respiratory Volume Equals Respiratory Rate Times Tidal Volume

The minute respiratory volume is the total amount of new air moved into the respiratory passages each minute; this is equal to the tidal volume times the respiratory rate per minute. The normal tidal volume is about 500 milliliters, and the normal respiratory rate is about 12 breaths per minute. Therefore, the minute respiratory volume averages about 6 liter/min.

Alveolar Ventilation

The rate at which new air reaches the alveoli, alveolar sacs, alveolar ducts, and respiratory bronchioles is called alveolar ventilation.

Rate of Alveolar Ventilation

Alveolar ventilation per minute is the total volume of new air entering the alveoli and adjacent gas exchange areas each minute. It is equal to the respiratory rate times the amount of new air that enters these areas with each breath.

$$A = Freq \times (VT–VD)$$

where A is the volume of alveolar ventilation per minute, Freq is the frequency of respiration per minute, VT is the tidal volume, and VD is the physiologic dead space volume. Thus with a normal tidal volume of 500 milliliters, a normal dead space of 150 milliliters, and a respiratory rate of 12 breaths per minute, alveolar ventilation equals 12 × (500 – 150), or 4200 ml/min.

46. VENTILATION/PERFUSION RATIO

ALVEOLAR VENTILATION (Fig. 7.18)

The entire air that enters the lungs does not reach the alveoli. Some amount of air fills the airway. This is called dead space.

The actual air that reaches the alveoli per minute is called alveolar ventilation. Pulmonary ventilation –dead space = alveolar ventilation. Tidal volume during quiet breathing is 500 ml. Dead space is about 150 ml. Only 350 ml of inspired air during quite breathing reaches the alveoli. Normal average alveolar ventilation is 2–2.5 liters.

Alveolar ventilation = F × (TV – DS).

- F = Frequency (breaths/min)
- TV = Tidal volume.

DS = Dead space

Dead Space

The air that does not take part in gas exchange is called dead space. It is of two types:

1. Anatomical dead space
2. Physiological dead space.

Anatomical Dead Space (Fig. 7.19)

It is the volume of air in the respiratory passage from the nose and the mouth to the terminal bronchioles. It can be measured by Fowler's method as follows:

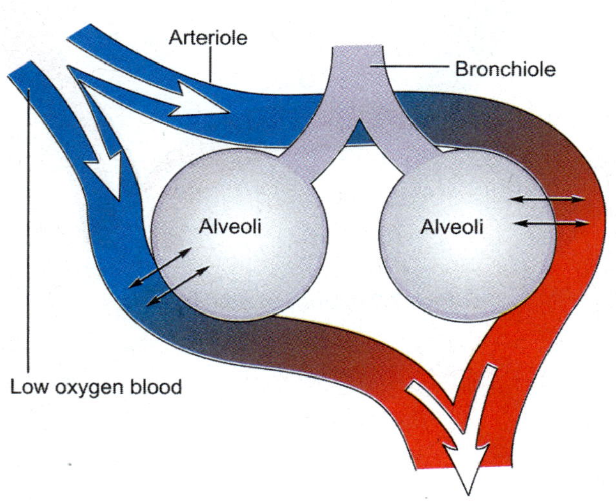

Fig. 7.18: Ventilation in alveoli

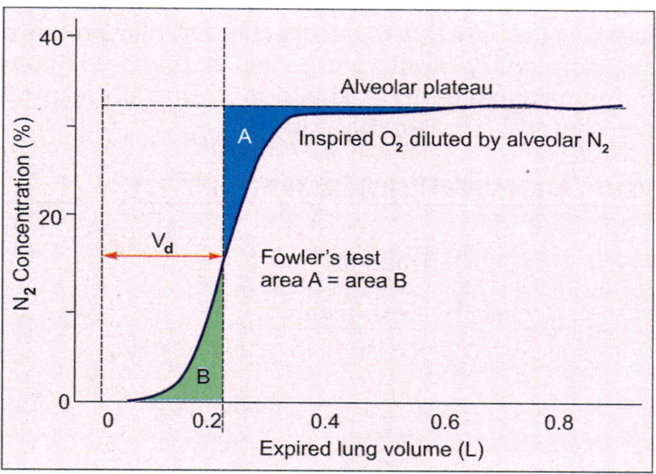

Fig. 7.19

Subject is asked to take a deep breath of pure oxygen and then to breath out into a nitrometer which measures the concentration of nitrogen. The first portion of air that comes out does not contain nitrogen and has only pure oxygen as it comes from upper airways. Then as the air from the alveoli starts coming out there is gradual increase in nitrogen concentration at the end of expiration nitrogen concentration reaches 60% and then levels off.

In the recording area in green represents dead space and area with blue represents alveolar air.

$$\text{Dead space} = \frac{\text{Area of green} \times \text{volume of expired air}}{100}$$

$$= \frac{30 \times 500}{100} = 150 \text{ ml}$$

Physiological Dead Space

This includes: Anatomical dead space, volume of air that ventilates under perfused alveoli and of air in the alveoli that in excess of the capillary blood. It can be measured by 'Bohr's equation;

$$\text{Dead space} = \text{Tidal volume} \times \frac{\text{PCO}_2 \text{ in alveolar air CO}_2 - \text{PCO}_2 \text{ in expired air}}{\text{PCO}_2 \text{ in alveolar air}}$$

$$= 500 \times \frac{40 - 28}{40}$$

$$= 150 \text{ ml}$$

7

PERFUSION OF LUNGS

Lungs are perfused with venous blood about 5 liters per minute. It gets affected by gravitational influences. The perfusion gradually increases from the apex towards the base due to the effect of alveolar pressure and pulmonary capillary pressure as discussed in the pulmonary circulation. This non uniformity can be detected by ^{133}Xe isotope study.

VENTILATION/PERFUSION RATIO (Fig. 7.20)

The ratio between alveolar ventilation (V) and perfusion (Q) is termed as:

$$\frac{\text{Ventilation}}{\text{Perfusion ratio}} \text{ or } \frac{V}{Q}$$

$$\text{Normal } \frac{V}{Q} \text{ is } \frac{4.2}{5} \text{ which is } 0.84.$$

Each lung displays the same ratio. But within the lung, the ratio differs in different parts as displayed below. At the apex the ratio is 3.4 due to under perfusion and at the base it is 0.63 due to over perfusion in relation to their ventilation. Normally, this physiological mismatch is corrected by autoregulation of the local blood flow, that is diverting the blood from under ventilated alveoli to normally ventilated alveoli.

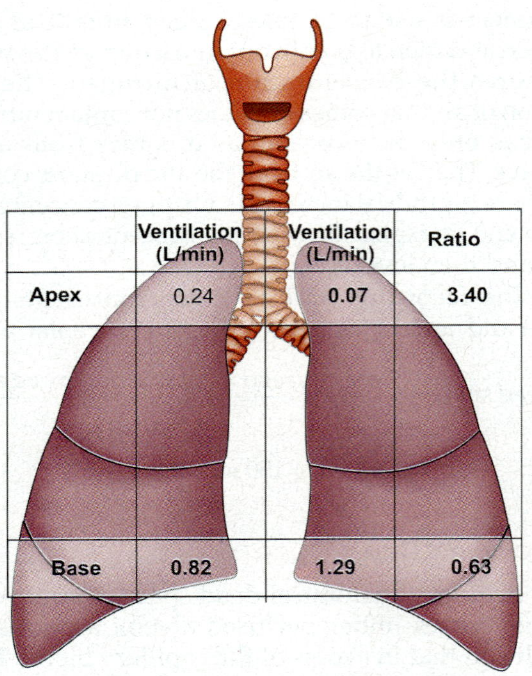

Fig. 7.20: Ventilation/perfusion ratio

Causes of Abnormal V/Q Ratio

Uneven Ventilation

- Asthma
- Pneumothorax
- Emphysema
- Pulmonary fibrosis.

Uneven Perfusion

- Anatomical shunts
- Pulmonary embolism
- Reduction in pulmonary vascular bed.

V/Q ratio influences the diffusion of oxygen and CO_2 in the alveoli (Fig. 7.21). In areas of high ratio ventilation is wasted and in areas with low ratio hypoxemia develops. This ultimately results in hypoxic hypoxia. Management depends on the cause.

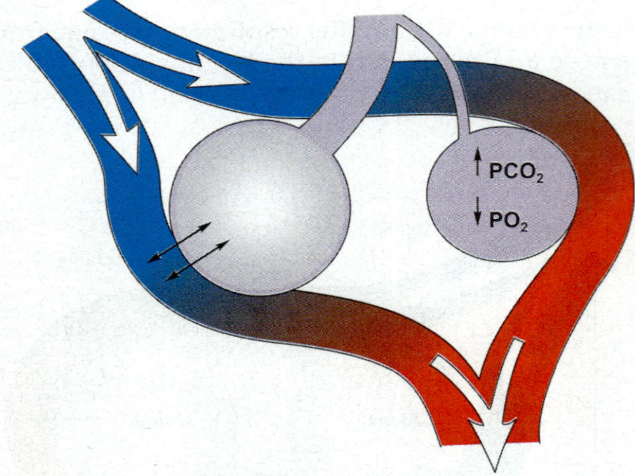

Fig. 7.21: Uneven ventilation

47. DIFFUSION OF GASES IN THE LUNGS

DIFFUSION

After the alveoli are ventilated with fresh air, the next step is diffusion of O_2 from alveoli to the blood and the diffusion of CO_2 from the blood to the alveoli. Oxygen and carbon dioxide cross the alveolar and pulmonary capillary membrane by diffusion. These two membranes are collectively called as 'Respiratory membrane'.

Diffusion: The gas molecules are free to move among one another by their own kinetic motion from the high concentration area to the low concentration area.

Partial pressure: In a mixture of gases the pressure caused by one particular gas alone is called as the partial pressure of that gas. It also depends on the solubility coefficient of that gas.

Diffusion coefficient: It is the product of solubility and molecular weight of that gas. If we take diffusion coefficient of oxygen is 1, CO_2 is 20 and nitrogen is 0.5.

Alveolar air and the atmospheric air do not have the same composition, because

- Alveolar air is only partially replaced by atmospheric with each breath
- O_2 is constantly absorbed into the pulmonary blood
- CO_2 is constantly diffuse into alveoli from blood
- Humidification of air in the respiratory passages adds to the water vapor pressure (Fig. 7.22).

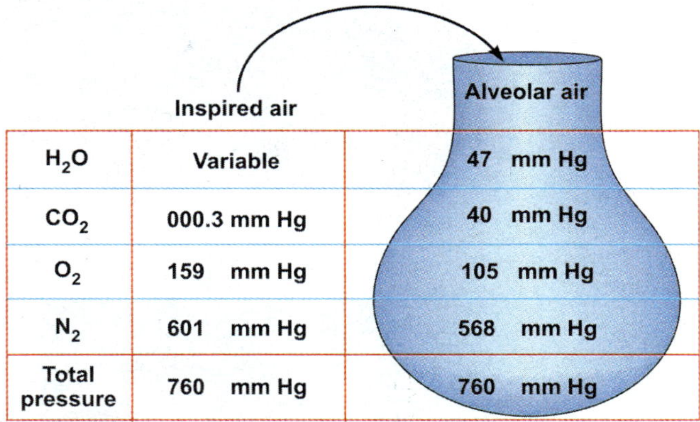

Fig. 7.22: Composition of atmospheric air and alveolar air

The overall thickness of the respiratory membrane is as little as 0.2 micrometer; total surface area of the respiratory membrane is about 70 square meters in the normal adult human male.

Factors that affect the rate of gas diffusion through the respiratory membrane

- Characteristics of respiratory membrane
- Pressure gradient
- Solubility of gas
- Molecular weight of the gas
- Diffusion coefficient
- Diffusion capacity

DIFFUSION OF GAS THROUGH RESPIRATORY MEMBRANES (Figs 7.23, 7.24b)

Respiratory Membrane

The following are the different layers of the respiratory membrane:

1. A layer of fluid lining the alveolus and containing surfactant that reduces the surface tension of the alveolar fluid.
2. The alveolar epithelium composed of thin epithelial cells.
3. An epithelial basement membrane.
4. A thin interstitial space between the alveolar epithelium and the capillary membrane.
5. A capillary basement membrane that in many places fuses with the alveolar epithelial basement membrane.
6. The capillary endothelial membrane.

Characteristics of Respiratory Membrane

i. *Thickness:* Diffusion is inversely related to thickness. Increase in thickness as in fibrosis and edema decreases the diffusion.

ii. *Permeability of the membrane:* Diffusion is directly related to permeability.

iii. *Surface area:* Diffusion directly is affected by the surface area.

Pressure Gradient

Diffusion is better when there is higher pressure gradient.

Solubility of Gas

Increase in solubility of gas in water increases diffusion. CO_2 can diffuse faster than O_2 because of better solubility.

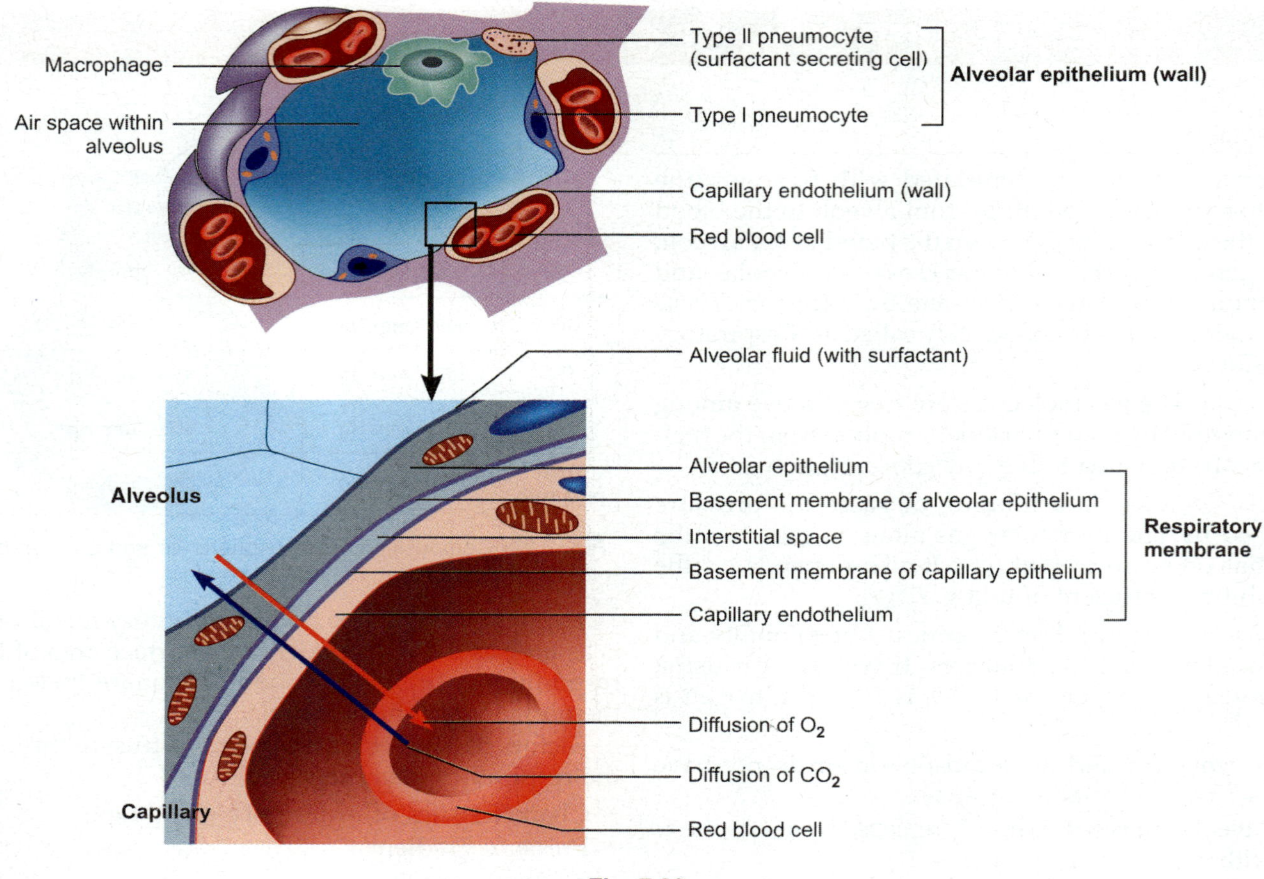

Fig. 7.23

Fig. 7.24: Structure of the bronchi and alveoli

Molecular Weight of the Gas

Diffusion is inversely proportional to molecular weight.

Diffusion Coefficient

It is defined as the volume of gas measured in ml that diffuses through one cm^2 of the membrane when there is a pressure gradient of 1 cm across the membrane (ml/cm^2/min/mm Hg). Diffusion coefficient of oxygen is 1, CO_2 is 20 and nitrogen is 0.5.

Diffusion Capacity

Diffusing capacity of the lung is the amount of gas that diffuses from the lung into the blood/minute when the pressure is 1 mm Hg across (ml/min/mm Hg) for oxygen is 21 ml/min/mm Hg for CO_2 is 20 times of O_2. So, 400–450 ml/min/mm Hg.

48. TRANSPORT OF CARBON DIOXIDE

DIFFUSION OF CO_2 FROM THE TISSUES TO THE BLOOD

CO_2 can diffuse about 20 times as rapidly as oxygen. Therefore, the pressure difference required is far less than that required for oxygen diffusion.

Decrease in blood flow increases the peripheral PCO_2 from 45 mm Hg to 60 mm Hg (Fig. 7.25).

Increase in tissue metabolic rate elevates the interstitial fluid PCO_2 to ten-fold from the tissues 3.7 ml CO_2/dl is added. So, the pH drops from 7.4 to 7.36.

TRANSPORT IN BLOOD

CO_2 is Transported in Three Forms in the Plasma

1. Dissolved form
2. *Carbaminocompounds:* CO_2 combined with plasma proteins
3. HCO_3^-

CO_2 in the RBC

1. Combines with Hb and forms carbamino Hb
2. Combines with other proteins and forms carbamino-compounds
3. Dissolved form in cytoplasm.

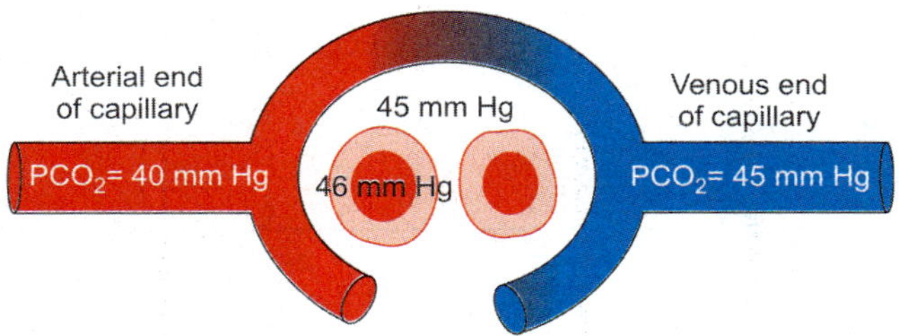

Fig. 7.25: Diffusion of CO_2 from tissues

Chloride shift: CO_2 gets hydrated in the presence of cabonic anhydrase and forms carbonic acid. This splits up into H^+ and HCO_3^-. HCO_3^- concentration increases inside the cells. So, it diffuses out of the RBC. To maintain the electroneutrality Cl^- ion enters the RBC from the plasma. This exchange is brought about by band three protein present in the RBC membrane (Fig. 7.26).

Because of this, chloride-bicarbonate shift, RBC gains more number of ions. H_2O also moves into the RBC to maintain tonicity. RBC volume increases. That is why, hematocrit of venous blood is more. This is also called Hamberger phenomenon.

Each 100 ml blood picks up 4 ml of CO_2

Forms	Arterial blood	Venous blood
Dissolved	2.6 ml	3 ml
Carbamino	2.6 ml	3.4 ml
HCO_3	42.8 ml	45.6 ml
Total	*48.0 ml*	*52.0 ml*

Delivery of CO_2 to the Lungs

Venous blood delivers the CO_2 to the lungs where the following factors influence the dissociation of CO_2.

Pressure gradient: Venous blood 45 mm Hg and alveoli is 40 mm Hg. This gradient favors CO_2 diffusion into the alveoli. PO_2^- increase in PO_2 in the alveoli facilitates CO_2 diffusion.This is called 'Haldane effect'.

Reverse chloride shift: CO_2 diffuse into the alveoli and O_2 diffuse from the alveoli into the RBC and combines

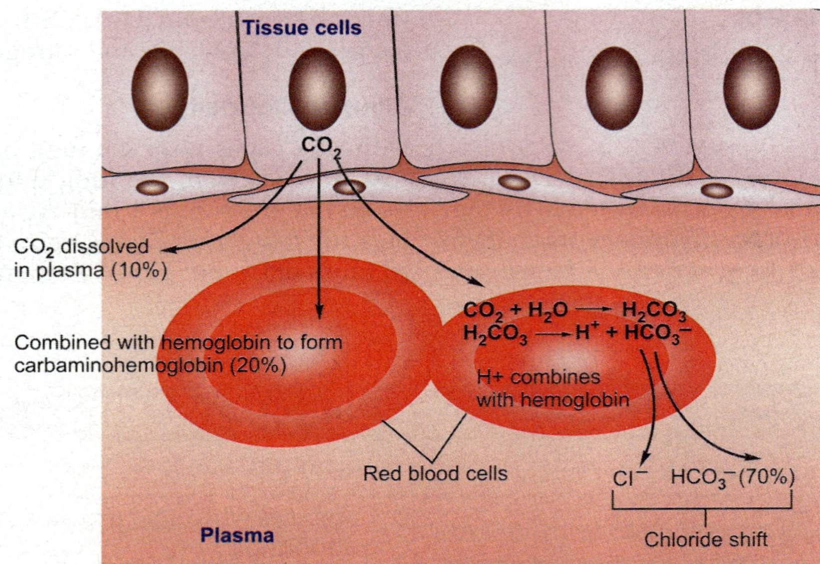

Fig. 7.26: Chloride shift

with Hb displacing H^+ and CO_2. Now, the Cl moves out in exchange for HCO_3. The HCO_3 which entered the RBC combines with H^+ and forms H_2CO_3, which splits into H_2O and CO_2, both diffuse into the plasma and into the alveoli. The size of RBC comes back to normal (Fig. 7.27).

7

CO_2 Dissociation Curve

The effect of PCO_2 and PO_2 on the CO_2 uptake and release by the blood can be studied through CO_2 dissociation curve (Fig. 7.28).

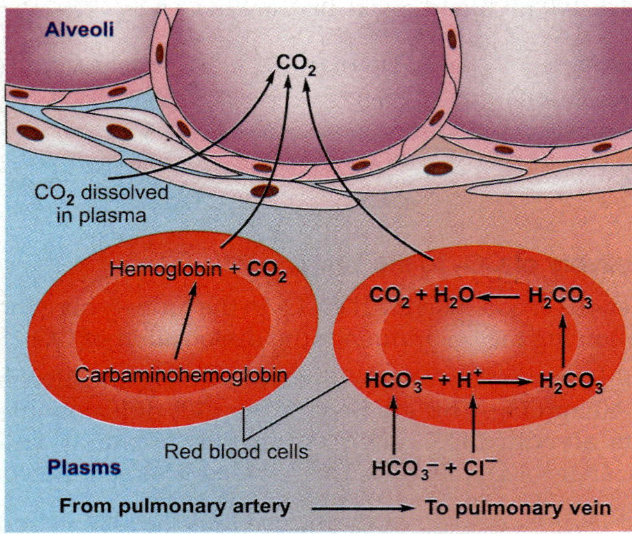

Fig. 7.27: Reverse chloride shift

From the graph it is clear that CO_2 content is proportional to CO_2 tension. With increased tension there is linear increase in CO_2 in the dissolved form. 200 ml of CO_2 per minute at rest. The CO_2 content of blood depends on the PCO_2 and PO_2 content of that blood. In the graph the lower curve is when the PO_2 is 100 mm Hg in the lung capillaries and the lower curve denotes the case in tissue capillaries when the PO_2 is 40 mm Hg. Point A shows the normal PCO_2 of 45 mm Hg in tissues and point B represents the fall in PCO_2 on entering the lungs as the PO_2 rises to 100 mm Hg. This Haldane effect doubles the amount of CO_2 released into the lungs and so, doubles the CO_2 pick up from the tissues.

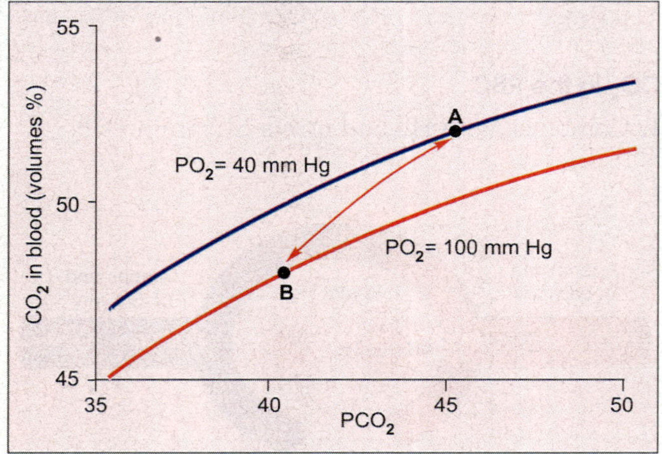

Fig. 7.28: CO_2 dissociation curve

49. TRANSPORT OF OXYGEN

OXYGEN DELIVERY SYSTEM

Oxygen delivery system comprises:
1. Lungs
2. Cardiovascular system.

STEPS OF TRANSPORT OF OXYGEN

Uptake: The PO_2 of the gases oxygen in the alveolus averages 104 mm Hg. PO_2 entering the pulmonary capillary at its arterial end is only 40 mm Hg. The initial pressure difference that causes oxygen to diffuse into the pulmonary capillary is 104 – 40 = 64 mm Hg. Oxygen reaches equilibrium with the pulmonary capillary blood in about 0.3 secs, i.e. before the blood crosses 1/3rd distance of the capillary.

Transport in arterial blood: It occurs in two forms:
  i. Dissolved form in simple solution
  ii. In combination with Hb.

Dissolved form in simple solution: (3%) oxygen dissolves in plasma and transported in negligible amount. It is 0.3 ml/100 ml. This form is very important in situation-like exercise when demand for oxygen is very high. But if this dissolved form exceeds the limits then oxygen toxicity ensues. In combination with Hb – 97%.

Reversible combination with Hb: Heme is a protein made up of four subunits, each of which contains a heme moiety attached to the polypeptide chain. Heme is a complex made up of porphyrin and iron in ferrous form at four corners. On the whole one oxygen molecule attaches with each iron molecule. So, each Hb reacts with four oxygen molecules. This takes only 0.01 sec and is reversible.

Oxygen affinity: The quaternary structure of Hb decides the affinity for oxygen. In deoxy form of Hb the globin units are tightly bound in a tense 'T' configuration which reduces its affinity for O_2. When the first molecule of oxygen binds with it the bond holding the globin units are relaxed, 'R' configuration, which exposes more binding sites and oxygen then binds vividly. Amount of oxygen that combines with Hb–in a normal person, Hb = 15 gm. Each 1 gm combines with 1.34 ml of O_2. So, 15 gm can bind to 20.1 ml of O_2, which is known as 20 volume percent. This is termed as HB is 100% saturated. But arterial blood is only 97% saturated due to physiological shunts (19.4 ml of O_2 is bound to Hb).

OXYGEN DISSOCIATION CURVE (ODC) (Fig. 7.29)

This curve relates the percentage saturation of Hb with PO_2. This curve is sigmoid in shape, due to T-R configuration. It demonstrates the progressive increase in percentage of Hb bound with O_2 as blood PO_2 increases which is known as percent saturation of Hb. The partial pressure of O_2 at which Hb is 50% saturated with O_2 is P50 at PO_2 of 26 mm Hg Hb is 50% saturated. This is P50. At 40 mm Hg Hb is 75% saturated. At 60 mm Hg, it is 90% saturated. The working range under

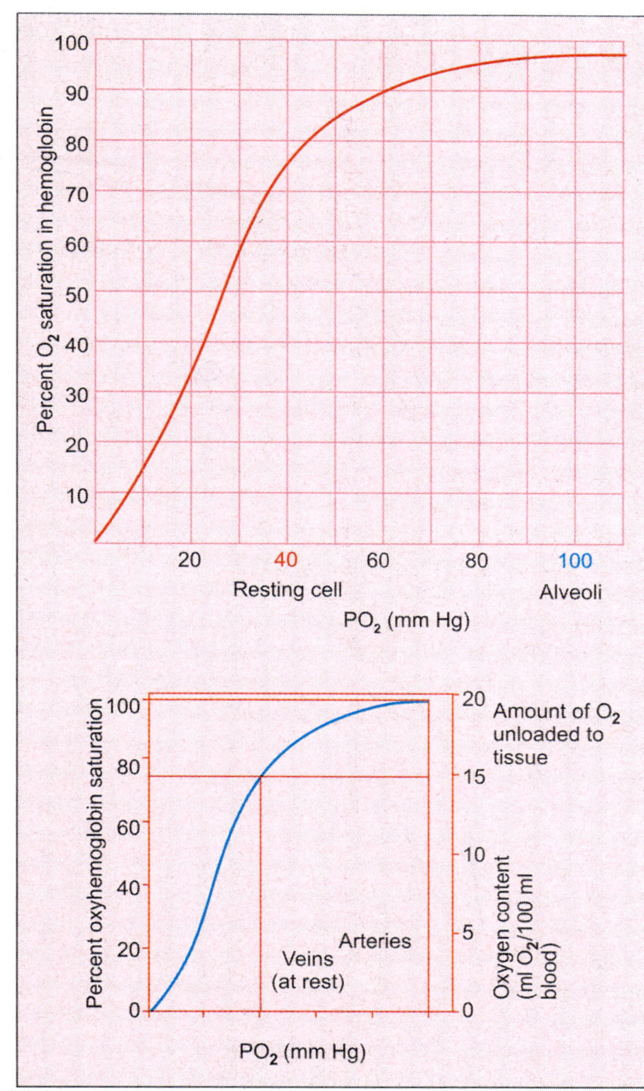

Fig. 7.29: Oxygen dissociation curve and its working range

resting condition is between 97% and 75%. That is arterial blood is saturated 97% and after delivery to the tissues when it comes to venous end it is 75% saturated. Factors which affect the Hb affinity (ODC) shift the curve either to the right (release of oxygen) or to the left (combines with oxygen).

Factors that Shift the Curve to the Right (Fig. 7.30)

- *pH:* When the blood becomes slightly acidic (decrease in pH), decreasing from 7.4 to 7.2 the curve shift to the right. Deoxy Hb binds to H^+ more actively than oxy Hb.
- *Decreased PO_2:* Because of increased in pressure gradient more oxygen dissociates from Hb.
- *Increased PCO_2:* This decreases the pH and cause release of O_2. CO_2 and H^+ enhances the release of O_2 from the blood to the tissues and from lung into the blood which is called Bohr's effect.
- *Increased temperature:* Increases diffusion and tissue demand for O_2.
- *Increased 2, 3-DPG:* It is formed from 3-phosphoglyceraldehyde, which is a product of Embden-Meyerhof pathway. It is highly charged anion that binds to the β chains of deoxy Hb displacing O_2. Increase in 2, 3-DPG shift the curve to the right causing liberation of more O_2. Its level decreases in acidosis and in stored blood. 2, 3-DPG increases in exercise, ascent to high altitude, under the influence of thyroid hormone, GH, and androgen.

Factors that Shift the Curve to the Left

In reverse state of all the above conditions the curve shift to the left.

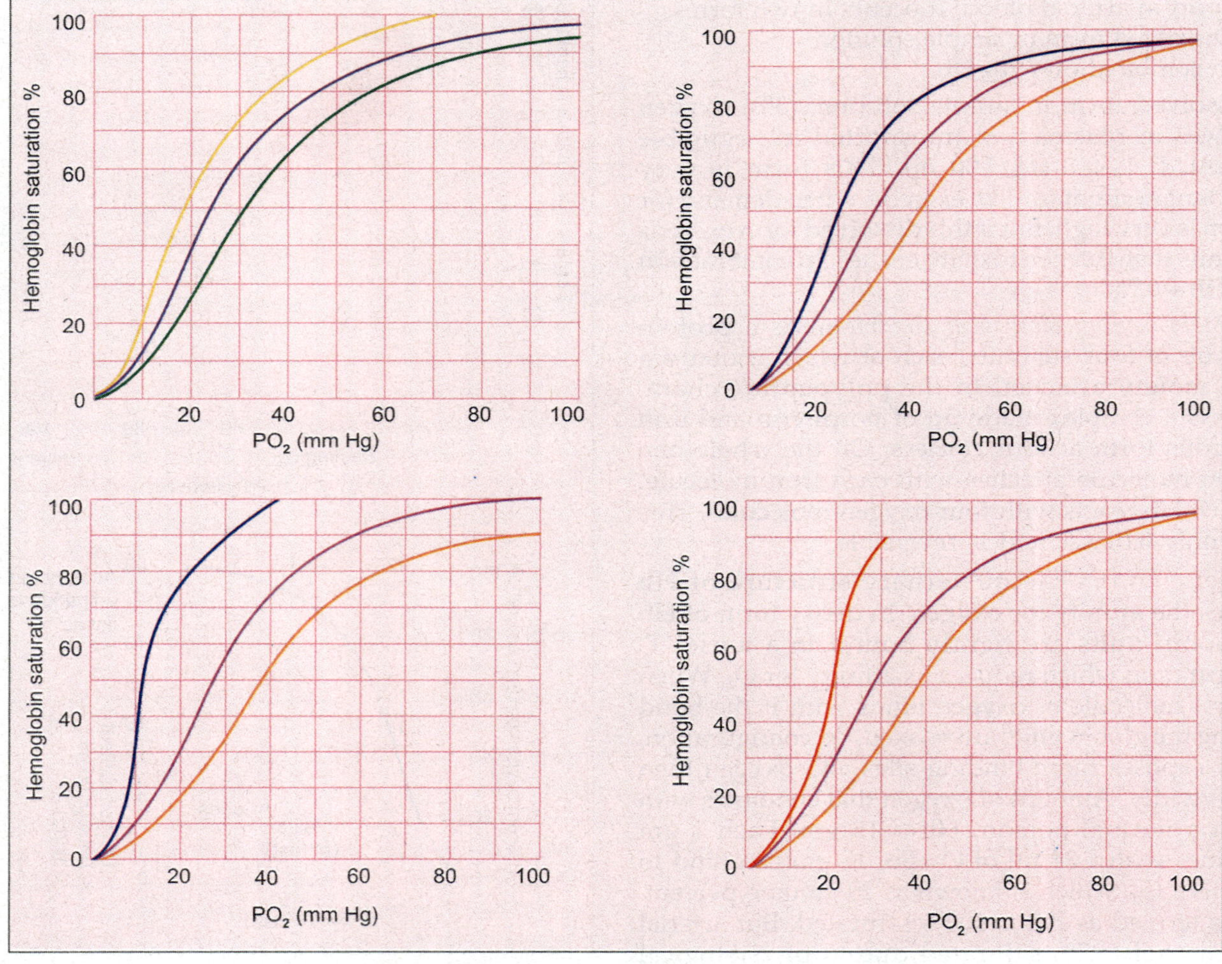

Fig. 7.30: Shift of ODC due to various factors

Fetal Hb: The affinity of HbF (Fetal) for O_2 is much greater than HbA (Adult), facilitating the movement of O_2 from the mother to the fetus. 2, 3-DPG also binds poorly with HbF favoring O_2 binding.

O_2 Uptake by the Tissues (Fig. 7.31)

Blood leaving the lungs is 97% saturated (19.8 ml/dl). In venous blood the Hb is 75% saturated (15.2 ml/dl). Thus at rest tissues remove 4.6 ml/dl. So, on the whole 250 ml of O_2 is delivered to the tissues per minute at rest. This tissue uptake depends on:

- Rate of energy expenditure by the cells
- Diffusion distance from the capillary
- Blood flow to the tissues.

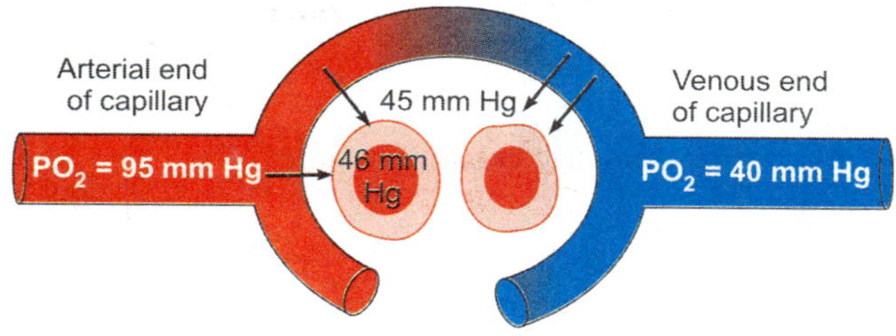

Fig. 7.31: O_2 diffuses into tissues

50. REGULATION OF RESPIRATION

Respiration is regulated by two mechanisms:
1. Neural
2. Chemical

NEURAL REGULATION OF RESPIRATION (Fig. 7.32)

Two separate neural mechanism regulate respiration: Voluntary and Involuntary (automatic system).

Voluntary Control

This is located in the cerebral cortex and sends impulses to the respiratory muscles through the corticospinal tract. This system remains quiescent but becomes active during:

a. Exercise
b. Defecation

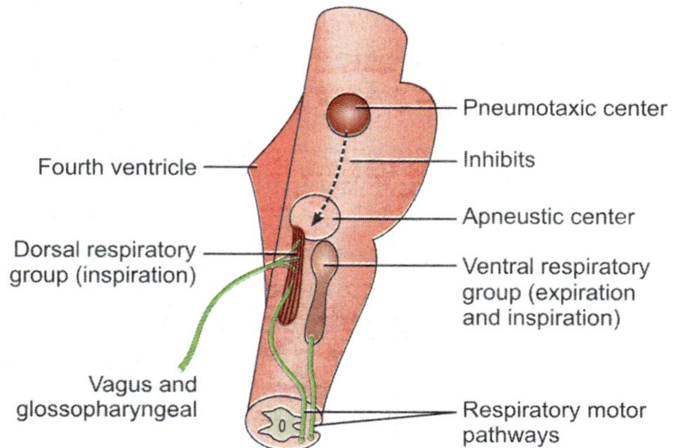

Fig. 7.32: Respiratory centers

The Automatic System/Involuntary System

These are a bilateral structure located in the pons and medulla and are well interconnected. It is divided into four major collection of neuron:

1. *Pneumotaxic center:* Located in the pons
2. *Apneustic center:* Located in the pons
3. *Dorsal respiratory group:* Located in the medulla
4. *Ventral respiratory group:* Located in the medulla.

7

Pacemaker Cells

It now seems that rhythmic respiration is initiated by a small group of cells, synaptically coupled in the pre-Botzinger complex on either side in the medulla between nucleus ambiguous and lateral reticular nucleus. These are like SA nodal cells having unstable RMP, hence fire spontaneously. There are NK-1 receptors and μ opiod receptors on these neurons. Substance-P stimulates and opioid inhibits their action. These neurons produce rhythmic discharge in:

- Phrenic motor neurons
- Hypoglossal nuclei
- Tongue

The spontaneous activity is brought to an end by the network connection with DRG neurons in which one set excites and the other inhibits the first and this cycle continues.

Pneumotaxic Center

This group of neurons is located in the nucleus parabrachialis in the upper pons. They do not have spontaneous activity, but on stimulation limits the action of DRG, either:

- Directly
- Through apneustic center.

Functions

- When pneumotaxic center activity is stronger duration of inspiration is shortened
- When pneumotaxic center activity is weaker: prolongs the inspiration.

So, the primary functions of this center is to increase the rate of breathing by shortening the respiratory cycle. By limiting the inspiration it plays a role in switching between inspiration and expiration.

Apneustic Center

This group of neurons is in the lower pons. The function of this center is to provide extra drive to the DRG neurons to cause a better filling off the lungs. But normally pneumotaxic neuron and the vagus override this drive in order to maintain normal respiration. So, when pneumotaxic center and vagus are cut, the effect is prolonged inspiratory spasm resembling breath holding called 'apneusis'.

Dorsal Respiratory Group (DRG) of Neurons

These are present in the nucleus tractus solitarius and to some extent in the adjacent reticular substance of the medulla. It is the sensory termination of vagal and glossopharyngeal nerves. These nerves transmit sensory signals from:

i. Peripheral chemoreceptor
ii. Baroreceptor
iii. Several types of receptors in the lungs.

DRG neurons are interconnected with pre-Botzinger complex and emit repetitive inspiratory neuron action potentials.

Inspiratory Ramp Signal

The nervous signal that are transmitted to the inspiratory muscles mainly the diaphragm is not an instantaneous burst of action potential. Instead it begins weakly and then increases steadily for about 2 seconds. Then it ceases abruptly for approximately the next 3 seconds, which turns off excitation of the diaphragm and allows elastic recoil of the lungs and chest wall. This causes expiration passively. The cycle repeats again and again. Based on the shape of recording activity this is termed as 'Ramp signal.'

Advantages of Ramp

- Steady increase in lung volume during inspiration rather than gasps.
- During heavy respiration the rate of increase in ramp is rapid, so that the lung volume is not affected.
- Earlier the ramp ceases it shortens the duration of inspiration and thereby the frequency of respiration is increased.

Ventral Respiratory Group (VRG) of Neurons

This group is located 5 mm lateral and ventral to DRG. Nucleus ambiguous rostrally and nucleus retro-ambiguous caudally. This contains both inspiratory and expiratory neurons. They do not have spontaneous rhythmic discharge.

Functions

1. They are inactive during quiet breathing. But in forced breathing they stimulate both inspiratory and expiratory muscles.
2. They do not participate in basic rhythmic oscillations.
3. When the input to DRG is strong the impulse spills onto VRG and then VRG contributes to the extra-respiratory drive especially to abdominal muscles for expiration.
4. Electrical stimulation of some neurons in VRG causes inspiration and other neurons cause expiration.

MECHANISM OF BREATHING

The pre-Botzinger complex fire spontaneously on the DRG of neurons, which steadily discharge in a crescendo manner for about 2 seconds. This is called inspiratory ramp. Now these neurons are facilitated by the Apneustic center causing sustained contractions of the inspiratory muscles for about 2–3 seconds. Chest wall and along with the lungs expands. Air enters the lungs causing inspiration. The lung stretch receptors through the vagus and impulses from the Pneumotaxic center arrest the discharge from the inspiratory neurons. Inspiratory muscles relax and chest recoils. Air from lungs expired out. The vagal afferents and pneumotaxic center are inactive now causing the onset of second cycle of inspiratory ramp. There is reciprocal activity noted in the inspiratory and expiratory neurons. When inspiratory neurons are active the expiratory neurons are inactive.

The pneumotaxic center and the vagal inputs check the activity of the DRG neurons causing increase in rate of respiration. On the other hand the effect of apneutic center is to prolong the inspiratory drive to aid in better filling of the lungs.

EXPERIMENTAL EVIDENCE

- Complete transection of the brainstem above the pons with all the cranial nerves cut—regular breathing continues.
- Section at midpontine level with bilateral vagotomy—DRG discharges continuously, arrest in inspiration-apneusis.
- Section at midpontine level with vagus intact (AC action is override by vagus)—regular respiration.
- Section between pons and medulla with or without vagi—continuous irregular respiration (pre-Botzinger complex and DRG discharge).
- Complete transection below the medulla—stops all respiration.

FACTORS AFFECTING THE RESPIRATORY CENTER

The activity of the respiratory center is affected by various mechanisms.

- Afferents from higher centers
- Afferent impulses from the peripheral receptors
- Reflexes
- Drugs

Afferents from Higher Centers

a. Cerebral cortex—has voluntary control. Automatic control gets sometimes disrupted without loss of voluntary control, clinically called as 'Ondine curse'. Patients with bulbar polio and disease that compress the medulla suffer with this clinical condition.

b. The ventilatory changes during emotions are controlled by limbic system.

c. Hypothalamus influences the ventilatory changes associated with temperature variations of the body.

Afferent Impulses from the Peripheral Receptors

- *Pulmonary stretch receptors:* These slow adapting myelinated nerve fibers are present among the airway smooth muscle cells and participate in Hering-Breuer reflex.
- *Fast adapting receptors (irritant receptors):* They participate in bronchoconstriction, hyperapnea, cough and sneezing.
- *J-receptor:* These are present between the alveolar wall and the capillaries . They are stimulated when fluid gets accumulated between capillary and alveolus in conditions like exercise, pulmonary embolism, edema, etc. stimulation of this receptor causes dyspnea and hyperpnea.
- *Pulmonary chemoreflex:* These receptors gets stimulated by nicotine like substances causing rapid breathing, hypotension and bradycardia.
- *Joint receptors:* The tendon, joint and joint capsule receptors stimulate breathing during exercise.
- *Inspiratory muscle spindle:* They maintain the tidal volume by detecting the load on the muscles.
- *Pain receptors:* Sudden painful stimulation causes reflex apnea. But, prolonged pain causes deeper respiration.
- *Thermoreceptors:* Sudden cold stimuli cause apnea. During diving this prevents entry of water into the airway. Warm stimuli increases rate of breathing.
- *Choking reflex:* Stimulation of receptors in pharynx and larynx by irritating chemicals cause temporary apnea to prevent aspiration.
- *Baroreceptor:* Baroreceptor stimulation inhibits respiration.

Reflexes that Modify Respiration

- *Sneezing:* Irritation of nasal mucosa causes deep inspiration followed by explosive expiration through the mouth and the nose.
- *Coughing:* Irritation of tracheobronchial mucosa causes deep inspiration followed by explosive expiration through the mouth only.
- *Swallowing:* A reflex apnea during swallowing prevents aspiration.
- *Vomiting:* A reflex apnea during vomiting prevents aspiration.
- *Speech:* Deep inspiratory effort followed by slow expiratory process.
- *Yawning:* Deep inspiration and stretching the body opens the under ventilated alveoli to prevent them from collapsing. This may be due to slight rise in PCO_2.
- *Hiccup:* Spasmodic contraction of the diaphragm produces inspiration and sudden glottic closure.

Drugs

Catecholamine, nicotine, caffeine stimulates breathing.

Anesthetic agents, sedatives inhibit breathing.

51. CHEMICAL REGULATION

Pulmonary ventilation is increased or decreased depending on the level of chemicals in the plasma, CSF and interstitial fluid of the brain. This, influence of chemicals on the respiratory center is called as chemical regulation.

Chemicals that alter respiratory activity

i. CO_2
ii. O_2
iii. H^+ (pH) of arterial blood.

These chemicals act through the chemoreceptors (Fig. 7.33):

i. Peripheral chemoreceptors
ii. Central chemoreceptors

Excess CO_2 or excess H^+ in the blood mainly acts directly on the respiratory center causing increased inspiratory and expiratory signals to the respiratory muscles. But, oxygen does not have direct effect on the respiratory center. It acts entirely on the peripheral chemoreceptors which transmit appropriate signals to control the respiratory center.

7

PERIPHERAL CHEMORECEPTORS

These are present in the 'Carotid body' and 'Aortic body'. Carotid body is present in the bifurcation of carotid artery and aortic body are present in the arch of aorta. These are made up of two kinds of cells.

Type-I: Glomus cells—contains dopamine, which modulates the response to hypoxia (Fig. 7.34). This is possible by the oxygen sensitive K channel in these cells which prevents K efflux during hypoxia, causing depolarization Ca influx excitation of the neurons innervating them.

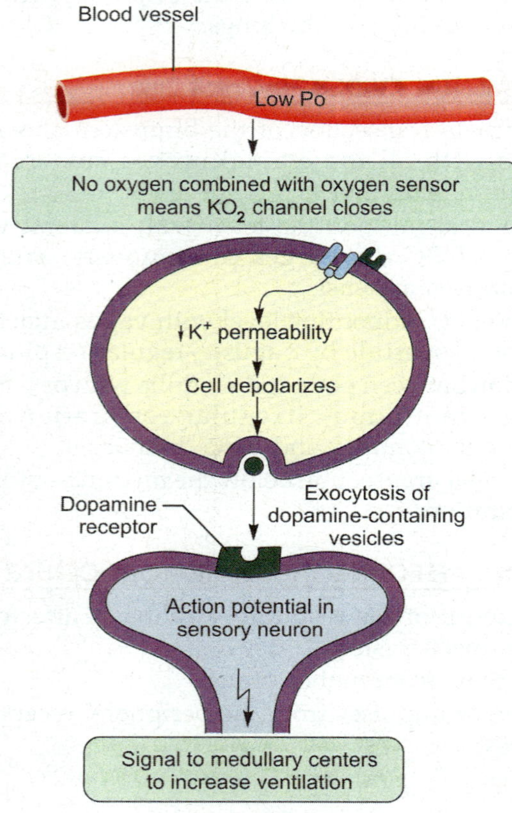

Fig. 7.34: Response to hypoxia

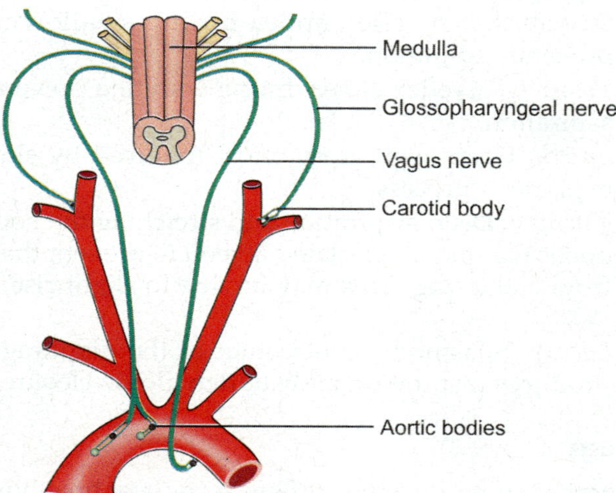

Fig. 7.33: Chemoreceptors

Type-II: Glial cells: they surround the type I cells and support them.

Functions

Both the carotid and aortic bodies have similar functions. They have enormous blood supply. They weigh about 2 mg but receives a blood flow of about 2000 ml/100 gm/min. They take dissolved oxygen from the blood that is why in anemia where the total oxygen is less but the dissolved oxygen is normal, these receptors are not stimulated. But sympathetic stimulation cause decreased blood flow and so, stimulates them.

PULMONARY AND MYOCARDIAL CHEMORECEPTORS

Injection of nicotine and like chemicals produce apnea, hypotension and bradycardia followed by tachypnea, which are due to the stimulation of chemoreceptors present in the coronary and pulmonary vessels. This is called Bezold-Jarish reflex which is not normal.

CENTRAL CHEMORECEPTORS

These are located in the ventral surface of the medulla, separate from the respiratory center. They monitor H^+ concentration of CSF and interstitial fluid of the brain. So, an increase in H^+ concentration stimulates them. But H^+ ion cannot readily cross the blood brain barrier. Hypercapnia (CO_2) is a potent stimulus. CO_2 readily cross the BBB as if barrier does not exists. The CO_2 that enters the brain and CSF is hydrated to H_2CO_3. This, then dissociates rising the local H^+ ion concentration. Blood CO_2 level has only an acute effect on the control of respiratory center. Because, this rise in CO_2 in taken care of by the renal system (Fig. 7.35).

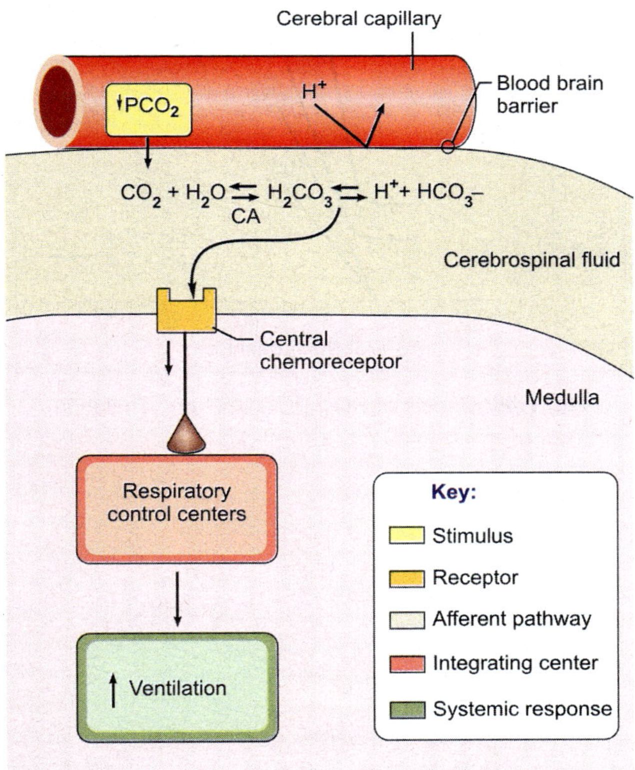

Fig. 7.35: Central chemoreceptor action to PCO_2

Role of Chemoreceptors on the Respiratory Center

Mechanism of Action of PCO_2 on Ventilation

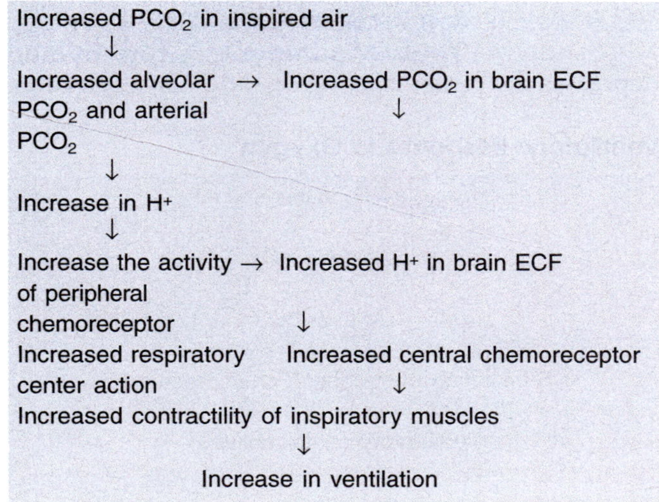

Effect of Different Level of ↑ Arterial PCO_2 (Carbon Dioxide Narcosis)

Mild 1.5% increase in PCO_2: CO_2 reaches the medulla and increase the rate and depth of respiration eliminating excess CO_2. No toxic symptoms.

Moderate 6% level: Arterial PCO_2 remains elevated and ventilation gets elevated 3–4 times the normal.

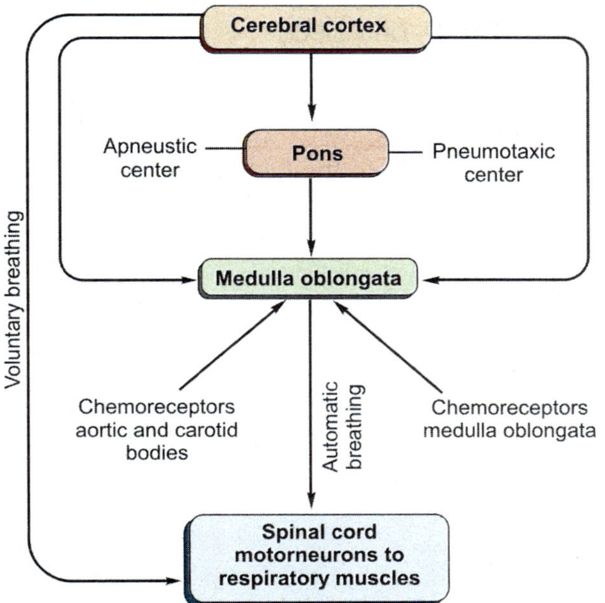

Fig. 7.36: Co-ordination of neural and chemoreceptors

Severe 10% level: PCO_2 begins to rise abruptly in spite of elevated ventilation and stimulates respiratory center tremendously. There wil be dyspnea, dizziness and headache.

Very severe >15%: CO_2 accumulates rapidly and depresses the center causing cessation of respiration.

Ventilatory Response to Oxygen

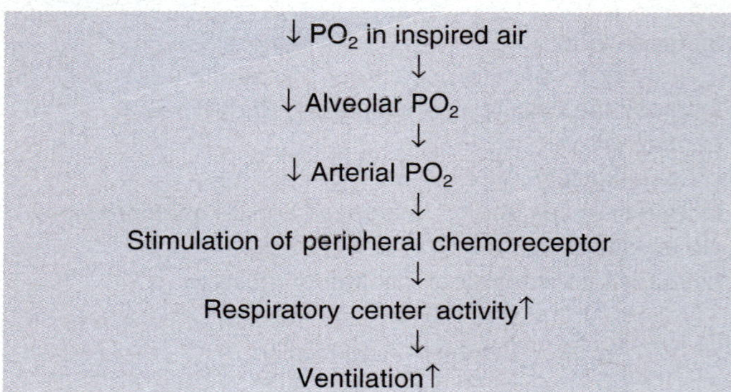

This rise is not noticed until the PO_2 drops less than 60 mm Hg. But slight change in ventilation is noticed even at 100 mm Hg which is not that much stimulatory. Because increase in ventilation washes out CO_2, the potent stimulus for the center (Fig. 7.37).

7

Effect of ↑ PCO_2 and ↑ H^+ Ion

Both the increase has an additive effect. 60% by CO_2 and the remaining 40% by the rise in H^+.

Effect of ↑ PCO_2 and ↓ PO_2

When there is hypoxia is always PCO_2 and acidosis. But it cannot be said they cause additive effect. The pulmonary ventilation at any time is due to the combined effect of all the factors on the respiratory center. Hypoxia makes an individual more sensitive to an increase in PCO_2 (Fig. 7.38).

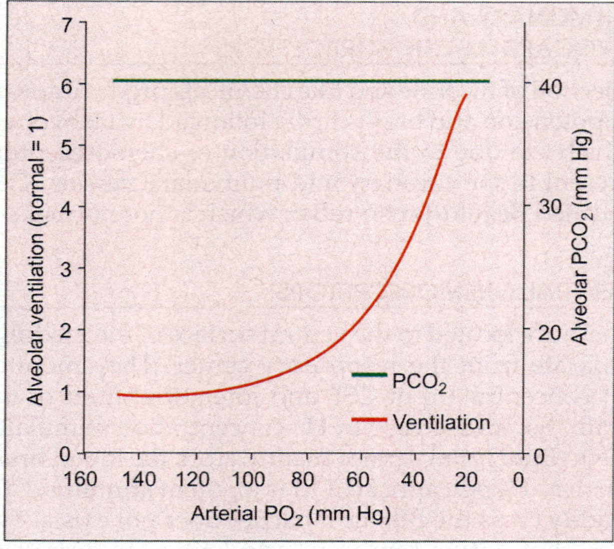

Fig. 7.37: Ventilatory response to O_2 and CO_2 levels

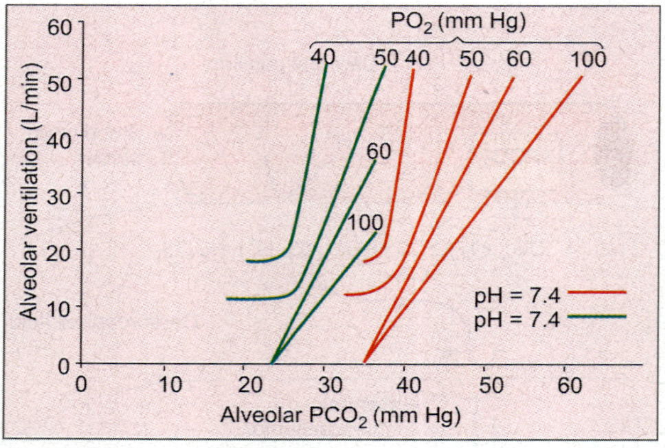

Fig. 7.38: Effects of PO_2, PCO_2, pH on ventilation

52. RESPIRATORY ADJUSTMENT DURING SLEEP

Respiration during Sleep

Respiration is less rigorously controlled during sleep than in wakeful state. During slow wave sleep the breathing is regular, slow and deeper. In REM sleep breathing is less deeper, rapid and irregular.

SLEEP APNEA

Apnea means absence of spontaneous breathing. Occasional apnea occurs in normal sleep. In sleep apnea the cessation of breathing is increased to 300–500 times each night with prolonged duration.

Causes

- Obstruction in upper airway
- Impaired respiratory drive.

Obstruction in Upper Airway
(Obstructive Sleep Apnea)

During sleep the muscles of pharynx relax. But the airway passage normally remains open enough to permit adequate airflow. Some have an exceptionally narrow passage. So that, during sleep the muscle relaxation completely closes the pharynx, preventing the airflow into the lungs. This causes loud snoring, labored breathing, interrupted by a long silent period during which no breathing occurs. This decreases PO_2 and increases PCO_2, which stimulates respiration, causing sudden attempt to breathe leading to loud snore. This gets repeated several hundred times during night resulting in restless sleep.

Effects

- Day time drowsiness
- Increased sympathetic activity
- Increased heart rate
- Pulmonary and systemic hypertension
- Risk of cardiovascular diseases.

Management

- Mostly occurs in obese persons. So, surgery to remove excess fat at the back of the throat can be done (uvulopalatopharyngoplasty)
- Opening in trachea (tracheostomy)
- Nasal ventilation with CPAP
- Removal of enlarged tonsils and adenoids.

Central Sleep Apnea

Occurs in:

- Damage to central respiratory centers
- Neuromuscular abnormalities.

These conditions cause cessation ventilatory drive during sleep. Patients with such problem will be able to manage with the assistance from voluntary breathing when they are awake. Cause is not known. Medications that stimulate respiratory center can sometimes help. But artificial ventilation (CPAP) is usually necessary at night.

Sudden Infant Death Syndrome (SIDS)

Central apnea in premature babies leads to death. Lack of maturation of respiratory center could be the cause.

PERIODIC BREATHING

It is a type of breathing in which breathing is interrupted by apneic periods. It is not seen normally.

7

Conditions

- Voluntary hyperventilation
- Premature infants
- Unacclimatized person at high altitude
- Heart failure
- Renal failure
- Increase in intracranial pressure
- Morphine poisoning
- Brainstem damage

Types

- Cheyne-Stokes respiration
- Biot's
- Kussmaul's
- Gasp

Cheyne-Stokes Respiration (Fig. 7.39)

Characterized by gradual waxing and waning, followed by a period of apnea, occurring about every 40–50 secs. This type of breathing is seen in:

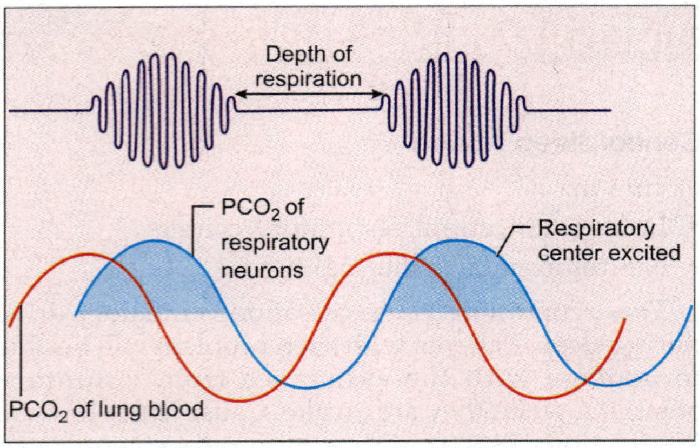

Fig. 7.39: Cheyne-Stokes pattern

i. Premature infants
ii. Unacclimatized person at high altitude
iii. During deep sleep
iv. Voluntary hyperventilation
v. Heart failure
vi. Renal failure

Mechanism: Hypoxia → hyperventilation → washes off CO_2 → respiratory center inhibited → apnea → CO_2 builds up → stimulates respiratory center → cycle repeats. Normally, this mechanism is damped.

Biot's (Fig. 7.40)

In this type apnea and hyperpnea are abrupt. Seen in:

i. Increase in intracranial pressure
ii. Morphine poisoning
iii. Brainstem damage

Mechanism: Over reaction of the center to a normal stimulus.

Rise in intracranial pressure → decrease in blood flow → ischemia of brain → increase in CO_2 accumulation → simulation of respiratory and vasomotor center → rise in BP → increase in cerebral blood flow → ischemia relieved → depression of respiratory center → apnea → cycle repeats.

Kussmaul's–Air Hunger

In metabolic acidosis increase in H^+ concentration stimulates the respiratory center through peripheral chemoreceptor.

Gasp: Occasional inspiratory effort seen in premature babies and in brain damage.

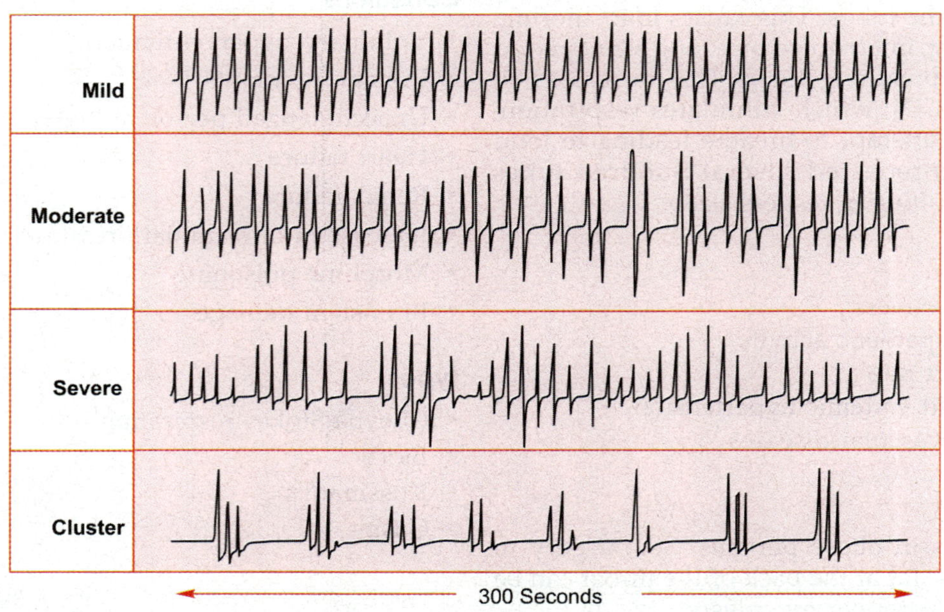

Fig. 7.40: Grading of Biot's

53. RESPIRATORY INSUFFICIENCY

Respiratory Diseases Results

- Inadequate ventilation
- Abnormalities of diffusion through pulmonary membrane
- Abnormal blood transport of gases between the lungs and tissues.

SPECIFIC PULMONARY ABNORMALITIES

Emphysema

The lungs lose their elasticity as a result of disruption of elastic tissue. The walls between alveoli breakdown and are replaced by large sacs.

Causes

Cigarette smoking, α_1-antitrypsin deficiency, etc.

Effects

- Increase in physiologic dead space, uneven alveolar ventilation } → hypoxia
- Perfusion of under ventilated alveoli → hypoxia.

Hypoxia leads to polycythemia which increases pulmonary resistance thereby causing pulmonary hypertension. This results in right ventricular hypertrophy, called as cor pulmonale.

Cystic Fibrosis

Congenital recessive condition in which the function of a Cl^- channel is depressed [cystic fibrosis transmembrane conductance regulator (CFTR)].

Effects

- Na^+ and Cl^- reabsorption is decreased
- Secretions become thick and lead onto recurrent respiratory tract infection especially with *Pseudomonas pneumonia.*
- This inspissated secretion blocks the spermatic duct and cause sterility.

Asphyxia

Acute lack of O_2 (hypoxia) and CO_2 excess (hypercapnia) when developed together is labeled as Asphyxia. It happens in conditions like drowning, strangulations, foreign body in trachea, etc.

Stages

- Exaggerated breathing
- Convulsions
- Collapse

Pulmonary Hypertension

Like systemic hypertension, it is a syndrome with multiple causes like:

- Hypoxia
- Cocaine inhalation
- Repeated use of appetite suppressing
- Systemic lupus erythematoses (SLE).

All these lead to increase in pulmonary vascular resistance and cause right ventricular hypertrophy, failure and death.

Pneumonia

This term includes any inflammatory condition of the lung in which some of the alveoli are filled with fluid and blood. Common pathogens are bacteria. Inflammation starts in the alveoli and later spreads to lobe or the whole of the lungs. Now, the condition is called as consolidation.

Atelectasis

It means collapse of the alveoli. Caused by:

- Total obstruction of airway
- Lack of surfactant in the alveolar lining [hyaline membrane disease (HMD)]
- Presence of air in pleural space (pneumothorax)
- Fluid in pleural space (hydrothorax)
- Blood in pleural space (hemothorax).

Asthma

Asthma is characterized by episodic or chronic wheezing, cough and a feeling of tightness in the chest as a result of bronchoconstriction. Fundamental cause unknown but a link to allergy has been recognized and plasma IgE level is often elevated.

The following abnormalities have been identified:

1. Partially reversible airway obstruction
2. Airway inflammation
3. Airway hyper-responsiveness to a variety of stimuli.

Pathophysiology

Leucotrienes from eosinophil and mast cells cause bronchoconstriction. Numerous amines, neuropeptides and interleukins damage the airway epithelium. Proteins from eosinophils contribute to airway hyper responsiveness. Asthma attacks are more severe in the late night and early morning which is the period of maximum constriction of bronchus (circadian rhythm).

Respiratory Failure

Whenever, the respiratory system fails to maintain normal PaO_2 and $PaCO_2$, it is referred to as respiratory failure.

Causes

- Increased work of breathing
- Decreased efficiency of gases
- Weakness of respiratory muscles
- Reduced respiratory center response to neural and chemical stimuli.

Types

- *Type I:* PaO_2 is less, $PaCO_2$ and pH is normal.
- *Type II:* PaO_2 is less, $PaCO_2$ is increased and pH is decreased.

54. HYPOXIA AND OXYGEN THERAPY

Hypoxia is oxygen deficiency at tissue level.

CLASSIFICATION

Hypoxia is classified based on the following factors:

- Oxygen tension in the arterial blood
- Oxygen carrying capacity
- Blood flow rate to the tissues
- Oxygen utilization by the tissues.

7

Based on the above factors hypoxia is classified as follows:

1. Hypoxic hypoxia
2. Anemic hypoxia
3. Stagnant hypoxia
4. Histotoxic hypoxia.

Hypoxic Hypoxia

It causes decrease in arterial PO_2 and decrease in oxygen delivery to the tissues. It occurs in the following conditions:

i. Low PO_2 in the inspired air (mines, high altitudes)
ii. Hypoventilation (airway obstruction, respiratory center depression)
iii. Diffusion defect (fibrosis, pulmonary edema)
iv. Abnormal V/Q ratio (atelectasis, collapse, large shunts).

Anemic Hypoxia

Arterial PO_2 is normal but the amount of Hb available to carry oxygen is reduced. It occurs in:

i. Anemia (increased 2, 3-DPG)
ii. Hemorrhage
iii. Carbon monoxide poisoning
iv. Abnormal hemoglobin.

Stagnant Hypoxia

Arterial PO_2 is normal, the amount of Hb available to carry oxygen is also normal. But the rate of blood flow to the tissues is reduced. It occurs in:

i. Shock
ii. Heart failure
iii. Intravascular obstruction.

Histotoxic Hypoxia

Arterial PO_2 is normal, the amount of Hb available to carry oxygen is normal, the rate of blood flow to the tissues is also normal. But the tissue is not able to utilize the oxygen delivered to it due to the presence of toxic agents. It is seen in:

i. Cyanide, sulfide poisoning
ii. Diphtheria
iii. Beriberi

EFFECTS OF HYPOXIA

On Cells

Hypoxia causes production of transcription factors named Hypoxia Inducible Factors (HIF), which are made of α and β subunits. In normally, oxygenated tissues the α subunits are destroyed. In hypoxic cells factor α dimerize with β and activate genes that produce angiogenic factors and erythropoietin.

On Brain

In generalized hypoxia brain gets affected first. Less severe hypoxia causes impaired judgment, drowsiness dulled pain sensation, excitement, disorientation, loss of time sense and headache. A sudden drop in inspired PO_2 to 20 mm Hg causes loss of consciousness in 10–20 secs and death in 4–5 minutes.

Other Tissues

- Nausea
- Vomiting
- Tachycardia
- Hypertension
- Reduced work capacity of muscles
- Fatigue
- Increase in ventilation in proportion to severity of hypoxia.

OXYGEN THERAPY (Fig. 7.41)

Oxygen can be delivered by various routes:

1. *Tent:* Placing patients head in a tent that contains air fortified with oxygen.
2. *Mask:* Allowing patient to breathe in oxygen from a mask connected with an oxygen cylinder.
3. *Intranasal tube:* Administering oxygen through intranasal tube.

In hypoxic hypoxia: Oxygen therapy increases PO_2 in alveoli from normal 100 mm Hg to as high as 600 mm Hg. This creates an increase in pressure gradient for diffusion.

In anemic hypoxia: In this type oxygen therapy is of limited value because oxygen is already available in the alveoli. But can be used to increase the dissolved form of oxygen in blood.

In stagnant hypoxia: Oxygen therapy is of little help in this form of hypoxia. Little extra oxygen given might increase the dissolved oxygen and may be beneficial.

In histotoxic hypoxia: Tissues are not able to utilize the oxygen even if supplied. However, hyperbaric oxygen therapy may benefit the individual.

Hyperbaric Oxygen Therapy

Administration of 100% oxygen at increased pressure increases the onset of oxygen toxicity. On the other hand, exposure to 100% oxygen at 2–3 atmospheres can increase dissolved oxygen in arterial blood, and oxygen toxicity is not a problem. This form of oxygen delivery is called *hyperbaric oxygen therapy*. It is of marked use in the following conditions:

- Carbon monoxide poisoning
- Radiation induced tissue injury
- Gas gangrene
- Very severe blood loss anemia
- Diabetic leg ulcers
- Slow healing wounds

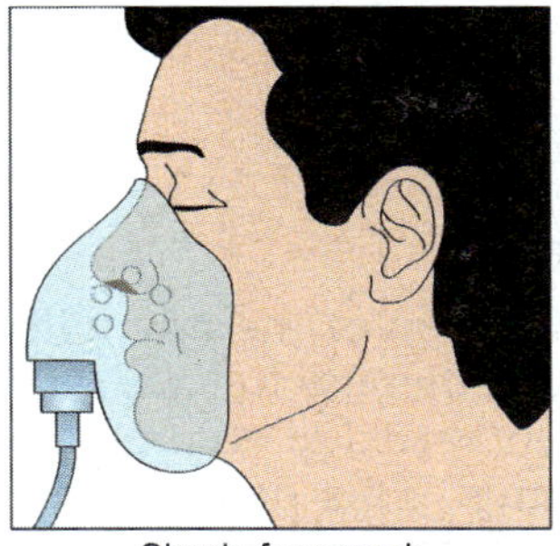

Simple face mask

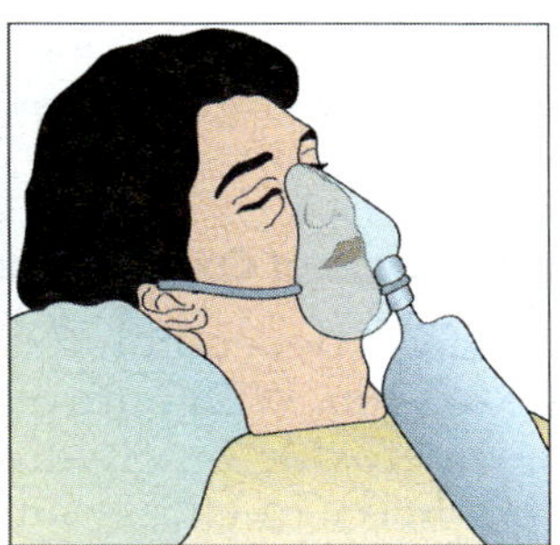

Partial rebreather mask

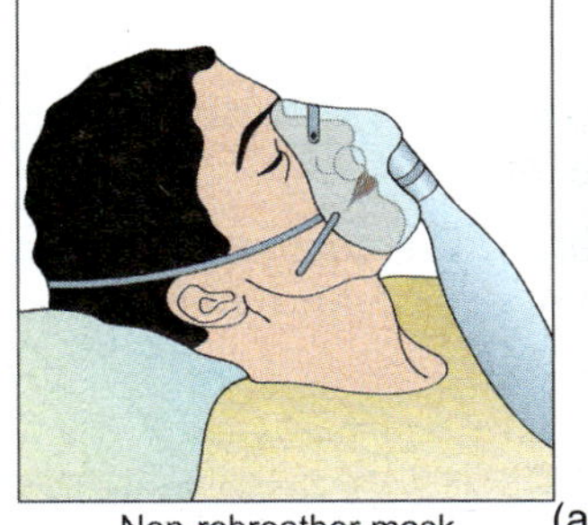

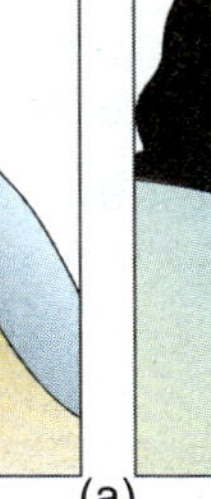

Non-rebreather mask

(a)

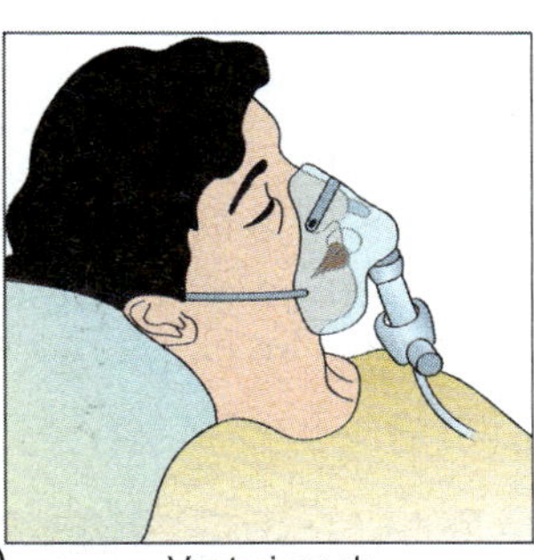

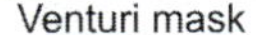

Venturi mask

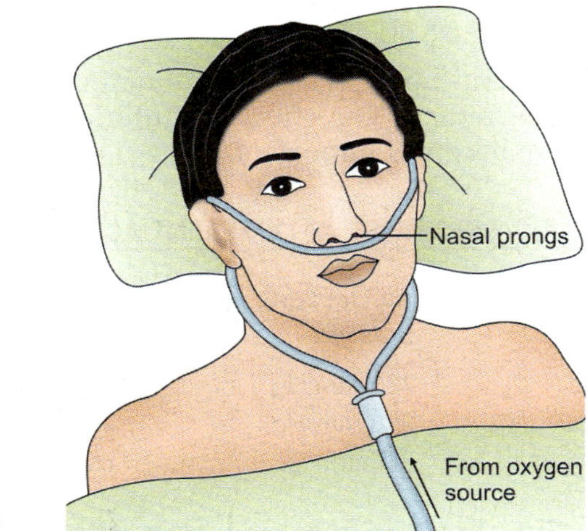

(b)

Figs 7.41a and b: Oxygen therapy. (a) Mask, (b) Intranasal tube

- Rescue of skin grafts and flaps
- Decompression sickness
- Air embolism

Toxic Effects of Oxygen Therapy

The effects depend on the duration of therapy with pure oxygen. With pure oxygen therapy free radicals like superoxide O_2^-, hydrogen peroxide accumulate in the body in excess amounts. This oxidizes the polyunsaturated fatty acids and destroys the cellular enzymes. As a result toxic effects due to oxygen therapy develop.

CNS: Nausea, irritability, dizziness, disorientation, facial twitching and convulsions.

RS: Congestion and irritation of the airway decrease in surfactant level, pulmonary edema and atelectasis.

Special senses: Spontaneous ringing (tinnitus) in the ear, loss of equilibrium, blurring of vision and retrolental hyperplasia in newborn.

Summary

Parameters	*Hypoxic hypoxia*	*Anemic hypoxia*	*Stagnant hypoxia*	*Histotoxic hypoxia*
PO_2 in blood	↓	Normal	Normal	Normal
O_2 carrying capacity	Normal	↓	Normal	Normal
O_2 content in blood	↓	↓	Normal	Normal
Blood flow rate	Normal	Normal	↓	Normal
Tissue utilization of oxygen	Normal	Normal	Normal	↓
Oxygen therapy	Very useful	Much useful	Can be useful	Doubtful

55. HIGH ALTITUDE AND SPACE PHYSIOLOGY

When we ascend up in aviation, mountain climbing and in space vehicles the effect of altitude and low gas pressure becomes important.

7

BAROMETRIC PRESSURES AT DIFFERENT ALTITUDES

Altitude	*Atmospheric pressure*	*PO_2 in the atm.*
Sea level	760 mm Hg	159 mm Hg
10000 ft	523 mm Hg	–
50000 ft	87 mm Hg	18 mm Hg

From the above it becomes clear that as the atmospheric pressure raises the PO_2 decreases (21% of the total pressure). PO_2 is also affected by the PCO_2 and water vapor pressure.

For Instance, at the Top of Mount Everest (20,028 ft)

Barometric pressure	253 mm Hg
Water	–47
All the other gases:	206 mm Hg
PO_2	–07
	199 mm Hg

Of which 1/5 is PO_2 (40 mm Hg) and 4/5 is N 2.5 mm Hg is normally being absorbed. So, at anytime only 35 mm Hg is the PO_2 in the alveoli with which a person cannot survive at that altitude. Therefore, it becomes essential to breathe pure O_2 for survival.

EFFECT OF BREATHING PURE OXYGEN

Altitude in feet	*Atmospheric pressure in mm Hg*	*PO_2 in air in mm Hg*	*PO_2 in alveoli in mm Hg*	*Arterial O_2 saturation in %*	*Breathing pure O_2*	
					PO_2 in mm Hg	*Arterial O_2 saturation in %*
Sea level	760	159	104	97	673	100
10,000	523	110	67	90	436	100
20,000	349	73	67	90	262	100
30,000	226	47	18	24	139	99
40,000	141	29	–	–	58	84
50,000	87	18	–	–	16	15

ACCLIMATIZATION

When a person ascends high altitude and stays there for longer periods, he slowly gets adapted to the new environment. The body mechanisms that undergo changes to bring an adaptation in, the new environment of low PO_2, so that it causes few deleterious effect on the body is termed as *acclimatization*.

It can appear in a few hours and may take several days. Maximum height to which adaptation occurs is 18,000 ft. Beyond which a person needs oxygen inhalation for survival (*see* above table).

Systemic Changes

Respiratory System

- ↑ in pulmonary ventilation due to stimulation of chemoreceptors, increasing rate and depth of respiration
- ↑ in diffusing capacity
- Respiratory muscles hypertrophy.

Kidney

- Excretes more HCO_3^- in urine
- Produces erythropoietin in large amounts.

Blood

- Erythropoietin stimulates bone marrow causing in RBCs
- Polycythemia
- ↓ Hb
- ↓ PCV
- Hypoxia and alkalosis ↓ 2, 3-DPG shifting the oxygen dissociation curve to the right, facilitating O_2 release.

Cardiovascular System

- Rise in heart rate, cardiac output and blood pressure
- ↑ in tissue blood flow and coronary flow
- Activation of sympathetic system initially but later parasympathetic system takes over and restores cardiovascular functions.

Tissues

- ↑ in capillary density
- ↑ in oxidative enzyme activity
- ↑ in number of mitochondria
- ↑ angiogenesis
- ↑ in myoglobin
- ↑ in cytochrome oxidase

ACUTE MOUNTAIN SICKNESS (AMS)

A small percentage of people who ascend rapidly to high altitude become sick, because of nonadaptation to hypoxia. The signs and symptoms which develop in these people are collectively called as *acute mountain sickness.*

Events of AMS

Acute cerebral edema: Hypoxia causes local cerebral vasodilatation → increase in blood flow into the cerebral capillaries → increase in pressure → fluid leak into cerebral tissues → causing headache, irritability, loss of coordination and memory.

GIT: Nausea, vomiting and diarrhea due to gaseous distension of GIT.

Respiratory system: Hypoxia stimulates respiration causing hyperpnea and dyspnea.

Acute Pulmonary Edema

In severe hypoxia, the pulmonary arteries constrict potently in some parts of lungs than in the other areas. So, more and more blood is forced through unconstricted vessels causing increase in capillary pressure and leakage into interstitial space causing pulmonary edema. Progression of this sometimes leads to severe respiratory dysfunction and becomes lethal.

CHRONIC MOUNTAIN SICKNESS (MONGE'S DISEASE)

This is seen in long-term residents of high altitude, e.g. Aldes.

Events of Monge's

- ↑ in red cell mass and hematocrit
- ↑ in pulmonary arterial pressure
- Enlarged right heart
- ↑ in peripheral arterial pressure
- Congestive heart failure
- Death unless brought back to low altitude.

Causes

1. ↑ in red cell mass and hematocrit → increase in blood viscosity ↓ tissue blood flow leading to tissue hypoxia.
2. Pulmonary vasoconstriction increases pulmonary arterial pressure.
   This increase right heart size and later leads to right heart failure.
3. Alveolar arterial spasm leads to increase in pulmonary shunt.

Most of these recover within a few days or weeks when they are moved to lower altitude.

56. DEEP SEA PHYSIOLOGY

EFFECT OF INDIVIDUAL GAS HIGH PRESSURE

When a person descends beneath the sea, the pressure around him increases tremendously. To keep the lung from collapsing due to this increased external pressure air must be supplied to the lung at high pressure. This exposes the lung blood to high alveolar gas pressure, a condition termed as hyperbarism.

Level	*Atmospheric pressure*
Sea level	1
33	2
66	3
100	4
133	5
166	6
200	7
300	10

Pressure in Relation to Sea Depth

For every 33 ft depth the pressure increases by 1 atmospheres.

7

For example, a person 33 ft beneath the sea level is exposed to 2 atmospheric pressures, i.e. one caused by weight of air above water and one caused by weight of water itself. Another important effect of depth is compression of gases to smaller volume. The volume to which a given quantity of gas is compressed is inversely proportional to the pressure (Boyle's law). This is very important drawback in diving physiology because increased pressure can collapse the air chambers especially the lungs.

Effect of Individual Gas High Partial Pressures on the Body

Gases to which a diver is exposed when breathing air are:

- Nitrogen
- Oxygen
- Carbon dioxide

The inhaled gases dissolves in the body fluids during deep sea diving and causes:

- Nitrogen narcosis
- Oxygen toxicity
- HPNS
- Dysbarism
- Air embolism

Nitrogen Narcosis

About 4/5th of air is nitrogen. When a diver remains beneath the sea for an hour or more and is breathing compressed air the first symptom of high nitrogen pressure called nitrogen narcosis appear at 120 ft.

At 150 ft he becomes drowsy

250 ft: Clumsy and weak to perform action

>250 ft: Becomes useless. As these effects are similar to alcohol intoxication effects it is also called as *'Rapture of depth'.*

Pathophysiology: Nitrogen dissolves in fatty substances in neuronal membrane causing alteration in ionic conductance and reduces neuronal excitability.

Prevention: By replacing nitrogen with helium.

Oxygen Toxicity

On oxygen transport: In the normal range of alveolar PO_2 (<20 mm Hg) almost none of total oxygen is accounted for dissolved form. But as PO_2 rises to 1000 mm Hg a large portion gets dissolved in the water of the blood.

On tissues: As this blood with highly dissolved oxygen passes through the capillaries to the tissues, oxygen is delivered to tissue at extremely high pressure. Molecular oxygen has little capability of oxidizing other chemical compound, for it must be converted to an active form of oxygen which are collectively called as 'oxygen free radicals'. Important of them are:

- Superoxide
- Hydrogen peroxide

Even normally at 40 mm Hg PO_2, small amount of free radicals are formed from dissolved oxygen. But they are rapidly removed by peroxidases, catalase and superoxide dismutase. Above a critical PO_2 the tissue oxygen rises to hundred or thousand times the normal. The amount of enzymes to neutralize, then formed free radicals becomes insufficient. So, the free radicals are free to cause serious effects by oxidizing cell membrane (especially neurons) and cellular enzymes.

Symptoms of Acute Oxygen Poisoning

- Nausea
- Dizziness
- Muscle twitching
- Disturbance of vision
- Irritability
- Disorientation
- Seizure
- Coma

Chronic Oxygen Poisoning Effects

>12 hours of >1 atmosphere of oxygen exposure causes

- Airway congestion
- Pulmonary edema
- Atelectasis

Carbon Dioxide Toxicity

Depth does not increase the rate of CO_2 production in the body as long as the diver breathe at normal tidal volume and expires CO_2 as it is formed. Sometimes, such as diving helmets and with some rebreathing apparatus, CO_2 builds up in the dead space and is again rebreathed by the diver. Up to 80 mm Hg of PCO_2 (twice normal) he can tolerate by eliminating the excess CO_2 by increasing the minute ventilation. Beyond 80 mm Hg respiration gets depressed and then fails due to respiratory acidosis. Finally, even anesthesia develops as discussed in CO_2 narcosis.

Decompression sickness (dysbarism/caisson's disease/bends/divers palsy).

Dysbarism is a condition which occurs when a subject is exposed to high atmospheric pressures and is suddenly brought to low atmospheric pressure. It occurs in:

- Deep sea divers
- Workers in caisson (caisson-water tight chamber used for carrying out construction under water).

Pathophysiology

Amount of nitrogen that is dissolved in body fluids is proportional to the depth. Nitrogen is carried to all the tissues of the body equal to breathed in nitrogen. It is lipid soluble but not metabolized by the body. So it remains in the dissolved state until the nitrogen pressure in the comes down to lower level. Then the nitrogen is removed by reverse respiratory process. But this removal should happen slowly. Because as long as the person remains beneath the sea the pressure outside his body compresses all the tissues and the nitrogen in the tissues are kept compressed in dissolved state. When he suddenly rises to sea level the gas escapes from dissolved state and forms bubbles of nitrogen.

Small bubbles of nitrogen coalesce → block large vessels → tissue ischemia → tissue death.

Symptoms

i. Presence of bubbles in the myelin sheath of sensory fibers produce severe pain in joints and muscles of limbs
ii. Bubbles in motor nerves and cerebral vessels cause paralysis and brain damage
iii. Coronary vessel block cause myocardial infarction
iv. Dyspnea, cyanosis and chocking
v. Loss of consciousness
vi. Even death

High Pressure Nervous Syndrome (HPNS)

As dissolved nitrogen causes narcotic effect a mixture of helium and oxygen are preferred in deep sea divers. The reasons are:

- Narcotic effect of helium is 1/5th of nitrogen
- Air flow resistance is less, so reduces work of breathing
- Less soluble in body fluids.

However, it causes HPNS due to its anesthetic effect. High pressure nervous syndrome (HPNS) is characterized by:

- Tremors
- Drowsiness
- Lack of co-ordination
- Impairment of manual dexterity.

Management

- Subject should be slowly decompressed to the surface (not more han 3 m/hour).
- If he started developing symptoms he has to be first recompressed and then decompressed.
- It should follow the decompression table chart framed by US Navy, which takes about 3 hours.
- If he has reached the surface with symptoms he is put into a pressurized tank and then the pressure is slowly brought down to normal atmospheric pressure.

- Helium can be used instead of nitrogen to prevent such hazards.

SCUBA

In 1943 Jacques Cousteau popularized the self contained under water breathing apparatus (SCUBA) for underwater diving (Fig. 7.42).

Components

1. One or more tanks of compressed air or some other breathing mixture.
2. Reduction valve for reducing high pressure from the tank to low pressure level.
3. Inhalation and exhalation valve that allows air to be pulled into the lungs and then exhaled to sea.
4. Mask and tube with small dead space.

With each inspiration air from the tank enters the lungs through the mask. On expiration air goes out into the sea.

Disadvantage

SCUBA can be used for only stipulated time depending upon the depth and the quantity of air required.

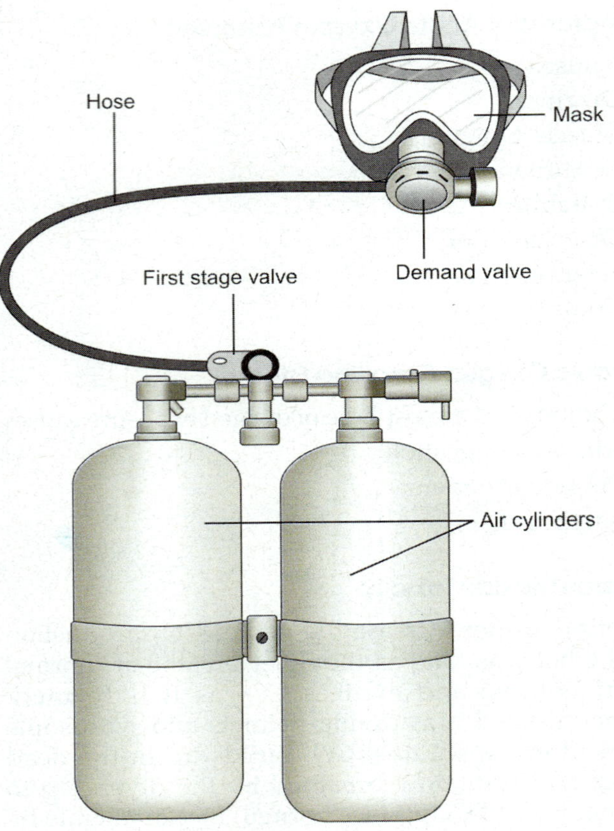

Fig. 7.42: SCUBA

7

57. AVIATION PHYSIOLOGY

Rapid change in velocity and direction in airplanes and space craft affect the body with several acceleratory forces.

- *Beginning of flight:* Linear acceleration
- *End of flight:* Deceleration
- *When vehicle turns:* Centrifugal acceleration.

'G' ACCELERATORY FORCE

When an aviator is simply sitting in his seat, the force with which he is pressing against the seat is due pull of gravity. This force is said to be +1 G (positive G). If the plane goes through a loop the person lifts off the seat and needs to be held down by seat belt. This force with which he is held down by his belt is – 1 G (negative G).

Effects of Positive G

CVS: Blood is mobile and therefore gets translocated to lowermost part of the body. So, the pressure in leg veins greatly increases. As the pressure increase, the vessels dilate and so venous return decreases which reduces the cardiac output. So, when the G becomes +3.3 both systolic pressure and diastolic pressure goes below 22 mm Hg at the initial acceleration then SP becomes 55 and DP is 20 mm Hg in another 10–15 seconds due to baroreceptor reflex. Acceleration >4–6 G can cause 'Black out' of vision within a few sec and become unconscious. If this continues the person will die.

Vertebrae: high positive G causes fracture of vertebrae. The maximum +G a person can withstand in sitting position before vertebra fracture occurs is about +20 G.

Effects of negative G: Negative G effects are less dramatic acutely but more damaging permanently than +G. Up to – 4 to – 5 G no harm occurs. Although it causes intense momentary hyperemia of head and psychotic disturbances, lasting for 15–20 minutes due to brain edema. If it becomes >–20 G centrifugation of blood into the head becomes so great that cerebral BP becomes 300–400 mm Hg causing small vessels to rupture. But the increase in CSF pressure acts as a cushion to prevent intracerebral vascular rupture. Because eyes are not protected by the cranium the intense hyperemia causes temporary blindness termed as 'Red out'.

Protection of Body Against G Forces

1. *Procedure:* Aviator tightens his abdominal muscles to maximum, leans forward to compress abdomen and increase the venous return so as to delay the black out.
2. *Anti-G suit:* This suit applies positive pressure to the leg and abdomen by inflating compression bags as the G increases. But even this cannot prevent displacement of heart, lung and diaphragm beyond 10 G.

ZERO G (MICRO GRAVITY/WEIGHTLESSNESS)

A person in an orbiting space craft experiences weightlessness. This means the person floats within the space craft which is due to the action of gravity on both the space craft and the person at the same time, in the same direction and with the same force. So, the person is not attracted anywhere and floats (Fig. 7.43).

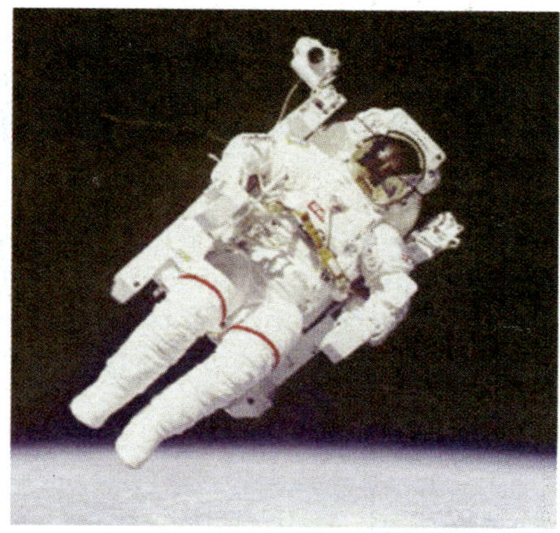

Fig. 7.43: Astronaut wearning space suit

Physiological Problems due to Weightlessness

- Motion sickness during first 2–5 days
- ↓ in blood volume
- ↓ in red cell mass
- ↓ in muscle strength and atropy
- ↓ in cardiac output
- Lose of calcium and phosphorus from bones
- When the stay is prolonged cardiovascular deconditioning happens causing impaired baroreceptor reflexes
- Bone fractures due to loss of bone mass.

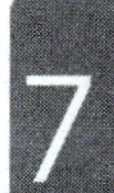

Counter measures to zero G effects

1. Exercise during prolonged stay
2. Intermittent artificial gravity of 2–3 G for short periods.

58. ARTIFICIAL RESPIRATION

Artificial respiration is given to a subject whenever, there is respiratory deficiency or arrest, as the brain cannot survive long in the absence of oxygen.

INDICATIONS

- Drowning
- Gas poisoning
- Electric shock
- Anesthesia
- Accidents
- Poliomyelitis
- During surgery
- Head injury

METHODS

Two artificial methods are in practice:
1. Instrumental
2. Manual

Instrumental

This method is used when a person requires artificial respiration for prolonged periods as in tetanus or polio.

1. Positive Pressure Method

Lung is inflated by air or air + O_2 mixture from a Boyle's apparatus at positive pressures either continuously or intermittently. It is used in operation theaters. But this cannot be used for prolonged periods as it impairs venous return.

2. Negative Pressure Method

This is achieved by artificially compressing and relaxing the chest wall

a. *Drinkers' (iron lung chamber) method (Fig. 7.44):* The patient is placed inside an airtight chamber in which the pressure can be increased or decreased alternatively from outside. When pressure inside is ↑ expiration occurs and when pressure inside is ↓ inspiration is caused.
b. *Braggpaul method:* A hollow elastic rubber bag is wrapped around the chest. When the bag is inflated chest is compressed and the air is expelled.

Manual

7

1. *Holger-Neilson method (back pressure–arm lift method):* Subject is placed in prone position and head turned to one side. Shoulder abducted and arm flexed at elbow with hands placed under cheeks of the patient. The operator kneels down at the head end of the subject, bends forward and presses the back for expiration. Then the operator lifts the abducted shoulder of the subject and approximates the elbows for expanding the chest.
2. *Eve's rocking method:* Subject is placed on a stretcher in prone position and rocked up and down like a seesaw. When the head is down the abdominal viscera pushes the diaphragm down and expiration occurs. In heel down position diaphragm is pulled down so that air is drawn in.
3. *Mouth-to-mouth breathing:* The patient is placed in supine position and is airways cleaned placing a handkerchief or clean fine cloth covering the mouth of the subject, operator places his mouth over-the- mouth of the subject and exhales into the subjects mouth covering his nose to prevent air leak. This inflates subjects lung. Then expiration happens passively. This procedure is repeated at the rate of 12 times a minute.

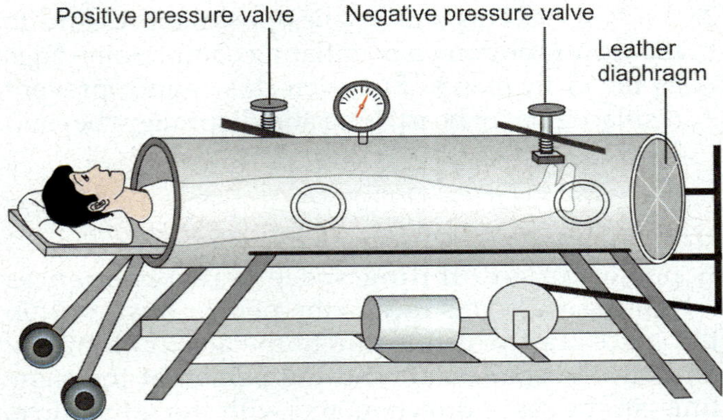

Fig. 7.44: Iron lung chamber

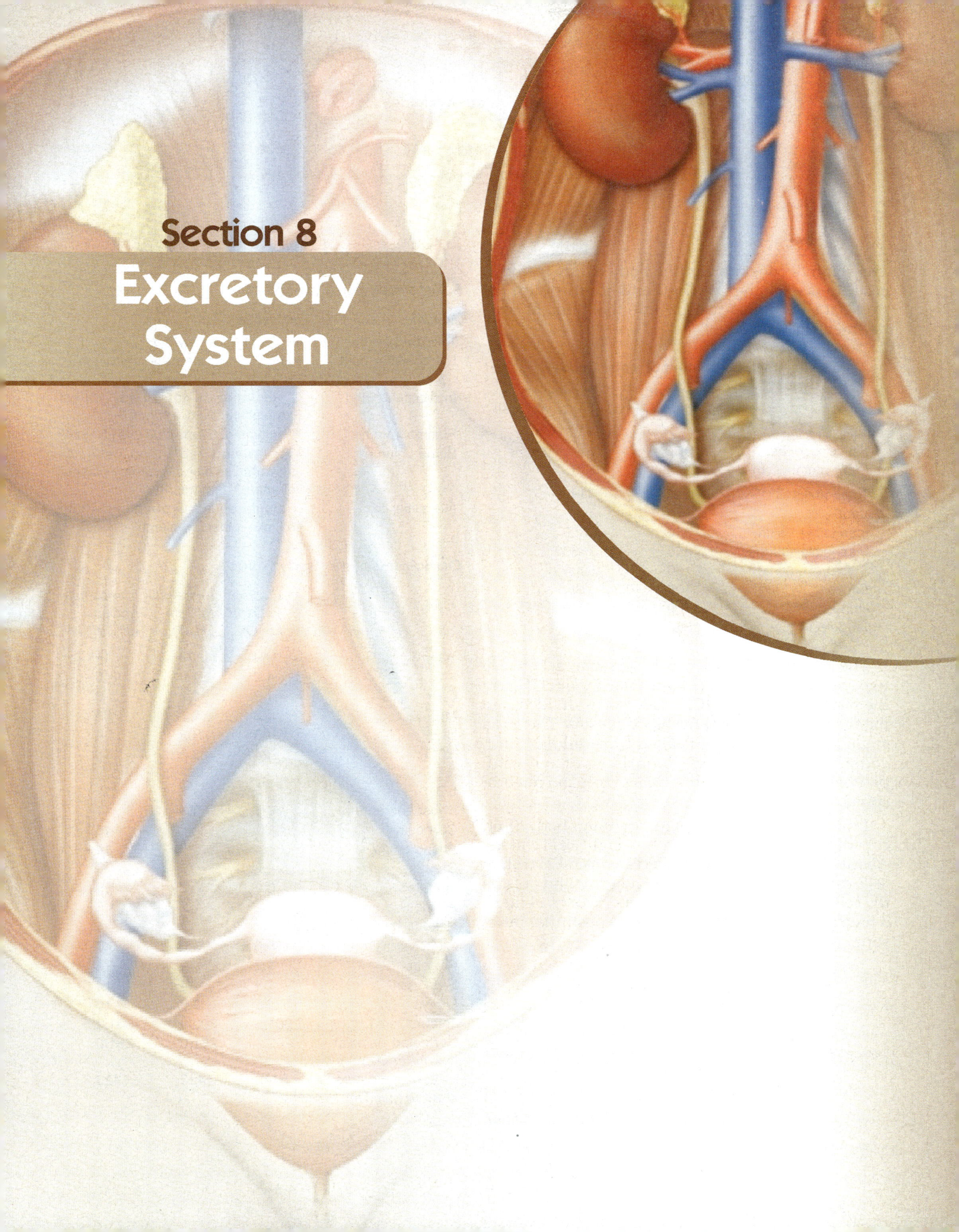

Section 8

Excretory System

59. THE BODY FLUID COMPARTMENTS

INTRODUCTION

The relative constancy of the body fluids is due to continous exchange of fluid and solutes with the external environment and within the different compartments of the body.

Daily intake and output of water (ml/day)		
	Normal	*Prolonged heavy exercise*
Intake		
Fluids ingested	2100	Variable
From metabolism	200	200
Total intake	2300	Variable
Output		
Insensible—skin	350	350
Insensible—lungs	350	650
Sweat	100	5000
Feces	100	100
Urine	1400	500
Total output	2300	6600

The total body fluid is distributed mainly between two compartments, the extracellular fluid (ECF) and the intracellular fluid (ICF). The ECF is divided into the interstitial fluid and the blood plasma. There is a small fluid compartment called transcellular fluid, constituting 1 to 2 liters comprising of synovial, peritoneal, pericardial, intraocular spaces and cerebrospinal fluid.

In an average adult weighing 70 kg, body fluid constitutes about 60% of body weight or 42 liters. About 28 liters of 42 liters of fluid are inside 75 trillion cells called intracellular fluid. 14 liters of fluid outside the cells are called extracellular fluid. Out of 14 liters, 3 liters constitutes plasma, 11 liters constitutes interstitial fluid.

Total body water (TBW) **42 liters**

Intracellular fluid (ICF) **28 liters** Extracellular fluid (ECF) **14 liters**

Plasma **3 liters** Interstitial fluid **11 liters**

MEASUREMENT OF FLUID VOLUMES IN THE DIFFERENT BODY FLUID COMPARTMENTS

Substances Used in Estimation

Volume	*Indicators*
Total body water	^3H_2O, ^2H_2O, Antipyrine
Extracellular fluid	^{22}Na, ^{125}I-iothalamate, thiosulfate, inulin
Intracellular fluid	(Calculated as total body water: Extracellular fluid volume)
Plasma volume	^{125}I-albumin, Evans blue dye (T-1824)
Blood volume	^{51}Cr-labeled red blood cells, or calculated as blood volume = plasma volume/(1-hematocrit)
Interstitial fluid	(Calculated as extracellular fluid volume—plasma volume)

Osmolarity of the Body Fluids

	Plasma (mOsm/ LH_2O)	*Interstitial (mOsm/ LH_2O)*	*Intracellular (mOsm/ LH_2O)*
Na^+	142	139	14
K^+	4.2	4.0	140
Ca^{++}	1.3	1.2	0
Mg^+	0.8	0.7	20
Cl^-	108	108	4
HCO_3^-	24	28.3	10
SO_4^-	2	2	11
Phosphocreatine	0.5	0.5	1
Carnosine			45
Amino acids			14
Creatine	2	2	8
Lactate	0.2	0.2	9
Adenosine triphosphate	1.2	1.2	1.5
Hexose monophosphate			5
Glucose	5.6	5.6	3.7
Protein	1.2	0.2	4
Urea	4	4	4
Others	4.8	3.9	10
Total mOsm/L	301.8	300.8	301.2
Corrected osmolar activity (mOsm/L)	282.0	281.0	281.0
Total osmotic pressure at 37°C (mm Hg)	5443	423	5423

The total osmolarity of each compartment is about 300 mOsm/L. The corrected osmolar activity of the body fluids is about 282 mOsm/L. The corrections is that molecules and ions in solution exert interionic and intermolecular attraction or repulsion from one solute molecule to the next, and these two effects can cause respectively, a slight decrease or an increase in the osmotic activity.

Total Osmotic Pressure Exerted by the Body Fluids

For each milliosmole concentration, 19.3 mm Hg osmotic pressure is exerted across the cell membrane totalling to about 5443 mm Hg.

EDEMA

Refers to the excess fluid in the body tissues mainly in the ECF, may be in ICF also.

ICF Edema

Two Conditions

a. Depression of the metabolic systems of the tissues.
b. Lack of adequate nutrition to the cells.

ECF Edema

Two Conditions

a. Abnormal leakage of fluid from the plasma to the interstitial fluid.
b. Failure of the lymphatics to return fluid from the interstitium back into the blood.

Factors that can Increase Capillary Filtration

$$\text{Filtration} = K_f \times (P_c - P_{if} - \pi_C + \pi_{if})$$

- K_f is the capillary filtration coefficient (the products of the permeability and surface area of the capillaries)
- P_C is the capillary hydrostatic pressure.
- P_{if} is the interstitial fluid hydrostatic pressure.
- π_C is the capillary colloid osmotic pressure.
- π_{if} is the interstitial fluid colloid osmotic pressure.
  - Increased capillary filtration coefficient
  - Increased capillary hydrostatic pressure
  - Increased plasma colloid osmotic pressure. All these factors ultimately increase the filtration.

Causes of ECF Edema

1. Increased capillary pressure as in acute or chronic kidney failure.

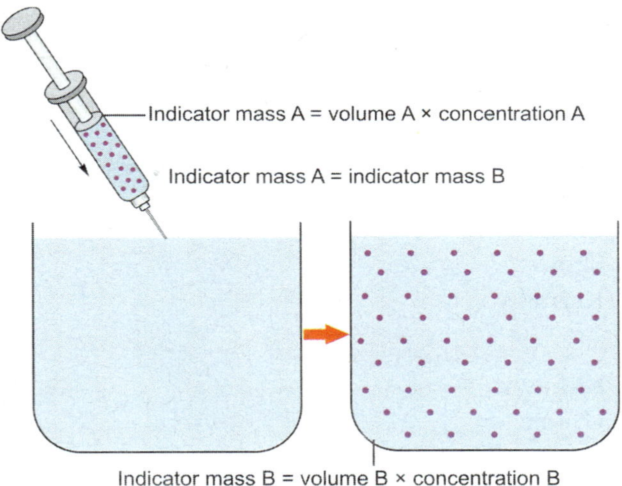

Indicator dilution method

2. Decreased plasma proteins:
   a. Loss of proteins in urine (nephrotic syndrome).
   b. Loss of protein from denuded skin, cause being burns and wounds.
   c. Failure to produce proteins, cause being cirrhosis.
3. Increased capillary permeability due to toxins, bacterial infections and histamine.
4. Blockage of lymph return due to cancer, filaria, surgery or congenital absence of lymphatic vessels.

Safety Factors that Normally Prevent Edema

1. Low compliance of the interstitium in the negative pressure range about –3 mm Hg prevents edema. Once the interstitial fluid pressure rises above 0 mm Hg the compliance of the tissues increases markedly allowing large amounts of fluid to accumulate in the tissues.
2. Increased lymph flow by 10 to 15-fold produces 7 mm Hg. The function of lymphatic system is to return to the circulation the fluid and proteins filtered from the capillaries into the interstitium. Without this continuous return the plasma volume would be rapidly depleted and edema would occur.
3. "Wash-down" of the interstitial fluid protein against edema—increased lymph flow and interstitial fluid colloid osmotic pressure caused by the proteins decreases the protein concentration. This is about 7 mm Hg.

The total safety factor against edema is about 17 mm Hg. The capillary pressure in a peripheral tissue should rise above 17 mm Hg to produce edema.

60. STRUCTURE AND FUNCTIONS OF KIDNEY

The main excretory organs of human body are

a. Lungs
b. Liver
c. Skin
d. Kidneys

Organs of the urinary system are

a. Kidneys
b. Ureter
c. Urinary bladder
d. Urethra

EXTERNAL ANATOMY OF KIDNEY (Fig. 8.1)

- Paired kidney: Bean shaped organ
- 4–5 inches long
- 2–3 inches wide
- 1 inch thick
- Found just above the waist between the peritoneum and posterior wall of abdomen.
- Retroperitoneal along with adrenal glands and ureters.
- Protected by 11th and 12th ribs with right kidney at lower level.

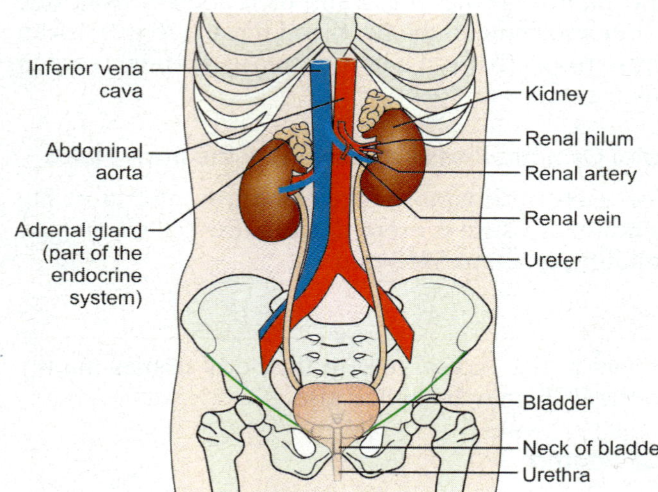

Fig. 8.1: External anatomy of kidney

Kidneys account for less than 1% body weight, but they receive about 25% of resting cardiac output.

STRUCTURE OF KIDNEY (Fig. 8.2)

- Three layers of tissue surround each kidney.
- The deep renal capsule is a smooth, transparent fibrous membrane that provides a barrier against

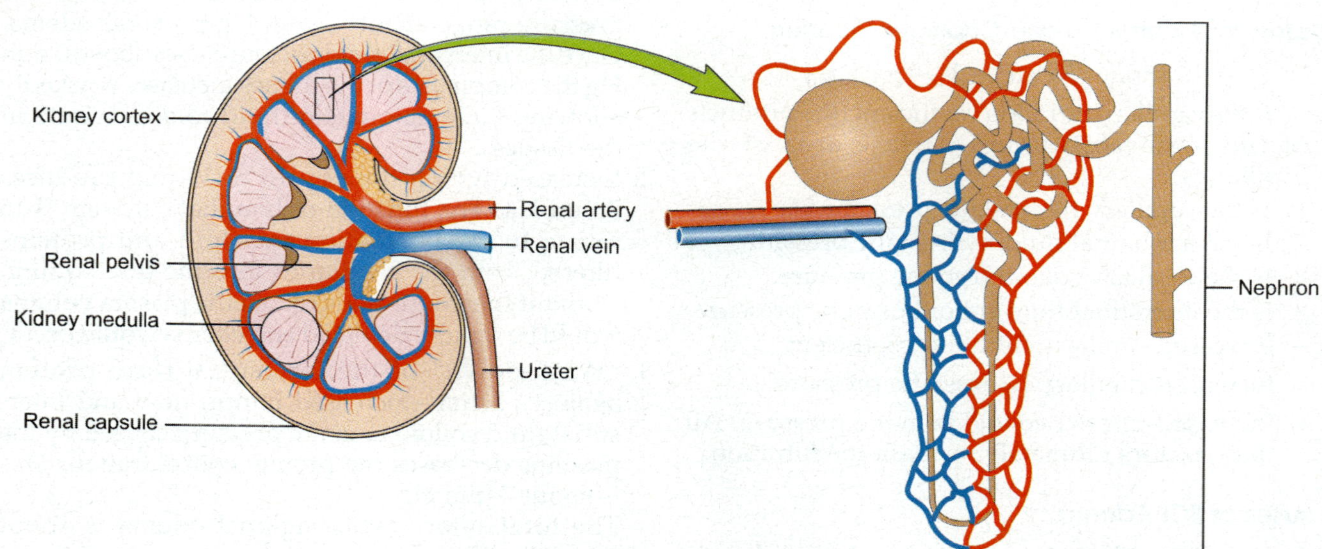

Fig. 8.2: Coronal section through the kidney

trauma and helps to maintain the shape of the kidney.

- The intermediate adipose capsule (perirenal fat) is a mass of fatty tissue that also protects the kidney from trauma and holds it securely in position within the abdominal cavity.
- The superficial renal fascia is a thin dense, irregular layer that anchors the kidney to its surrounding structures and the abdominal wall.
- Kidneys have 2 distinct regions:
  - Cortex contains the nephrons.
  - Medulla houses tubules leading to the papillae.

INTERNAL ANATOMY OF THE KIDNEY

Functional Anatomy (Fig. 8.3)

A medial depression in the kidney leads to a hollow renal sinus into which blood vessels, nerves, lymphatics and the ureter enter. Inside the renal sinus lies a renal pelvis that is subdivided into major and minor calyces, small renal papillae project into each minor calyx. Each major calyx is fed by 4–5 minor calyces. Urine leaves renal pelvis to ureter.

STRUCTURE OF NEPHRON

Nephrons are functional and structural unit of kidney (Fig. 8.2). There are about 1 to 1.5 million nephrons in each kidney.

Nephron consists of a renal corpuscle and a renal tubule. Renal corpuscle is the filtering portion. It is made up of a ball of capillaries called the glomerulus and a Bowman's capsule (Fig. 8.4) that receives the filtrate.

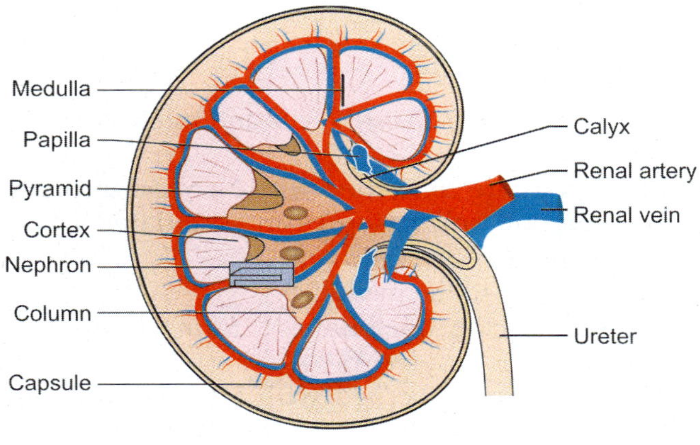

Fig. 8.3

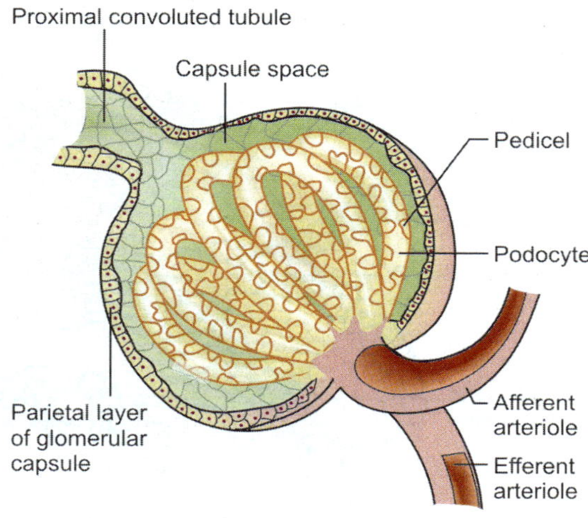

Fig. 8.4

Bowman's capsule is the outer epithelial wall of the corpuscle (parietal layer). Bowman's space is the space within Bowman's capsule.

Glomerulus (Fig. 8.4)

- Glomerular capillaries have an endothelium that is fenestrated.
- The capillaries are wrapped by podocytes (visceral layer of Bowman's capsule).
- The fitration membrane is found between the podocytes and capillary endothelium.
- Fluid leaving the glomerular capillaries enter the Bowman's space and is called filtrate.

Renal Tubules

The renal tubules (Fig. 8.5) leads away from the glomerular capsule and first becomes a proximal tubule made up of highly coiled portion, proximal convoluted tubule (PCT) and straight portion, pars recta. This leads to loop of Henle (LOH) and finally to distal tubule (DT) which then becomes collecting duct (CD). The renal tubules receives filtrate from the glomerulus and processes it into urine. The total length of the nephrons including the collecting ducts ranges from 45 to 65 mm.

Proximal Tubule (PT)

- It is about 15 mm long
- Arise from Bowman's capsule
- Longest and most coiled walls of the PCT consists of cuboidal epithelium with innumerable microvilli (brush border). They are united by apical tight junctions.

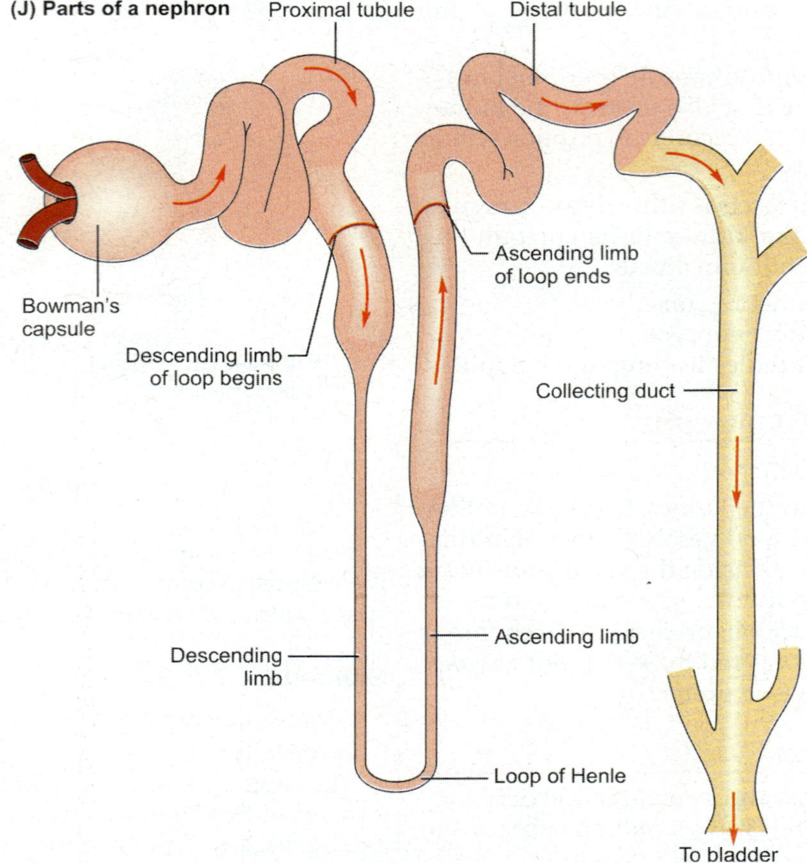

Fig. 8.5: Juxtamedullary nephron

Loop of Henle (LOH)

- U-shaped structure.
- First part the descending limb passes from the cortex to the medulla.
- The ascending limb returns from the medulla to the cortex.
- Thick segment of about 12 mm in the length form the first part of the descending and most of the ascending limbs, lined with simple cuboidal epithelium and numerous mitochondria.
- Thin segment about 2 to 14 mm forms the lower part of the loop and is lined with simple squamous epithelium.

The Distal Convoluted Tubule (DCT)

When the nephron loop returns to the cortex it is coiled again and forms the DCT.

- About 5 mm long.
- It is lined by simple cuboidal epithelium.
- Shorter and less convoluted than PCT.
- No distinct brush border and few microvilli.

The Collecting Ducts (CDs)

- About 20 mm long.
- Collects many DCTs.
- Made up of principal (P) cells and intercalated (I) cells.
- The P cells are concerned with Na^+ reabsorption, K^+ secretion and vasopressin stimulated water reabsorption.
- Passes down to the medulla.
- Several collecting ducts unites to form the papillary duct.
- The cells are concerned with H^+ secretion and reabsorbs K^+ and HCO_3 ions (Fig. 8.6).

Two Types of Nephron (Fig. 8.6)

- Cortical nephrons
  - 85% of all nephrons.
  - Located in the cortex.
  - Relatively short loops that dip only slightly in the medulla.
  - Fluid flows fast.
- Juxtamedullary nephrons
  - 15% of all nephrons.
  - Loop of Henle is very long and extends deep into renal pyramids.
  - Almost solely responsible for the medullary gradient and takes part in countercurrent mechanism.
  - Fluid flows slowly.

JUXTAGLOMERULAR APPARATUS (JGA)

Introduction

To perform the function of autoregulation, the kidneys have a feedback mechanism through a complex called juxtaglomerular apparatus (JGA) (Fig. 8.7).

Components

1. Juxtaglomerular cells (JG cells)
2. Macula densa
3. Lacis cells.

JG Cells (Fig. 8.7)

Juxtaglomerular cells are modified granular cells of afferent and efferent arterioles. They secrete renin in response to various stimuli like decreased arterial pressure, low GFR and reduced blood volume.

The renin plays an important role in renin-angiotensin-aldosterone mechanism for maintaining blood pressure.

Macula Densa

The macula densa is a specialized group of epithelial cells in the distal tubules that comes in close contact with afferent and efferent arterioles. They act as sensors for detecting the changes in sodium and chloride load in distal tubule.

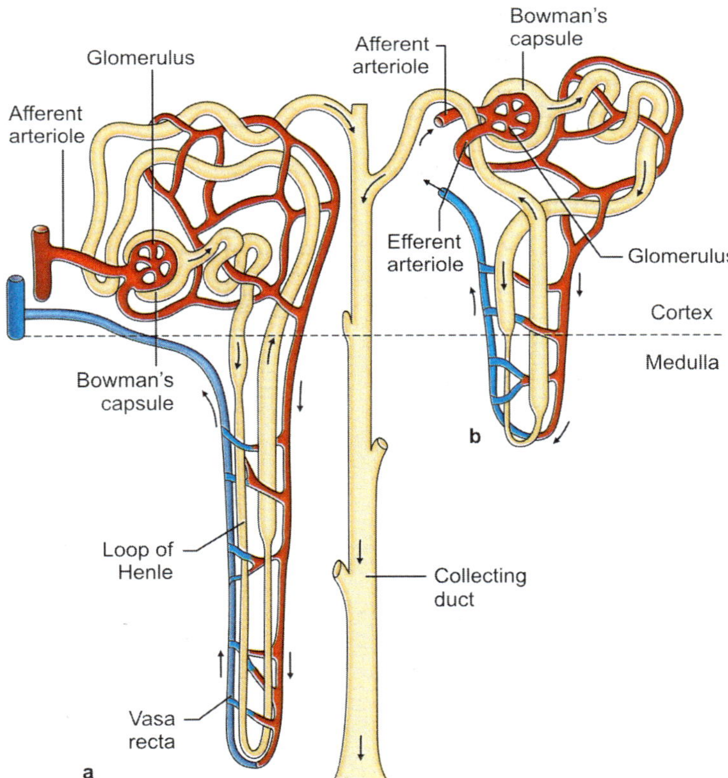

Figs 8.6a and b: Renal circulation: (a) Juxtamedullary nephron; (b) cortical nephron

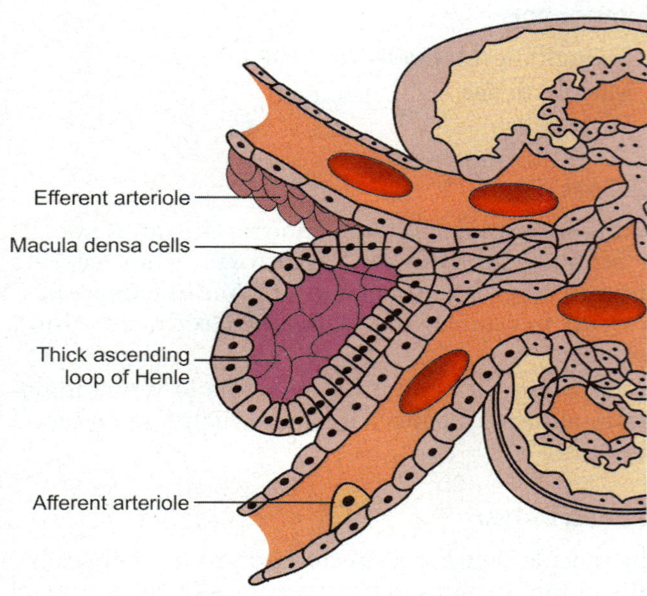

Fig. 8.7: Juxtaglomerular apparatus

Lacis Cells

Lacis cells are mesangial cells. They are similar to pericytes which are found in the walls of the capillaries elsewhere in the body. They are contractile and influence blood flow and glomerular filtration. They also secrete various substances like renin, take up immune complexes and are involved in the production of glomerular disease.

Functions of JGA

1. Autoregulation of GFR and renal blood flow.

Decreased GFR
↓
Slow flow of tubular fluid
↓
Increased reabsorption of Na^+ and Cl^- in LOH
↓
Decreased NaCl delivery to DT
↓
Macula densa sends signals to JG cells producing following effects

   a. Decrease resistance to blood flow in afferent arteriole → increased glomerular hydrostatic pressure → return of GFR to normal.
   b. Release of renin → AT II formation → constriction of efferent arteriole → increased glomerular hydrostatic pressure → return of GFR to normal.
2. Regulation of ECF volume and hence BP.

FUNCTIONS OF KIDNEY

Excretory Functions of Kidney

- Filters wastes and produce urine by glomerular filtration, tubular reabsorption and secretion.
- Maintains acid–base balance by reabsorbing biocarbonate ions and excreting hydrogen ions.
- Maintains plasma osmolarity 282 mOsm/L by varying water excretion.
- Maintains plasma concentration of electrolytes.
- Excretes nitrogenous end-products from protein metabolism, i.e. urea, uric acid and creatinine.

Nonexcretory Functions

1. *Endocrine Functions* (Fig. 8.8)
   a. *Erythropoietin:* It is a glycoprotein hormone secreted by interstitial cells in the peritubular capillary bed of the kidneys (80%) and hepatocytes (20%). This regulates erythropoiesis by enhancing all the steps of erythropoiesis.
   b. *1, 25-dihydroxycholecalciferol (calcitriol):* This is the active form of vitamin D formed from inactive

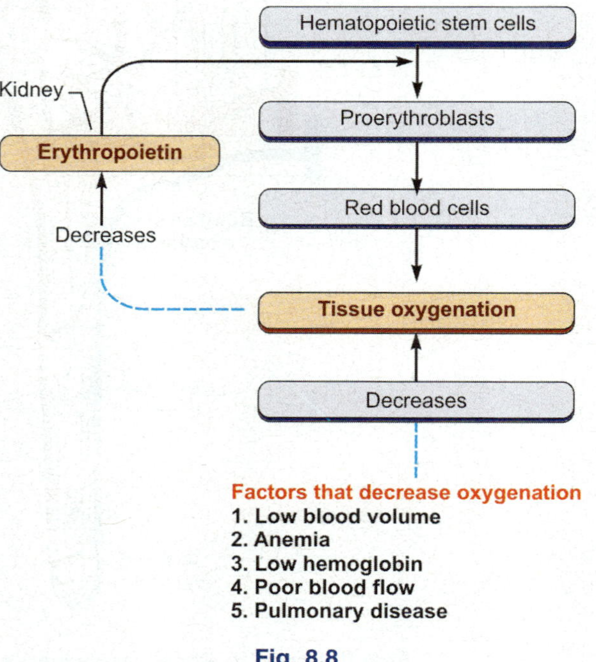

Fig. 8.8

8

25-hydroxycholecalciferol (calcidiol) in the cells of the proximal tubules of the kidneys. It increases Ca^{2+} reabsorption in the kidneys and the intestines which is essential for normal calcification of bone matrix (Fig. 8.9).

c. *Renin:* It is a small protein enzyme released by the JG cells of the kidney. It maintains normal ECF volume and BP through renin-angiotensin mechanism (Fig. 8.10).

d. *Prostaglandins:* They are produced by medullary interstitial type I cells and cells of collecting tubule. They increase rennin secretion and cause vasodilatation.

e. *Kallikrein:* Renal kallikrein-kinin system acts as local hormone and produces vasodilatation and Na^{+} excretion.

2. Gluconeogenesis

The kidneys synthesize glucose from amino acids and other precursors during prolonged fasting by a process called gluconeogenesis.

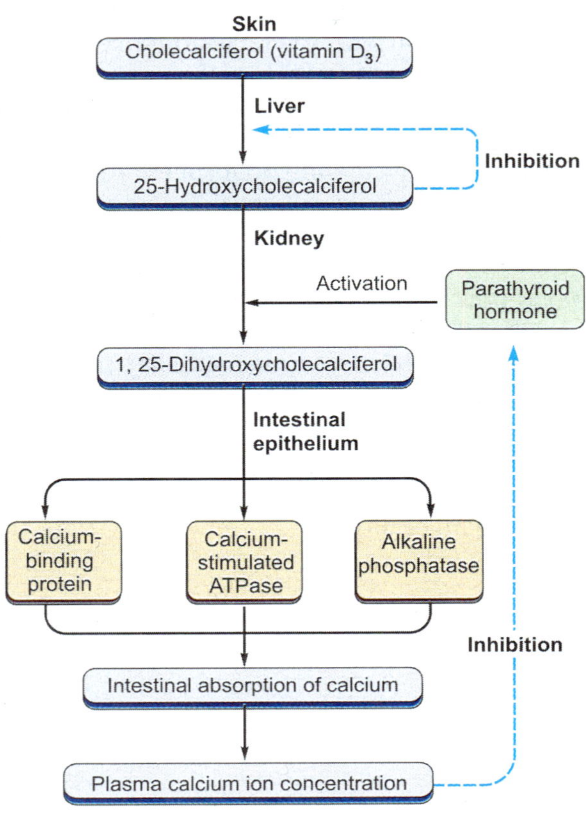

Fig. 8.9

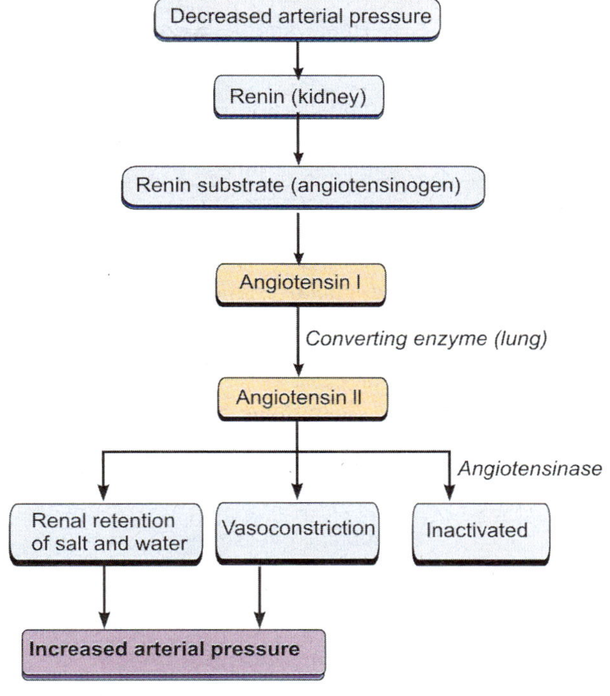

Fig. 8.10

BLOOD SUPPLY TO THE KIDNEYS (Fig. 8.11)

- Blood travels from afferent arteriole to capillaries in the nephron called glomerulus.
- Blood leaves the nephron via the efferent arteriole.
- Blood travels from efferent arteriole to peritubular capillaries and vasa recta.

8

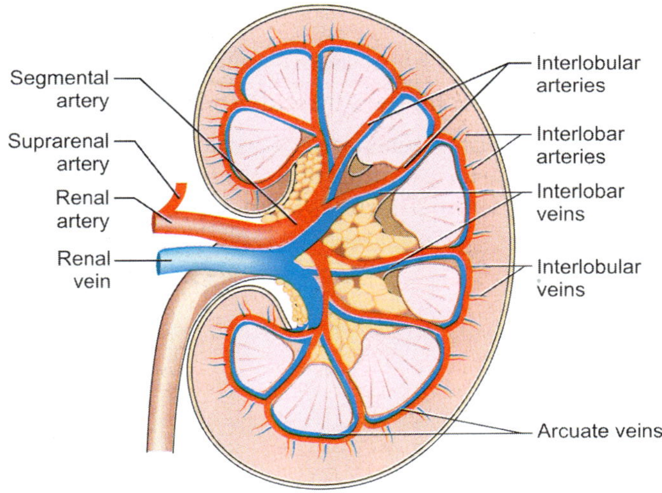

Fig. 8.11

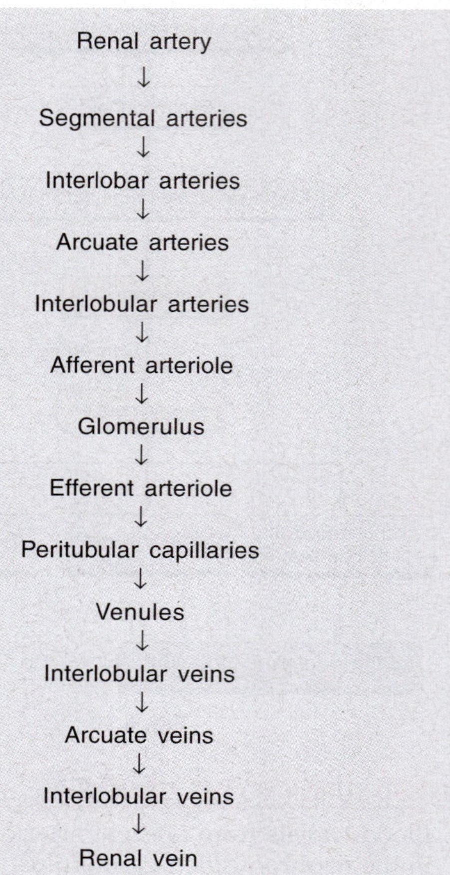

Renal Blood Flow

Blood flow through both the kidneys in an adult is 1200 ml/min which is about 25% of cardiac output. Kidneys being the second organ next to liver receiving the highest blood flow.

$$\text{RBF} = \frac{\text{Renal artery pressure} - \text{renal vein pressure}}{\text{Total renal vascular resistance}}$$

Renal vascular resistance is mainly offered by interlobular arteries, afferent and efferent arterioles. The size of efferent arterioles is smaller in comparison to afferent arteriole which creates a higher pressure in glomerulus to enhance glomerular filtration.

Measurement of Renal Blood Flow

1. Direct method by electromagnetic flow meters and Doppler method.
2. Indirect method by using Fick's principle. The substances commonly used are para-aminohippuric acid (PAH).

$$\text{RBF} = \frac{\text{Amt. of substance taken in a unit time}}{\text{Arteriovenous difference}}$$

Peculiarities of Renal Circulation

1. Each kidney weighing about 150 gm, have very high blood supply about 25% of cardiac output. (1200 ml/min).
2. As the renal arteries arise at right angles from abdominal aorta, their arterial pressure is high. Glomerular capillaries has high hydrostatic pressure of about 60 mm Hg elsewhere capillary pressure is only 32 mm Hg.
3. The efferent arteriole is of much smaller diameter than afferent arteriole which offers considerable resistance to blood flow.
4. It is like the portal system of circulation having two sets of capillaries one of them is the glomerular capillaries, they combine to form efferent arteriole which in-turn breaks into peritubular capillaries in cortical nephrons and vasa recta in juxtamedullary nephrons.
5. Blood flow through vasa recta is sluggish and only 1 to 2% of blood flows through it which is helpful to minimize solute loss from medullary interstitium.
6. Renal circulation is autoregulated between the systemic blood pressure of 80 and 140 mm Hg.
7. The arteriovenous oxygen difference is low 1.7 ml/100 ml of blood when compared to normal 4 to 5 ml/100 ml of blood.

61. FORMATION OF URINE—GLOMERULAR FILTRATION

The rate at which different substances are excreted in the urine represents the sum of three renal processes.

1. Glomerular filtration.
2. Tubular reabsorption of substances from the renal tubules into the blood.
3. Tubular secretion of substances from the blood into the renal tubules.

Excretion = Filtration – Reabsorption + Secretion

URINE FORMATION RENAL HANDLING OF SUBSTANCES (Fig. 8.12)

Four classes of substances:

a. Filtered, not reabsorbed (creatinine, inulin, uric acid)
b. Filtered, partly reabsorbed (Na^+, Cl^-, bicarbonate)
c. Filtered, totally reabsorbed (amino acids, glucose)
d. Filtered, totally secreted (organic acids and bases).

GLOMERULAR FILTRATION (Fig. 8.13)

It is the first step in urine formation.

Glomerular filtrate is produced from blood plasma. It must pass through the glomerular membrane which is relatively impermeable to proteins. So the filtrate is similar to plasma in terms of concentrations of salts and of organic molecules (e.g. glucose, amino acids) except it is essentially protein-free and devoid of cellular elements including red blood cells.

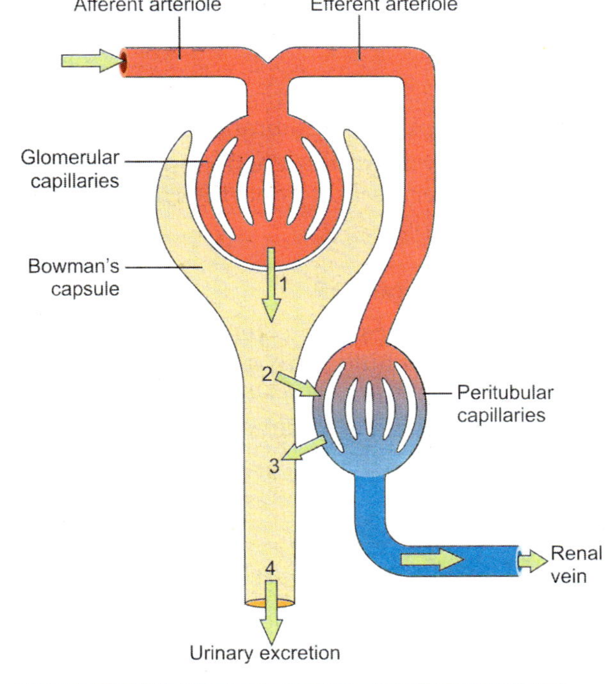

Fig. 8.12

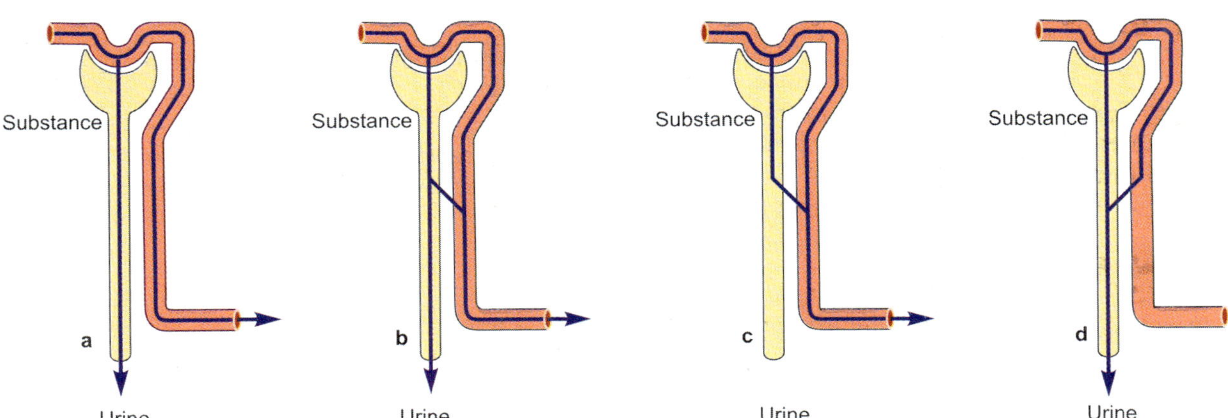

Figs 8.13a to d: (a) Filtration only; (b) filtration, partial reabsorption; (c) filtration, complete reabsorption; (d) filtration, secretion

GLOMERULAR FILTRATION RATE (GFR)

Amount of filtrate formed by both kidneys together in unit time is called GFR. It is about 20% of the renal plasma flow.

Normal value is 125 ml/min or 180 L/day. GFR is determined by:

a. The balance of hydrostatic and colloid pressures across the capillary membrane
b. The capillary filtration coefficient (Kf). It is the product of permeability and filtering surface area of the capillaries.

Advantages of High GFR

- High GFR is necessary to remove waste products that are filtered but poorly reabsorbed.
- High GFR makes it possible for entire plasma volume to be filtered 60 times per day, if plasma is 3 L with GFR 180 L/day.

FILTRATION FRACTION (FF)

It is the fraction of renal plasma flow that is filtered at the glomerulus.

$$FF = \frac{GFR}{RPF} = 0.20$$

Glomerular Capillary Membrane

This membrane is similar to any other capillary membrane having three layers:

a. *The endothelium of the capillary:* This is perforated by thousands of small holes called fenestrae which are large but negatively charged hindering the passage of plasma proteins.
b. *A basement membrane:* It consists of a meshwork of collagen and proteoglycan that have large spaces through which solutes and water pass through.
c. *A layer of epithelial cells:* These cells are not continuous but have long foot like processes (podocytes). The foot processes are separated by slit pores through which glomerular filtrate moves.

The glomerular capillary membrane is thicker but more porous filtering more fluid at a higher rate. The filterability of solutes is inversely proportional to the size. Normally, molecules with 4 nm diameter passes easily. Between 4–8 nm filtered with difficulty. Above 8 nm molecules are not filtered. A filterability of 1.0 means substance is freely filtered as water. If it is 0.75 means substance is filtered only 75%. Na^+ and glucose are freely filtered.

The electrical charges affect the filtration. The negatively charged large molecules are filtered less easily than positively charged molecules of equal size, e.g. albumin which is 6 nm in diameter is not filtered due to its negative charge. Neutral dextrans are filtered better than negatively charged dextrans the reason being negativity of the basement membrane repels negatively charged molecules.

Determinants of GFR (Fig. 8.14)

It is determined by:

1. The sum of hydrostatic and colloid osmotic pressures across the glomerular membrane which gives net filtration pressure (NFP).
2. The filtration coefficient (kf).

$$GFR = K_f \times NFP$$

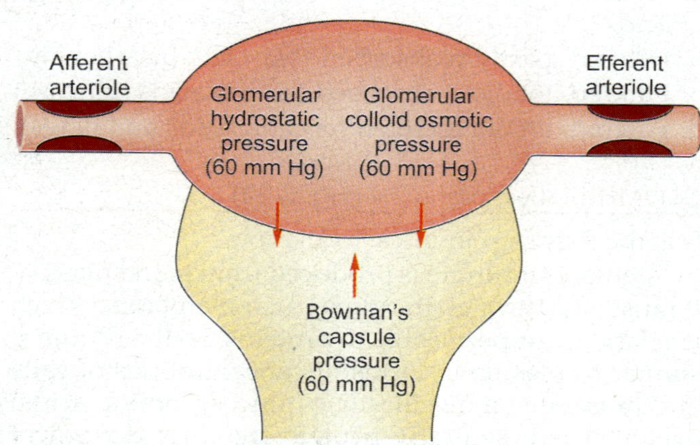

Fig. 8.14

FORCES AFFECTING FILTRATION

Favoring filtration	*Opposing filtration*
Glomerular hydrostatic pressure 60 mm Hg (P_G)	Glomerular capillary colloid osmotic pressure (π_G) 32 mm Hg
Bowman's capsule colloid osmotic pressure (π_B) 0 mm Hg	Bowman's capsule hydrostatic pressure (P_B) 18 mm Hg

$$NFP = +10 \text{ mm Hg}$$

$$K_f = \frac{GFR}{NFP}, \text{ where kf} \rightarrow \text{filtration coefficient}$$

$$GFR = K_f \times NFP\ (PG - P_B - \pi_G + \pi_B)$$

SUMMARY OF FACTORS THAT CAN DECREASE GFR

1. Filtration Coefficient (K_f)

Since the GFR is 125 ml/min and NFP is 10 mm Hg, normal K_f is calculated as 12.5 ml/min/mm Hg.

Decreased K_f	→	Decreased GFR	→	In renal disease, diabetes mellitus, hypertension
Increased P_B	→	Decreased GFR	→	In urinary tract obstruction, e.g. kidney stones
Increased π_G	→	Decreased GFR		Decreased renal blood flow
Arterial pressure	→	Angiotensin II	→	Sympathetic activity
Decreased P_G	→	Decreased GFR		Increased plasma proteins

Factors Affecting Glomerular Filtration

- Filtering membrane—size, pores and charge.
- Particle—size, shape, charge.
- Filtering forces.
- Amount of blood flow.

When there is a rapid rate of blood flow effective filtration pressure and GFR increases. Conversely, slow rate of blood flow reduces GFR.

- Autoregulation
  - a. Tubuloglomerular feedback
  - b. Myogenic mechanism.
- *Mesangial cells:* The contraction of mesangial cells compresses the glomerulus and reduces the surface area of glomerular membrane which is normally 0.8 m^2.
- *Sympathetic nerves:* Strong stimulation of sympathetic system constricts the renal arterioles and decreases renal blood flow and GFR. Mild and moderate stimulation has little influence.
- Other factors like high protein diet and increased blood glucose increases renal blood flow and GFR.

REGULATION OF GLOMERULAR FILTRATION AND RENAL BLOOD FLOW

- Autoregulation.
- Sympathetic nervous system.
- Hormonal control.

Autoregulation

Two Mechanisms

a. Myogenic mechanism.
b. Tubuloglomerular feedback.

Myogenic Mechanism (Fig. 8.15)

When blood flow to the kidneys increases, it stretches the smooth muscle lining the blood vessel wall.

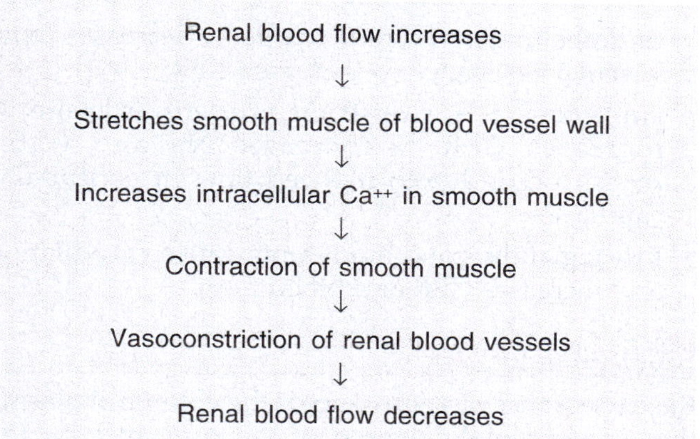

Tubuloglomerular Feedback (TGF) Mechanism

Alteration of tubular flow NaCl is sensed by the macula densa of the Juxtaglomerular apparatus and produces a signal renin that alters GFR.

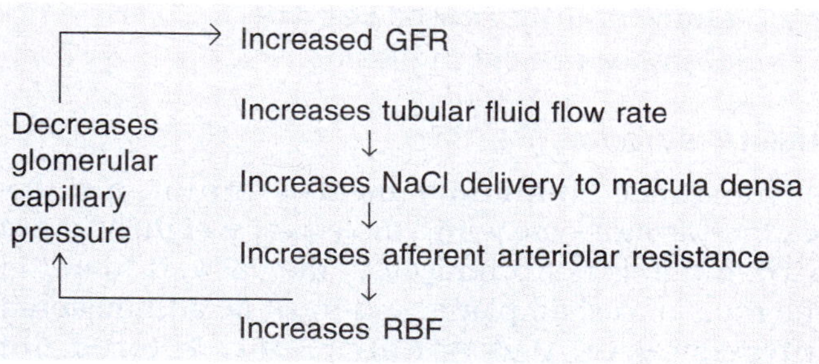

Sympathetic Nervous System

Sympathetic stimulation → constriction of renal arterioles → decreases RBF and GFR.

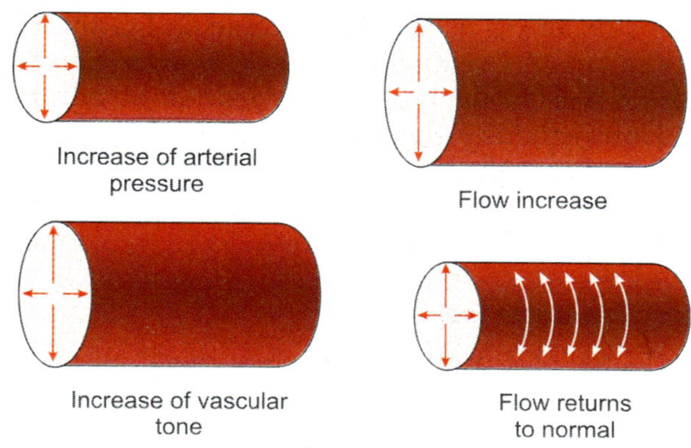

Fig. 8.15

Hormonal Control

- Norepinephrine, epinephrine and endothelin → constricts afferent and efferent arterioles causing decreased GFR and RBF.
- Endothelin derived nitric oxide → decreases renal vascular resistance → increases GFR.
- Angiotensin II: Constricts efferent arteriole → increases GFR → increases Na and water reabsorption due to reduced flow in peritubular capillaries.
- Prostaglandins and bradykinin cause vasodilation and increases GFR and blood flow.

ESTIMATION OF GFR

Renal clearance of a substance is the volume of plasma that is completely cleared of the substance by the kidneys per unit time.

$$C_s = \frac{U_s \times V}{P_s}$$

C_s = Clearance of the substance
U_s = Substance present in urine
V = Volume of urine passed per day
P_s = Substance present in plasma.

Inulin Clearance (Fig. 8.16)

8

A substance commonly used is inulin, a polysaccharide molecule with a molecular weight of about 5200. Inulin is not produced in the body, is found in the roots of certain plants and must be administered intravenously. It is nontoxic, only filtered not reabsorbed. It is costly and not easily available. Inulin clearance is taken as gold standard since its value almost equals GFR value.

Creatinine Clearance Test

Other substances used are creatinine and radioactive iodothalamate. Creatinine is synthesized from muscle creatine with in the body so it need not be administered intravenously. Since creatinine is secreted in pars recta, it over estimates GFR. The range of creatinine clearance is wide between 70 and 140 ml/min depending on the muscle mass.

Urea Clearance Test

Urea is the end-product of protein metabolism. It is partly reabsorbed by the renal tubules, so urea clearance is less than GFR. It is influenced by the protein content of the diet.

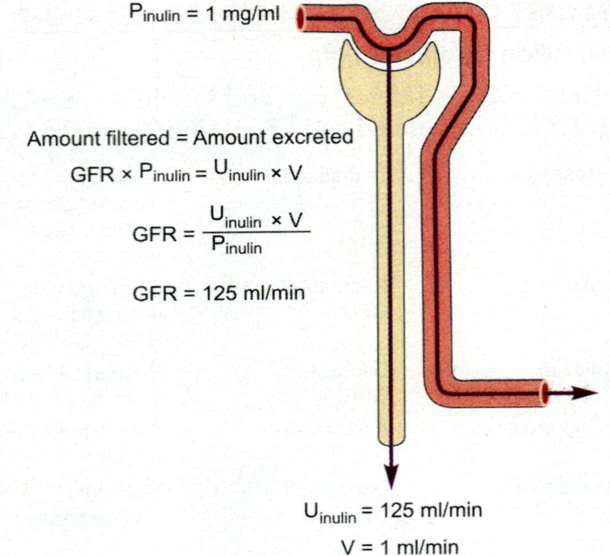

Fig. 8.16

Maximal Urea Clearance

$$\frac{U \times V}{P} \quad \text{Normal values} = 75 \text{ ml/min.}$$

This is applicable when urine output is more than 2 ml/min.

U = Urea concentration in urine (mg/ml)
V = Volume of urine excreted (ml/min)
P = Urea concentration in plasma (mg/ml)

Standard Urea Clearance

$$\frac{U \times \sqrt{V}}{P} \quad \text{Normal values} = 54 \text{ ml/min.}$$

This is applicable when the urine volume is less than 2 ml/min.

Comparisons of Inulin Clearance with Clearance of Different Solutes

1. If the clearance rate of the substance equals that of inulin, the substance is only filtered and not reabsorbed or secreted.
2. If the clearance of the substance is less than inulin clearance, the substance must have been absorbed by the nephron tubules.
3. If the clearance is greater than that of inulin clearance, substance must have been secreted by the tubules.

62. FORMATION OF URINE—TUBULAR REABSORPTION AND TUBULAR SECRETION

INTRODUCTION

Tubular reabsorption and tubular secretion are selective and quantitatively large. It includes both passive and active transport mechanisms. Water and solutes can be transported through all membranes themselves (transcellular route) or through the junctional spaces between the cells (paracellular route). From the cells into interstitial fluid, water and solutes are transported by ultrafiltration (bulk flow) mediated by hydrostatic and colloid osmotic forces.

TUBULAR REABSORPTION (Fig. 8.17)

Sodium: Potassium ATPase, hydrogen ATPase, hydrogen-potassium ATPase and calcium ATPase are examples of primary active transport. It moves solutes against an electrochemical gradient. The energy is provided by the membrane bound ATPase.

In secondary active cotransport of glucose and amino acids, sodium diffuses down its electrochemical gradient, the energy released is used to drive another substance, that is glucose/amino acid.

Secondary active countertransport: Sodium hydrogen countertransport. The energy liberated from the downhill of one of the substances (e.g. sodium) enables uphill of a second substance (hydrogen) in the opposite direction.

Pinocytosis: Reabsorption of proteins occur by this process. In this, protein gets attached to the brush border of the luminal membrane which invaginates into the interior of the cell until it completely pinches off and a vesicle is formed.

Solvent Drag

As water moves across the tight junctions by osmosis, it can also carry with it some of the solutes a process called solvent drag.

Transport maximum (Tm) for substances that are actively reabsorbed or secreted. There is a limit to the rate at which the solute can be transported, termed as transport maximum. This is due to the saturation of the specific transport systems involved when the tubular load of solutes exceed the capacity of the carrier proteins involved in the transport process.

Tm for glucose average	320 mg/min
	375 mg/min for males
	300 mg/min for females

There is a relation between tubular load of glucose, Tm for glucose and rate of glucose loss in the urine. when tubular load is 125 mg/min, there is no loss of glucose in urine (Fig. 8.17). When tubular load rises

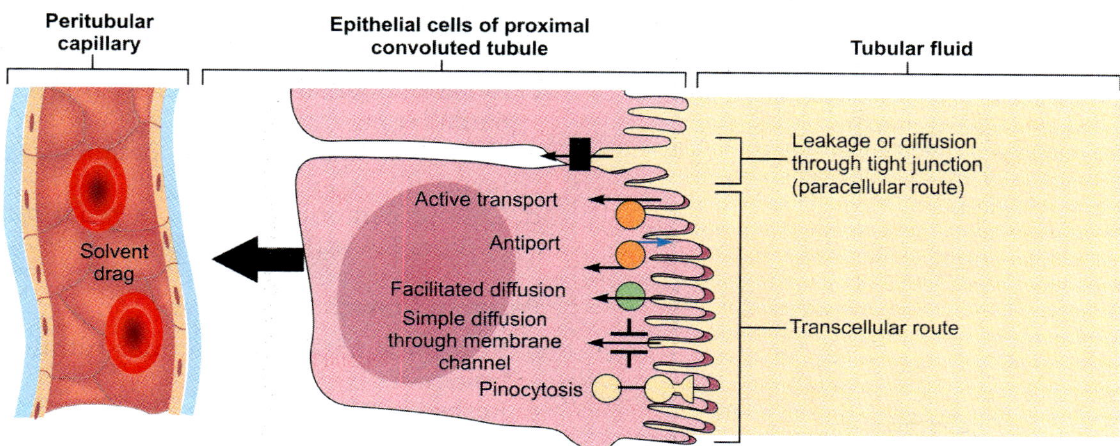

Fig. 8.17

above 180 mg/min, a small amount appears in the urine, that is called renal threshold for glucose. This appearance of glucose occurs even before Tm is reached. The reason being not all nephrons have same Tm for glucose.

Splay

The ideal curve shown in this diagram (Fig. 8.18) is obtained if the Tm_G in all the tubules was identical. This is not the case in humans, the actual curve is rounded and deviates from the ideal curve. This deviation is called splay. The magnitude of the splay is inversely proportionate to the avidity with which the transport mechanism binds the substance it transports. Tm for actively secreted substances.

For example Creatinine : 16 mg/min
PAH : 80 mg/min

Gradient Time Transport

It is for passively reabsorbed substances which depends on the electrochemical gradient and the time that the substance is in the tubule which in turn depends on the tubular flow rate.

Regulation of Tubular Reabsorption

Nervous: Sympathetic nervous system stimulation decreases.

a. Sodium and water excretion by constricting the renal arterioles.
b. Increase Na reabsorption in proximal tubule and thick ascending limb of LOH.
c. Increases renin and angiotensin II release.

8

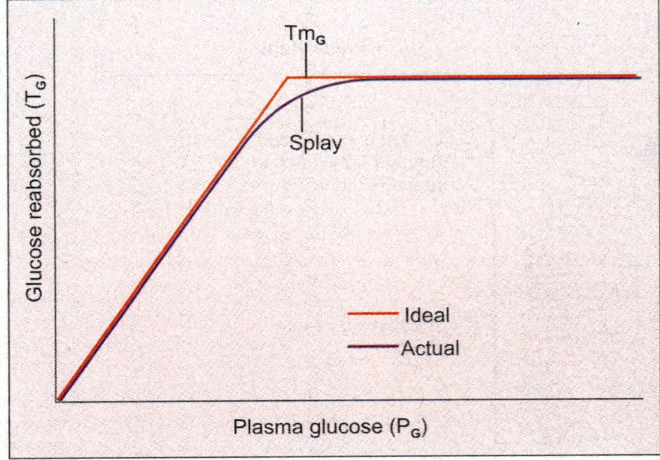

Fig. 8.18

1. *Hormonal*

Hormones that regulate tubular reabsorption:

Hormone	*Site of action*	*Effects*
a. Aldosterone	Collecting duct	Increases NaCl, H_2O reabsorption Increases K^+ secretion
b. Angiotensin II	Proximal convoluted tubule, thick ascending limb of loop of Henle	Increases NaCl, H_2O reabsorption and H^+ secretion
c. ADH	Distal tubule/Collecting duct	Increases H_2O reabsorption
d. ANP	Distal tubule/Collecting duct	Increases NaCl reabsorption
e. Parathormone	Proximal tubule, thick ascending limb, distal tubule	Decreases PO_4^- reabsorption in proximal tubule Increases Ca^{++} releases in loop of Henle Increases Mg^+ reabsorption in loop of Henle

2. *Local Control*

a. Glomerulotubular balance: Increased GFR increases the tubular load thereby increasing tubular reabsorption.
b. Peritubular capillary and renal interstitial forces. Reabsorption = $K_f \times$ Net reabsorption force (NRF).

The NRF represents the sum of hydrostatic and colloid osmotic forces which favor or oppose reabsorption across peritubular capillaries. These forces are (Fig. 8.19):

a. Peritubular hydrostatic (P_c) pressures oppose RA = 13 mm Hg.
b. Renal interstitial hydrostatic (P_{if}) favoring RA = 6 mm Hg.
c. Colloid osmotic pressure in peritubular capillaries favors RA (π_C) = 32 mm Hg.
d. Colloid osmotic pressure in renal interstitium opposes RA (π_{if}) = 15 mm Hg.

Proximal Convoluted Tubules

- Reabsorbs 65% of glomerular filtrate by active transport.
- Reabsorbs Na^+, Cl^-, HCO_3 , K^+, Ca^+, H_2O, glucose, amino acids, vitamins, uric acid and phosphates. Pars recta secretes substances like creatinine,

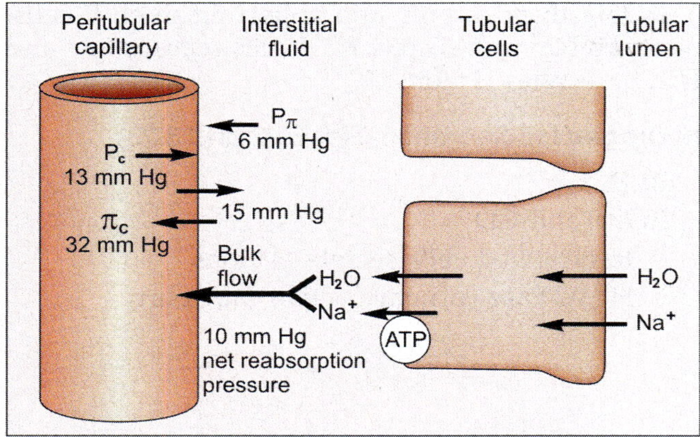

Fig. 8.19

phenolphthalein dyes, PAH, acids, bases, drugs like penicillin, sulphonamides (Fig. 8.18).

Loop of Henle

Descending thin segment is highly permeable to water. Water moves out of nephron reducing the volume of filtrate and increasing its osmolarity.

Ascending thick segment is not permeable to water but is permeable to solutes. 25% of filtered solutes are reabsorbed.

Distal Tubule (Fig. 8.20)

The very first portion of the distal tubule forms part of JG apparatus. The next early part is highly convoluted and has same reabsorptive characteristics as that of ascending limb of loop of Henle. Na^+, Cl^- H_2O, HCO_3, Ca^+ and K^+ are reabsorbed but impermeable to water and urea. This is also known as diluting segment because it dilutes the tubular fluid.

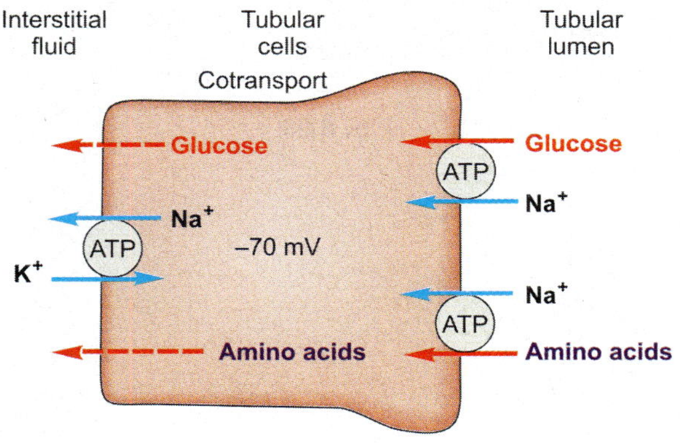

Fig. 8.20

Collecting Tubule

The second part of the distal tubule is the late distal tubule continues as cortical collecting tubule having principal cells and intercalated cells. The tubular membranes are impermeable to urea is concerned with Na^+, Cl^- reabsorption, HCO_3 secretion, HCO_3 reabsorption, secretion of K^+ and H^+ secretion. The permeability of the tubules to water is controlled by antidiuretic hormone (ADH) (Fig. 8.21).

Medullary Collecting Duct

They are the final site for processing urine. The permeability to water depends on presence of ADH. They are permeable to urea and secretes H^+ against a large concentration gradient. 15% of solutes are reabsorbed in distal tubule and collecting duct.

Sodium and Chloride Reabsorption

Na^+ is reabsorbed in PCT, thick segment of LOH and distal nephron except in thin segment.

Mechanisms

In PCT: 65–70%

Unidirectional Na transport

Movement of Na^+ against concentration gradient–glucose, amino acids and phosphate are transported with it.

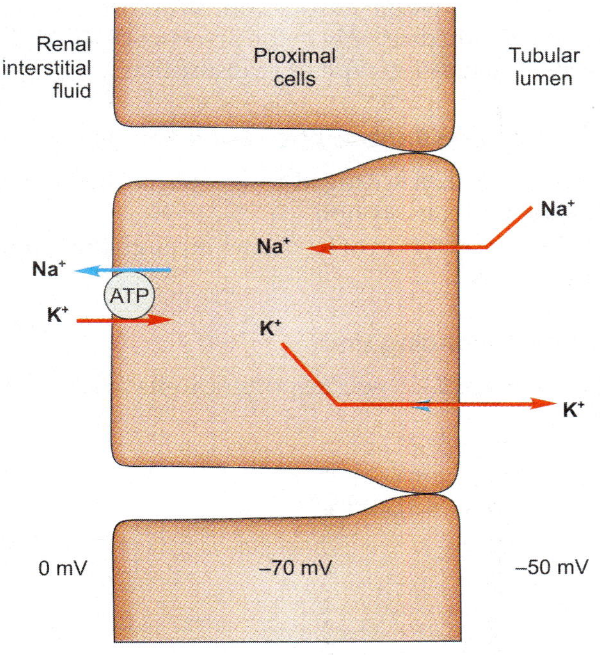

Fig. 8.21

8

Na^+ — H^+ exchange (antiport)

In thick ascending limb–25%

1 Na^+ — 1 K^+ — 2 Cl^- symporter.

Distal nephron–10%

Unidirectional Na^+ transport but under the influence of aldosterone.

Glucose and Amino Acid Reabsorption

- Reabsorbed in PCT.
- Na^+ cotransport mechanism.

Sodium dependent glucose transporter (SGLT) on luminal (apical) membrane and glucose transporter on the basolateral membrane (GLUT).

Water Reabsoption

- *PCT:* 65 to 70%
  - Passive transport by osmosis (couples to Na reabsorption)
  - Solvent drag through paracellular route—water takes Na^+, Cl^-, K^+, Ca^+, Mg^+ along with it. As the substances are absorbed proportionally, the fluid remains isotonic at the end of PCT. This passive reabsorption of water is called obligatory type of reabsorption.
- *DT and CD:* Under ADH control.

ADH introduces water channels called aquaporins which allows water absorption. Water is absorbed from collecting duct only in the presence of ADH. This is called facultative type of reabsorption.

8

Potassium and Reabsorption Secretion (Fig. 8.21)

- *In PCT:* Solvent drag through paracellular route cause K^+ reabsorption.
- Minimal secretion of K^+ occurs through the luminal membrane.

In Thick Ascending Limb

1 Na^+ — 1 K + 2 Cl^- cotransporter causes reabsorption.

In late distal tubule and collecting duct, P cells, reabsorb Na^+ and secrete K^+. I cells reabsorb K^+ and HCO_3, secretes H^+ ions.

Hydrogen Ion Secretion (Figs 8.22 and 8.23)

- In PCT
- In DT and CD
  - Intercalated cells secrete H^+ ions
  - H^+ ATPase (primary active transport).

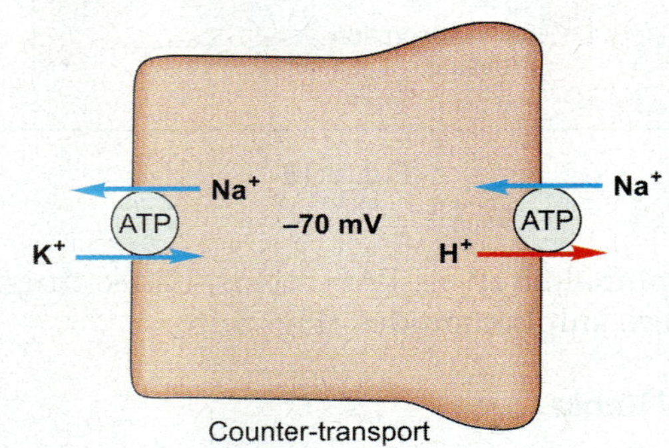

Fig. 8.22

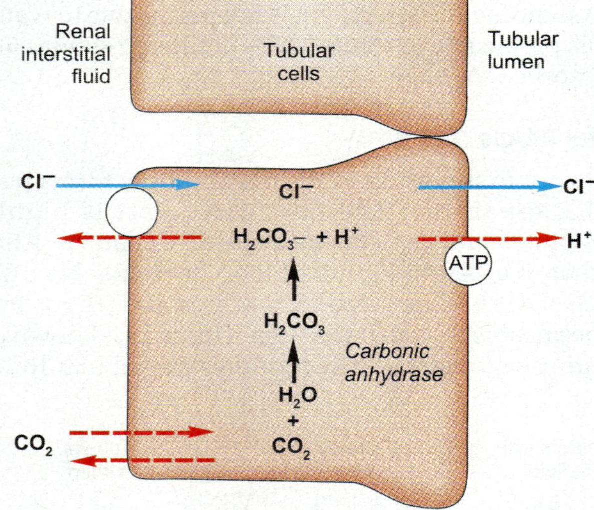

Fig. 8.23

63. CONCENTRATION AND DILUTION OF URINE

INTRODUCTION

The normal kidney has tremendous capability to vary the relative proportions of solutes and water in the urine. They can excrete urine with an osmolarity as low as 50 mOsm/L, when there is excess water in the body and ECF osmolarity low. They can also excrete urine with a concentration of 1200–1400 mOsm/L, when there is a deficit of water and extracellular fluid osmolarity high.

OBLIGATORY URINE VOLUME (OUV)

The maximal concentrating ability of the kidney depends on how much urine volume must be excreted each day, to void the body of waste products of metabolism and ions that are ingested. A normal 70 kg human must excrete about 600 mOsm of solute each day. If maximum urine concentrating ability is 1200 mOsm/L, the minimal volume of urine is OUV can be calculated as:

$$\frac{600 \text{ mOsm/day}}{1200 \text{ mOsm/L}} = 0.5 \text{ L/day}$$

REQUIREMENTS FOR EXCRETING A CONCENTRATED URINE

1. High ADH levels
2. Hyperosmotic renal medulla.

High ADH Levels

When osmolarity of the body fluids increases above normal the posterior pituitary secretes more ADH.

This increases the permeability of the distal tubule and collecting duct to water. So, more water is reabsorbed and concentrated urine is formed.

When there is excess water and ECF osmolarity is reduced, ADH from posterior pituitary decreases, thereby reducing permeability of distal tubule and collecting duct to water causing a dilute urine.

Hyperosmotic Renal Medulla

Hyperosmotic renal medulla is produced by countercurrent mechanism and urea.

The renal medullary interstitium surrounding the collecting duct is very hyperosmotic. So, when ADH levels are high, the water moves through the tubular membrane by osmosis into the renal interstitium, from there into vasa recta back into blood.

The countercurrent mechanism depend on the special anatomical arrangement of the long loops of Henle of juxtamedullary nephrons and the vasa recta, the specialized peritubular capillaries of the renal medulla. Loop of Henle is called as countercurrent multiplier and vasa recta as countercurrent exchanger.

The corrected osmolar activity which accounts for intermolecular attraction and repulsion is about 282 mOsm/L. The osmolarity of renal interstitium is about 1200 to 1400 mOsm/L in the tip of medulla.

The major factors that contribute to high solute concentration into the renal medulla are:

1. Active transport of sodium ions and cotransport of potassium chloride out of the thick ascending limb of LOH into medullary interstitium.
2. Active transport of ions from the collecting ducts into the medullary interstitium.
3. Passive diffusion of large amounts of urea from inner medullary CD into the medullary interstitium.
4. Diffusion of only small amounts of water from tubules into interstitium.

COUNTERCURRENT MULTIPLIER SYSTEM IN THE LOOP OF HENLE (Fig. 8.24)

Step 1: Assume the loop of Henle (LOH) is filled with fluid with a concentration of 300 mOsm/L, the same concentration as in proximal tubule.

Step 2: The active transport of Na^+ and other ions out of thick ascending limb of LOH reduces the concentration of solute inside tubule but raising in interstitium.

Step 3: The tubular fluid in the descending limb of LOH and interstitium reaches osmotic equilibrium because of osmosis of water out of descending limb. The osmolarity in interstitium maintained at 400 mOsm/L.

Step 4: It is additional flow of fluid into LOH from proximal tubule which causes hyperosmotic fluid in descending limb to move into ascending limb.

Step 5: When fluid is in ascending limb, additional ions are pumped into interstitium with water remaining behind until a 200 mOsm/L osmotic gradient is reached, with interstitium fluid osmolarity raising to 500 mOsm/L.

8

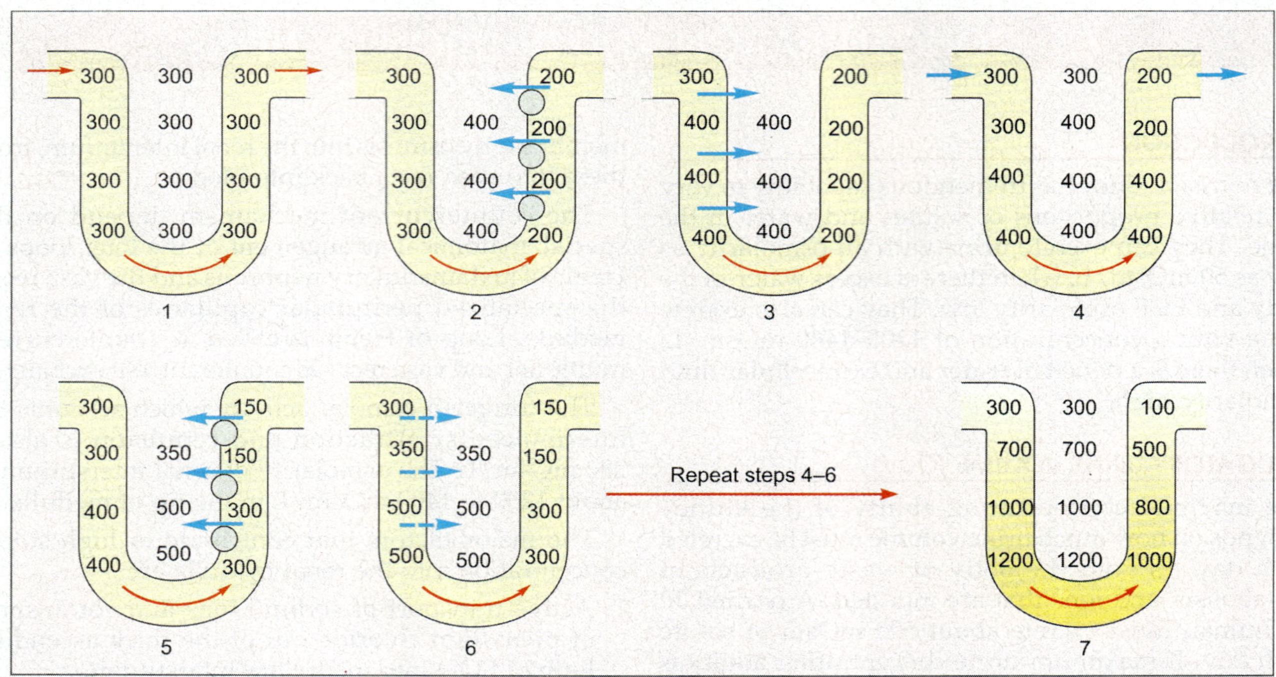

Fig. 8.24: Operation of loop of Henle as a countercurrent multiplier producing a gradient of hyperosmolarity in the medullary interstitium

Step 6: Once again the fluid in descending limb reaches equilibrium with hyperosmotic interstitial fluid. This fluid moves from descending limb to ascending limb so more solute is pumped out of the tubules and deposited in interstitium. These steps are repeated again and again till interstitium osmolarity reaches 1200–1400 mOsm/L.

UREA CONTRIBUTION TO HYPEROSMOTIC RENAL MEDULLARY INTERSTITIUM (Fig. 8.25)

Urea contributes about 40% (500 mOsm/L) of osmolarity of the renal medullary interstitium. When there is water deficit and ADH levels in blood are high, large amounts of urea are passively released from inner medullary collecting duct into interstitium which is highly permeable to urea.

Urea can also be recirculated from collecting duct into interstitium. The thick ascending limb of LOH, distal tubule and cortical collecting duct are impermeable to urea. A person usually excretes 40–60% of filtered urea. Excretion depends on two factors:

a. Concentration of urea in plasma

b. GFR.

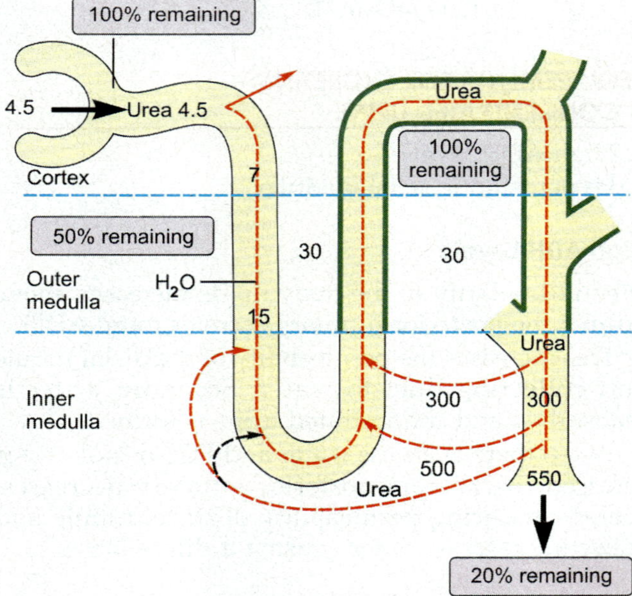

Fig. 8.25

COUNTERCURRENT EXCHANGE IN THE VASA RECTA PRESERVES HYPEROSMOLARITY (Fig. 8.26)

The vasa recta are highly permeable to solutes in the blood, except for the plasma proteins. Plasma flowing

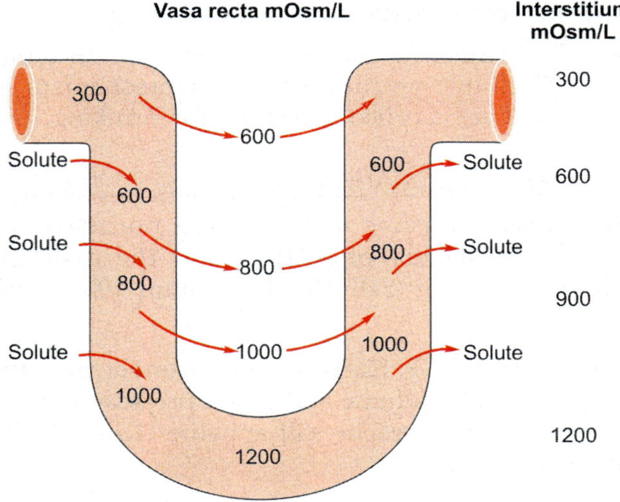

Fig. 8.26: Operation of the vasa recta as counter exchanger in the kidney

down the descending limb of vasa recta becomes more hyperosmotic because of diffusion of solutes from interstitial fluid into blood. In the ascending limb LOH, solutes diffuse back into interstitial fluid and water diffuses back into vasa recta.

Osmolar Clearance (C_{osm})

It is the volume of plasma cleared of solutes each minute. It is expressed in ml/min.

$$C_{osm} = \frac{U_{osm} \times V}{P_{osm}}$$

U_{osm} is urine osmalarity. V is urine flow rate. P_{osm} is plasma osmolarity.

Free Water Clearance (C_{H_2O})

The rate at which solute-free water is excreted by the kidneys. It is expressed in ml/min.

$$C_{H_2O} = V - C_{osm} = V - \frac{(U_{osm} \times V)}{(P_{osm})}$$

It is calculated as the difference between urine flow rate and osmolar clearance. When C_{H_2O} is positive, excess water is being excreted by kidney. When C_{H_2O} is negative excess solutes are being removed from the blood by kidneys.

Disorders of Urine Concentrating Ability

It can be due to:

1. Inappropriate secretion of ADH as in central diabetes insipidus, cause being congenital infections or head injuries.
2. Impairment of countercurrent mechanisms.
3. Inability of DT, CD to respond to ADH: In conditions like nephrogenic diabetes insipidus and in usage of various drugs like lithium and tetracyclines, even if ADH is produced in normal amounts, abnormality of kidneys makes them to fail to respond to ADH.

8

64. CONTROL OF ECF OSMOLARITY AND SODIUM CONCENTRATION

$$\text{Osmolarity} = \frac{\text{Number of osmoles}}{\text{Liter of solution}}$$

Three mechanisms by which ECF osmolarity and sodium concentration maintained are:

1. The osmoreceptor: ADH feedback system
2. Thirst mechanism
3. Salt appetite mechanism.

Plasma sodium = 140 – 145 mEq/L
Plasma osmolarity = 300 mOsm/L ± 2 to 3%

Na and other ions HCO_3, Cl constitutes for about 94% of solute in ECF, with glucose and urea contributing 3 to 5% of the total osmoles.

OSMORECEPTOR ADH SYSTEM

Water deficit
↓
ECF osmolarity ↑
↓
↓ Osmoreceptors senses
↓
↑ ADH secretion (postpituitary)
↓
↑ Plasma ADH
↓
↑ H_2O permeability in DT, CD
↓
↑ H_2O reabsorption
↓
↓ H_2O excreted

The opposite sequence of events occurs when ECF is hypo-osmotic, ADH secretion decreased, renal tubules decrease their permeability for water, less water is reabsorbed and a large volume of dilute urine is formed.

THIRST MECHANISM

The thirst centers are located along the anteroventral wall of the third ventricle (AV3V), preoptic nucleus and organum vasculosum of the lamina terminalis (OVLT). The stimuli for increasing thirst sensation are increased osmolarity, decreased blood volume, decreased blood pressure, increased angiotensin II and dryness of mouth. Angiotensin II acts on subfornical organ and on OVLT of the lamina terminalis.

Threshold for Osmolar Stimulus of Drinking

When the sodium concentration increases even about 2 mEq/L above normal, the thirst mechanism is activated. This is called threshold for drinking.

SALT APPETITE MECHANISM

Humans can survive and function normally on 10 to 20 mEq/day of sodium but the average sodium intake for individuals is about 100 to 200 mEq/day.

Decreased ECF fluid sodium concentration, decreased blood volume and blood pressure are the primary stimuli to excite salt appetite center, AV3V region of the brain.

65. INTEGRATION OF RENAL MECHANISMS FOR CONTROL OF BLOOD VOLUME AND ECF VOLUME

INTRODUCTION

Extracellular fluid volume is determined by the balance between intake and output of water and salt. Sodium excretion is controlled by altering glomerular filtration or tubular reabsorption of sodium.

8

1. Pressure Natriuresis and Diuresis

These are key components of a renal body fluid feedback for regulating blood and ECF volume.

Step 1: An increase in fluid and sodium intake causes temporary accumulation of fluid in the body.

Step 2: As long as fluid intake exceeds urine output, fluid accumulates in the blood and interstitial spaces causing ECF and blood volume to increase.

Step 3: An increase in blood volume raises mean circulatory filling pressure.

Step 4: This increases the pressure gradient for venous return.

Step 5: These changes elevates cardiac output.

Step 6: An increased arterial pressure occurs.

Step 7: This causes pressure diuresis and natriuresis which means raised arterial pressure makes water and sodium to be more excreted in the urine.

Step 8: The increased fluid excretion compensates for increased fluid intake and accumulation of fluid is prevented.

2. Nervous Factors

During hemorrhage when blood volume is reduced, pressures in blood vessels is also decreased and decreased stretch of arterial wall receptors which in-turn stimulates the sympathetic nervous system. The ultimate effect is to increase sodium and water reabsorption by:

a. Constriction of renal arterioles causing decreased GFR.
b. Stimulation of renin, angiotensin II and aldosterone formation.

3. Hormonal Factors

a. Angiotensin II increases the effectiveness of pressure natriuresis in addition to the action of increasing the tubular reabsorption of sodium and water.
b. *Aldosterone:* Angiotensin II increases the aldosterone secretion, which in-turn increases sodium reabsorption.

   Aldosterone escape: In patients with tumors of the adrenal gland (Conn's syndrome) increased aldosterone causes sodium, water retention causing the ECF to rise by 10–15% and also the blood pressure. This causes pressure diuresis and natriuresis resulting in sodium and water excretion, so the kidneys "escape" from sodium water retention.

c. *ADH:* Excess ADH causes only small increase in ECF but large decreases in sodium concentration. Due to increased water reabsorption of kidney which dilutes the ECF sodium and also small increase in BP causes increased sodium loss cause ECF sodium to decrease largely.

d. ANP is released by the cardiac atrial muscle fibers. Excess of blood volume causes over stretch of atria which is a stimulus for release of ANP. High sodium intake also activates natriuretic systems. This cause increased sodium excretion.

Regulation of Potassium in ECF

Normal ECF potassium concentration is about 4.2 mEq/L and ICF potassium concentration being 140 mEq/L. Potassium intake is around 100 mEq/L per day which equals to potassium output.

Factors that can Regulate K^+ Distribution between the ICF and ECF

Factors that shift K^+ into cells (decrease ECF K^+)	*Factors that shift K^+ out of cells (increase ECF K^+)*
Insulin	Diabetes mellitus
Aldosterone	Addison's disease
Adrenergic stimulation	Adrenergic blockers
Alkalosis	Acidosis
Decreased osmolarity	Strenuous exercise

Factors that Regulate K^+ Excretion

1. The rate of K^+ filtration (GFR × plasma K^+ concentration).
2. The rate of K^+ reabsorption.
3. The rate of K^+ secretion from principal cells of late distal and cortical collecting tubules. The intercalated cells can reabsorb K^+ and secrete H^+ ions. The factors that increases K^+ secretion are:
   a. Increased ECF K^+ concentration
   b. Increased aldosterone.
   c. Increased tubular flow rate.

One factor which decreases K^+ secretion is increased H^+ ion concentration that is acidosis.

Regulation of Calcium in ECF

ECF calcium normally remains at 2.4 mEq/L. About 50% exists in the ionized form, 40% bound to plasma proteins, 10% as nonionized form with phosphate and citrate. When calcium ion decreases there is increase in excitability of nerve and muscle cells called hypocalcemic tetany. When calcium concentration increases it results in depression of neuromuscular excitability which can lead to arrhythmias.

Regulation of Phosphate and Magnesium

When PTH is increased, it promotes bone resorption of phosphates so there is increased ECF phosphates. PTH also decreases transport maximum for phosphates, thereby increasing phosphate excretion in urine. Magnesium excretion is increased by increased ECF magnesium concentration and increased ECF Ca concentration.

66. MICTURITION

INTRODUCTION

It is the process by which the urinary bladder empties when it becomes filled. When bladder fills progressively and pressure in its walls rises above threshold level, it causes a nervous reflex called the micturition reflex. It is an autonomic spinal cord reflex.

ANATOMY OF URINARY BLADDER

The urinary bladder is a smooth muscle chamber composed of detrusor muscle which is made up of body and neck. On the posterior wall of the bladder there is a small triangular area called trigone above the bladder neck. At the lower most part of the trigone, the bladder neck opens into the posterior urethra and two ureters enter the bladder at the uppermost angles of the trigone. The inner lining of the bladder is smooth in trigone part, when it is folded to form rugae in other parts of bladder mucosa.

The bladder neck is 2 to 3 cm long and is composed of detrusor muscle and elastic tissue. The muscle in this area is called internal sphincter. The tone in internal sphincter keeps the bladder neck and posterior urethra empty of urine. Beyond the posterior urethra, the urethra passes through the urogenital diaphragm which contains a skeletal muscle layer called external sphincter, this is under voluntary control.

INNERVATION OF URINARY BLADDER

Parasympathetic Innervation (Fig. 8.27)

Motor Innervation

The PS efferent fibers (nerve erigentes) are derived from the second, third and fourth sacral segments. These fibers carry impulses to cause contraction of detrusor muscle and emptying of bladder. These fibers are inhibitory to the internal sphincter.

Sympathetic Innervation

These fibers arise from 11th thoracic to 2nd lumbar segments. These fibers are inhibitory to detrusor muscle. It causes filling of bladder so fullness and in some instances pain.

Somatic Motor Innervation

The somatic pudendal nerve (S_2, S_3, S_4) supplies external sphincter which is voluntary.

8

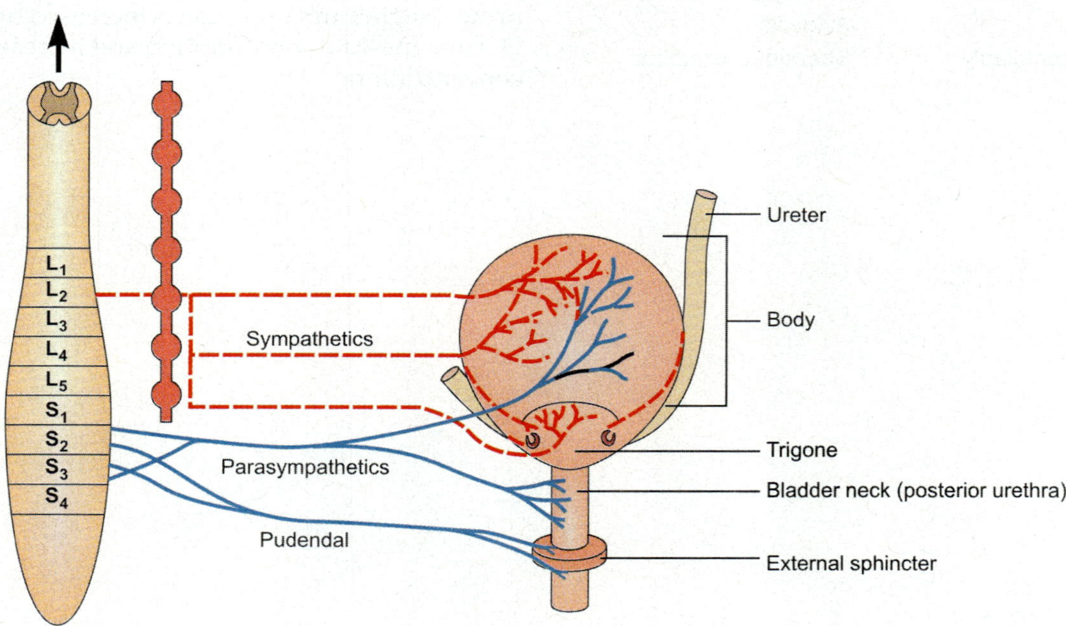

Fig. 8.27: Innervation of the bladder

Sensory Innervation

Afferents from the detrusor stretch receptors travel to the spinal cord via the nerve erigentes from the bladder neck and trigone, the afferents travel through the hypogastric plexus to spinal cord segments T11 to L2.

Physiology of Micturition

The main physiological events in the micturition process are:

1. Filling of the bladder
2. Emptying of the bladder.

The physiological capacity of bladder is 600 ml in adults. The anatomical capacity which is never approached under normal physiological conditions is 1 liter, beyond which bladder ruptures.

The relation between intravesical pressure and volume known as cystometrogram can be studied by inserting a catheter and emptying the bladder, then recording, the pressure while the bladder is filled with 50 ml increments of water or air. This is known as cystometry.

CYSTOMETROGRAM

There are three components in this curve. 1a, 1b and II (Fig. 8.28).

1a: The first urge to void urine is felt at a bladder volume of 150 ml and a sense of fullness at about 400 ml.

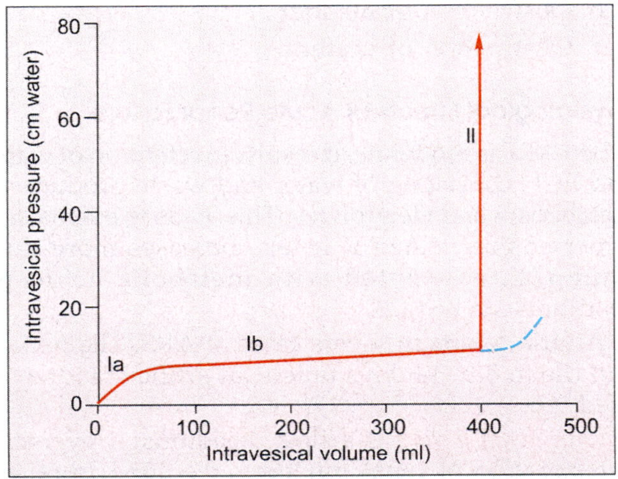

Fig. 8.28: Cystometrogram in a normal human

1b: The flatness of curve is due to manifestation of the law of Laplace. The law states that the pressure in a spherical viscus is equal to twice the wall tension divided by the radius.

II: The tension increases as the organ fills, but also the radius increases so the pressure increase is slight until the bladder is full.

FACILITATION OR INHIBITION OF MICTURITION BY THE BRAIN

The micturition reflex is a completely autonomic spinal cord reflex being controlled by centers in pons and cerebral cortex. The micturition reflex is the basic cause of micurition but the higher centers normally exert final control.

1. The higher centers usually have partial inhibition except when micturition is desired.
2. The higher centers can even prevent micturition even if micturition reflex occur by continual contraction of external sphincter.
3. When it is time to urinate, the cortical centers can facilitate sacral micturition centers to initiate a micturition reflex by relaxing the external sphincter.

ABNORMALITIES OF MICTURITION

1. *Atonic bladder:* It is caused by destruction of sensory nerve fibers when there is crush injury to the sacral region of the spinal cord or syphilis involving bladder called tabetic bladder. This prevents stretch signals transmission from the bladder to the spinal cord. Instead of emptying periodically, the bladder fills to capacity and overflows a few drops at a time through the urethra. This is called overflow incontinence.
2. *Automatic bladder:* It is caused by spinal cord damage above the sacral region. The micturition reflexes are initially suppressed because of spinal shock caused by the sudden loss of facilitatory impulses from brainstem and cerebrum. Later micturition reflexes return, then periodic but unannounced bladder emptying occurs.
3. *The uninhibited bladder/Neurogenic bladder:* It is caused by lack of inhibitory signals from the brain. The facilitatory signals keep the sacral centers, so excitable that even a small volume of urine elicit an uncontrollable micturition reflex and frequent micturition. This is common in infants where brain has not still well-developed.

67. DIURETICS

INTRODUCTION

They are substances which cause diuresis. Diuresis means increased water excretion in urine, most diuretics also increases sodium output in urine called natriuresis. Since sodium loss decreases ECF volume which is of much clinical use in diseases with edema and hypertension. Decreased ECF volume is also important to reduce arterial pressure and GFR.

CLASSIFICATION

Class of diuretic	*Mechanism of action*	*Tubular site of action*
Osmotic diuretics, e.g. mannitol, glucose	Inhibit solute and water reabsorption by increasing osmolarity of tubular fluid	Proximal tubule
Loop diuretics, e.g. furosemide, ethacrynic acid	Inhibit Na^+ K^+ Cl^- cotransport in luminal membrane	Thick ascending limb of LOH
Thiazide diuretics, e.g. chlorthiazide	Inhibit $NaCl^-$ cotransport in luminal membrane	Early distal tubule
Carbonic anhydrase inhibitors (Acetazolamide)	Inhibit H^+ secretion and HCO_3 reabsorption which reduces Na^+ reabsorption	Proximal tubule
K^+ sparing diuretics competitive inhibitors of aldosterone, e.g. water, ethanol spironolactone	Inhibit action of aldosterone decrease Na^+ reabsorption, ↓ K secretion	Collecting tubules
Sodium channel blockers (Amiloride and triamterene)	Block entry of Na^+ into Na^+ channels of luminal membrane, decrease Na reabsorption and ↓ K^+ secretion	Collecting tubules

68. APPLIED ASPECTS

8

Polyuria: Normal urine output per day is 1 liter to 2.5 liters. If urine output is more than 3 liters. This is known as polyuria.

Nocturia: Excessive urine excretion at night.

Dysuria: Burning sensation during micturition.

Enuresis means involuntary passage of urine at night or during sleep. It is also called bedwetting or nocturnal enuresis.

Oliguria: If urine output is less than 500 ml/day.

Anuria: Not passing urine or less than 50 ml/day.

Acute renal failure(ARF): Where GFR decreases suddenly over a period of days or weeks and there is rise in urea and non-nitrogenous substances in the blood causes:

1. Prerenal causes
   a. hemorrhage
   b. Anaphylactic shock
   c. Burns
2. Intrarenal causes
   a. Acute glomerulonephritis
   b. Acute pyelonephritis
   c. Vasculitis
3. Postrenal causes
   a. Bilateral obstruction of ureter or renal pelvis by large stones or blood clots
   b. Obstruction of bladder
   c. Obstruction of urethra.

Physiological Effects of Acute Renal Failure

When ARF is moderate, it results in retention of water and ECF, consisting of water and waste products of metabolism and electrolytes. This leads to edema and hypertension. When K levels increases more than 8 mEq/L, associated with metabolic acidosis, condition can be fatal.

Anuria occurs in severe cases of ARF. The patient will die in 8 to 14 days unless an artificial kidney is used.

Chronic renal failure is a slow, insidious, irreversible deterioration of renal functions resulting in raised blood urea levels. It results from irreversible loss of large numbers of functioning nephrons.

Causes

Chronic pyelonephritis TB, polycystic kidney, benign enlargement of prostate, diabetes mellitus and atherosclerosis.

Vicious cycle that can occur with kidney disease. Loss of nephrons because of disease may increase GFR and blood flow in the reviving glomerular capillaries, which in turn may eventually injure these normal capillaries as well, thus causing progressive sclerosis and eventual loss of these glomeruli (Fig. 8.29).

Effects of Renal Failure

1. *On the body fluids*
   - Generalized edema resulting from water and salt retention.
   - Acidosis: Failure of kidney to get rid of acidic products.
   - High concentration of nonprotein nitrogens like urea, creatinine and uric acid. They are all metabolic end-products of proteins.
   - High concentrations of other substances excreted by the kidneys like phenols, sulfates, phosphates, potassium and guanidine bases. This total condition is called uremia (Azotemia) because of high concentration of urea in the body fluids.
2. Anemia in CRF caused by decreased erythropoietin secretion.
3. *Osteomalacia* in CRF caused by decreased production of active vitamin D and by phosphate retention of kidneys.
4. *Hypertension and kidney disease*
   - Increased renal vascular resistance.
   - Decreased glomerular capillary filtration co-efficient.
   - Excessive tubular sodium reabsorption. All these conditions lead to hypertension.

Specific Tubular Disorders

1. *Renal glycosuria:* Failure of the kidneys to reabsorbs glucose results in presence of glucose in urine. In this, the blood glucose concentration may be normal but transport maximum for glucose is limited.
2. *Aminoaciduria:* Failure of kidneys to reabsorbs amino acids. The cause being deficiency of specific carrier systems.
3. *Renal tubular acidosis:* Failure of the tubules to secrete hydrogen ions.
4. *Nephrogenic diabetes insipidus:* Failure of the kidneys to respond to antidiuretic hormone.
5. *Fancon's syndrome:* A generalized reabsorptive defect of the renal tubules. There is increased urinary excretion of amino acids, glucose, phosphate, potassium and calcium. In severe cases there is also metabolic acidosis and nephrogenic diabetes insipidus.

The proximal tubular cells are especially affected due to hereditary defects in cell transport mechanisms or due to toxins, drugs and ischemia.

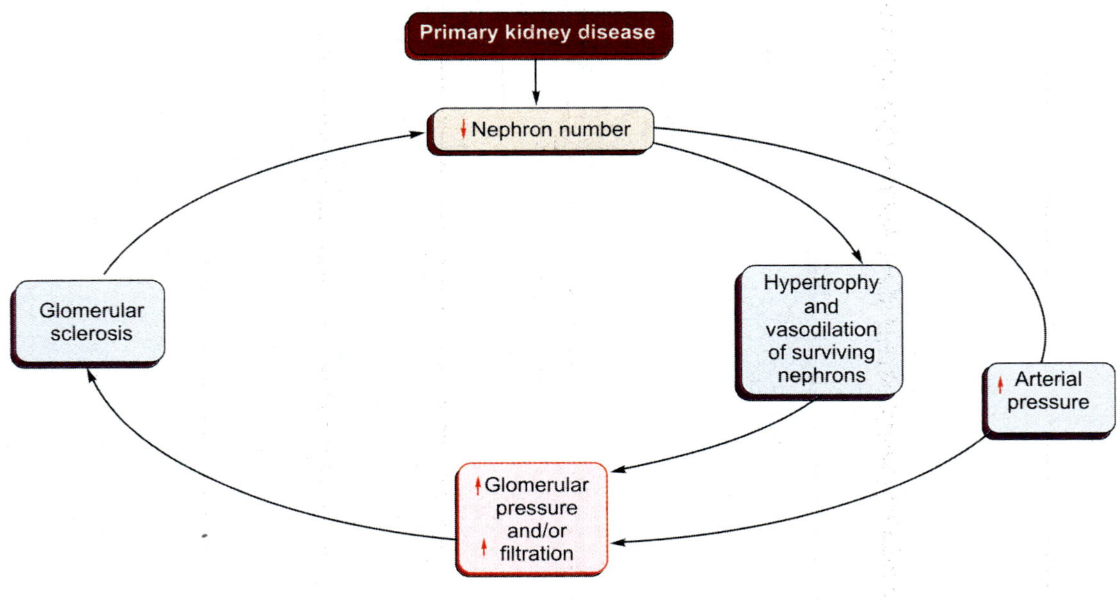

Fig. 8.29

8

69. DIALYSIS/ARTIFICIAL KIDNEY

INTRODUCTION

An artificial kidney is used to tide the patient over until the kidneys resume their function. If the loss is irreversible, it is necessary to perform dialysis chronically to maintain life but still dialysis cannot maintain completely normal body fluid composition. So, a better treatment for permanent loss of kidney function is kidney transplant.

Types of Dialysis

There are two types of dialysis:

1. Hemodialysis (Fig. 8.30)
2. Peritoneal dialysis (Fig. 8.31).

The basic principle of the artificial kidney is to pass blood through minute blood channels bounded by a thin membrane. On the other side of the membrane is a dialysing fluid into which unwanted substances in blood pass by diffusion.

In artificial kidney blood flows continually between two thin membranes of cellophane, outside the membrane is a dialysing fluid. The cellophane is porous which allows all the constituents to diffuse in both directions except the plasma proteins.

There is a net transfer of the substance from the plasma into the dialysing fluid if the concentration of the substance is greater in the plasma than in the dialysing fluid. The solute movement across the dialysis membrane depends on:

a. The concentration gradient of the solute between the two solutions.
b. The permeability of the membrane to the solute.
c. The surface area of the membrane.
d. The length of time, that the blood and fluid remain in contact with the membrane.

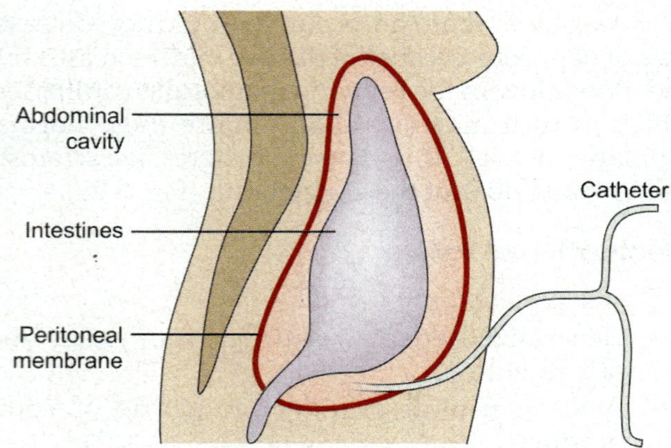

Fig. 8.31: Peritoneal dialysis

8

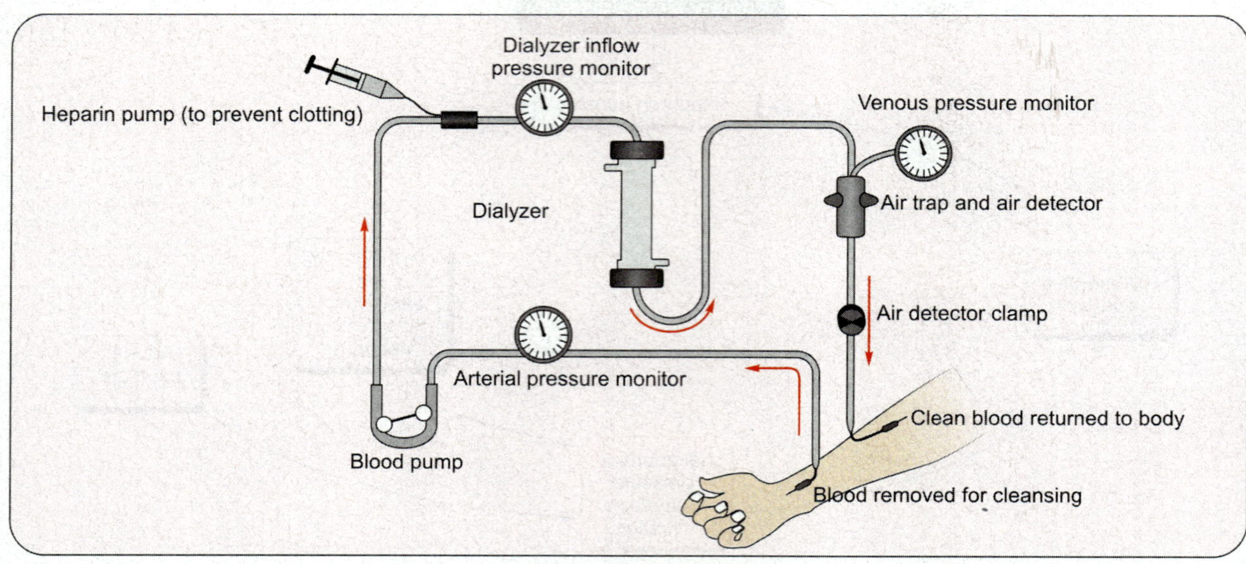

Fig. 8.30: Hemodialysis

The total amount of blood in the artificial kidney is usually less than 500 ml at one time. The total diffusion surface area is between 0.6 and 2.5 square meters. A small amount of heparin is added as an anticoagulant.

In addition to diffusion of solutes, mass transfer of solutes and water can be produced by applying a hydrostatic pressure to force them by the process of filtration called bulk flow. The artificial kidney is used for only 4 to 6 hours per day, three times a week. They can clear urea from the plasma at a rate of 100 to 225 ml/min. But still overall the plasma clearance is limited, cannot replace some of functions of the kidneys, such as secretion of erythropoietin.

70. RENAL FUNCTION TESTS

INTRODUCTION

1. Urine Analysis

The initial and cost effective laboratory evaluation of kidney function is the routine analysis of urine.

Routine examination	Volume/24 hrs, of color, chemical examination of protein, glucose, blood and bile. Microscopy–RBC, WBC, casts
Special tests on urine	Urine pH, osmolarity, specific gravity, protein/creatinine ratio

2. Examination of Blood

Blood: Urea, creatinine, Na^+, K^+, calcium, phosphate, uric acid, H^+, HCO_3^- creatinine clearance, inulin clearance, 24 hours output: Na^+, K^+, calcium, phosphate, urea and amino acids.

a. Tests for Renal Blood Flow

15 minute phenol sulphone phthalein (PSP) excretion test.

Reagents: Phenol red, 6 mg/ml in water.

Techniques

1. Breakfast is with held.
2. Ask patient to drink 500 ml of water.
3. After 20–30 minutes inject intravenously 1 ml of phenol red.
4. Collect urine specimen at intervals of 15, 30, 60 and 120 minutes.

Estimation of PSP

Add a few ml of 10% NaOH to urine until reddish purple color develops.

Interpretation: Volume of urine after 15 min should be over 100 ml. Normal kidney excretes 30–50% of the dye.

Excretion of less than 23% of dye in the 1st 15 min indicates impaired kidney.

b. Tests for Glomerular Function

- Urea clearance test
- Creatinine clearance
- Inulin clearance
- PAH clearance.

c. Tests for Tubular Function

An early sign of impaired tubular function is decreased ability to concentrate urine. Nephrosclerosis and other diseases which diminishes blood flow in kidney, causes inability to concentrate or dilute the urine with resultant isothenuria (fixation of specific gravity at 1.010).

8

Concentration Test

This test of impairment of water reabsorption is based on the ability of tubule to concentrate urine.

Clearance rate (C_s)

$$C_s = \frac{U_s \times V}{P_s} \text{ ml/min}$$

Glomerular filtration rate (GFR)

$$GFR = \frac{U_{inulin} \times V}{P_{inulin}}$$

Clearance ratio

$$\text{Clearance ratio} = \frac{C_s}{C_{inulin}}$$

Effective renal plasma flow (ERPF)

$$ERPF = C_{PAH} = \frac{U_{PAH} \times V}{P_{PAH}} \text{ ml/min}$$

Renal plasma flow (RPF)

$$RPF = \frac{C_{PAH}}{E_{PAH}}$$

$$= \frac{(U_{PAH} \times V / P_{PAH})}{(P_{PAH} - V_{PAH})/P_{PAH}} \text{ ml/min}$$

$$= \frac{U_{PAH} \times V_1}{P_{PAH} - V_{PAH}}$$

Renal blood flow (RBF)

$$RBF = \frac{RPF}{1 - \text{Hematocrit}} \text{ ml/min}$$

Water deprivation: Maximum concentration is attained when the patient is deprived of water for 24 hours. The specific gravity of urine passed during last 12 hours should not be less than 1.022 but may increase up to 1.040 in normal young adults.

Dilution Test

It is a less sensitive test.

1. Patient withholds breakfast.
2. Patient drinks 1200 ml of water during an interval of 30 min.
3. Urine is collected hourly thereafter for 4 hours.
4. Largest part is passed during first 2 hours. Specific gravity should fall to 1.003.
5. In kidney diseases, quantity of urine voided in the 4 hour period is smaller and specific gravity may not fall below 1.010.

Other Methods of Study

1. Micropuncture technique to analyze tubular fluid.
2. Microcryoscopic studies of renal tissue.
3. Microelectrode studies to measure membrane potential.
4. Radiology imaging
   a. Plain radiograph of abdomen in identifying calcium–radiopaque renal stones.
   b. Intravenous pyelography is performed by injecting a dye like urographin IV and taking X-ray after 1, 5, 10 and 30 min.
   c. Ultrasonography–quick, noninvasive, inexpensive.
   d. Computed tomography.
   e. Radionuclide studies by using gamma camera.
   f. Renal biopsy is done by using Vem-Silverman needle.

71. ACID-BASE HOMEOSTASIS

Definition

Acid–base homeostasis is the part of human homeostasis concerning the proper balance between acids and bases, in other words, the pH. The body is very sensitive to its pH level, so strong mechanisms exist to maintain it. Outside the acceptable range of pH, proteins are denatured and digested, enzymes lose their ability to function, and death may occur.

What is pH?

The term pH refers to the negative log of hydrogen ion concentration

$$pH = \log 1/H^+ = -\log [H^+]$$

Normal H^+ is 40 nEq/L.

Normal pH is

$pH = -\log [0.00000004]$

$pH = 7.4$

The normal range of blood pH falls between 7.35 and 7.45 and our Acid–base balance has to maintain pH within this normal range.

pH of Some Body Fluids

Arterial blood	7.4
Venous blood	7.35
Interstitial fluid	7.35
ICF	6–7.4
Urine	4.5–8
Gastric HCl	0.8
Survival range of pH is	6.8 to 8.0

ACID

An acid is a molecule containing hydrogen atom that can release hydrogen ions in solutions, e.g.

$$HCl \rightarrow H^+ + Cl^-$$
$$H_2CO_3 \rightarrow H^+ + HCO_3$$

There is always a constant production of acid by the body's metabolic processes and to maintain balance, these acids need to be excreted or metabolized. The various acids produced by the body are classified as respiratory (or volatile) acids and metabolic (or fixed) acids.

Respiratory Acid

The acid is more correctly carbonic acid (H_2CO_3) but the term 'respiratory acid' is usually used to mean carbon dioxide. Carbon dioxide is the end-product of complete oxidation of carbohydrates and fatty acids. It is called a volatile acid meaning in this context it can be excreted via the lungs. Of necessity, considering the amounts involved there must be an efficient system to rapidly excrete CO_2.

Metabolic Acids

This term covers all the acids the body produces which are nonvolatile. Because they are not excreted by the lungs they are said to be 'fixed' in the body and hence the alternative term fixed acids. All acids other than H_2CO_3 are fixed acids.

For Acid–base balance, the amount of acid excreted per day must equal the amount produced. The routes of excretion are the lungs (for CO_2) and the kidneys (for the fixed acids).

Acid–base imbalance: Acid–base imbalance occurs when a significant insult causes the blood pH to shift out of the normal range (7.35 to 7.45). An excess of acid is called acidosis (pH less than 7.35) and an excess of base is called alkalosis (pH greater than 7.45). The process that causes the imbalance is classified based on the etiology of the disturbance (respiratory or metabolic) and the direction of change in pH (acidosis or alkalosis). There are four basic processes: (i) Metabolic acidosis, (ii) Respiratory acidosis, (iii) Metabolic alkalosis, (iv) Respiratory alkalosis. One or a combination may occur at any given time.

Response to an Acid-base Imbalance

The body's response to a change in Acid–base status has three components:

1. *First defence:* Buffering
2. *Second defence:* Respiratory compensation by alteration in arterial PCO_2
3. *Third defence:* Renal compensation by alteration in HCO_3^- excretion.

BUFFER

Body Fluid

A buffer is any substance that can reversibly bind H^+.

Buffer + $H^+ \leftrightarrow$ H buffer

80 mEq of H^+ are produced per day.

1. *Bicarbonate buffer system:* The major buffer system in the ECF is the CO_2–bicarbonate buffer system. This is responsible for about 80% of extracellular buffering but it cannot buffer respiratory Acid–base disorders.
2. *The phosphate buffer systems* are not important blood buffer as its concentration is too low. It plays an important role in renal tubular system.
3. *Hemoglobin:* Protein buffers in blood include hemoglobin (150 g/l) and plasma proteins (70 g/l). Buffering is by the imidazole group of the histidine residues. Hemoglobin is quantitatively about 6 times more important then the plasma proteins as it is present in about twice the concentration and contain about three times the number of histidine residues per molecule. For example, if blood pH changed from 7.5 to 6.5, hemoglobin would buffer 27.5 mmol/l of H^+ and total plasma protein buffering would account for only 4.2 mmol/l of H^+. Deoxyhemoglobin is a more effective buffer than oxyhemoglobin.

The major body buffer systems

Site	*Buffer system*	*Comment*
Blood	Bicarbonate	Important for metabolic acids
	Hemoglobin	Important for carbon dioxide
	Plasma protein	Minor buffer
	Phosphate	Concentration too low
ICF	Proteins	Important buffer
	Phosphates	Important buffer
Urine	Phosphate	Responsible for most of 'Titrable acidity'
	Ammonia	Important formation of NH_4^+

ISOHYDRIC PRINCIPLE

'Whenever, there is a change in H^+ concentration in the ECF, the balance of all the buffer systems changes at the same time'.

$H^+ = K1 \times HA1/A1 = K2 \times HA2/A2 = K3 \times HA3/A3$.

K1, K2 and K3 are dissociation constants of 3 respective acids.

Respiratory Regulation of Acid-base Balance

- Regulates H^+ concentration through CO_2 in ventilation.
- $\uparrow [H^+] \rightarrow \uparrow$ alveolar ventilation
- Buffering power of respiratory system is 1–2 times greater than chemical buffers.
- Lung diseases decrease the efficacy of the buffering power. Respiratory regulation refers to changes in pH due to PCO_2 changes by altering the ventilation. This change in ventilation can occur rapidly with significant effects on pH. Carbon dioxide is lipid soluble and crosses cell membranes rapidly, so changes in PCO_2 result in rapid changes in $[H^+]$ in all body fluid compartments.

Control system for respiratory regulation of acid–base balance

Control element	*Physiological or anatomical correlate*	*Comment*
Controlled variable	Arterial PCO_2	A change in arterial PCO_2 alters arterial pH
Sensors	Central and peripheral chemoreceptor	Both respond to changes in arterial PCO_2
Central integrator	The respiratory center in the medulla	
Effectors	The respiratory muscles	An increase in minute ventilation increases alveolar ventilation and thus decreases arterial PCO_2 (the controlled variable). The net result is of negative feedback which tends to restore the PCO_2 to the 'set point'

Renal Regulation of Acid-base Balance

There are three systems that regulate H^+ concentration in the body fluids to prevent acidosis or alkalosis.

1. The chemical Acid–base buffer systems which combine with acid or base to prevent excessive changes in H^+ concentration.
2. The respiratory centers which regulates the removal of CO_2 from ECF.
3. The kidneys regulate blood pH by three mechanisms.
   i. The chemical Acid–base buffer systems which combine with acid or base to prevent excessive changes in H^+ concentration.
   ii. The respiratory centers which regulates the removal of CO_2 from ECF.
   iii. $CO_2 + H_2O \leftrightarrow H_2CO_3$ (Fig. 8.31)

$H_2CO_3 \xrightarrow{CA} H^+ + HCO_3$ the kidneys regulate blood pH by three mechanisms:

a. Excretion of acid in the form of titrable acid and ammonium ions.
b. Reabsorption of the filtered HCO_3
c. Generation of new $NaHCO_3$

Mechanism of H+ Secretion by PT

- Formation of carbonic acid
- Secretion of H^+ into the lumen via Na^+ H^+ counter-transport in luminal membrane—an example of secondary active transport.
- H^+ secreted in the lumen combines with filtered HCO_3 and helps in reabsorption.
- HCO_3 formed in the cell diffuses into interstitial fluid through basolateral membrane. This is done by Na HCO_3 transport and Cl HCO_3 exchanger. Thus for each H^+ secreted one Na^+ and one HCO_3 ion enter the interstitial fluid (Fig. 8.32).

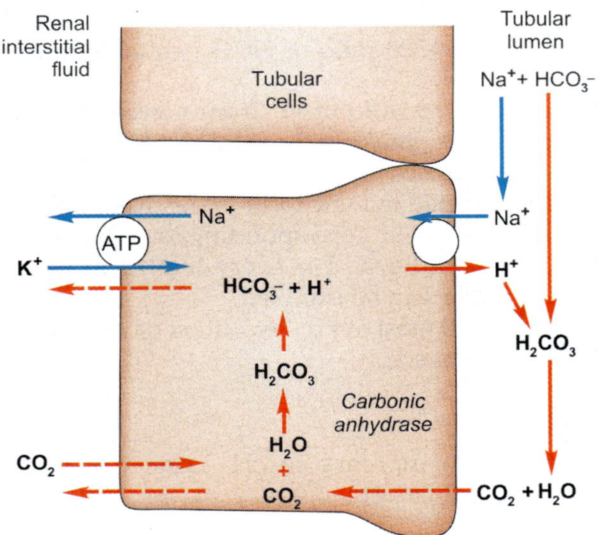

Fig. 8.32: Reabsorption of filtered bicarbonate

Fate of H ion into the Lumen

1. Nontitrable acidity
2. Titrable acidity

Nontitrable acidity: H^+ ion combines with HCO_3 and NH_3 producing nontitrable acids. The reactions are:

$$\text{Glutamine} \xrightarrow{\text{glutaminase}} \text{glutamic acid} + NH_3$$

$$\text{Glutamic acid} + NH_3 \xrightarrow[\text{dehydrogenase}]{\text{glutamic}} \alpha\text{-ketoglutaric acid} + NH_3$$

$$\text{Amino acid} \xrightarrow{\text{deamination}} \text{Ketoacid} + NH_3$$

$$NH_3 + H^+ \longrightarrow NH_4$$

The process by which NH_3 is secreted into the urine and then changed to NH_4 maintaining the concentra-tion gradient for diffusion of NH_3 is called nonionic diffusion.

Ammonium Ion Secretion

Glutamine is metabolized in PCT cells yielding ammonium and bicarbonate. The NH_4^+ is actively secreted by Na^+ NH_4^+ pump and bicarbonate is returned to blood (Fig. 8.33).

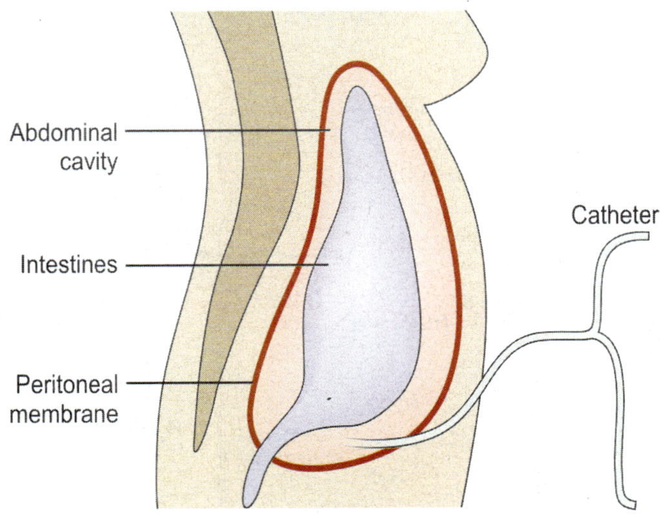

Fig. 8.33: Ammonium formation

Ammonium Ion Secretion in CD

The CD are permeable to NH_3 which diffuses into tubular lumen but less permeable to NH_4, therefore, NH_4 is trapped in the tubular lumen and excreted in the urine (Fig. 8.34)

TITRABLE ACIDITY

The H^+ ions that combine with dibasic phosphate produces monobasic phosphate which contributes titrable acidity (Fig. 8.35).

Net acid secretion = Titrable acidity + urinary NH_4 – urinary HCO_3

Total acid excreted by the kidney = 50 to 100 mEq/day.

8

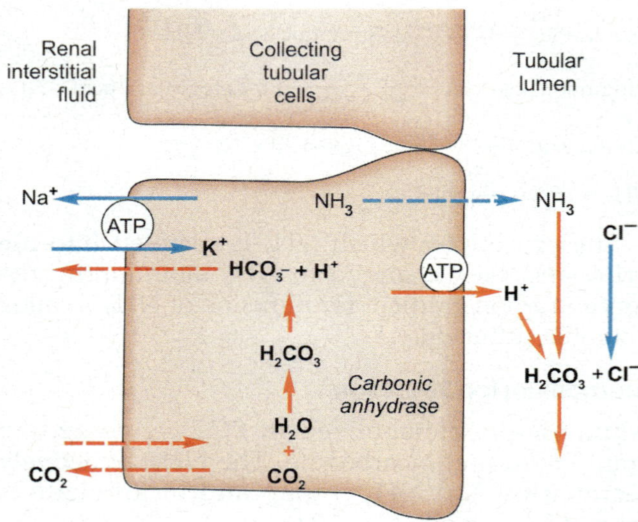

Fig. 8.34

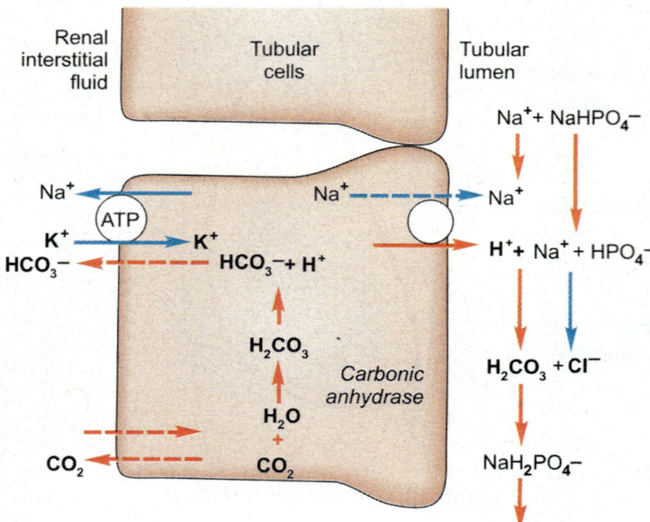

Fig. 8.35: Formation of monobasic phosphate

Mechanism of H^+ Secretion by DT and CD is independent of Na^+

- ATP driven pumps increases H^+ concentration by 1000 times. Aldosterone acts on this pump to increase H^+ secretion.
- H^+ K^+ ATPase is also responsible.

Reabsorption of Filtered HCO_3

PT reabsorbs 80% of filtered HCO_3, H^+ secreted in lumen of PT combines with HCO_3 to form H_2CO_3. It is converted to CO_2 and H_2O. CO_2 diffuses into tubular cells. CO_2 combines with H_2O to form H_2CO_3 which dissociates into H^+ and HCO_3.

The H^+ ion is secreted into tubule and HCO_3 ion diffuses into interstitial fluid. When each molecule of HCO_3 is reabsorbed into lumen, one molecule of HCO_3 diffuses into blood even though it is not the same molecule. The pH of fluid in proximal tubule is very little altered since the H^+ ion secretion is neutralized by HCO_3 ion reabsorption.

LOH reabsorbs 15% of filtered HCO_3.

DT and CT reabsorbs only 5% of the filtered HCO_3.

Generation of new $NaHCO_3$ ions: Phosphate and ammonia buffers in the tubule carries excess H^+ ions to generate new $NaHCO_3$ ions. Therefore, whenever H^+ ion secreted into the tubules combine with a buffer other than HCO_3, the net effect is addition of a new bicarbonate to the blood. For examples if H^+ reacts with NH_3 to form NH_4, NH_4 is trapped in the tubular lumen and eliminated in the urine. For each NH_4 excreted, a new HCO_3 is generated and added to the blood.

Kidneys filter 4320 mEq of HCO_3^-/day.

(180 L × 24 mEq/L)

To reabsorb 4320 mEq of HCO_3, equal amount of H^+ are secreted.

In addition, 80 mEq of H^+ from nonvolatile acids are also secreted, making the total of 4400 mEq of H^+ to be secreted/day. Only a small amount of excess H^+ can be secreted in ionic form in the urine. Minimal urine pH is about 4.5 corresponding to an H^+ concentration of 0.03 mEq/L. For every liter of urine only 0.03 mEq of H+ can be excreted.

To excrete 80 mEq of H^+, 2667 liters of urine would have to be formed.

Acidosis

Defined as an increase in H^+ concentration or decrease in pH (<7.4) .

Alkalosis

Defined as a decrease in H^+ concentration or increase in pH (>7.4).

Metabolic

Any disturbance of Acid–base balance resulting from changes in HCO_3^- concentration in ECF.

Metabolic acidosis: Decrease in plasma HCO_3^-

Metabolic alkalosis: Increase in plasma HCO_3^-.

Respiratory

Disturbances in Acid–base balance due to changes in PCO_2.

Respiratory acidosis: Increase in PCO_2

Respiratory alkalosis: Decrease in PCO_2.

Renal Correction

Alkalosis: Either a decrease in tubular secretion of H^+ or increased excretion of HCO_3^-.

Acidosis: Either a increase in excretion of H^+ or by generation of new HCO_3^-.

Respiratory Acidosis

Any factor that decreases the rate of pulmonary ventilation increases the PCO_2 of ECF $\rightarrow \uparrow H_2CO_3 \rightarrow \uparrow H^+$.

Causes

- Damage to respiratory center
- Obstruction of passages of the respiratory tract
- Pneumonia
- Emphysema

Respiratory Alkalosis

Caused by

- Hyperventilation
- Physiologically at high altitudes
- Psychoneurosis

Metabolic Acidosis

Causes

- Failure of kidneys to excrete metabolic acids
- Formation of excess quantities of metabolic acids
- Addition of metabolic acids to the body
- Loss of base from the body.

Renal Tubular Acidosis

- Chronic renal failure
- Addison's disease
- Fanconi's syndrome
- Diarrhea
- Vomiting of intestinal contents
- Diabetes mellitus
- Ingestion of acids (aspirin, methyl alcohol).

Metabolic Alkalosis

Causes

- Excess retention of HCO_3^-
- Loss of H^+ from the body
- Use of diuretics (except carbonic anhydrase inhibitor)
- Excess aldosterone
- Vomiting of gastric contents
- Ingestion of alkaline drugs
- Treatment of acidosis
- Oral $NaHCO_3$
- Infusion of sodium lactate and sodium gluconate.

Treatment of Alkalosis

- Oral ammonium chloride
- Lysine monohydrochloride.

Renal Correction

$\downarrow$ Tubular section of H^+ ions

$\uparrow$ Excretion of HCO_3 ions.

Acid–base Nomogram (Fig. 8.36)

To dignose acid–base disorders quickly and to find out the severity. pH, PCO_2 and HCO_3 values are used. Sufficient time should be given for compensatory response. 6–12 hours for lungs and 3–5 days for kidneys.

Nomogram

Anion Gap

It is the measure of difference between unmeasured anions and cations.

$= (Na^+) - (HCO_3^-) (Cl^-)$

$= 144 - 24 - 108$

$= 12$ mEq/L

Unmeasured cations are Ca^{++}, Mg^{++} and K^+.
Unmeasured anions are albumin, PO_4, SO_4, etc.
Normal range is 8–16 mEq/L.

Conditions Associated with Increased Anion Gap

- DM
- Lactic acidosis
- Chronic renal failure
- Starvation
- Aspirin poisoning

Conditions associated with Decreased Anion Gap

- Diarrhea
- Renal tubular acidosis
- Carbonic anhydrase inhibitors
- Addison's disease

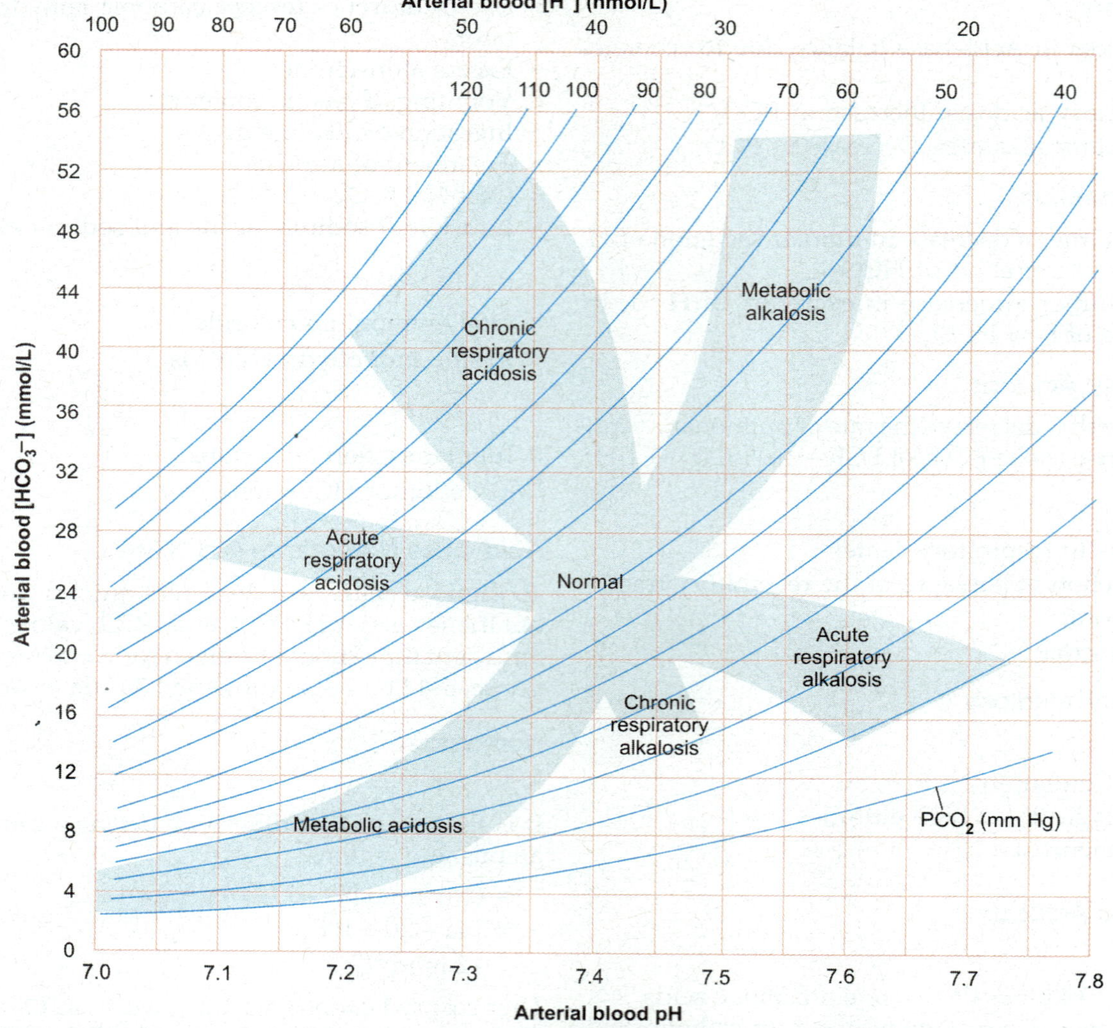

Fig. 8.36: Acid–base nomogram showing changes in the CO_2 plasma. HCO_3^- and pH of arterial blood in the respiratory and metabolic acidosis

		Disorder					
		Acidosis		Alkalosis			
Analyte	*Normal*	*Metabolic*	*Respiratory*	*Metabolic*	*Respiratory*	*RDS*	*Renal failure*
pH	7.4	↓	↓	↑	↑	↓	↓
PCO_2	40@	↓*	↑	↑*①	↓	↑	N*
PO_2	90@	N	↓	N	↓	↓	
HCO_3	24#	↓	↑*	↑	↓*	N	↓

*Initial stages are normal, but abnormal changes occur later.

RDS = Respiratory distress syndrome

① May be due to body compensation by hypoventilation

mmol/L @ mm Hg

Note: Arrows do not quantitate. Changes may be slight, moderate, or large.

72. THE SKIN AND ITS APPENDAGES

The skin and its derivatives forms the covering of body to constitute integument. Its average thickness is 1–2 mm where as it is 5 mm in interscapular region and sole of the foot. It is thin as 0.5 mm in eyelids.

The superficial layer (epidermis) and deeper layer (dermis) are two layers of skin. The epidermis is formed by 4 layers namely, stratum corneum, stratum lucidium, stratum granulosum and stratum germinativum. The dermis is a dense network of collagen fibers, fibroblasts and histiocytes. There are a lot of smooth muscles in the skin around the hair bulbs known as rector pili. Glands of the skin are sweat glands and sebaceous glands.

SWEAT GLANDS (Fig. 8.37)

The sweat glands are present all over the skin except in lips, eardrums, inner surface of prepuce and glans penis. They are coiled tubular glands 2 types namely eccrine or merocrine type and apocrine type. The eccrine glands are most common type in thick skin, are simple tubular glands.

The apocrine glands about 1 mm in diameter are mostly located in the axilla, umbilicus, areola of the breast, in eyelid and external auditory meatus.

The sweat glands have rich blood supply, are innervated by sympathetic cholinergic nerves.

The eccrine secretion is odorless and does not contribute to the body odor, which is absolutely due to apocrine secretion.

SEBACEOUS GLANDS

These are simple or branched alveolar glands whose secretions are poured through ducts into the neck of the hair follicle.

The secretion is holocrine type, secretory cells with secretory material extruded into the exterior which is known as sebum.

Appendages of Skin

They are hair, nails, sweat and sebaceous glands.

Hair

There are various types of hairs.

Lanugo Hair

Present in human fetus.

Vellus Hair

Of infants and facial hair of adult women.

Terminal Hair

Long, coarse and pigmented present all over the body, moustache, beard, axilla, limbs and head.

Nails

Each nail has a body portion, a free margin and nail root. The skin lying beneath the nail is known as nail bed. The nails grow about 0.1 mm per day. The nails become brittle and rough in iron deficiency anemia.

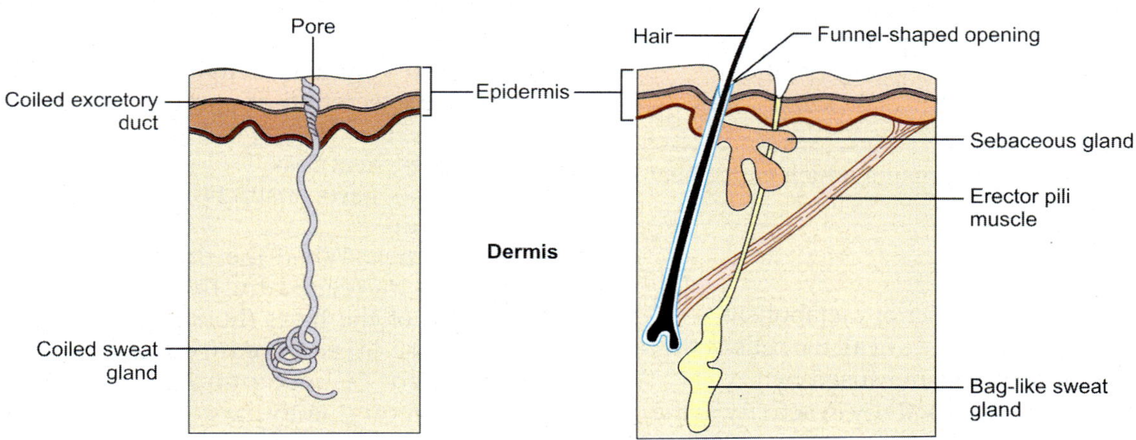

Fig. 8.37: Sweat glands

Functions of Skin

1. *Protective function:* Skin gives a protective covering to the delicate structures underneath it.
2. *Sensory function:* Contains thze cutaneous receptors. These sensory end organs communicate the message to central nervous system.
3. *Secretory function:* Sebaceous glands secrete sebum.
4. *Heat regulatory function:* It helps in temperature regulation by conduction, convection, evaporation and radiation.
5. *Excretory function:* Water, salts and fatty substances are excreted through skin.
6. *Synthetic function:* The cholesterol of the skin is converted into 7-dehydrocholesterol, the natural vitamin D_3 by sun's ultraviolet rays. The skin manufactures the pigment melanin from tyrosine, responsible for skin coloration.

73. BODY TEMPERATURE AND ITS REGULATION

INTRODUCTION

Man is warm blooded animal (homeothermic). The body temperature recorded in the mouth is oral temperature ranges between 35.8° and 37.3°C. The rectal temperature is 0.5° to 0.6°C (1°F) higher than oral temperature. The axillary temperature is 0.5° to 0.6°C lower than oral temperature. The shell or skin temperature is much lower than body temperature. It is about 29.5° to 33.9°C.

The core temperature is the body tissue temperature (critical body core temperature) is highest about 37.1°C. At temperatures above this level, the rate of heat loss is greater than heat gain, so the body temperature falls and approaches 37.1°C. At temperature below this level, the rate of heat production is greater than that of heat loss, so the body temperature rises and approaches 37.1°C. This critical temperature level is called "set point" of the temperature control mechanism.

Physiological factors influencing body temperature are age, sex, diurnal changes, diet, muscular activities, climate, menstruation, sleep and emotions.

THERMAL BALANCE

There are various mechanisms which cause heat gain and heat loss.

Heat Gain

It is a principal by-product of metabolism

1. Basic metabolic processes of all the cells of the body.
2. Extra rate of metabolism caused by:
   a. Increased chemical activity in activity in the cells.
   b. Food ingestion: Fat emits more energy than proteins and carbohydrates (specific dynamic action).
   c. Epinephrine, TSH and thyroid overactivity increase heat production.
   d. Increased muscular activity includes muscle contractions caused by shivering.

Heat Loss

By processes like conduction, convection, radiation, evaporation and sweating. These physical factors like conduction and radiation account for nearly 70% of the heat loss. Vaporization of sweat 27%, respiration 2%, urination and defecation 1%.

TEMPERATURE REGULATING MECHANISMS

Mechanisms Activated by Cold

1. *Shivering:* When subject is exposed to cold involuntary muscular activities are seen which is due to increased muscle tone and contraction of muscles.
2. Hunger
3. Increased voluntary activity
4. Increased secretion of epinephrine and norepinephrine
5. Decreased heat loss
6. Cutaneous vasoconstriction
7. Curling up
8. *Horripilation:* When the thickness of the trapped layer is increased by fluffing the features or erection of the hairs (horripilation), heat transfer across the layer is reduced and heat losses are decreased. "Goose pimples" are the result of horripilation due to the cold induced contraction of the piloerector muscles.

8

Mechanisms Activated by Heat

- Increased heat loss
- Cutaneous vasodilatation
- Sweating
- *Panting:* The rapid, shallow breathing greatly increases the amount of water vaporization in the mouth and respiratory system. Increased respiration decreases heat production mechanisms.

Composition of Sweat

- 0.5% solid (sodium, urea, potassium, calcium)
- 99.5% water

Critical Temperature of Sweating

Sweating begins at 29°C of environmental temperature and at skin temperature of 34°C. Approximately, 500–1000 ml is secreted per hour in a hot day.

Gustatory sweating: Spicy food and condiments can produce sweating during hot climate.

Hyperhydrosis: Sweat glands in palm of hand and sole of foot are overactive to provide sweat in these regions.

Fever is the most universal known hall mark of disease. It occurs not only in mammals but also in birds, reptiles, amphibian and fish. When it occurs in homeothermic animals, the thermoregulatory mechanisms behave as if they were adjusted to maintain body temperature at a higher than normal level that is, "as if the thermostat had been reset" to a new point above 37°C. The temperature receptors then signal that the actual temperature is below the new set point and the temperature raising mechanisms are activated.

Pathogenesis of Fever

a. Toxins from bacteria such as endotoxin act on monocytes, macrophages, and Kupffer cells to produce cytokines that act as endogenous pyrogens. IL–1β, IL–6, β–IFN, λ–IFN and TNF–α can also produce fever.
b. These cytokines are polypeptides which penetrate brain and act on OVLT.
c. This activates preoptic area of the hypothalamus, prostaglandins are released from hypothalamus which raises the temperature set point to produce fever. Aspirin the drug of choice for fever inhibits prostaglandin synthesis–PGE_2, is one of the prostaglandins that causes fever. It has got 4 subtypes of receptors–EP_1, EP_2, EP_3 and EP_4.

Hyperthermia slows the growth of some tumors. A rectal temperature over 41°C for prolonged periods results in permanent brain damage. When the temperature is over 43°C, heat stroke and death results.

Malignant Hyperthermia

Various mutations of the gene coding for the ryanodine receptor lead to excess Ca^{2+} release during muscle contraction. This in turn leads to contractures of the muscles, increased muscle metabolism and a great increase in heat production in muscle causes a marked rise in body temperature is fatal if not treated.

Hypothermia

When the skin or the blood is cooled enough to lower the body temperature in humans, metabolic and physiologic processes slow down. Respiration and heart rate are very slow, blood pressure is low and consciousness is lost. At rectal temperature of 28°C, the ability to spontaneously return the temperature to normal is lost, but the individual can survive if rewarmed with external heat. Humans can tolerate body temperatures between 21 and 24°C without permanent ill-effect, so induced hypothermia is used in surgery.

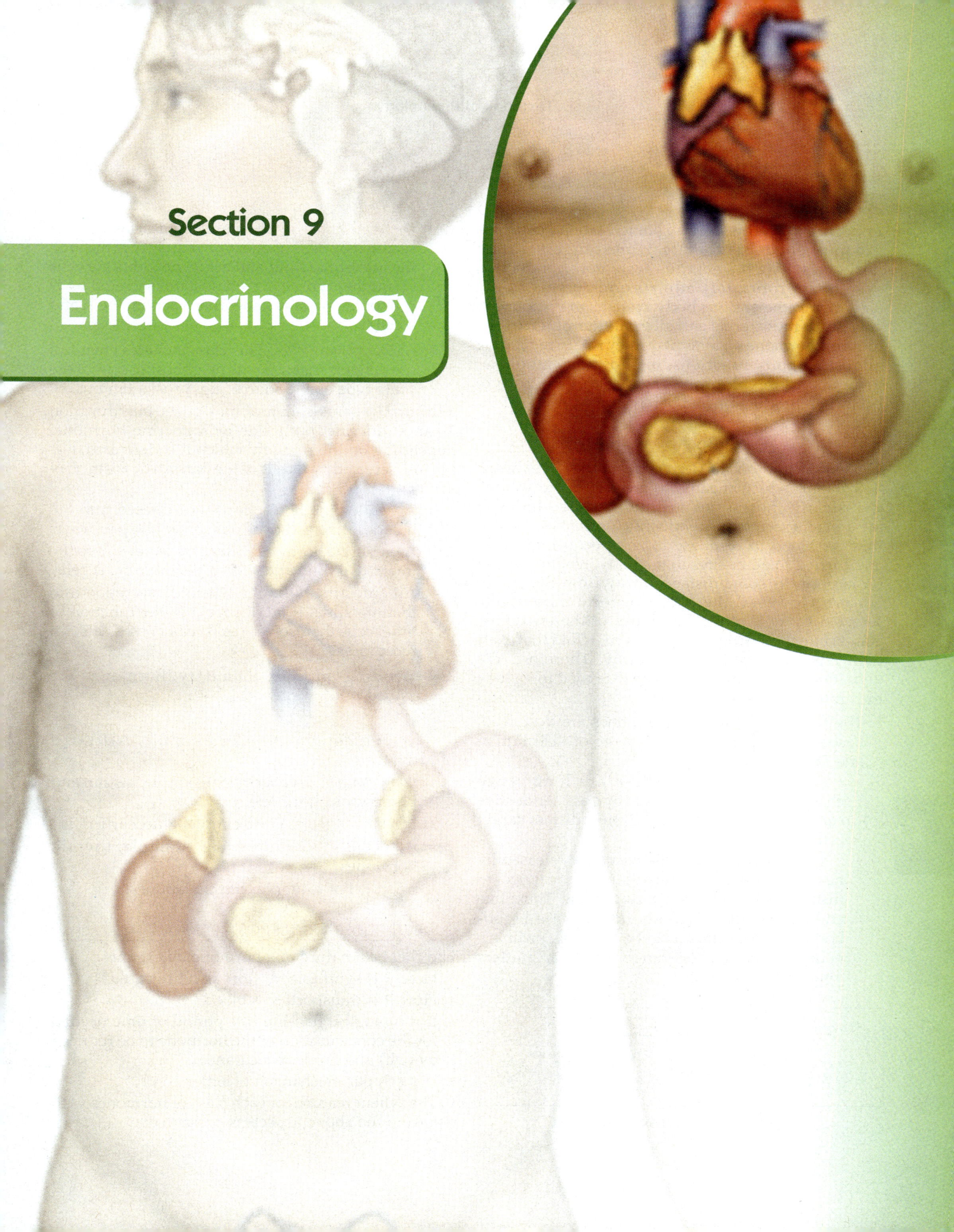

Section 9

Endocrinology

74. INTRODUCTION

Endocrinology is the study of homeostatic adjustments accomplished by chemical messengers called hormones. Like the nervous system, the endocrine system appropriately adjusts and correlates the activities of the various body systems in response to changes in the external and internal environment. The multiple hormone systems play a key role in regulating almost all body functions, including metabolism, growth and development, water and electrolyte balance, reproduction and behavior.

HORMONES: DEFINITION AND CLASSIFICATIONS

The word 'hormone' is derived from the Greek word 'hormaein' which means 'to arouse' or 'to excite'. Classically, hormones are defined as chemical messengers secreted by endocrine or ductless glands into the blood in response to an appropriate signal and carried to other sites in the body, where they act on target cells some distance away from the site of release. However, there are chemical messengers secreted by cells other than those of the endocrine glands into the surrounding interstitial fluid that exert their effects on target cells nearby. Therefore, the definition of a hormone has been extended to include the aforementioned categories.

1. The following classes of hormones are described, based on the cellular source, route of distribution and target cell (Fig. 9.1):
   - *Endocrine hormones:* These are long-range chemical messengers secreted by classic endocrine cells into the blood that act on a distant target cell.
   - *Neurohormones:* These chemicals are released by neurons into the bloodstream and carried to distant target cells, e.g. vasopressin. Thus, like endocrine cells, these neurons release blood-borne chemical messengers, whereas ordinary neurons secrete short-range neurotransmitters into a confined space.

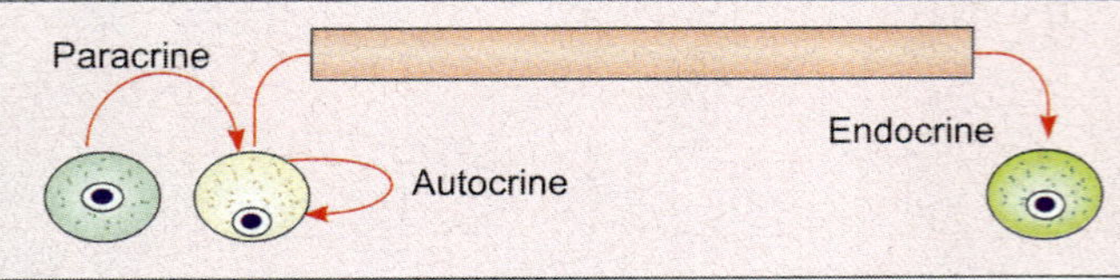

Fig. 9.1: Various classes of hormones

   - *Paracrine hormones:* These are chemical messengers secreted by cells of one type that diffuse through the interstitial fluid and act on neighboring cells of another type, e.g. somatostatin secreted by D cells of the islets of Langerhans acts on the A and B cells.
   - *Autocrine hormones:* This class includes chemical messengers that regulate neighboring cells of the same type as the source, e.g. prostaglandins.

   Note: The same chemical messenger may function as an endocrine, paracrine or autocrine hormone, depending on the route by which it is delivered, e.g. insulin, secreted by B cells of the pancreatic islets, may act as:
   - An endocrine hormone when released into the blood, influencing various metabolic pathways.
   - A paracrine hormone when it is secreted into the interstitial fluid and acts on neighboring A cells.
   - An autocrine hormone when, on secretion into the interstitial fluid, it regulates the function of the B cells themselves (as B cells possess insulin receptors).
2. Depending on their chemistry, hormones are classified into:
   - *Proteins*

     Short-chain peptides: For example, ADH and oxytocin.

     Long-chain polypeptides: For example, insulin and parathyroid hormone.
   - *Steroid hormones:* For example, glucocorticoids
   - *Amino acid derivatives:* For example, thyroid hormones.
   - *Amines:* For example, catecholamines.

GENERAL CHARACTERISTICS OF HORMONES

The chemical nature of a hormone determines:

- How it is synthesized, stored and released?
- How it is transported in blood?
- It is biological half-life (the period of time needed for the concentration of the hormone to be reduced by half) and mode of clearance.
- It is cellular mechanism of action.

The salient features of each class of hormones with regard to the above aspects is presented:

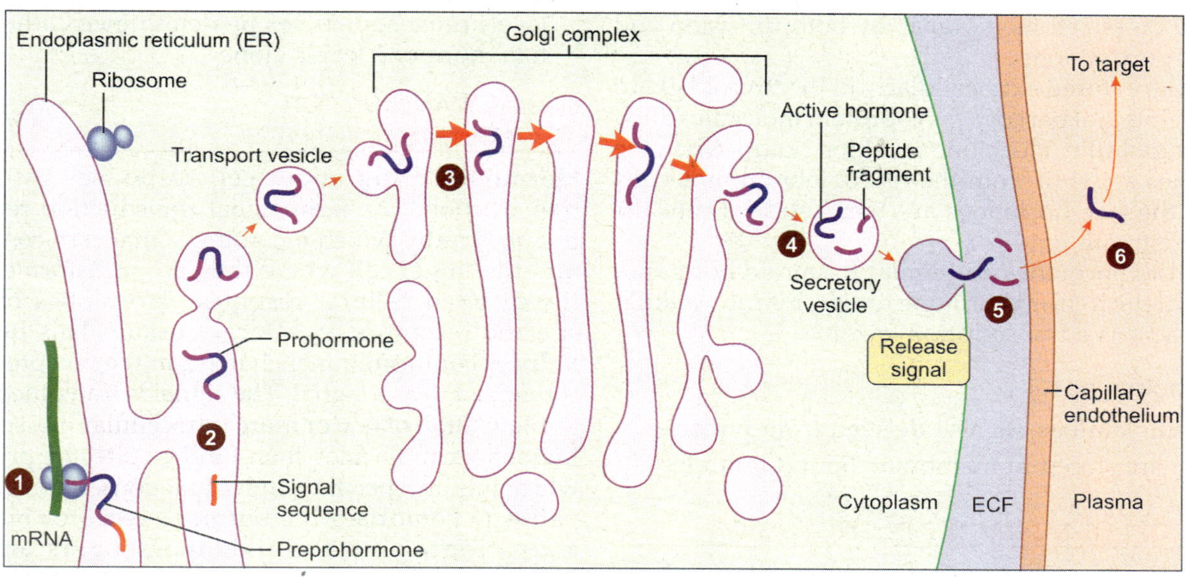

Fig. 9.2: Synthesis of protein hormones

(1) Messenger RNA on the ribosomes binds amino acids into a peptide chain called a preprohormone. The chain is directed into the ER lumen by a signal sequence of amino acids, (2) enzymes in the ER chop off the signal sequence, creating an inactive prohormone, (3) the prohormone passes from the ER through the Golgi complex, (4) secretory vesicles containing enzymes and prohormone bud off the Golgi. The enzymes chop the prohormone into one or more active peptides plus additional peptide fragments, (5) the secretory vesicles releases its contents by exocytosis into the extracellular space and (6) the hormone moves into the circulation for transport to its target

Protein/Peptide Hormones

- Protein/peptide hormones are synthesized on polyribosomes as large preprohormones. The preprohormones are processed by removal of a signal peptide in the endoplasmic reticulum to produce the hormone or the prohormone, which requires further cleavage to form the mature hormone. This final cleavage occurs while the prohormone is in the Golgi apparatus or the secretory granule (Fig. 9.2).
- They are stored in the gland in membrane-bound secretory granules and are released by regulated exocytosis in response to a stimulus.
- Being water-soluble, they circulate predominantly in the unbound form. Therefore, they tend to have short biological half-lives.
- Protein hormones are readily digested if administered orally. Hence, they are administered through parenteral routes.
- As they do not cross cell membranes readily, they signal through membrane receptors.

Steroid Hormones

- Steroid hormones are synthesized from cholesterol and contain the cyclopentanoperhydrophenanthrene ring (Fig. 9.3).

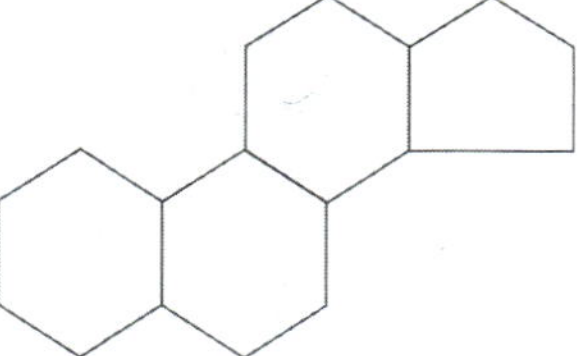

Fig. 9.3: Cyclopentanoperhydrophenanthrene ring

- They usually circulate bound to transport proteins as they are not readily soluble in blood.
- Being hydrophobic, steroid hormones pass through cell membranes easily and are not stored. Instead, the hormone precursors are stored as lipid droplets in steroidogenic cells.
- Steroid compounds are absorbed readily in the gastrointestinal tract and therefore, are administered orally.
- The receptors of steroid hormones are intracellular and the hormones act by regulating gene expression.

Thyroid Hormones

- Thyroid hormones are derived from tyrosine.
- They are sparingly soluble in blood and 99% of circulating thyroid hormone is transported bound to serum binding proteins.

- They cross cell membranes by both diffusion and transport systems.
- They are stored extracellularly in the thyroid gland as an integral part of a glycoprotein molecule called thyroglobulin. Hormone secretion occurs when the amines are split from the thyroglobulin molecule, and the free hormones are then released into the bloodstream.
- Thyroid hormones are similar to steroid hormones in that the thyroid hormone receptor is intracellular and acts as a transcription factor.

Catecholamines

- Catecholamines are also derived from tyrosine.
- They are stored in membrane-bound granules.

TRANSPORT OF HORMONES IN CIRCULATION

- There is an equilibrium between the concentrations of protein-bound hormone and free hormone. If free hormone levels drop, hormone is released from the transport proteins. Thus, bound hormone represents a "reservoir" of hormone and serves to "buffer" acute changes in hormone secretion.
- The free form is the biologically active form for target organ action and feedback control. Therefore, when evaluating hormonal status, free hormone levels must sometimes be determined rather than total hormone levels alone.

SIGNAL TRANSDUCTION (INTRACELLULAR SIGNALING)

Hormones bring about cell responses by signal transduction. The term signal transduction refers to the process by which incoming signals are conveyed into the target cell where they are transformed into the dictated cellular response. Hormones bind to specific receptors on a target tissue. This binding induces conformational changes in the receptor. This is referred to as a signal. The signal is transduced into the activation of one or more intracellular messengers. Messenger molecules then bind to effector proteins, which modify specific cellular functions. The signaling pathway comprises the hormone-receptor binding, activation of intracellular messengers and the regulation of one or more effector proteins. The final outcome is referred to as the cellular response.

Signaling from Membrane Receptors

Binding of a hormone (also known as the first messenger) to its specific surface membrane receptor brings response by three general means (Fig. 9.4):

1. By activating second messenger pathways via G protein-coupled receptors

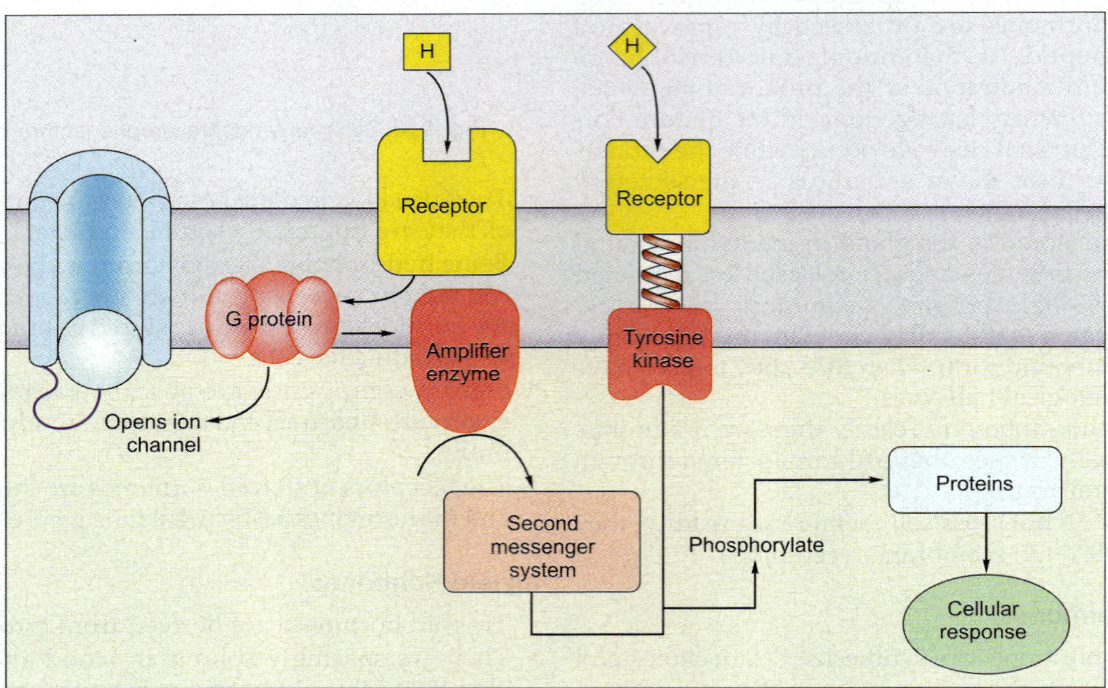

Fig. 9.4: Mechanism of action of hormone

2. By activating receptor enzymes
3. By opening or closing chemically gated receptor channels.

G Protein-Coupled Receptors (Fig. 9.5)

The G protein-coupled receptors represent the largest family of hormone receptors. The intracellular portions of the receptor are coupled to G proteins. G proteins are molecular switches that are active when bound to GTP and inactive when bound to GDP. They have intrinsic GTPase activity. The G proteins that directly interact with the receptors are termed heterotrimeric G proteins as they are composed of an α subunit (G_α) and a β/γ subunit dimer. The G_α is bound to GDP. On hormone binding, GDP is exchanged for GTP, thereby activating G_α. The G_α subunit separates from the β/γ subunit and brings about biologic effects. The intrinsic GTPase activity of the G_α subunit then converts GTP to GDP and this leads to reassociation of the α subunit with the β/γ subunit and termination of the effector activation.

There are many types of G_α proteins:

- $G_{s\alpha}$ stimulates the membrane enzyme, adenylyl cyclase, which generates cAMP from ATP. cAMP activates protein kinase A, which phosphorylates numerous proteins and thereby, alters cell function. cAMP is called a *second messenger* because it is not the hormone (the first messenger) itself that directly brings about the intracellular changes.
- $G_{i\alpha}$ inhibits adenylyl cyclase.
- $G_{q\alpha}$ activates phospholipase C, which generates diacylglycerol (DAG) and inositol triphosphate (IP_3) from the membrane lipid, phosphatidylinositol bisphosphate (PIP_2) (Fig. 9.6).

Diacylglycerol activates protein kinase C, which then phosphorylates a large number of proteins, leading to cellular response.

IP_3 binds to its receptor, which is a large complex including a Ca^{2+} channel, on the endoplasmic reticulum membrane and promotes Ca^{2+} efflux from the endoplasmic reticulum into the cytoplasm. Calcium ions have their own second messenger effects, such as smooth muscle contraction and changes in cell secretion.

Receptor Tyrosine Kinases

This family of receptors has intrinsic tyrosine kinase activity. Binding of the hormone to its receptor induces this tyrosine kinase activity and tyrosine residues in the receptor are phosphorylated, genera-

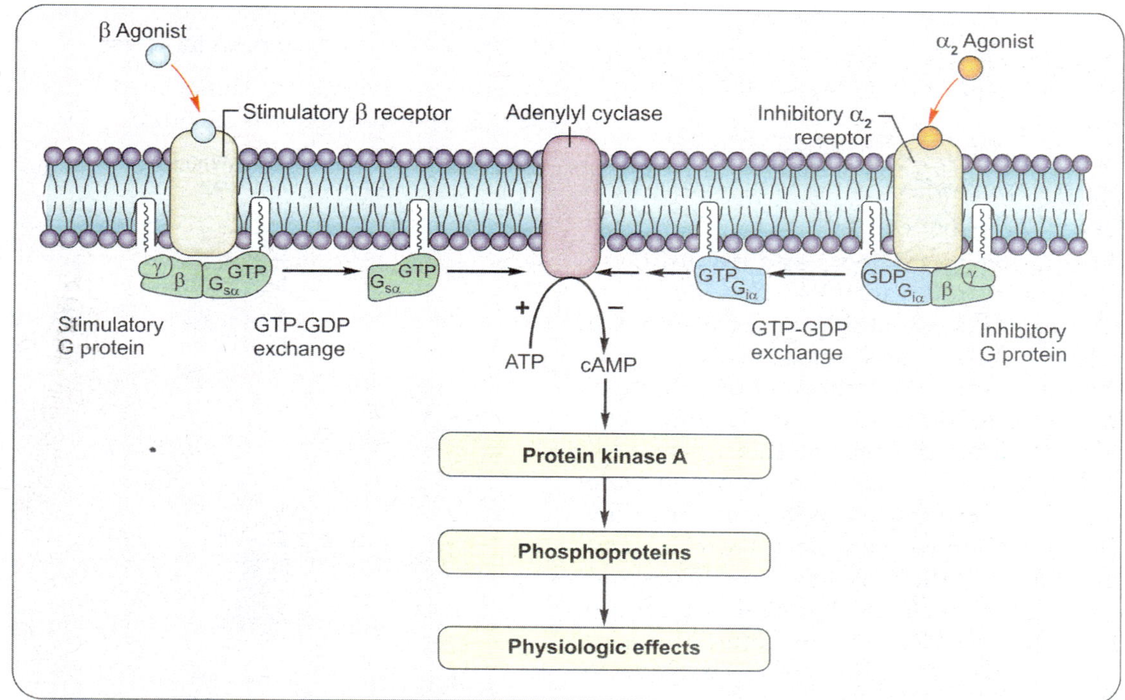

Fig. 9.5: G_{sa} (stimulatory) and $G_{\alpha i}$ (inhibitory) pathway of β and α_2 agonist respectively

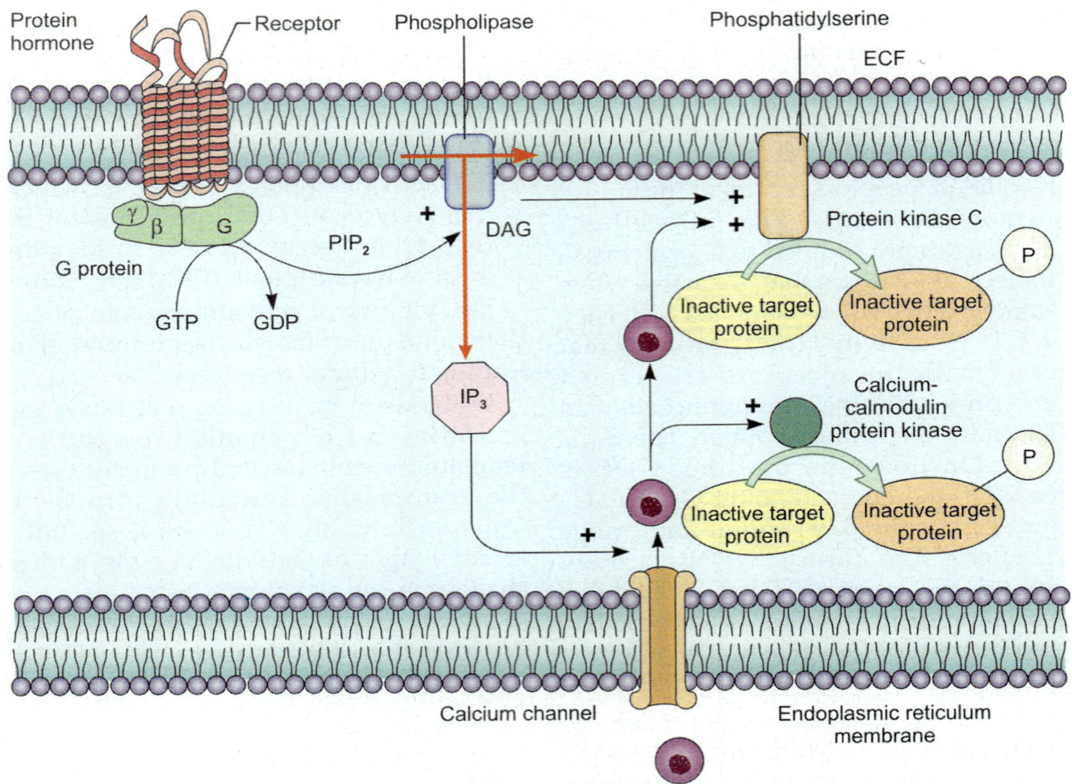

Fig. 9.6: Phospholipase IP_3–DAG pathway

ting phosphotyrosines. The phosphotyrosines function to recruit intracellular proteins that specifically recognize them.

Receptors associated with Cytoplasmic Tyrosine Kinases

These receptors exist as dimers and do not have intrinsic tyrosine kinase activity. Instead, their cytoplasmic domains are stably associated with tyrosine kinases of the Janus kinase (JAK) family. Hormone binding induces a conformational change, bringing the two JAKs associated with the dimerized receptor closer together and causing their transphosphorylation and activation. JAKs then phosphorylate tyrosine residues on the cytoplasmic domains of the receptor. The phosphotyrosine residues recruit latent transcription factors called signal transducers and activators of transcription (STAT) proteins. STATs are phosphorylated by JAKs, which cause them to dissociate from the receptor, dimerize and translocate to the nucleus, where they regulate gene expression (Fig. 9.7).

Receptor Serine/Threonine Kinases

These receptors exist as dissociated heterodimers in the unbound state. Hormone binding to the receptors

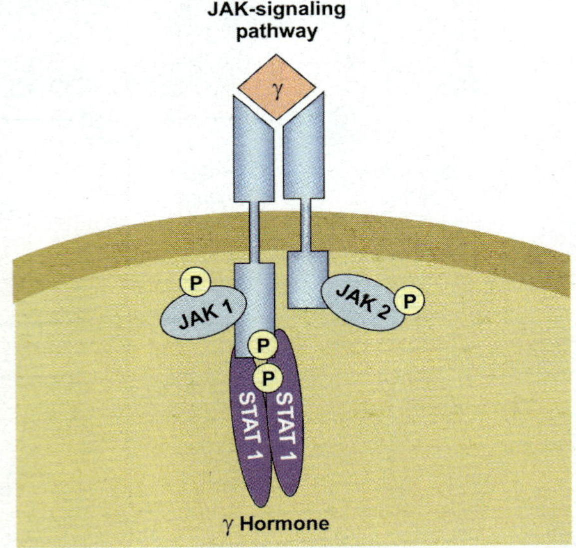

Fig. 9.7: JAK-STAT signaling pathway

induces dimerization and activation of the receptor by phosphorylation.

Receptors Regulating Ion Channels

Hormone binding to these receptors opens ion channels, the most common of which are calcium channels.

Signaling from Intracellular Receptors

Intracellular receptors act as transcription regulators. They may be located in the cytoplasm or the nucleus.

- *Cytoplasmic receptors:* In the absence of hormone, the cytoplasmic receptors are held in an inactive state through interactions with chaperone proteins (also called 'heat-shock proteins' because their levels increase in response to elevated temperatures and other stresses). Hormone binding induces a conformational change in the receptor, causing the hormone-receptor complex to dissociate from heat-shock proteins. This exposes the nuclear localization signal and the dimerization domains, so that the receptors dimerize and enter the nucleus. Once in the nucleus, these receptors bind to specific DNA sequences called hormone-response elements (HREs). Bound to their respective HREs, the receptors recruit other proteins called coactivators, that activate gene transcription (Fig. 9.8).
- *Nuclear receptors:* They are bound to corepressors in the absence of hormone. The receptor-corepressor complexes are bound to the specific hormone-response elements and keep the expression of neighboring genes repressed.

REGULATION OF HORMONE SECRETION

Negative Feedback

Secretion of most hormones is regulated by negative feedback. Negative feedback means that the hormone secreted acts directly or indirectly on the secretory cell in a negative way to inhibit further secretion, e.g. a rise in blood glucose detected by the B cells of the pancreas causes them to release insulin, which stimulates glucose uptake into tissues and thereby decreases blood glucose concentration. With restoration of blood glucose to the set-point level, the B cells are not stimulated any further and secretion of insulin is inhibited (Fig. 9.9).

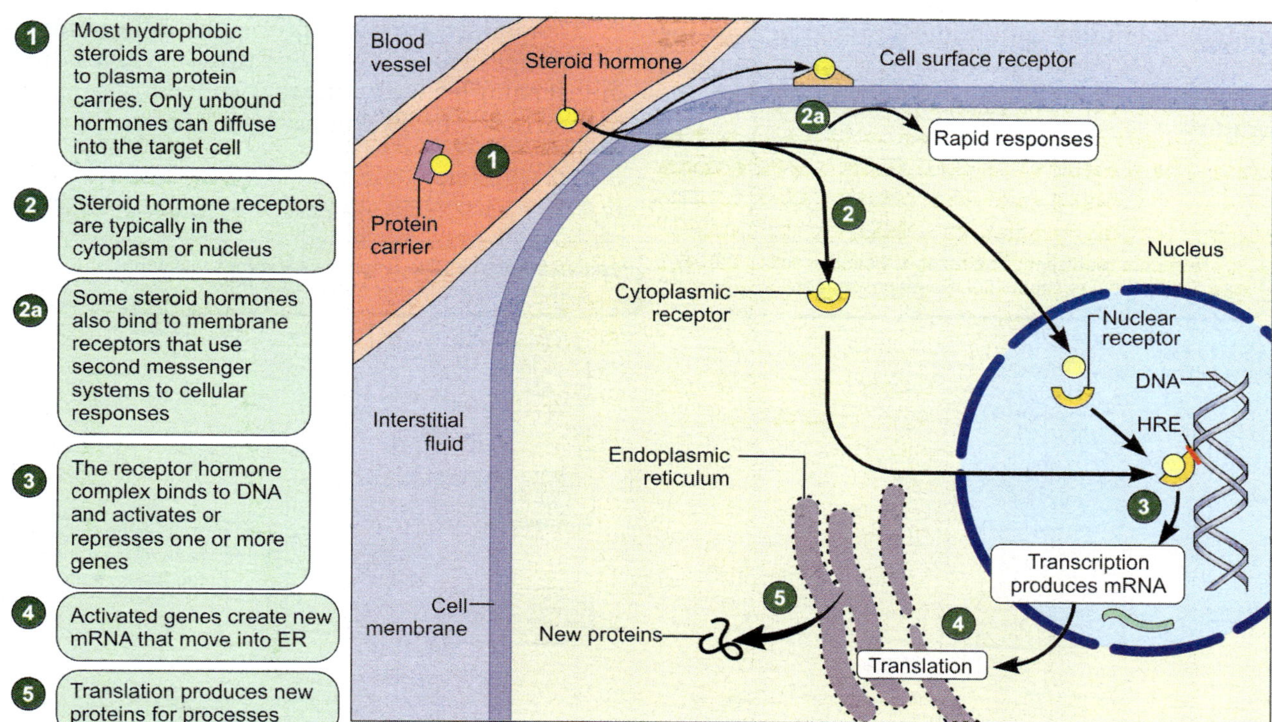

Fig. 9.8: Mechanism of action steroid hormones

Positive Feedback

Positive feedback means that the hormone secreted brings about stimulation of further secretion by its actions, e.g. effect of oxytocin on uterine muscle during childbirth. In this case, the stimulus for oxytocin secretion is dilation of the uterine cervix. Sensory nerves transmit this information to the brain and the brain signals release oxytocin from nerve endings in the posterior pituitary gland. Enhanced uterine contraction in response to oxytocin results in greater dilation of the cervix, which strengthens the signal for oxytocin release and so on until the infant is expelled from the uterine cavity (Fig. 9.9).

MEASUREMENT OF HORMONE CONCENTRATIONS IN BLOOD

As most hormones are present in extremely minute quantities in blood, they cannot be measured by the usual chemical means. An extremely sensitive method employed to measure hormones, their precursors and their metabolic end-products is called radioimmuno-assay.

Radioimmunoassay

Principle

This method employs antibodies formed against the hormone whose concentration is to be determined and a radioactively labeled hormone prepared in the laboratory.

Method

A small quantity of the antibody and an appropriate amount of the radioactive hormone are simultaneously mixed with the fluid sample containing the hormone to be measured. One specific condition to be met is that there must be too little antibody to bind completely both the radioactive hormone and the natural hormone in the fluid to be assayed. Therefore, the natural hormone in the assay fluid and the radioactive hormone compete for the binding sites of the antibody. In the process of competing, the quantity of each of the two hormones, the natural and the radioactive, that is bound to the antibody is proportional to its concentration in the assay fluid.

After binding has reached equilibrium, the antibody-hormone complex is separated from the remainder of the solution and the quantity of radioactive hormone bound in this complex is measured by radioactive counting techniques. If a large amount of radioactive hormone is bound with the antibody, it is clear that there was only a small amount of natural hormone to compete with the radioactive hormone; conversely, if only a small amount of radioactive hormone has bound, it is clear that there was a large amount of natural hormone to compete for the binding sites.

A "standard curve" is plotted by determining the percentage of antibody bound to radioactive hormone in test samples with different concentrations of the natural hormone. By comparing the radioactive counts

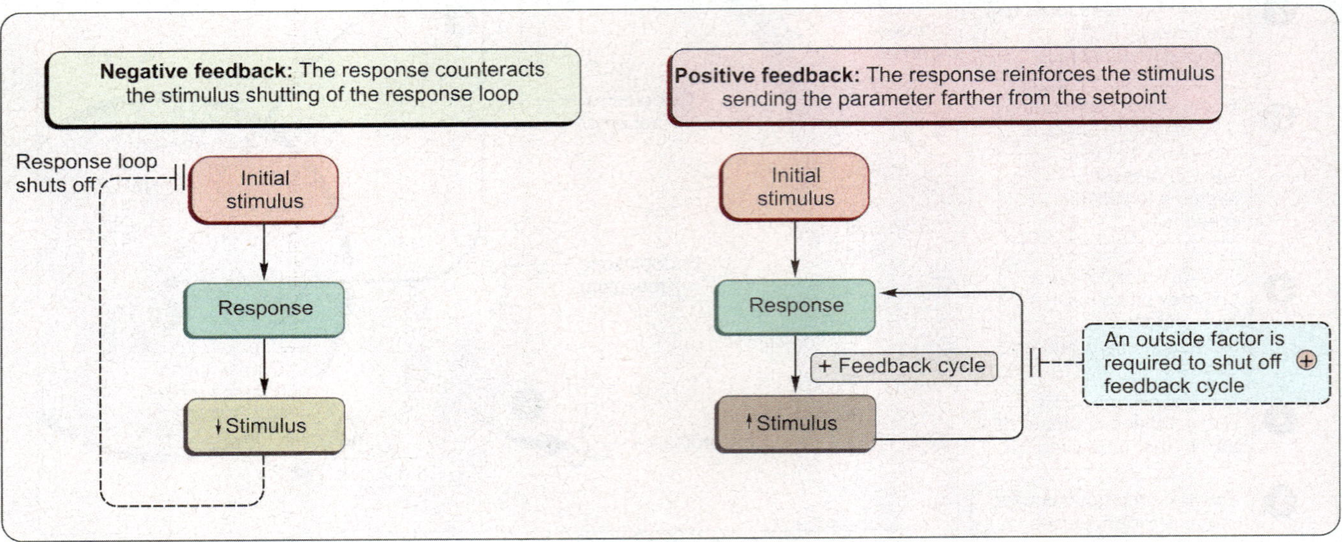

Fig. 9.9: Negative and positive feedback

9

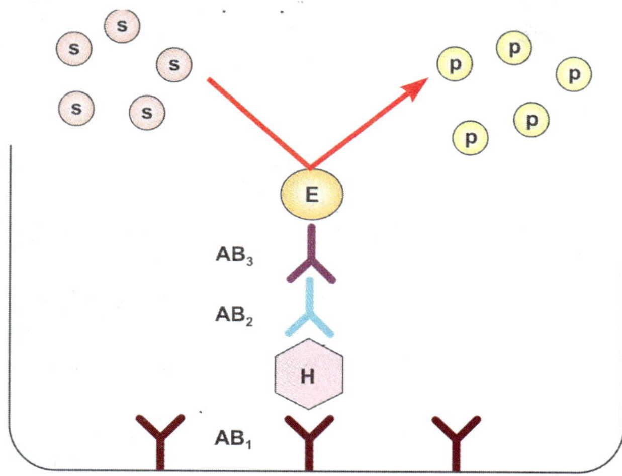

Fig. 9.10: Basic principles of the ELISA method

recorded from the unknown assay procedure with the standard curve, one can determine the concentration of the hormone in the unknown assayed fluid.

Enzyme-Linked Immunosorbent Assay (ELISA) (Fig. 9.10)

This highly sensitive method can be used to measure almost any protein. It is performed on plastic plates that each have 96 small wells. Each well is coated with and antibody (AB_1) that is specific for the hormone being assayed. Samples or standards are added to each of the wells, followed by a second antibody (AB_2) that is also specific for the hormone but binds to a different site of the hormone molecule. A third antibody (AB_3) is added that recognizes AB_2 and is coupled to an enzyme that converts a suitable substrate to a product that can be easily detected by colorimetric or fluorescent optical methods.

In contrast to competitive radioimmunoassay methods, ELISA methods use excess antibodies so that all hormone molecules are captured in antibody-hormone complexes. Therefore, the amount of hormone present in the sample or in the standard is proportional to the amount of product formed.

HORMONAL RHYTHMS

Most living cells have rhythmic fluctuations in their function that are about 24 hours in length; these rhythms are called circadian (diurnal; circa "about" + dia "day") rhythms. Rhythms with a periodicity of less than 24 hours are referred to as ultradian rhythms.

Biological rhythms are set by an internal clock or pacemaker and persist even in the absence of cues. The internal clock that drives a circadian rhythm can be synchronized to time cues in the environment, such as the light/dark cycle. This process of synchronization to an external stimulus is called entrainment. A rhythm that runs at a frequency that is independent of external cues is called a free-running rhythm. If a free-running nocturnal animal is exposed to periodic light and dark, the onset of activity soon becomes synchronized to the beginning of the dark period. The shift of activity produced by a synchronizing stimulus is referred to as a phase shift, and the process of shifting the rhythm is called entrainment.

Circadian rhythms are entrained (synchronized to the day-night cycle in the environment) by the paired suprachiasmatic nuclei (SCN) above the optic chiasm. These nuclei receive information about the light-dark cycle via the retinohypothalamic fibers that pass from the optic chiasm to the SCN. Efferents from the SCN initiate neural and humoral signals that entrain a wide variety of circadian rhythms. These include the sleep-wake cycle, the rhythms in the secretion of ACTH and other pituitary hormones and the secretion of the pineal hormone melatonin. The nocturnal peaks in melatonin secretion appear to be an important hormonal signal entraining other cells in the body.

75. ENDOCRINE PANCREAS

The islets of Langerhans constitute the endocrine portion of the pancreas and secrete two important hormones, insulin and glucagon, that are crucial for normal regulation of carbohydrate, lipid and protein metabolism. The other hormones secreted by the islets are somatostatin and pancreatic polypeptide. Somatostatin regulates islet cell secretion and pancreatic polypeptide is concerned primarily with gastrointestinal function.

Histology

There are about 1 million islets making up about 2% of the total pancreatic mass. They are ovoid collections of cells scattered throughout the pancreas but are more plentiful in the tail region.

Types of Cells

The cells in the islets are divided into four types on the basis of their staining properties and morphology: A, B and D cells are also called α, β and δ cells.

1. The A cells secrete glucagon.
2. The B cells secrete insulin and amylin.
3. The D cells secrete somatostatin.
4. The F cells secrete pancreatic polypeptide.

The B cells are the most common and make up about 75% of all the islet cells. They are generally located in the center of each islet and are surrounded by the A cells, which make up about 10–20% of the total, and the less common D and F cells.

Link: The close interrelations among the cell types in the islets allow cell-to-cell communication and direct control of secretion of some of the hormones by the other hormones: Insulin inhibits glucagon secretion, amylin inhibits insulin secretion, and somatostatin inhibits the secretion of both insulin and glucagon.

Embryology

The body, tail and anterior portion of the head of the pancreas arise from the dorsal pancreatic bud and contain islets that have many A cells and few F cells in the outer rim. The islets in the posterior part of the head of the pancreas, which arises from the ventral pancreatic bud, have F cell-rich islets. The ventral and dorsal pancreatic buds arise separately from the duodenum.

Blood Supply

Each islet has a copious blood supply and blood from the islets drains into the hepatic portal vein. Blood flows through the islets from B cells in the center of the islet to A and D cells in the periphery.

Link: Consequently, the first cells affected by circulating insulin are the A cells, in which insulin inhibits glucagon secretion.

INSULIN

Insulin was first isolated from the pancreas by Banting and Best in 1922.

Chemistry of Insulin

Insulin is a polypeptide with a molecular weight of 5808, containing two chains of amino acids, A and B (or α and β) that are linked by two disulfide bridges. A third disulfide bridge is contained within the A chain. There are minor differences in the amino acid composition of insulin from species-to-species. Pork insulin differs from human insulin by only one amino acid residue. Human insulin is now produced in bacteria by recombinant DNA technology.

Biosynthesis and Secretion (Fig. 9.11)

The gene for insulin is located on the short arm of chromosome 11 in humans and encodes preproinsulin. This molecule has a 23 amino acid signal peptide removed as it enters the rough endoplasmic reticulum of the B cells to form proinsulin. Proinsulin is packaged in the Golgi apparatus into membrane-bound secretory granules. Proinsulin contains the amino acid sequence of insulin plus the 31 amino acid C (connecting) peptide. Proteases involved in processing the proinsulin are packaged with proinsulin within the secretory granule.

Normally, 90–97% of the product released from the B cells is insulin along with equimolar amounts of C peptide. The rest is mostly proinsulin. When insulin secretion is rapid, the percentage of proinsulin secreted tends to rise. Proinsulin has about 7 to 8% of the biological activity of insulin and C peptide has no known biological activity.

Link: C peptide can be measured by radioimmunoassay, and its level provides an index of B cell function in patients receiving exogenous insulin.

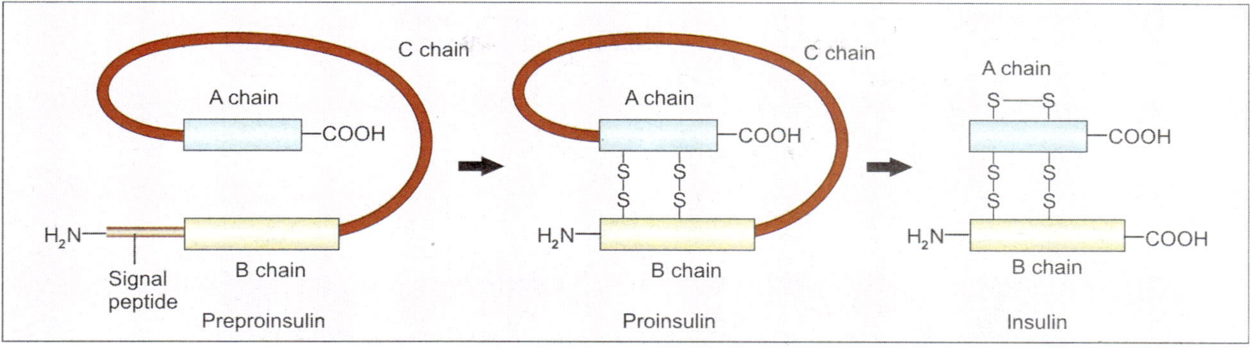

Fig. 9.11: Structure of preproinsulin, proinsulin and insulin

Insulin is stored in secretory granules as polymers or zinc aggregates. On stimulation of the B cells, the contents of the granules are released to the outside of the cell by exocytosis. The process is calcium-dependent and requires a functional microtubular system (Fig. 9.16).

Metabolism

Insulin circulates in an unbound form and is cleared rapidly from the circulation; it has a half-life of about 5 minutes. Insulin is bound to insulin receptors and some of it is internalized. Except for the insulin that combines with receptors in the target cells, the remainder is degraded by the enzyme insulinase mainly in the liver and to a lesser extent in the kidneys and muscles. Because insulin is secreted into the portal vein, it is exposed to the liver before it enters the peripheral circulation. Almost one half of the insulin is degraded before leaving the liver. Consequently, the peripheral tissues are exposed to only one half the serum insulin concentrations as the liver.

Mechanism of Action (Fig. 9.12)

The insulin receptor is an example of an enzyme-linked receptor. It is a member of the receptor tyrosine kinase family. It is a tetramer made up of two α and two β glycoprotein subunits. The extracellular α subunits bind insulin and the β subunits penetrating the membrane have tyrosine kinase activity. Binding of insulin to the α subunits triggers the tyrosine kinase activity, producing autophosphorylation of the tyrosine residues in the β subunits. This autophosphorylation triggers phosphorylation of some cytoplasmic proteins, including a group called insulin-receptor substrates (IRS). Different types of IRS (IRS-1, IRS-2, IRS-3) are expressed in different tissues. These activated proteins mediate the effects of insulin on carbohydrate, lipid and protein metabolism.

Actions of Insulin

These can be divided into rapid, intermediate and delayed actions.

Rapid Actions (seconds)
Increased transport of glucose, amino acids and K^+ into insulin-sensitive cells
Intermediate Actions (minutes)
Stimulation of protein synthesis
Inhibition of protein degradation
Activation of glycolytic enzymes and glycogen synthase
Inhibition of phosphorylase and gluconeogenic enzymes
Delayed (hours)
Increase in RNAs for lipogenic enzymes

The metabolic effects of insulin bring about net storage of carbohydrate, protein and fat. Therefore, insulin is called the "hormone of abundance". The effects on individual metabolisms are elaborated below:

Effects on Carbohydrate Metabolism (Fig. 9.13)

- Increased glucose uptake in skeletal muscle and adipose tissue:

  Insulin increases the transport of glucose into skeletal muscle and adipose tissue by increasing the number of glucose transporters (GLUT 4) in the cell membranes. This is the primary way by which insulin increases the peripheral utilization of glucose. (The normal resting muscle membrane is only slightly permeable to glucose and muscle tissue depends on fatty acids for its energy during most of the day. It is only during the few hours after a meal, when blood

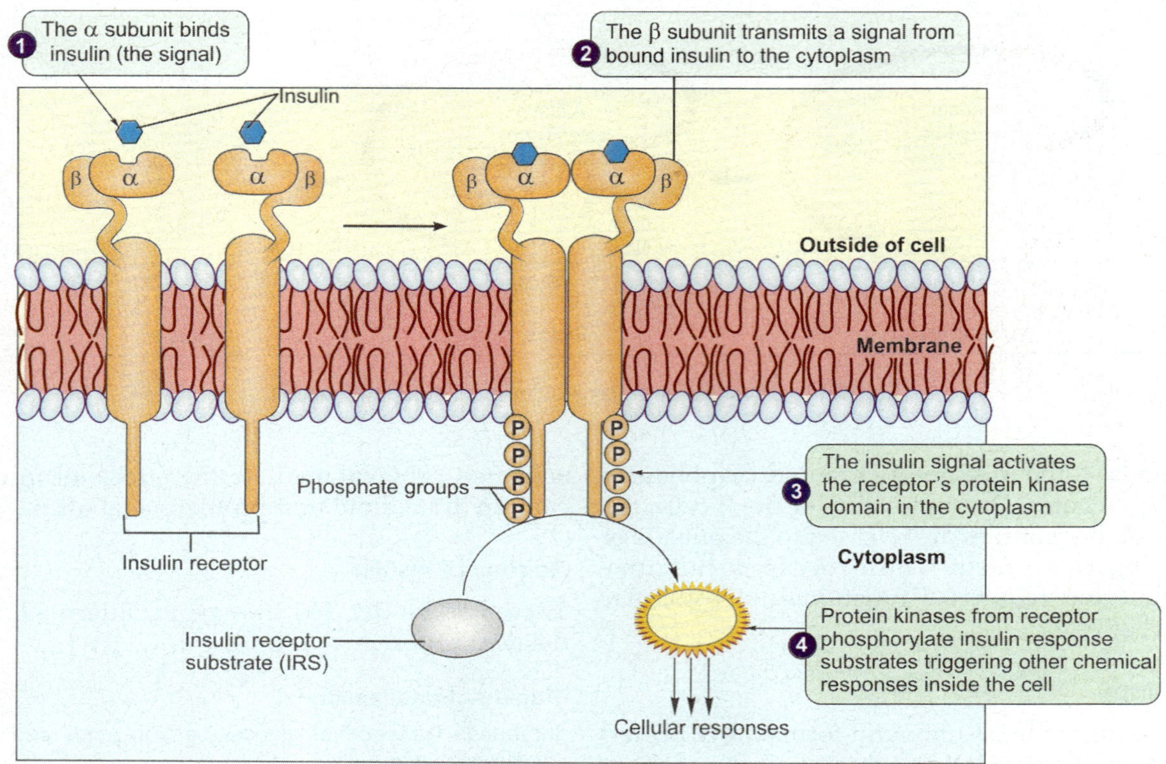

Fig. 9.12: Mechanism of action of insulin

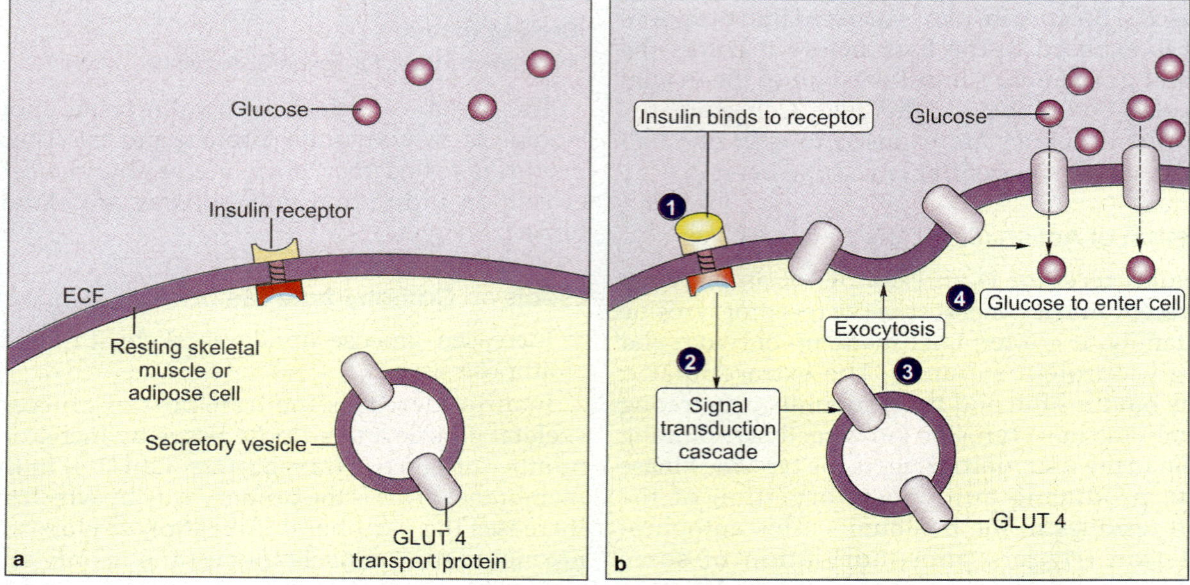

Figs 9.13a and b: (a) In the absence of insulin glucose cannot enter the cell; (b) insulin signals the cell to insulin GLUT 4 transporters into the membrane allowing glucose to enter cell

glucose levels are high and insulin is secreted in large quantities, that muscle uses glucose preferentially over fatty acids. In contrast, the brain cells are permeable to glucose and do not require insulin for glucose uptake.)

Glucose Transporters (GLUT)

Seven different glucose transporters, called in order of discovery GLUT 1–7, have been characterized. GLUT 4 is the transporter in muscle and adipose tissue that is stimulated by insulin. A pool of GLUT 4 molecules is maintained in vesicles in the cytoplasm of insulin-sensitive cells. When the insulin receptors of these cells are activated, the vesicles move rapidly to the cell membrane and fuse with it, inserting the transporters into the cell membrane. When insulin action ceases, the transporter-containing patches of membrane are endocytosed and the vesicles are ready for the next exposure to insulin.

Link: Glucose tolerance refers to the ability of an individual to minimize the excursions of blood glucose concentrations. A primary way in which insulin promotes glucose tolerance is the activation of glucose uptake in skeletal muscle.

- *Increased glucose uptake in the liver:* Glucose enters hepatocytes through the insulin-independent GLUT 2 transporter by facilitated diffusion. Insulin increases the intracellular trapping of glucose in the liver by increasing the expression of glucokinase, the enzyme which causes the initial phosphorylation of glucose after it diffuses into the liver cells. This maintains a low free glucose concentration in the hepatocytes, facilitating the entry of glucose into the cell. Insulin also represses gene expression of the enzyme, glucose-6-phosphatase. Thus, glucose is temporarily trapped inside the liver cells as phosphorylated glucose and cannot diffuse back through the cell membrane.
- *Increased glycogenesis in liver and skeletal muscle:* Insulin increases glycogenesis in the liver and skeletal muscle by increasing the activity of glycogen synthase, which is responsible for polymerization of glucose to form glycogen. Insulin also inactivates liver phosphorylase, the principal enzyme that causes liver glycogen to split into glucose. This prevents breakdown of the glycogen that has been stored in the liver cells. Once hepatic glycogen stores are replenished, insulin promotes the conversion of excess glucose to fatty acids, which are subsequently packaged as triglycerides in very-low-density lipoproteins (VLDLs).
- *Increased glycolysis in liver, muscle and adipose tissue:* Insulin brings about this effect by increasing the activity of certain glycolytic enzymes, namely, phosphofructokinase, pyruvate kinase and pyruvate dehydrogenase. Thus, insulin promotes utilization of glucose for energy needs of the cells. Adipose tissue utilizes glycolysis for energy needs and also for the generation of glycerol-3-phosphate, which is required for triglyceride synthesis.
- *Inhibition of gluconeogenesis:* Gluconeogenesis is inhibited by repression of the gluconeogenic enzymes, fructose-1, 6-bisphosphatase and phosphoenolpyruvate carboxykinase.

Distribution and characteristics of glucose transporters

Transporters	*Distribution*	*Characteristics*
GLUT 1	Ubiquitous	High affinity; transports basal levels of glucose
GLUT 2	Pancreatic B cell, liver small intestine kidneys	Low affinity; B cell glucose sensor; transports glucose out of intestinal and renal epithelial cells
GLUT 3	Ubiquitous	High affinity primary GLUT in neuronal tissue; transports basal levels of glucose
GLUT 4	Skeletal muscle Adipose tissue	Insulin dependent
GLUT 5	Small intestine Spermatozoa	Fructose transporter

Effects on Lipid Metabolism

1. Increased triglyceride synthesis in liver and adipose tissue:
   a. *Liver:* After the liver glycogen concentration reaches 5 to 6%, this in itself inhibits further glycogen synthesis. Then all the additional glucose entering the liver cells is converted to fat. The glucose is first split to pyruvate in the glycolytic pathway, and the pyruvate subsequently is converted to acetyl coenzyme A (acetyl CoA), the substrate from which fatty acids are synthesized. Insulin increases the activity of enzymes that favor FFA synthesis, including acetyl CoA carboxylase, and indirectly inhibits oxidation of FFAs by inhibiting the carnitine transport mechanism in the mitochondria. The FFAs synthesized are converted to triglycerides in the liver and are either stored or transported to adipose tissue in the form of VLDL.

b. *Adipose tissue:* Insulin is a fat sparer:
- Insulin stimulates the expression of lipoprotein lipase within adipocytes. This splits the triglycerides into fatty acids, a requirement for them to be absorbed into the adipose cells. They are again converted to triglycerides and stored.
- Insulin-enhanced glycolysis in adipocytes generates the glycerol-3-phosphate required for re-esterification of FFAs into triglycerides.
- Insulin also inhibits lipolysis by decreasing the activity of hormone-sensitive lipase, the enzyme that causes hydrolysis of triglycerides already stored in the fat cells, thereby preventing the release of FFAs from the adipose tissue into the blood.

Effects on Protein Metabolism

Insulin promotes protein synthesis and storage by:
- Promoting the transport of amino acids into cells
- Increasing the rate of transcription of selected DNA genetic sequences
- Increasing the translation of mRNA
- Inhibiting the catabolism of proteins
- Depressing gluconeogenesis in the liver.

Effects on Growth

As insulin is required for protein synthesis, it is as essential for growth as growth hormone. The two hormones function synergistically to promote growth. Figures 9.14 and 9.15 illustrate the actions of insulin versus the actions of growth hormone.

Regulation of Insulin Secretion

The amount of insulin secreted in the basal state is about 1 U/hour, with a fivefold to tenfold increase following ingestion of food. Therefore, the average amount secreted per day in a normal human is about 40 U. In response to sudden increase in blood glucose levels, insulin secretion increases markedly in two stages:

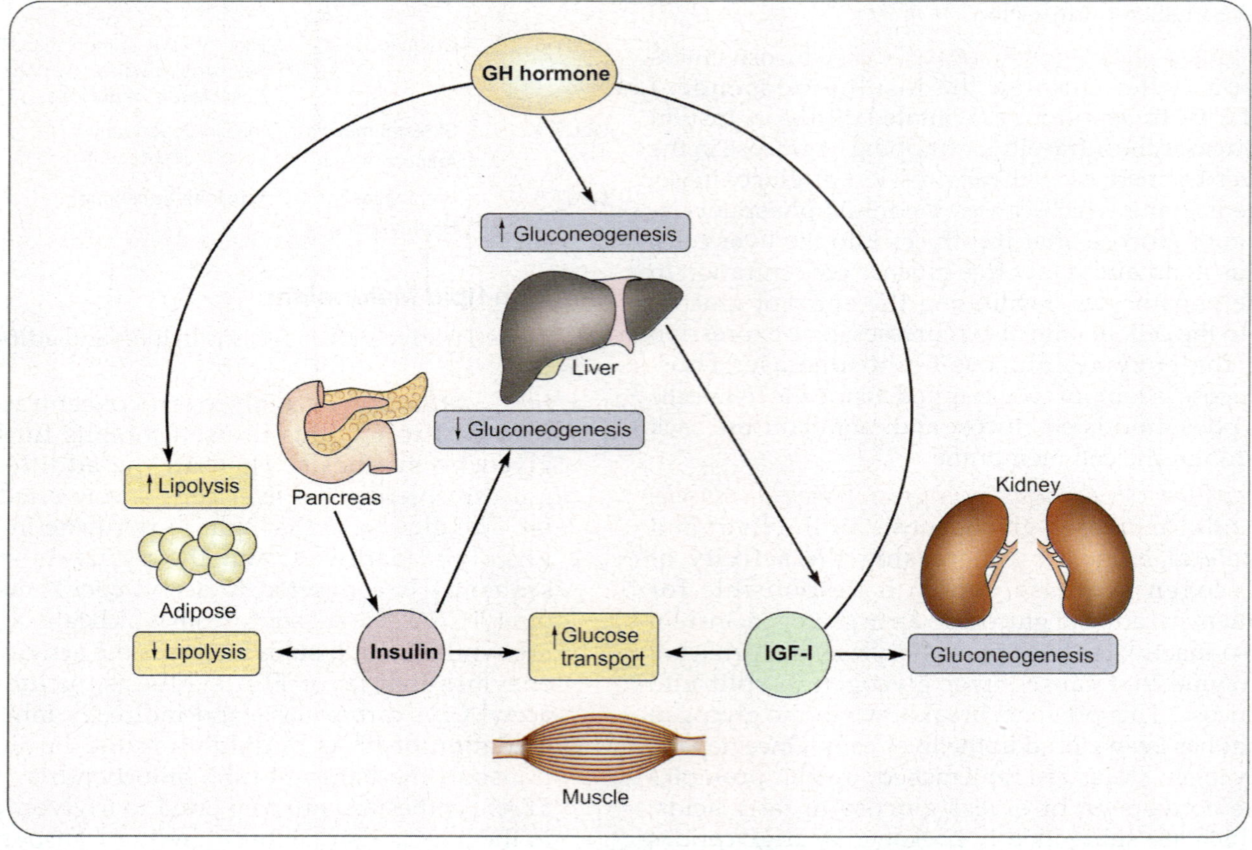

Fig. 9.14: A comparison of the actions of insulin, growth hormone and IGF on carbohydrate metabolism

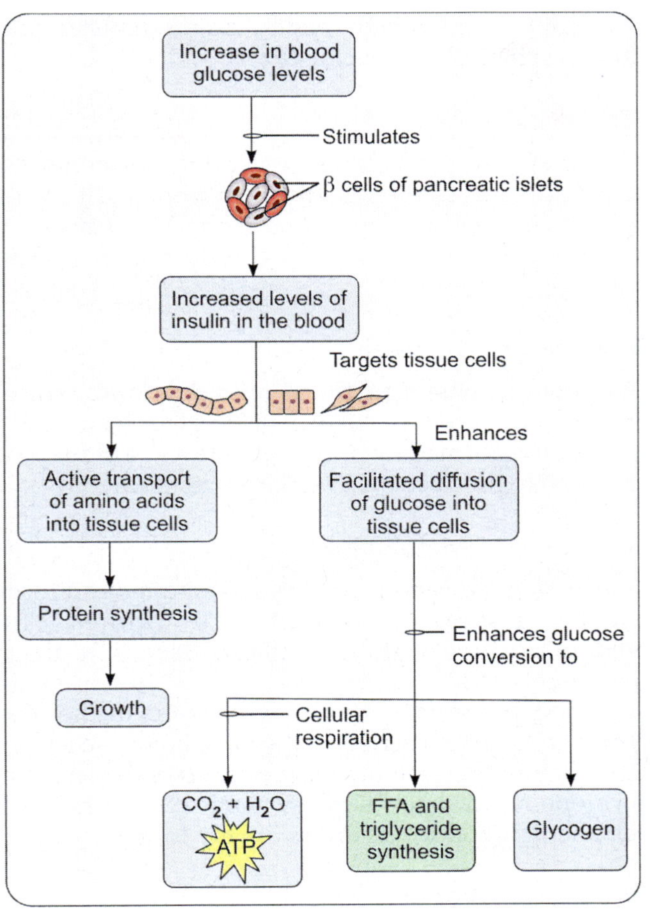

Fig. 9.15: Summary of the action of insulin

Plasma insulin concentration increases almost tenfold within 3 to 5 minutes after the acute elevation of blood glucose; this results from immediate release of preformed insulin from the B cells. However, this initial high rate of secretion is not maintained and the insulin concentration decreases about halfway back toward normal in another 5 to 10 minutes.

Beginning at about 15 minutes, insulin secretion rises a second time and reaches a new plateau in 2 to 3 hours, with a rate of secretion even greater than that in the initial phase. This secretion results both from additional release of preformed insulin and from activation of the enzyme system that synthesizes and releases new insulin from the cells.

Stimulators of Insulin Secretion (Fig. 9.16)

- Glucose acts directly on pancreatic B cells to increase insulin secretion. Glucose enters the B cells via GLUT 2 transporters. The rate of glucose influx is proportional to the blood concentration in the physiologic range. Once inside the B cell, glucose is phosphorylated by glucokinase. This step appears to be rate-limiting for glucose metabolism in the B cell and is considered as the major mechanism for glucose sensing. The glucose-6-phosphate is then metabolized to form ATP, which inhibits ATP-sensitive K^+ channels, reducing K^+ efflux. This depolarizes the B cell and Ca^{2+} enters through voltage-gated Ca^{2+} channels. The Ca^{2+} influx causes exocytosis of the insulin-containing granules.

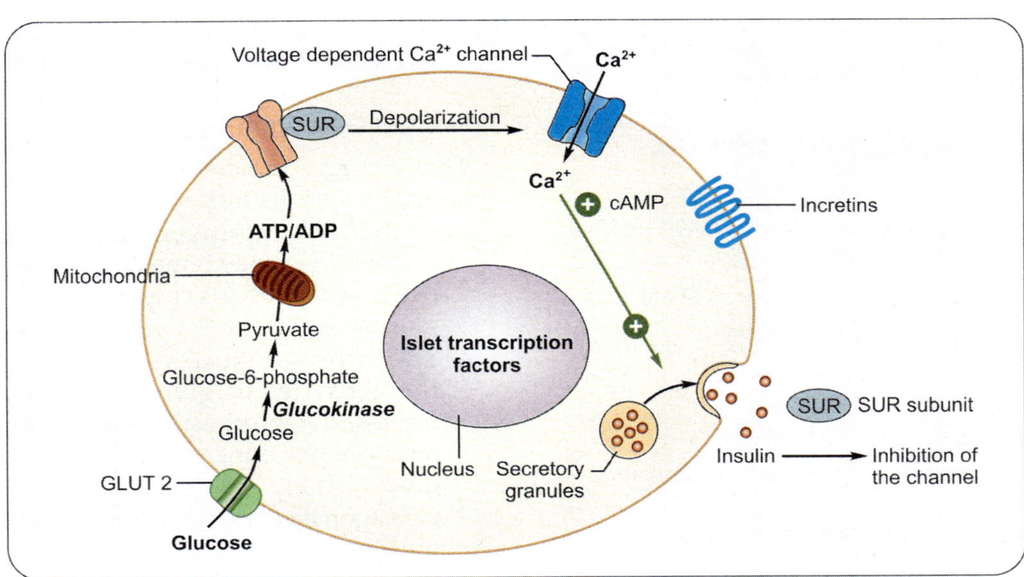

Fig. 9.16: Secretion of insulin through sulfonylurea receptors

9

- Certain amino acids, such as arginine, stimulate insulin secretion by generating ATP when metabolized; this closes the ATP-sensitive K^+ channels and depolarizes the B cells.
- Vagal stimulation (occurs in response to a meal) also stimulates insulin secretion as the acetylcholine released increases intracellular Ca^{2+} levels by activation of phospholipase C and formation of inositol triphosphate (IP_3).
- Free fatty acids also increase insulin secretion.
- Other hormones that increase insulin secretion include glucagon, growth hormone, cortisol and to lesser extent, progesterone and estrogen.
- Orally administered glucose exerts a greater insulin-stimulating effect than intravenously administered glucose as the gastrointestinal mucosa secretes hormones that stimulate insulin secretion (incretins).

Inhibitors of Insulin Secretion

- Catecholamines inhibit insulin secretion via α_2-adrenergic receptors. α_2-adrenergic receptors act by decreasing cAMP. This action serves to protect against hypoglycemia, especially during exercise.
- Somatostatin from the D cells of the islets inhibits the secretion of insulin.
- K^+ depletion decreases insulin secretion.
- Insulin may play an autocrine role in inhibiting its own production via insulin receptors on the pancreatic B cell. Insulin induces the down-regulation of its own receptors, i.e. it decreases its receptor concentration. When insulin binds to its receptors, they aggregate in patches and are taken into the cell by receptor-mediated endocytosis.

9

Factors affecting insulin secretion

Stimulators	*Inhibitors*
Increased blood glucose	Decreased blood glucose
Amino acids (arginine)	Somatostatin
Incretins: GIP and GLP 1	α-adrenergic stimulators
Acetylcholine	K^+ depletion
Glucagon	Leptin
cAMP and various cAMP generating substances	Insulin
β-adrenergic stimulation	β-adrenergic blockers

Long-term Changes in B Cell Responses

B cells respond to stimulation with hypertrophy like other endocrine cells; however, when the stimulation is marked or prolonged, they become exhausted and stop secreting (B cell exhaustion).

GLUCAGON

Glucagon is the primary hyperglycemic hormone that has functions diametrically opposed to those of insulin. Only a few micrograms of glucagon can cause the blood glucose level to double within a few minutes.

Structure and Synthesis

Glucagon is a member of the secretin gene family and is produced by A cells of the pancreatic islets. It is a linear polypeptide formed by proteolytic cleavage of preproglucagon to produce the 29 amino acid glucagon.

Transport and Metabolism

Like insulin, glucagon circulates in an unbound form and has a short half-life of 5–10 minutes. The predominant site of glucagon degradation is the liver. As much as 80% of the circulating hormone is degraded in one pass. As glucagon enters the hepatic portal vein and is carried to the liver before reaching the systemic circulation, a large portion of the secreted hormone never reaches the systemic circulation and peripheral blood levels are relatively low.

Mechanism of Action

The glucagon receptor is linked to Gs and on binding glucagon, increases intracellular cAMP levels in the liver. The increase in cAMP initiates the activation of various enzymes involved in the metabolic pathways.

Actions of Glucagon (Fig. 9.17)

- The hyperglycemic effect of glucagon is brought about by various mechanisms:
  - In the liver, glucagon activates the glycogen phosphorylase enzyme and therefore, increases breakdown of glycogen, increasing plasma glucose levels.
  - The increased glucagon/insulin ratio increases the activities of glucose-6-phosphatase and fructose-1, 6-bisphosphatase, while inhibiting the opposite reactions, thereby promoting release of glucose.
  - Glucagon increases gluconeogenesis by activating multiple enzymes, especially the enzyme system for conversion of pyruvate to phosphoenolpyruvate, a rate-limiting step in gluconeogenesis.

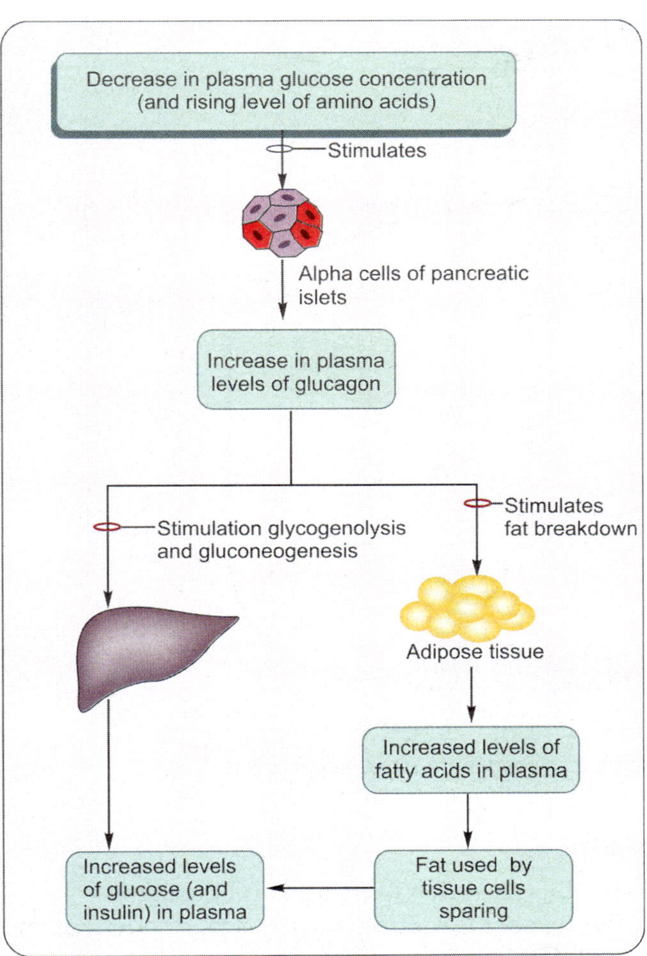

Fig. 9.17: Actions of glucagon

- Glucagon causes lipolysis in adipose tissue by activating the intracellular hormone-sensitive lipase enzyme, which catalyzes the breakdown of stored triglycerides into glycerol and fatty acids. Lipogenesis is inhibited by inhibition of acetyl CoA carboxylase and activation of the opposing enzyme malonyl CoA decarboxylase. The reduction of malonyl CoA also relieves inhibition on the carnitine transport mechanism, allowing more efficient transport of fatty acyl CoAs into the mitochondria and increasing beta oxidation of fatty acids.
- *Ketogenesis:* Increased beta oxidation of fatty acids results in the accumulation of acetyl CoA which is then utilized to form ketone bodies.

Thus, glucagon is glycogenolytic, gluconeogenic, lipolytic and ketogenic. It mobilizes energy stores and is a "hormone of energy release".

Action of insulin and glucagon on blood sugar levels are illustrated in Fig. 9.18.

Regulation of Glucagon Secretion

The principal factors that affect glucagon secretion are listed below.

Factors affecting glucagon secretion	
Stimulators	*Inhibitors*
Amino acids	Glucose
Cortisol	Somatostatin
Cholecystokinin (CCK), gastrin	FFA
Exercise	Insulin
Infections	GABA
β-adrenergic stimulators	α-adrenergic agonists

Stimuli that Increase Glucagon Secretion

- A major stimulus for glucagon secretion is a drop in blood glucose. When blood glucose levels are high, the B cells are stimulated to secrete insulin, which inhibits glucagon secretion. Also, the stimulated B cells release GABA that acts on the A cells to inhibit glucagon secretion by activating $GABA_A$ receptors. The $GABA_A$ receptors are Cl^- channels and the resulting Cl^- influx hyperpolarizes the A cells. Once blood glucose drops, insulin and GABA are not secreted; consequently, there is removal of the inhibition of A cells.
- Circulating catecholamines stimulate glucagon secretion via β_2-adrenergic receptors and inhibit glucagon secretion via α_2-adrenergic receptors. However, the effect of β-receptors predominates in the A cells and stimulation of sympathetic nerves increases glucagon secretion.
  Link: A diabetic patient will sometimes awaken with hyperglycemia even before eating. One cause of this preprandial hyperglycemia is the Somogyi effect, which results from nocturnal hypoglycemia that stimulates secretion of the stress or counter-regulatory hormones, i.e. glucagon, cortisol, growth hormone and epinephrine, that act to elevate glucose. People with this problem generally need a lower insulin dose at night time.
- Exercise, infection and other stresses possibly act via the sympathetic nervous system to increase glucagon secretion.
- Serum amino acids stimulate glucagon secretion. In this respect, the glucagon and insulin responses are not opposites. LINK: Hence, a protein meal will increase postprandial levels of both insulin and

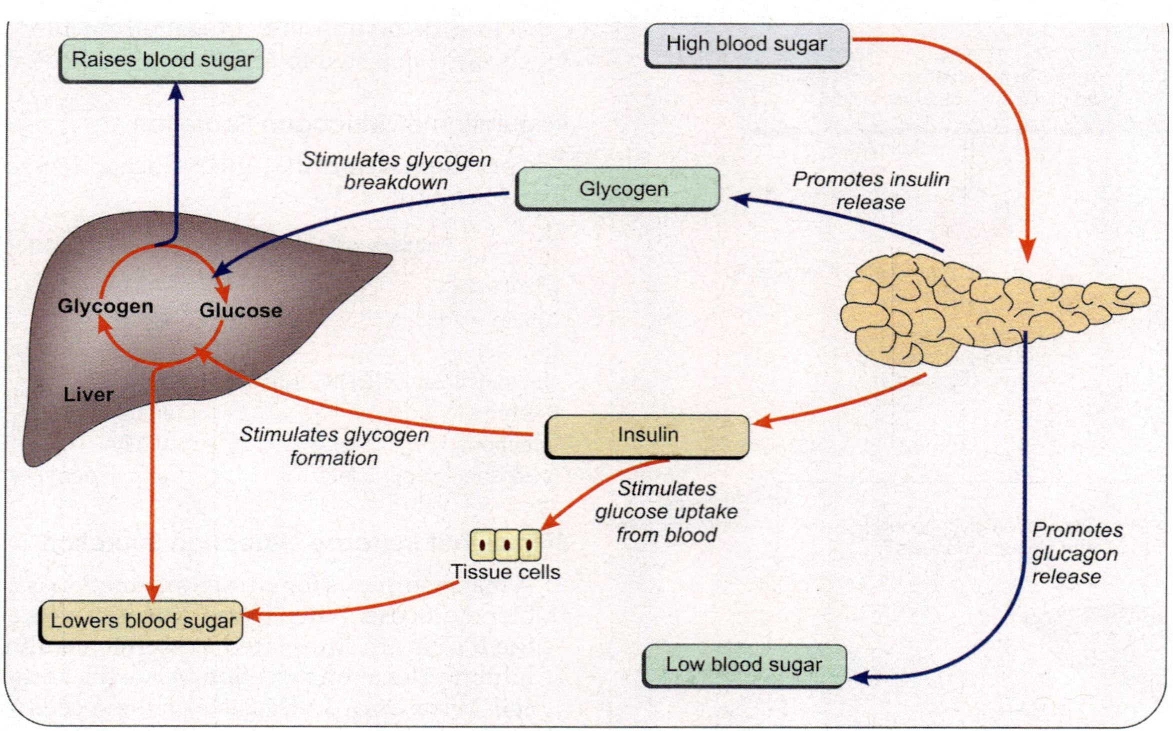

Fig. 9.18: Comparison of the actions of insulin and glucagon on blood sugar levels

glucagon, which protects against hypoglycemia, whereas a carbohydrate meal only stimulates insulin release.

- Orally administered amino acids produce greater glucagon secretion than intravenously administered amino acid because CCK and gastrin secreted by the intestinal mucosa stimulate glucagon secretion.

Stimuli that Inhibit Glucagon Secretion

- Glucose
- Somatostatin
- FFAs.

SOMATOSTATIN

Somatostatin is found in various tissues. It is secreted by the delta cells of islets of Langerhans. It is a polypeptide containing only 14 amino acids and has a short half-life of only 3 minutes. The secretion of pancreatic somatostatin is increased by several of the same stimuli that increase insulin secretion, i.e. glucose and amino acids, particularly arginine. It is also increased by CCK released from the upper gastrointestinal tract.

Actions

1. Inhibits secretion of insulin and glucagon
2. Decreases the motility of stomach, duodenum and gallbladder
3. Decreases both secretion and absorption in GIT.

PANCREATIC POLYPEPTIDE

Human pancreatic polypeptide is a linear polypeptide that contains 36 amino acid residues and is produced by F cells in the islets. Its exact physiologic function is still uncertain. Its secretion is increased by fasting, exercise and consumption of a protein meal and decreased by somatostatin. Pancreatic polypeptide slows the absorption of food in humans, and it may smooth out the peaks and valleys of absorption.

DIABETES MELLITUS

Diabetes mellitus is a syndrome of impaired carbohydrate, fat and protein metabolism caused by either lack of insulin secretion or decreased sensitivity of the tissues to insulin. It is characterized by hyperglycemia, polyuria, polydipsia, polyphagia (increased appetite) and weight loss (despite the polyphagia). There are widespread biochemical abnormalities due to two fundamental defects:

1. Reduced entry of glucose into peripheral tissues
2. Increased liberation of glucose into the circulation from the liver.

Thus, there is an extracellular glucose excess and in many cells, an intracellular glucose deficiency, a condition that has been described as "starvation in the midst of plenty". There are, in addition, features of disordered lipid and protein metabolism.

Physiological Basis of the Symptoms of Diabetes Mellitus

Hyperglycemia (Fig. 9.19)

High blood glucose levels are due to:

1. Decreased entry of glucose into cells, termed 'decreased peripheral utilization'. Without insulin, the entry of glucose into skeletal muscle and adipose tissue is decreased. Glucose uptake by the liver is also reduced as insulin facilitates glucose entry into hepatocytes by increasing the activity of the enzyme glucokinase. The intestinal absorption of glucose, glucose reabsorption by renal tubules and glucose uptake by the brain and red blood cells are insulin-independent processes and remain unaffected.
2. Increased hepatic production of glucose. The liver functions as a 'glucostat' that takes up glucose when its blood levels are high, storing it as glycogen and discharges glucose when its blood levels are low. Insulin facilitates glycogen synthesis and inhibits hepatic glucose output. When the plasma glucose is high, insulin secretion is normally increased and hepatic production of glucose is decreased. This effect is missing in diabetes.

Polyuria

Excessive urine production is called polyuria. As plasma glucose levels rise, glucose is presented to the renal tubules at a rate that exceeds the glucose tubular maximum (Tm). As the renal threshold is exceeded, glucose begins to appear in the urine (glycosuria).

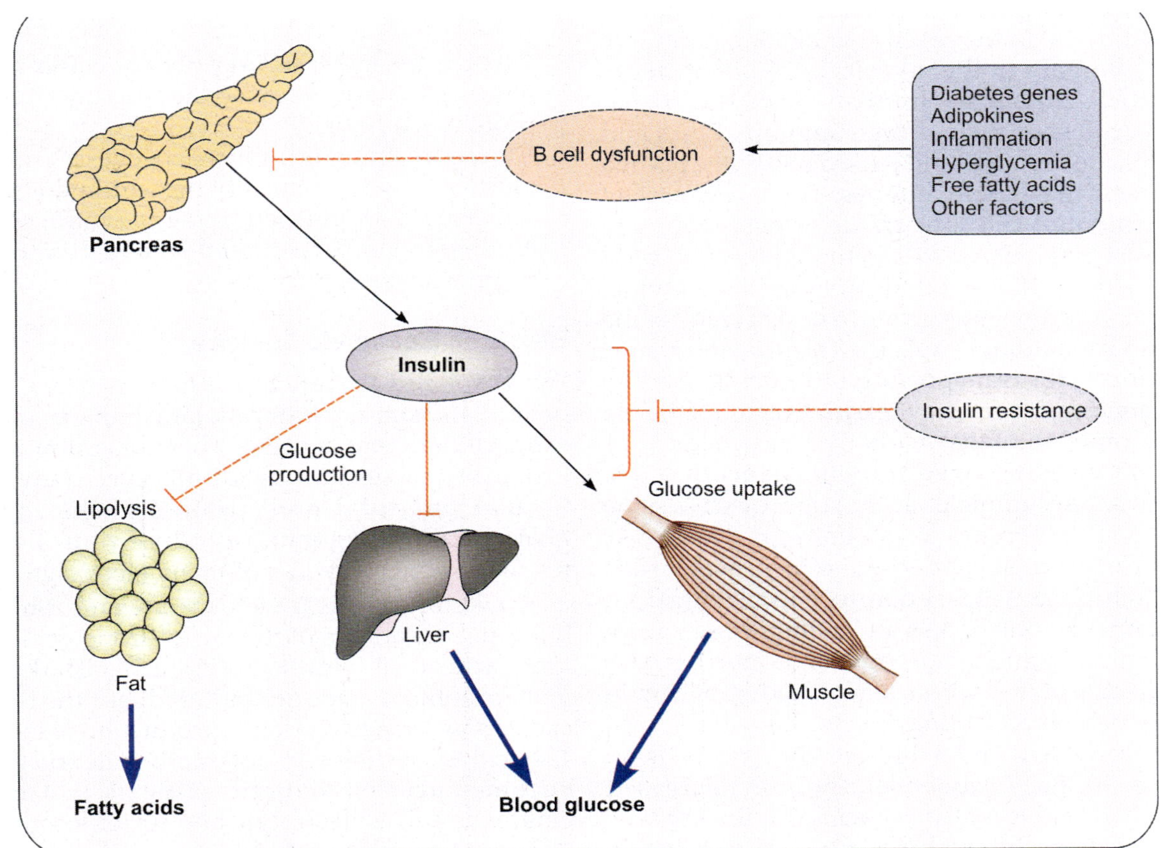

Fig. 9.19: Pathophysiology of hyperglycemia and increased free fatty acids in type 2 diabetes mellitus B

Since glucose is an osmotically active particle, it draws large amounts of water and acts as an osmotic diuretic.

Polydipsia

The dehydration that results as a result of osmotic diuresis activates the mechanisms regulating water intake, leading to increased thirst or polydipsia.

Polyphagia

Hypothalamic areas that regulate appetite have insulin-sensitive glucose transport systems. In the absence of insulin, intracellular glucose levels are low in the satiety center though plasma glucose levels remain high. This intracellular glucose deficit in the satiety area of the ventromedial nucleus decreases the activity of its cells and the lateral appetite area operates unopposed, increasing food intake.

Lipid Metabolism in Diabetes

The principal abnormalities in lipid metabolism in diabetes are:

- Increased lipolysis with excessive formation of ketone bodies. In the absence of insulin, hormone-sensitive lipase in the fat cells becomes strongly activated and causes hydrolysis of the stored triglycerides, releasing large amounts FFAs and glycerol into the blood and consequently, the plasma FFA levels rise within minutes. There is a marked impairment of the conversion of acetyl CoA to malonyl CoA, the first step in the synthesis of fatty acids. This is due to a deficiency of the enzyme, acetyl CoA carboxylase. In the liver, as a result of the decrease in malonyl CoA, the carnitine transport mechanism for transporting fatty acids into the mitochondria becomes increasingly activated. Beta oxidation of the fatty acids then proceeds very rapidly, releasing large amounts of acetyl CoA. Acetyl CoA accumulates as the supply exceeds, the capacity of the tissues to catabolize it. The excess acetyl CoA is then condensed to form acetoacetic acid, which is released into the circulation. Circulating ketone bodies are an important source of energy in fasting. As production is much greater than the rate of utilization, ketone bodies pile up in the bloodstream resulting in ketoacidosis.
- Decreased FFA and triglyceride synthesis in adipose tissue: In diabetes, there is decreased conversion of glucose to fatty acids in adipose tissue because of the intracellular glucose deficiency. Besides, there is a decreased supply of glycerol-3-phosphate, which is required for triglyceride synthesis.
- Increased plasma levels of triglycerides, FFA and cholesterol: In diabetes, decrease in the activity of lipoprotein lipase decreases the clearance of VLDL; consequently, plasma triglyceride levels rise. High plasma levels of FFAs reflect the increase in hormone-sensitive lipase activity and the resultant fat mobilization. The high FFA levels promote hepatic conversion of some of the fatty acids to phospholipids and cholesterol, which are discharged into blood in the lipoproteins. The rise in plasma cholesterol level is due to an increase in the plasma concentration of VLDL and LDL.

Protein Metabolism in Diabetes

In diabetes, there is net protein loss as insulin is required for normal amino acid uptake into cells. Further, as cellular glucose uptake is impaired, proteins are mobilized as an energy source resulting in muscle wasting. Protein depletion from any cause is associated with poor resistance to infections.

Gluconeogenesis is increased in diabetes mellitus as

- There is an increased supply of amino acids for gluconeogenesis (because they are not utilized for protein synthesis).
- Glucagon stimulates gluconeogenesis and hyperglucagonemia is generally present in diabetes.
- The activity of gluconeogenic enzymes, phosphoenolpyruvate carboxykinase and fructose-1, 6-bisphosphatase, is increased.

Effects on Electrolyte Balance

When insulin is deficient, there is a net shift of potassium from the intracellular compartment to the extracellular compartment. This potassium is lost in the urine, so serum potassium levels may appear normal but total body potassium is low. The glycosuria and ketonuria produce diuresis, which results in obligatory loss of many electrolytes.

The ketone bodies, acetoacetate and β-hydroxybutyrate, are anions of the fairly strong acids, acetoacetic acid and β-hydroxybutyric acids. The hydrogen ions from these acids are buffered, but the buffering capacity is soon exceeded if production is increased. The acidosis results in loss of bicarbonate and the urine becomes acidic. Diabetic acidosis is a medical emergency. The electrolyte and water losses lead to dehydration, hypovolemia and hypotension. The metabolic acidosis stimulates respiration, producing the rapid, deep respiration described by Kussmaul as "air hunger" and named Kussmaul breathing after him. Finally, the acidosis and dehydration depress consciousness to the point of coma. Independent of plasma pH, the hyperosmolarity of the plasma causes unconsciousness (hyperosmolar coma). Accumulation of lactate in the blood (lactic acidosis) may also complicate diabetic ketoacidosis if the tissues become hypoxic and may itself cause coma.

Link: When treating a patient with poorly controlled diabetes, insulin should not be administered too rapidly as it can produce hypokalemia by causing intracellular shift of potassium; this is the reason for administration of insulin with potassium supplemen-tation.

Long-term Sequelae of Diabetes Mellitus

In long-standing diabetes, in addition to the acute complications (acidosis and hyperosmolar coma), there are microvascular, macrovascular and neuropathic abnormalities. The ultimate cause of the microvascular and neuropathic complications is chronic hyperglycemia. Tight control of the plasma glucose levels reduces their incidence.

The microvascular abnormalities are proliferative scarring of the retina (diabetic retinopathy), leading to blindness; and renal disease (diabetic nephropathy), leading to renal failure.

The macrovascular abnormalities are due to accelerated atherosclerosis, which is secondary to increased plasma LDL levels. There is an increased incidence of stroke and myocardial infarction.

The neuropathic abnormalities (diabetic neuropathy) involve the autonomic nervous system and peripheral nerves. The neuropathy coupled with atherosclerotic circulatory insufficiency in the extremities and the reduced resistance to infection can lead to chronic ulceration and gangrene, particularly in the feet (diabetic foot).

Raised intracellular glucose levels alter cell function and contribute to pathological changes (glucotoxicity). The exact mechanisms by which cell function is altered are unclear. High intracellular glucose levels lead to nonenzymatic glycation of proteins forming advanced glycation end products (AGEs). The AGEs have altered function: secreted AGEs cross-link matrix proteins, damaging blood vessels; they interact with receptors on leucocytes and interfere with the leucocyte responses to infection, activation of endothelial receptors for AGEs leads to proinflammatory gene expression.

An important circulating product of nonenzymatic glycation is hemoglobin A_{1c} (HbA_{1c}). Once glycation occurs, the haemoglobin remains glycated for the remainder of the red blood cells lifespan. The proportion of HbA_{1c} is low in a nondiabetic person while a diabetic person who has had prolonged periods of hyperglycemia over the last two to three months will have elevated levels. Careful control of the diabetes with insulin reduces the amount of HbA_{1c} formed.

Link: HbA_{1c} levels are measured clinically as an integrated index of diabetic control for the 4 to 6 week-period before the measurement.

Types of Diabetes

Type 1 or insulin-dependent diabetes mellitus (IDDM) is due to insulin deficiency caused by autoimmune destruction or viral infection of the B cells in the pancreatic islets. Type 2 or noninsulin-dependent diabetes mellitus (NIDDM), is characterized by insulin resistance and impaired insulin secretion. Secondary diabetes is due to other diseases such as Cushing's syndrome and acromegaly.

Most of the cases of type 1 diabetes begin in childhood between 10 and 14 years of age, hence the term juvenile diabetes for this disorder. This term is no longer used because type 1 diabetes can present at any time of life. Patients with this disease are not obese and have a high incidence of ketosis and acidosis. About 50% of type 1 diabetes is related to problems with the major histocompatibility complex on chromosome 6.

Type 2 or noninsulin-dependent diabetes mellitus is the most common type of diabetes, accounting for 90% of the diagnosed cases. There is a genetic susceptibility as seen for type 1 diabetes. The vast majority of cases are polygenic in origin and the actual genes involved are still unknown. Type 2 diabetes usually develops after age 40 and is not associated with total loss of the ability to secrete insulin. It is usually associated with obesity and defects in the ability of target organs to respond to insulin (insulin resistance). The major features of obesity-induced insulin resistance are:

1. A decreased ability of insulin to increase GLUT 4-mediated glucose uptake.
2. A decreased ability of insulin to repress hepatic glucose production
3. An inability of insulin to repress hormone-sensitive lipase and/or increase lipoprotein lipase in adipose tissue. Type 2 diabetes is rarely associated with ketosis.

Maturity-onset diabetes of the young (MODY) accounts for 1% of the cases of type 2 diabetes. In this condition, loss-of-function mutations have been described in six different genes. Five of the genes code for transcription factors affecting the production of enzymes involved in glucose metabolism. The sixth is the gene for glucokinase, the enzyme that controls the rate of glucose phosphorylation in the B cells.

Diagnosis of Diabetes Mellitus

The diagnosis of diabetes mellitus is based primarily on plasma glucose.

Fasting Plasma Glucose Level

Normal fasting plasma glucose levels (fasting denotes no caloric intake for at least 8 hours) should be below 100 mg/dl. A patient is considered to have impaired glucose tolerance if the fasting plasma glucose is between 110 and 126 mg/dl, and the diagnosis of diabetes mellitus is made if the fasting plasma glucose exceeds 126 mg/dl on two successive days.

Presentation with the symptoms of diabetes and a nonfasting plasma glucose greater than 200 mg/dl also indicates the diagnosis of diabetes mellitus. (Yet to check the latest on diagnosis of DM).

Oral Glucose Tolerance Test

Another approach to the diagnosis of diabetes is the oral glucose tolerance test. After overnight fasting, the patient is given a bolus amount of glucose (75 g) orally, and blood glucose levels are measured at 2 hours. A 2-hour plasma glucose greater than 200 mg/dl on two consecutive days is sufficient to make the diagnosis of diabetes. In a normal, fasting person, the blood glucose level rises from about 90 mg/dl to 120 to 140 mgl/dl and falls back to normal in about 2 hours. In a person with diabetes, there is a much greater rise in blood glucose level and the glucose level falls back to normal only after 4 to 6 hours.

9

Plasma Insulin Level

Type I and Type II diabetes can be distinguished from each other by measurements of plasma insulin, with plasma insulin being low in type I diabetes and high in type II diabetes.

Urinary Glucose

A normal person loses undetectable amounts of glucose in urine, whereas a person with diabetes loses glucose in small to large amounts, depending on the severity of the disease and the intake of carbohydrates.

(*See* Chapter 70 in Section 8 for glycosuria).

Urinary Ketoacids

Ketoacids can be detected by chemical means in the urine. Small quantities of acetoacetic acid in the blood are converted to acetone. This is volatile and vaporized into the expired air. Consequently, one can frequently make a diagnosis of type I diabetes mellitus simply by smelling acetone on the breath of a patient.

OBESITY

Obesity can be defined as an excess of body fat. A surrogate marker for body fat content is the body mass index (BMI), which is calculated as:

$$BMI = \text{Weight in kg/Height in m}^2$$

In clinical terms, a BMI between 25 and 29.9 kg/m^2 is called overweight, and a BMI greater than 30 kg/m^2 is called obese. Obesity is caused by greater energy intake than energy expenditure. The causes of obesity are complex. Genetic factors, lifestyle, environmental factors and neurogenic abnormalities affect food intake and energy metabolism.

Obesity, Metabolic Syndrome and Type 2 Diabetes

Obesity has a special relation with disordered carbohydrate metabolism and diabetes. As body weight increases, there is increasing insulin resistance and so weight reduction decreases insulin resistance. Hyperinsulinemia, dyslipidemia and atherosclerosis are usually associated with obesity. The hyper-insulinemia could be a compensatory response to the increased insulin resistance. The dyslipidemia is characterized by high circulating triglycerides and low HDL. This cluster of findings: obesity, insulin resistance, dyslipidemia and atherosclerosis is commonly called the metabolic syndrome or syndrome X or insulin resistance syndrome. Some of the patients with metabolic syndrome are prediabetic, whereas others have type 2 diabetes.

HYPOGLYCEMIA

Glucose is the only fuel used in appreciable quantities by the brain but the carbohydrate reserves in neural tissue are very limited. When blood glucose levels fall, the metabolism of the central nervous system becomes depressed.

Clinical Features

As the plasma glucose level falls into the range of 50 to 70 mg/dl, the first symptoms are anxiety, palpitations, sweating, hunger, tremors and extreme nervousness because this degree of hypoglycemia sensitizes neuronal activity and there is autonomic discharge. The symptoms caused by autonomic discharge serve as a warning to seek glucose replacement but in long-term diabetics, the autonomic symptoms may not occur (hypoglycemia unawareness). As the blood glucose level falls to 20 to 50 mg/dl, neuroglycopenic symptoms appear. These include confusion and the other cognitive abnormalities. At even lower plasma glucose levels, lethargy, convulsions, coma and eventually death occur.

Causes

- "Insulin reactions" are common in type 1 diabetics. There is an increase in glucose uptake by skeletal muscle and an increased absorption of injected insulin during exercise.
- Infants born to diabetic mothers are at risk of developing hypoglycemia. They often have high birth weights and large organs (macrosomia). This condition is caused by excess circulating insulin in the fetus, which in-turn is caused by stimulation of the fetal pancreas by glucose from maternal blood.
- In liver disease, the glucose tolerance curve is diabetic but the fasting plasma glucose is low.
- In some thyrotoxic patients, glucose absorption is abnormally rapid. The plasma glucose rises to a high, early peak, but it then falls rapidly to hypoglycemic levels because the wave of hyperglycemia evokes a greater than normal rise in insulin secretion. Symptoms characteristically occur about 2 hours after meals.
- Rarely, excess insulin production occurs from an adenoma of the islets of Langerhans (insulinomas).

Compensatory Mechanisms

- One important compensation for hypoglycemia is cessation of the secretion of insulin. Inhibition of insulin secretion is complete at a plasma glucose level of about 80 mg/dl.
- Hypoglycemia triggers increased secretion of four counter-regulatory hormones: Glucagon, epinephrine, growth hormone and cortisol.
- Glucagon and Epinephrine increases hepatic output of glucose by increasing glycogenolysis. The keys to counter-regulation appear to be glucagon and epinephrine: if both fail to increase, there is little if any compensatory rise in the plasma glucose level. The actions of the other hormones are supplementary.
- Growth hormone and cortisol decrease the utilization of glucose in various peripheral tissues.

ADIPOSE TISSUE AS AN ENDOCRINE ORGAN

Following the link between adiposity and insulin resistance, the discovery of hormones secreted by adipose tissue has led to the emerging concept that adipose tissue is an endocrine organ. The hormones secreted by it are called adipokines. They include leptin, adiponectin, tumor necrosis factor-α (TNF-α) and resistin. Leptin and adiponectin decrease insulin resistance, whereas TNF-α and resistin increase insulin resistance.

There are two forms of adipose tissue: Brown adipose tissue (BAT) and white adipose tissue (WAT). BAT plays an important role in thermogenesis in the newborn but is much reduced in adults. WAT plays three roles: First, it is used for cushioning, as in the orbits around the eyeballs; second, it is used as a metabolic storage depot that can be called on to release FFAs and glycerol in times of fasting and third, it functions as a classic endocrine organ.

WAT is divided into subcutaneous and intra-abdominal (visceral) depots. The intra-abdominal depot refers primarily to omental and mesenteric fat, and is the smaller of the two depots. The two depots differ in their blood supply, innervation, regulation and hormone production. Venous return from the intra-abdominal depot leads into the hepatic portal system. Thus, intra-abdominally-derived FFAs are mostly cleared by the liver, whereas subcutaneous fat is the primary source of FFAs for muscle during exercise or fasting. These depots are innervated by distinct sets of autonomic nerves and are influenced differently by sex steroids. Men tend to gain fat in the visceral depot [android adiposity (apple-shaped)], whereas women tend to gain fat in the subcutaneous depot, particularly in the thigh and buttocks [gynecoid adiposity (pear-shaped)].

The established protein factors produced by WAT are leptin, adiponectin and TNF-α.

Leptin

Leptin (from the Greek word for 'thin') is a protein hormone secreted by adipocytes that acts on the hypothalamus to decrease food intake and increase energy consumption. It is structurally related to cytokines and is sometimes referred to as an adipocytokine. Leptin is a product of the ob gene; mice that are homozygous for a defective ob gene (*ob/ob mice*) do not become sated after eating and become obese and diabetic. Fasting decreases leptin concentrations sharply and conversely, sustained overfeeding increases plasma levels.

Leptin Receptor

The leptin receptor belongs to the class of transmembrane cytokine receptors that signals by activation of the cytosolic tyrosine kinase JAK2. Leptin receptors are found in various peripheral tissues as well as the brain.

Actions of Leptin (Fig. 9.20)

- The principal targets for leptin are neurons in the arcuate nuclei of the hypothalamus. Leptin appears to decrease the production and release of neuropeptide Y in the arcuate nuclei; neuropeptide Y increases appetite and lowers energy expenditure. Leptin also increases the activity of neurons that express pro-opiomelanocortin (POMC). POMC gives rise to α-melanocyte stimulating hormone (α-MSH), which is a potent negative regulator of food intake.
- Adipocytes express leptin receptors and respond to leptin in an autocrine manner with an increase in lipolysis.
- Insulin stimulates leptin secretion and in typical negative feedback fashion, leptin acts directly on pancreatic B cells to inhibit insulin secretion.

In summary, leptin operates as part of a feedback loop by which the size of the body fat depots can regulate food intake through a hormonal link.

Adiponectin

Adiponectin regulates metabolism in a manner similar to leptin, in that it decreases insulin resistance in terms of glucose uptake; however, it opposes insulin in terms of FFA utilization or storage. Adiponectin stimulates FFA oxidation and reduces intracellular triglyceride content; this effect is associated with enhanced insulin-dependent glucose uptake, i.e. increased insulin sensitivity. Adiponectin also increases FFA oxidation in the liver and decreases hepatic glucose output.

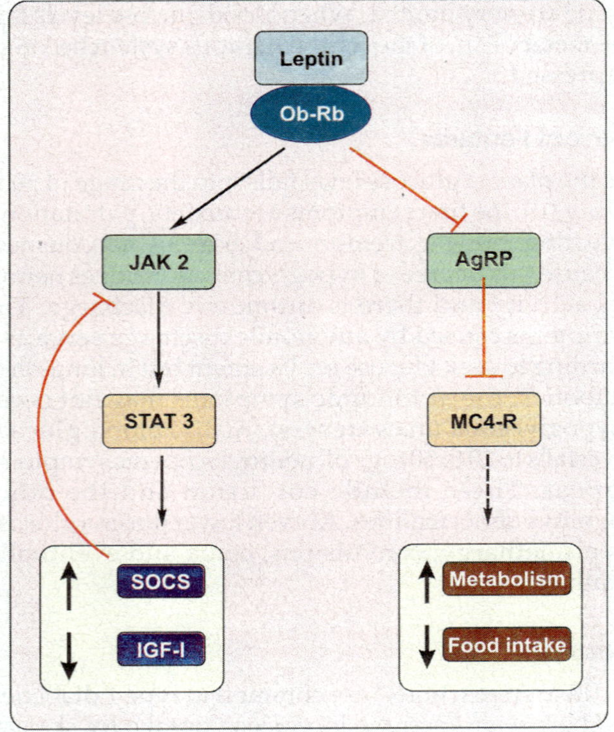

Fig. 9.20: Mechanism of action of leptin

Unlike leptin, adiponectin levels decrease with obesity. As adipocytes enlarge with stored triglycerides, they secrete less adiponectin. Weight loss increases adiponectin levels.

Tumour Necrosis Factor-α (TNF-α)

TNF-α production by adipose tissue increases with obesity. It acts in an autocrine/paracrine manner to repress the expression of genes that encode proteins involved in the uptake of FFAs and glucose, and in lipogenesis. It reduces insulin sensitivity by decreasing the expression of GLUT 4 and insulin receptor substrate-1.

76. PITUITARY GLAND

Introduction

The pituitary gland or hypophysis is a small endocrine gland located at the base of the forebrain just below the hypothalamus, encased in the sella turcica of the sphenoid bone. It is connected to the hypothalamus by the pituitary or hypophyseal stalk that emerges superiorly out of the sella turcica in the area where the optic nerves and optic chiasm are located (Fig. 9.21).

Embryology of the Pituitary Gland (Fig. 9.22)

The pituitary gland is a compound organ made up of two distinct types of tissues: epithelial and neural. The epithelial component which is derived embryologically from the primitive foregut is called the adenohypophysis (adeno = glandular) and the neural part derived from the brainstem is termed the neurohypophysis.

During development, a caudal extension of the diencephalon grows toward the roof of the primitive oral cavity. This neural down growth, called the infundibular process, secretes factors that induce the epithelium of the roof of the oral cavity to extend cranially toward the base of the developing brain. This extension of the oral ectoderm is called Rathke's pouch. As Rathke's pouch moves upward, it loses contact with the oral cavity and comes in direct contact with the infundibular process.

Link: Remnants of Rathke's pouch may persist and can give rise to craniopharyngiomas.

The cells on the ventral side of the pouch expand considerably and give rise to the anterior lobe or pars distalis. The intermediate lobe or pars intermedia develops from the dorsal half of the pouch that faces the infundibular process and is closely adherent to the posterior lobe in the adult. It is separated from the anterior lobe by the remains of Rathke's pouch, the residual cleft. A third division of Rathke's pouch develops into the pars tuberalis and is composed of a thin layer of cells that wrap around the infundibular stalk. The adenohypophysis is thus composed of the anterior lobe, the pars tuberalis and the intermediate lobe, which is rudimentary in adult humans.

The infundibular process expands at its lower end to give rise to a structure called the pars nervosa or the posterior lobe of the pituitary. At the superior end of the infundibular process, a funnel-shaped swelling develops called the median eminence. The rest of the infundibular process, which extends from the median eminence down to the pars nervosa, is called the

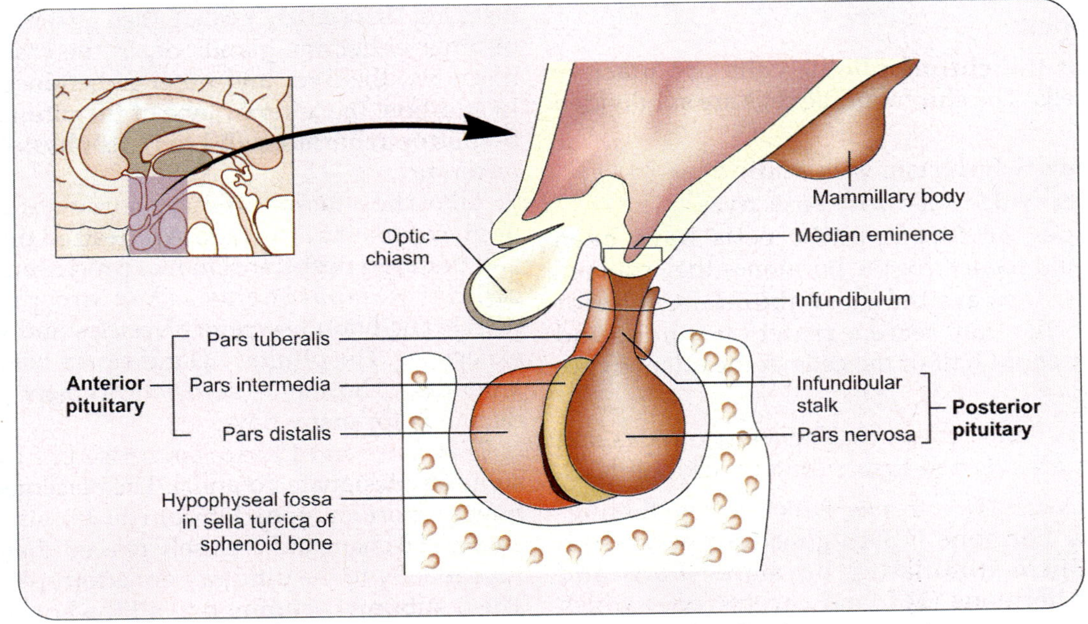

Fig. 9.21: Parts of the pituitary gland

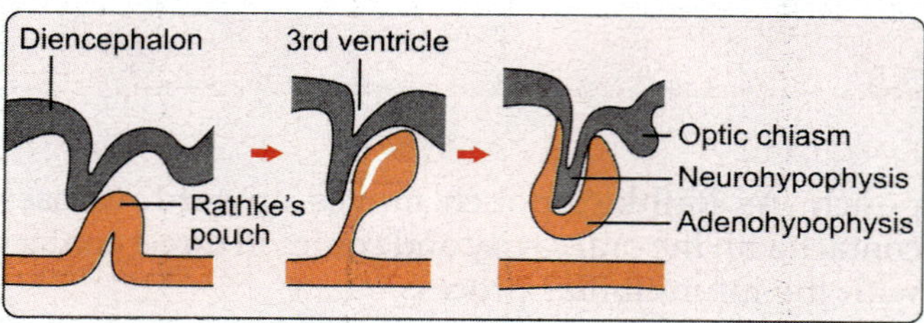

Fig. 9.22: Embryological development of pituitary gland

infundibulum. Thus, the neurohypophysis develops from a down growth of neural tissue at the base of the diencephalon and is made up of the posterior lobe, the infundibulum and the median eminence. The infundibulum and the pars tuberalis make up the pituitary stalk.

Histology and Morphology

The anterior pituitary is made up of large polygonal cells arranged in cords and surrounded by an extensive network of sinusoidal capillaries. The endothelium of the capillaries is fenestrated, like that in other endocrine organs. The cells contain granules of stored hormones that are extruded from the cells by exocytosis. The anterior lobe is sparsely innervated and lacks any secretomotor nerves.

The cells of the anterior pituitary have traditionally been divided on the basis of their staining reactions into:

a. Chromophobes
b. Chromophils.

Many of the chromophobic cells are inactive secretory cells. The chromophilic cells are subdivided into:

a. Acidophils, which stain with acidic dyes
b. Basophils, which stain with basic dyes.

Five types of chromophilic cells have been identified and named for the hormones they contain.

Somatotropes are the most abundant anterior pituitary cells; they secrete growth hormone and account for about half of the cells of the adenohypophysis.

Lactotropes secrete prolactin: The somatotropes and lactotropes are referred to as pituitary acidophils.

The basophils are: Thyrotropes, which secrete thyroid-stimulating hormone (TSH); gonadotropes, which secrete follicle-stimulating hormone (FSH) and luteinizing hormone (LH) and corticotropes which secrete adrenocorticotropin (ACTH).

The posterior pituitary is richly endowed with nonmyelinated nerve fibers that contain secretory vesicles stored in bulbous nerve endings. These axonal swellings can be observed by light microscopy with certain stains and are termed Herring bodies.

The anterior pituitary is linked to the brainstem by the hypothalamohypophyseal portal system through which it receives most of its blood supply. A portal system refers to a set of vessels that begins and ends in a capillary plexus. There is an intricate network of capillaries, the primary plexus, in the median eminence of the hypothalamus. Capillaries of the primary plexus converge to form long hypophyseal portal vessels, which course down the infundibular stalk to deliver their blood to the sinusoidal capillary network in the anterior lobe. Nearly all the blood that reaches the anterior lobe is carried in the portal vessels.

The portal arrangement of blood flow is important because blood that supplies the anterior pituitary first drains the hypothalamus. Portal blood can thus pick up chemical signals released by the hypothalamic neurons and deliver them directly to secretory cells of the anterior pituitary (Fig. 9.23).

ANTERIOR PITUITARY HORMONES

The six established hormones secreted by the anterior pituitary and their principal actions are listed. They have been called tropic or trophic hormones (from the Greek tropic , meaning "to turn toward" or trophos, meaning "to nourish"). Since, they govern the function of other endocrine glands or, in the case of growth hormone, the liver and other nonendocrine tissues. In addition, the anterior lobe of the pituitary secretes β-lipotropin hormone (β-LPH). Its physiologic role is uncertain.

All of the anterior pituitary hormones are proteins or glycoproteins. They are synthesized on ribosomes and undergo post-translational processing in various cellular compartments. They are packaged in membrane-bound secretory vesicles and secreted by exocytosis. The pituitary gland stores relatively large amounts of hormone, sufficient to meet physiologic demands for many days.

TSH, FSH and LH are comprised of two peptide subunits, designated α and β. The placental hormone, human chorionic gonadotropin (hCG), also consists of an α and β chain and is closely related chemically and functionally to the pituitary gonadotropic hormones. The α subunit is common to all the hormones, the β subunits confer physiologic specificity (Fig. 9.24).

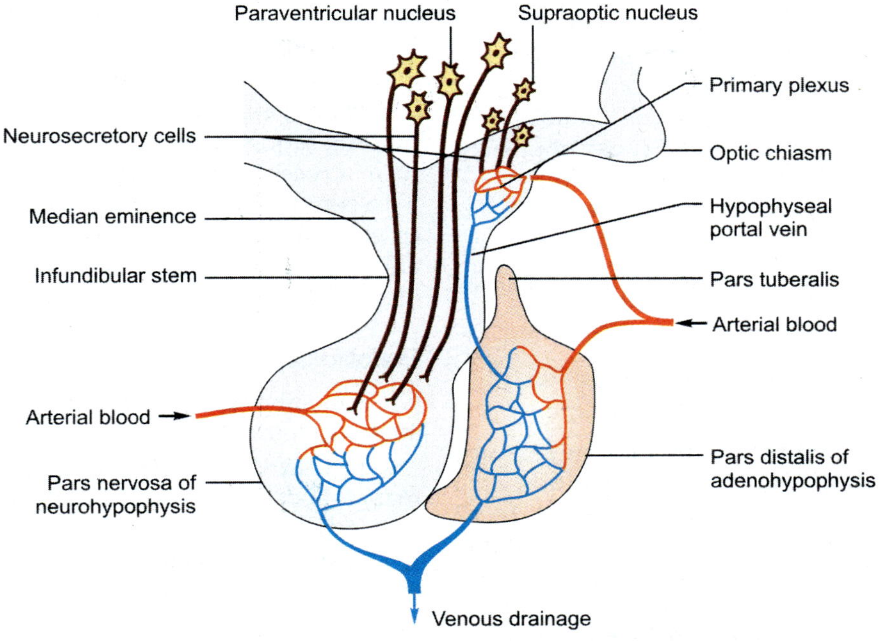

Fig. 9.23: Pituitary gland in hypothalamohypophyseal portal system

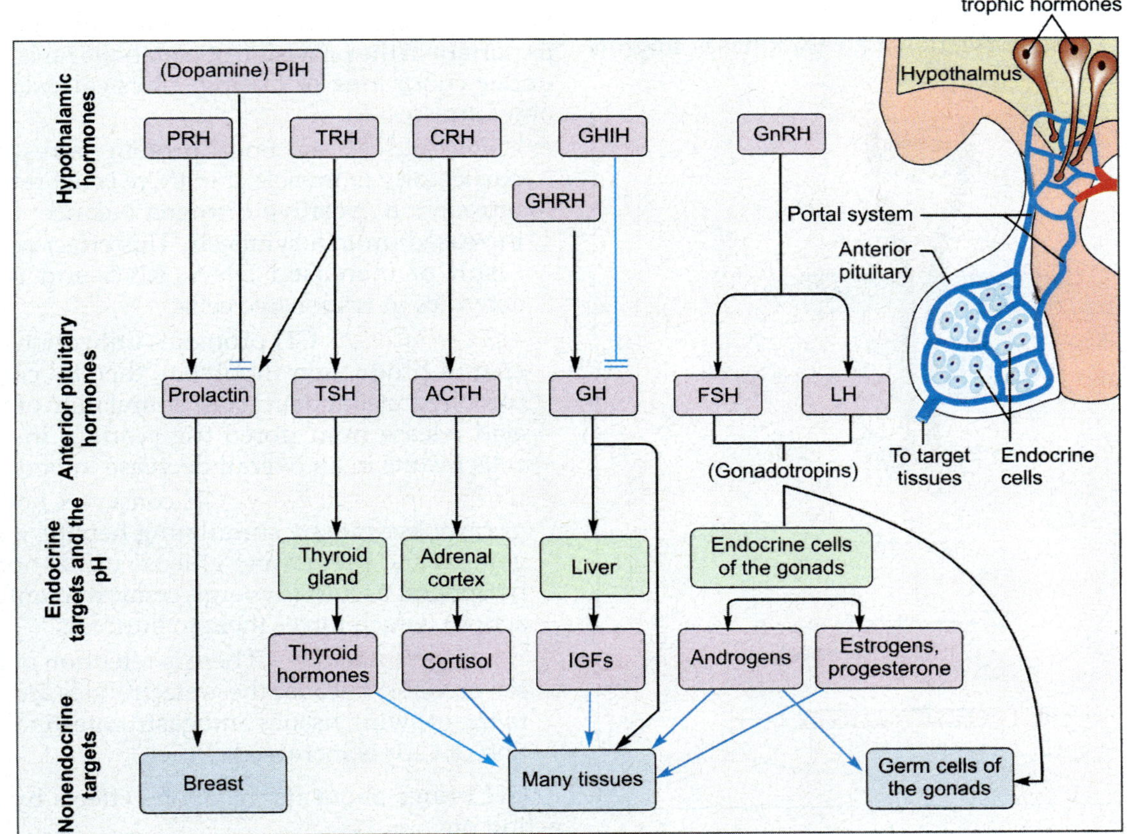

Fig. 9.24: Hypothalamic hormones, anterior pituitary hormones and their targets

GROWTH HORMONE

Growth hormone [GH or Somatotropin or Somatotropic hormone (STH); Greek soma = body], which is secreted throughout life, is the most abundant of the pituitary hormones. It is the single most important hormone for normal growth.

Chemistry of GH

GH is a polypeptide of 188 amino acids with two disulfide bonds.

Receptors and Mechanism of Action of GH (Fig. 9.25)

The GH receptor is a member of the cytokine receptor superfamily. It is a glycoprotein that binds to a cytosolic enzyme called Janus kinase 2 (JAK2). JAK2 is a member of the Janus family of cytoplasmic tyrosine kinases which catalyzes the phosphorylation of tyrosine residues on the receptor. Tyrosine phosphorylation provides docking sites for other proteins and facilitates their phosphorylation. STATs (signal transducers and activators of transcription) are a family of inactive cytoplasmic transcription factors that upon phosphorylation by JAK kinases migrate to the nucleus and activate various genes. The JAK-STAT pathways also mediate the effects of prolactin and various growth factors.

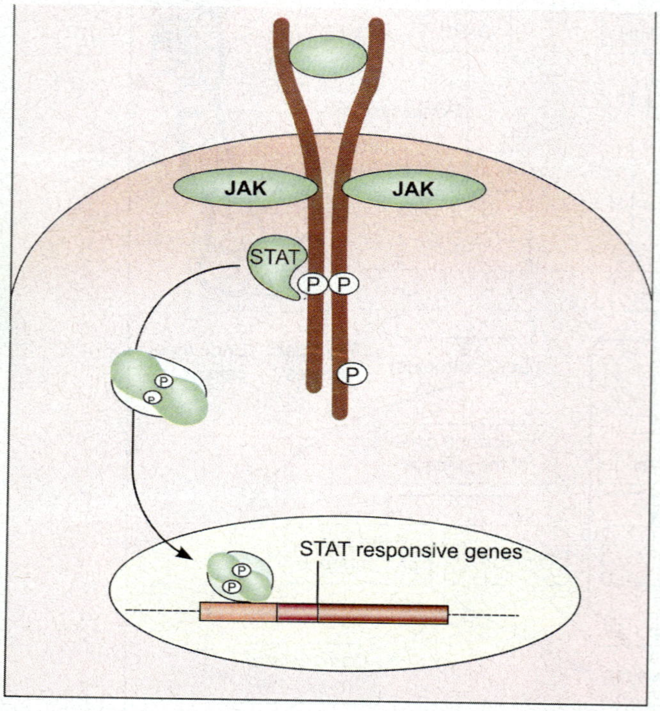

GH activates the JAK-STAT signaling pathway by binding sequentially to two GH receptor molecules to form a receptor dimer that sandwiches the hormone between the two receptor molecules. Dimerization is essential for receptor activation. Thus, GH produces its effects in various cells by stimulating the transcription of specific genes.

Fig. 9.25: Mechanism of action of growth hormone

Metabolism of GH

GH is metabolized rapidly; the half-life for GH is only about 20 minutes.

GH that crosses the glomerular membrane is reabsorbed and destroyed in the kidney, which is the major site of GH degradation. GH is also degraded in its various target cells following uptake by receptor-mediated endocytosis.

Actions of GH

Direct Actions

Direct actions of GH on cellular metabolism are important in the provision of metabolic fuels to tissues under conditions of fasting, physical exercise and other stresses.

- *Protein metabolism:* Body protein stores increase, particularly in muscle, and there is net retention of nitrogen: a positive nitrogen balance: reflecting increased protein synthesis. This effect occurs as a result of increased DNA, RNA and ribosome activities in responsive cells.
- *Lipid metabolism:* GH promotes utilization of fat for energy production (lipolytic), thereby conserving carbohydrates and proteins. Stimulation of free fatty acid release from stored triglycerides in white fat cells results in an overall decrease in body fat.
- *Carbohydrate metabolism:* GH conserves body stores of carbohydrate by stimulating hepatic gluconeogenesis and preventing glucose utilization by the peripheral tissues (hyperglycemic and anti-insulin action), which forces them to burn fats.
- *Electrolyte metabolism:* There is retention of Na^+ and K^+, probably because these electrolytes are diverted to the growing tissues and gastrointestinal absorption of Ca^{2+} is increased.

GH brings about its metabolic effects by directly acting on:

- Muscle

- Liver
- Adipose tissue

Liver: GH increases fatty acid uptake and oxidation in the liver. There is an increase in glucose output from the liver as the increase in fatty acid oxidation raises the levels of liver acetyl coenzyme A (acetyl CoA), which is utilized for gluconeogenesis.

Adipose tissue: GH activates hormone-sensitive lipase and therefore, mobilizes neutral fats from adipose tissue. As a result, serum fatty acid levels rise after GH administration. GH is ketogenic because it increases circulating free fatty acid levels and their oxidation. Glucose uptake is inhibited by the rise in serum free fatty acids. Thus, GH antagonizes the action of insulin in adipose tissue.

Skeletal muscle: GH inhibits protein breakdown and stimulates new protein synthesis in skeletal muscle. It increases fatty acid uptake and oxidation in skeletal muscle. Glucose uptake is inhibited by the raised serum free fatty acids (FFAs). Thus, GH exerts an anti-insulin effect (insulin promotes glucose utilization by skeletal muscle) and decreases insulin sensitivity (diabetogenic) in skeletal muscle. When secreted in excess, GH can cause diabetes mellitus: The hyperglycemic effect of GH is due to the inhibition of glucose uptake by tissues which secondarily stimulates the B cells to secrete insulin and causes their eventual exhaustion.

Indirect Actions

The indirect actions of GH are important in tissue growth and repair and development of the skeleton.

Skeletal Growth (Fig. 9.26)

The ultimate height attained by an adult is mainly determined by the length of the vertebral column and long bones of the legs. Growth of these bones occurs by a process called endochondral ossification, in which proliferating cartilage is replaced by bone.

- The ends of long bones are called epiphyses and arise from ossification centers that are separate from those responsible for ossification of the diaphysis, or shaft.
- In the growing individual, the epiphyses are separated from the diaphysis by cartilaginous regions called epiphyseal plates, in which continuous production of chondrocytes occurs at the epiphyseal border, providing for continual elongation of columns of chondrocytes. As they grow and mature, chondrocytes produce the mucopolysaccharides and collagen that constitute the cartilage matrix.
- Cartilage cells at the diaphyseal border degenerate as the surrounding matrix becomes calcified. In growth of blood vessels and migration of osteoblast progenitors from the diaphysis result in replacement of calcified cartilage with true bone.
- Proliferation of chondrocytes at the epiphyseal border of the growth plate is balanced by cellular degeneration at the diaphyseal end, so in the normally growing individual the thickness of the growth plate remains constant as the epiphyses are pushed further and further outward by the elongating shaft of bone.
- Eventually, progenitors of chondrocytes lose their capacity to divide; the epiphyseal plate becomes

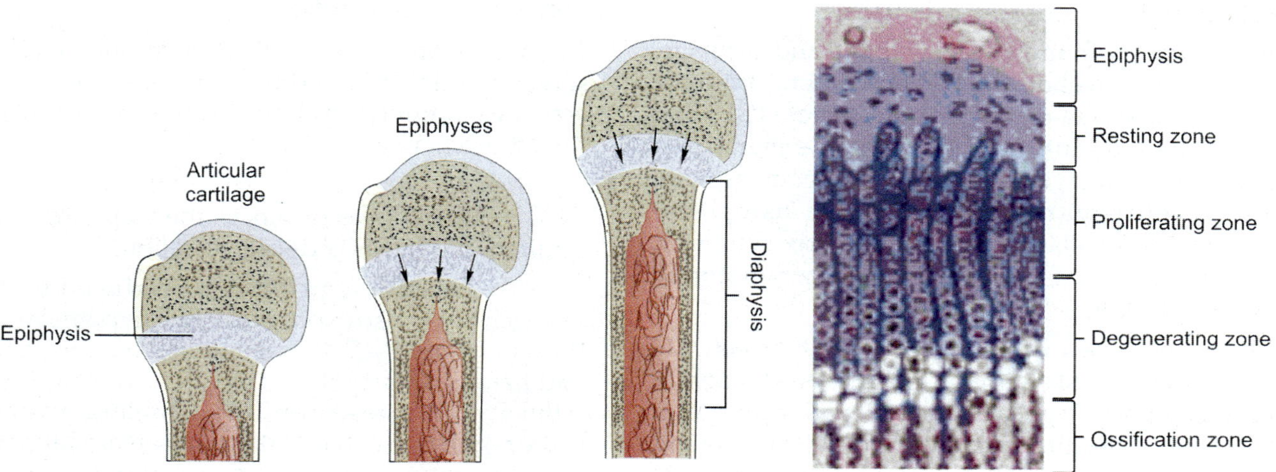

Fig. 9.26: Longitudinal section of bone showing various zones

progressively narrower and ultimately the bony epiphyses fuse with the diaphyseal bone (epiphyseal closure). With epiphyseal closure, the capacity for further growth is lost.

- Thickening of long bones is accomplished by proliferation of osteoblastic progenitors from the periosteum that surrounds the diaphysis.
- As it grows, bone is also subject to continual reabsorption and reorganization. Remodeling, which is an intrinsic property of skeletal growth, is accompanied by destruction and replacement of calcified matrix.

Insulin-like Growth Factors

Most of the actions of GH on skeletal growth: increased cartilage growth, long bone length and periosteal growth are mediated by a group of hormones called insulin-like growth factors (IGFs). These compounds were once called somatomedins because they mediate GH (somatotropin) action on cartilage and bone growth.

These multifunctional peptide hormones resemble insulin in structure and function. Of the two hormones in this family, IGF-I (somatomedin C; sulphation factor because it stimulates the incorporation of sulfate into cartilage) is the major form produced in most adult tissues that mediates the actions of GH, IGF-II is the major form in the fetus and is considered a fetal growth regulator. Though liver is the principal source of IGF in blood, it is now known that GH acts directly on a wide variety of tissues to promote IGF-I production. GH cannot stimulate IGF production in the absence of insulin.

9

IGFs have profound effects on bone and cartilage. GH stimulates prechondrocytes and other cells in the epiphyseal plates to synthesize and secrete IGFs that act locally in an autocrine or paracrine manner to stimulate chondrocyte maturation and bone growth. IGFs are mitogenic; they stimulate osteoblast replication and collagen and bone matrix synthesis. Parathormone and estradiol are also effective stimuli for osteoblastic IGF-I production.

The current view of the relationship between GH and IGF-I is that GH stimulates IGF-I production in liver and epiphyseal growth plate. Hepatic production of IGF-I stimulates circumferential growth of bone and acts primarily as a negative feedback regulator of GH secretion.

Receptors for IGFs

Two receptors have been identified for the IGFs. The IGF-I receptor is remarkably similar to the insulin receptor and signals in a similar manner (tyrosine kinase activity). It binds IGF-I with greater affinity than IGF-II. The IGF-II receptor binds IGF-II with a very much higher affinity than IGF-I.

Pattern of GH Secretion

As is typical of anterior pituitary hormones, GH secretion is pulsatile. Frequent bursts of secretion occur throughout the day, with the largest being associated with the early hours of sleep. Pulsatility appears to be the result of intermittent secretion of both GHRH and somatostatin (Fig. 9.27).

GH secretion is most active during the adolescent growth spurt but persists throughout lifelong after the epiphyses have fused and growth has stopped. With age, the daily rate of secretion gradually decreases in both men and women.

Stimuli that affect growth hormone secretion	
Increase GH	*Decrease GH*
Hypoglycemia	Glucose
Exercise	Cortisol
Fasting	FFA
Certain amino acids	Growth hormone
Sleep	
Stressful stimuli	
Estrogens and androgens	

Regulation of GH Secretion

1. Growth hormone-releasing hormone (GHRH, somatoliberin) by hypothalamic neurons. GHRH activates adenylyl cyclase through a typical Gs-linked mechanism.
2. *Somatostatin (growth hormone-inhibiting hormone: GHIH, SST)* reduces or blocks the response of the pituitary to GHRH-induced secretion.
3. *Ghrelin:* Ghrelin is primarily produced by the stomach but is also expressed in the hypothalamus. It acts via the IP_3-DAG second messenger system and brings about release of calcium from intracellular stores in response to IP_3. Ghrelin is involved in the regulation of food intake; it increases appetite and may serve as a signal to coordinate nutrient acquisition with growth.

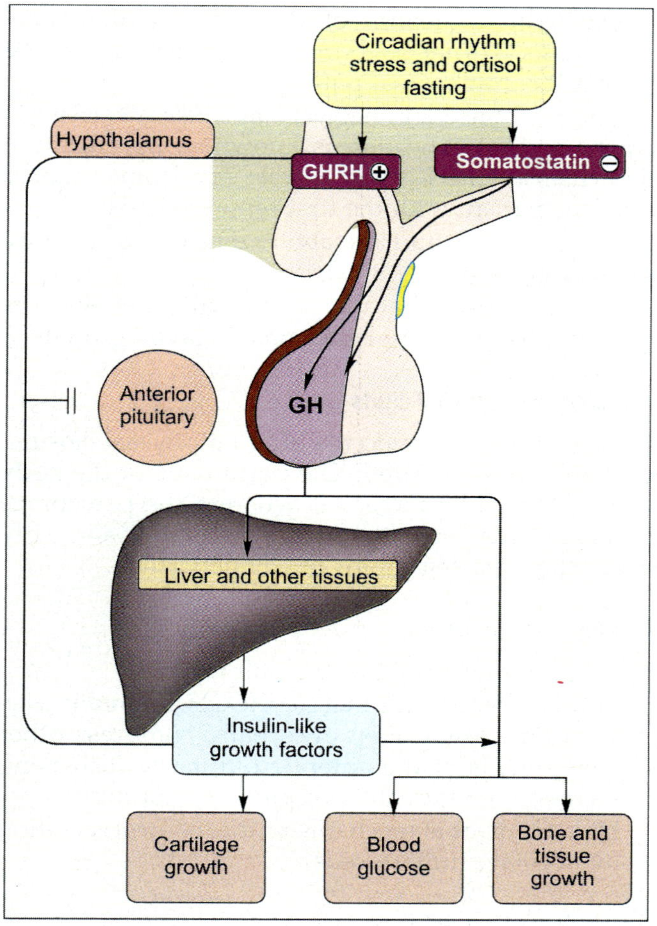

Fig. 9.27: Action of growth hormone

Physiology of Growth

Growth is a complex phenomenon affected by:

- Genetic factors
- Nutrition
- *Hormones:* Growth hormone, thyroid hormones, insulin, androgens, estrogens and glucocorticoids.

Growth involves an orderly sequence of maturational changes with accumulation of protein that manifests as an increase in length and size. In humans, there are two periods of rapid growth: the first in infancy and the second in late puberty.

The first period of accelerated growth is partly a continuation of the fetal growth period. Growth *in utero* is independent of fetal growth hormone. The second growth spurt, at the time of puberty, is due to growth hormone, androgens and estrogens. Estrogens then bring about epiphyseal closure and linear growth ceases. Thyroid hormones appear to have a permissive effect on the actions of growth hormone and are necessary for a normal rate of growth hormone secretion. Insulin stimulates protein synthesis from amino acids entering the cells and inhibits protein degradation, thereby fostering growth. Maximum insulin-induced growth is present only when a high-carbohydrate diet is supplied. Glucocorticoids are potent inhibitors of growth because of their direct action on cells and also inhibit secretion of growth hormone; however, they 'permit' growth in the sense that their effects on blood pressure and circulation are necessary to achieve normal growth.

Applied Aspects

Pituitary Dwarfism

Isolated GH Deficiency

Pituitary dwarfism is the failure of growth that results from lack of GH during childhood. Pituitary dwarfs typically are of normal weight and length at birth and grow rapidly and nearly normally during early infancy. Before the end of the first year, however, growth is noticeably below the normal rate. Left untreated, they may reach heights of around 4 feet. Individuals with this condition have normal intelligence. Typically, the pituitary dwarf retains a juvenile appearance because of the loss of GH-induced lipolysis and the disproportionately small size of maxillary and mandibular bones.

Panhypopituitarism

If the deficiency in GH is accompanied by deficiencies in other anterior pituitary hormones, the following features are present:

- The individuals do not mature sexually and remain infertile as the gonadotropins are deficient.
- Hypogonadism is manifested by amenorrhea in women, impotence in men and loss of libido in both men and women.
- TSH deficiency leads to hypothyroidism; some of the typical clinical manifestations are cold, dry skin, constipation, hoarseness and bradycardia.
- Adrenal insufficiency caused by the ACTH deficiency can result in weakness, mild postural hypotension, hypoglycemia and a loss of pubic and axillary hair.
- People with panhypopituitarism become particularly sensitive to the actions of insulin because of the decreased secretion of the insulin antagonists, GH and cortisol. They are prone to develop hypoglycemia, particularly when stressed.

- Patients tend to have sallow complexions because of the ACTH deficiency.
- The only symptom associated with the PRL deficiency is the incapacity for postpartum lactation.

Panhypopituitarism might result from:
  - A tumour that either destroys pituitary cells themselves or their connections to the hypothalamus
  - Traumatic injury to the pituitary gland
  - Defects in pituitary development
  - *Pituitary apoplexy:* It results from acute infarction of the pituitary gland due to tumor, trauma or postpartum necrosis. In women who have an episode of shock due to postpartum hemorrhage, the pituitary may become infarcted, with the subsequent development of postpartum necrosis. This condition is called Sheehan's syndrome. The blood supply to the anterior pituitary is vulnerable because it descends on the pituitary stalk through the rigid diaphragma sellae, and during pregnancy the pituitary is enlarged.
- Laron dwarfs are GH resistant because of a genetic defect in the expression of the GH receptor so that response to GH is impaired. Hence, although the serum GH levels are normal to high, they do not produce IGFs in response to GH. Treating patients afflicted by Laron dwarfism (also called growth hormone insensitivity) with GH will not correct the growth deficiency.
- The African pygmy represents another example of abnormal growth. Individuals with this condition have normal serum GH levels, but they do not exhibit the normal rise in IGF that occurs at puberty. They also may have a partial defect in GH receptors because IGF-I levels do not rise normally after GH is administered. Unlike the Laron dwarfs, they do not totally lack the IGF response to GH.

Other Causes of Dwarfism

Achondroplasia is the most common form of dwarfism. It is characterized by short limbs with a normal trunk. It is an autosomal dominant condition, caused by a mutation in the gene that codes for fibroblast growth factor receptor 3. This receptor is normally expressed in cartilage and the brain.

As thyroid hormones have widespread effects on the ossification of cartilage, the growth of teeth and proportions of the body, cretins are dwarfed and have infantile features.

Dwarfism is a feature of the syndrome of gonadal dysgenesis (Turner's syndrome) seen in patients who have XO chromosomal pattern.

Chronic abuse and neglect can cause dwarfism in children. This condition is known as psychosocial dwarfism or the Kaspar-Hauser syndrome, named after the patient with the first reported case.

Various bone and metabolic diseases also cause stunted growth.

In many cases there is no known cause and the condition is called 'constitutional delayed growth'.

GH Deficiency in Adults

If the GH deficiency occurs after epiphyseal closure, growth is not impaired. The percentage of the body weight that is fat increases, whereas the percentage that is protein decreases. Muscle weakness and early exhaustion are symptoms of GH deficiency.

GH Hypersecretion

Hypersecretion of GH may result from:

- Pituitary tumor cells that secrete GH autonomously. Tumour growth may eventually compress other components of the anterior pituitary, decreasing secretion of other anterior pituitary hormones.
- Derangement in mechanisms that control secretion by normal pituitary cells.

Gigantism (Fig. 9.28a)

Overproduction of GH before puberty results in gigantism. In this condition, an adult height in excess of 8 feet can be reached. Body weight is also increased.

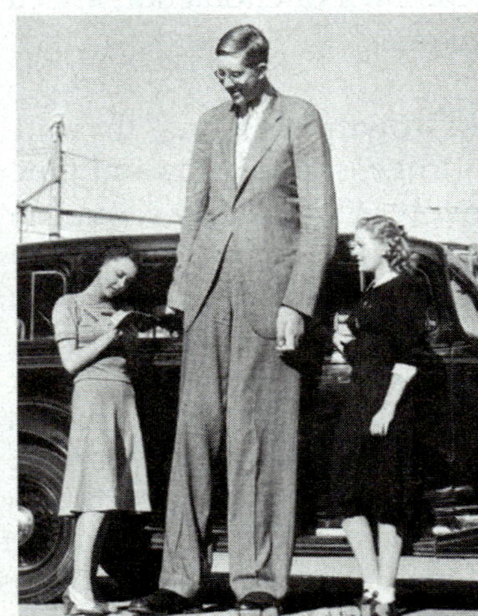

Fig. 9.28a

9

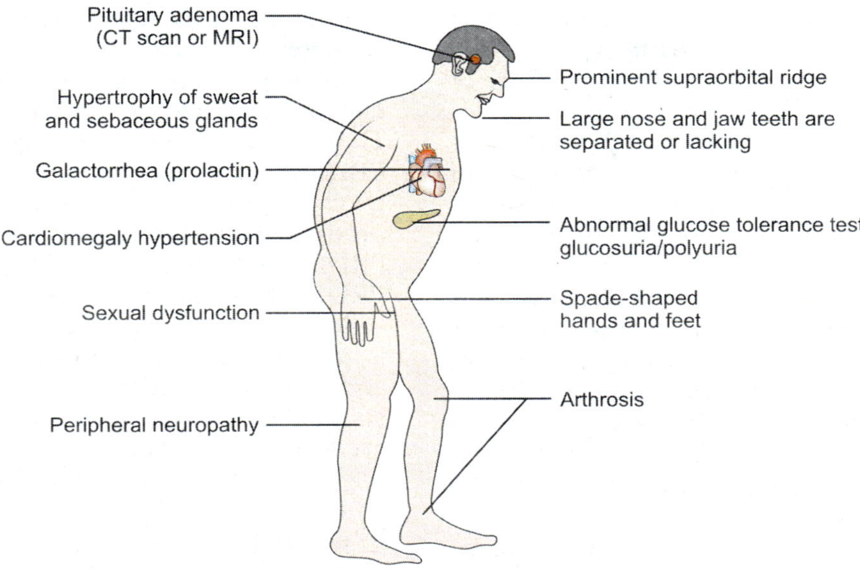

Fig. 9.28b: Acromegaly

Glucose intolerance and hyperinsulinism are frequent. Overt clinical diabetes can develop. There are cardiovascular problems including cardiac hypertrophy. All viscera increase in size (visceromegaly). There is increased susceptibility to infections than normal; and individuals rarely live past their 20s. People with gigantism eventually exhibit acromegaly if the condition is not corrected before puberty.

Acromegaly (Figs 9.28b and c)

Overproduction of GH during adulthood, after the growth plates of long bones have fused, produces growth only by stimulation of osteoblastic progenitor cells in the periosteum (appositional growth) and linear growth does not occur. Cartilage and membranous bones continue to grow and gross deformities can result.

There is thickening of the cranium and mandible: with the mandibular enlargement producing prognathism (protrusion of the lower jaw) and widely spaced teeth: as well as enlargement of the nose, ears and some facial bones. The calvarium thickens and the frontal sinuses enlarge, resulting in protrusion of the frontal ridge of the orbit of the eye. Overgrowth of the frontal and facial bones combines with prognathism to produce the coarse facial features called acromegalic facies. Enlargement of the hands and feet is the basis for the name acromegaly (acro = end or extremity, megaly = enlargement) to describe this condition. The excessive bone and cartilage growth can produce

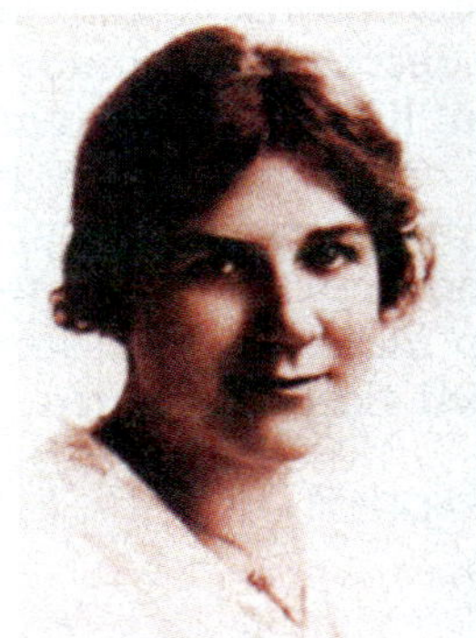
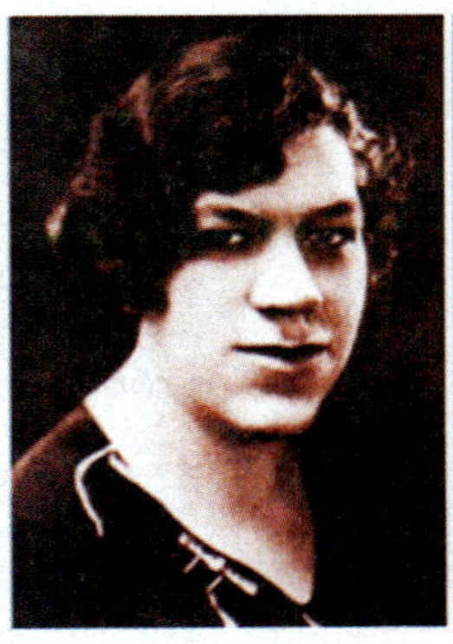
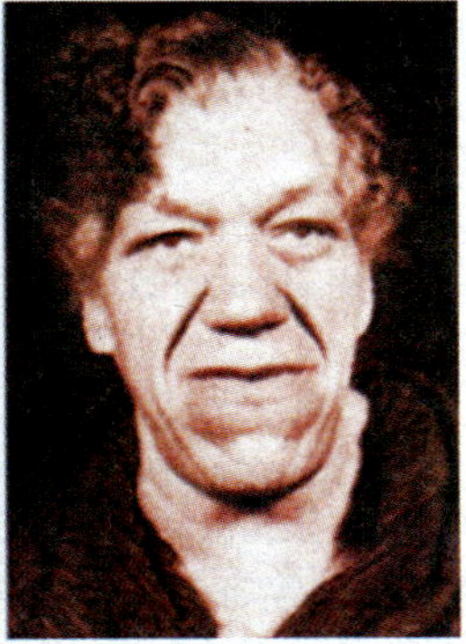

Fig. 9.28c: Acromegaly

carpal tunnel syndrome and joint problems. The skeletal changes predispose to osteoarthritis. The voice deepens because of laryngeal growth. Persistence of responsive cartilage progenitor cells in the costochondral junctions leads to elongation of the ribs to give a typical barrel-chested appearance. In addition, soft tissue growth increases and the abdomen protrudes as a result of visceral enlargement. Body hair is increased in amount (hirsutism).

The protein content of the body is increased and fat content is decreased. Abnormal glucose tolerance/diabetes mellitus is present in 25% of the patients with GH-secreting tumors of the anterior pituitary. Hypersecretion of GH is accompanied by hypersecretion of prolactin in 20 to 40% of patients with acromegaly about 4% of acromegalic patients develop lactation in the absence of pregnancy.

Local effects of the pituitary tumor include enlargement of the sella turcica, headache and visual field disturbances, such as bitemporal hemianopia (defective vision in the temporal halves of the visual fields).

As it is generally slow in onset, patients typically do not seek medical help for 13 to 14 years and by that time they have permanent physical deformities. A person with untreated acromegaly has a shortened life expectancy.

PHYSIOLOGY OF PROLACTIN

Prolactin

Chemistry

Prolactin (PRL) is a 199-amino acid single-chain protein and has considerable structural similarity to human growth hormone and hCS.

9

Receptor and Mechanism of Action

The PRL receptor resembles the GH receptor and belongs to the cytokine receptor superfamily. Therefore, PRL acts through a JAK/STAT signaling pathway.

Transport

PRL circulates unbound to serum proteins and thus has a relatively short half-life of about 20 minutes.

Actions

- During pregnancy, PRL levels increase steadily until term and under the influence of this hormone plus the high levels of estrogens and progesterone, full lobuloalveolar development of the breasts takes place.
- PRL causes milk secretion from the breast after estrogen and progesterone priming. After expulsion of the placenta at parturition, there is an abrupt decline in circulating estrogens and progesterone. The drop in circulating estrogen initiates lactation. PRL and estrogen synergize in producing breast growth but estrogen antagonizes the milk-producing effect of PRL on the breast. In addition, PRL facilitates the maternal behavior.
- PRL inhibits GnRH secretion and antagonizes the action of gonadotropins on the ovaries. Ovulation is inhibited, and the ovaries are inactive, so estrogen and progesterone output falls to low levels. Nursing stimulates PRL secretion; consequently, nursing is associated with lactational amenorrhea, which refers to cessation of menstrual periods in women who frequently and regularly nurse a baby. This effect of prolactin has been called "nature's contraceptive" and hence, nursing is a natural but unreliable method of birth control.
- The function of PRL in normal males is unsettled but hyperprolactinemia in men is associated with impotence and hypogonadism that disappear when PRL secretion is reduced.

Control of Secretion

PRL is unique among the anterior pituitary hormones in that its release is normally under tonic inhibition by the hypothalamus. This is exerted by dopaminergic tracts that secrete dopamine (prolactin-inhibiting hormone, PIH) at the median eminence. The cell bodies of these dopaminergic neurons are located in the arcuate nuclei. Dopamine binds to the D_2 receptor, which is linked to a Gi signaling pathway.

Lactotropes increase in size and number during pregnancy. The human pituitary enlarges two to three-folds in volume during pregnancy. The increase in lactotropes is due to stimulation by placental estrogen in response to estrogens.

PRL is secreted continuously at low basal rates throughout life, regardless of sex.

PRL is one of the many hormones released in response to stress. Surgery, fear, stimuli causing arousal and exercise are all effective stimuli. As with GH, sleep increases PRL secretion and PRL has a pronounced sleep-associated diurnal rhythm.

Applied Aspects

Hyperprolactinemia

The prolactinoma (PRL-secreting tumor) is the most common form of hormone-secreting pituitary tumor.

Hyperprolactinemia in women is associated with oligomenorrhea or amenorrhea and infertility. GnRH release, the gonadotrope response to GnRH and the ovarian response to LH all decrease. The hypogonadism produced by prolactinomas is associated with osteoporosis due to estrogen deficiency.

Hyperprolactinemia can produce infertility in men. While breast enlargement can occur, true gynecomastia (inappropriate growth of mammary glandular tissue) and galactorrhea (inappropriate flow of milk) are rare.

As PRL synthesis and secretion is predominantly under inhibitory control by the hypothalamus, disruption of the pituitary stalk and the hypothalamo-hypophyseal portal vessels (e.g. due to surgery or physical trauma) results in an increase in PRL levels.

Chiari-Frommel Syndrome

This is a rare condition in which there is persistence of lactation (galactorrhea) and amenorrhea in women who do not nurse after delivery. It is due to persistent prolactin secretion without the secretion of the FSH and LH necessary to produce maturation of new follicles and ovulation.

Prolactin Deficiency

The only pathologic problem known to be associated with a deficiency in PRL secretion is the inability to initiate postpartum lactation.

POSTERIOR PITUITARY HORMONES

Introduction

The posterior pituitary and the hypothalamus together form a neuroendocrine system. The cell bodies of the neurons that secrete the two posterior pituitary hormones, vasopressin and oxytocin, are located in the supraoptic and paraventricular nuclei of the hypothalamus. These magnocellular neurons project axons down the infundibular stalk as the hypothalamohypophyseal tract to end on capillaries in the posterior lobe. The posterior pituitary is thus made up of axon terminals of the hypothalamic neurons and supportive cells called pituicytes, which are modified astrocytes.

The magnocellular neurons in the supraoptic nuclei (SON) appear to be the major source of vasopressin, whereas cells in the paraventricular nuclei (PVN) may be the principal source of oxytocin. These neurohormones are packaged in secretory vesicles and transported by molecular motors down the axons in the infundibular stalk to the neuronal terminals in the posterior pituitary where they are stored until there is appropriate stimulation for release.

When a stimulatory input reaches the SON and PVN nuclei, primarily in the form of neurotransmitters released from hypothalamic interneurons, the neurons depolarize and propagate action potentials down the axons. At the axonal terminals, the action potentials trigger Ca^{2+}-dependent exocytosis of the secretory vesicles, releasing the hormones into the extracellular fluid of the posterior pituitary (Fig. 9.29).

Chemistry and Synthesis of ADH and Oxytocin

ADH and oxytocin are nanopeptides (nine amino acids) that differ by only two amino acids. Like other peptide hormones, they are synthesized on ribosomes as preprohormones called preprovasophysin and prepro-oxyphysin in the cell bodies of the hypothalamic neurons. Each preprohormone is composed of the nanopeptide hormone and a cosecreted peptide called neurophysin-neurophysin I (associated with ADH) or neurophysin II (associated with oxytocin).

Post-translational processing involves removal of the leader sequences in the endoplasmic reticulum and the prohormone is packaged in a membrane-bound secretory vesicle in the Golgi apparatus along with the enzymes that cleave it into the final secretory product. During the intra-axonal transit of the secretory vesicle, the prohormones are proteolytically cleaved, producing equimolar amounts of hormone and neurophysin. The neurophysins are cosecreted with ADH or oxytocin, but have no known hormonal actions. Secretory vesicles containing the fully

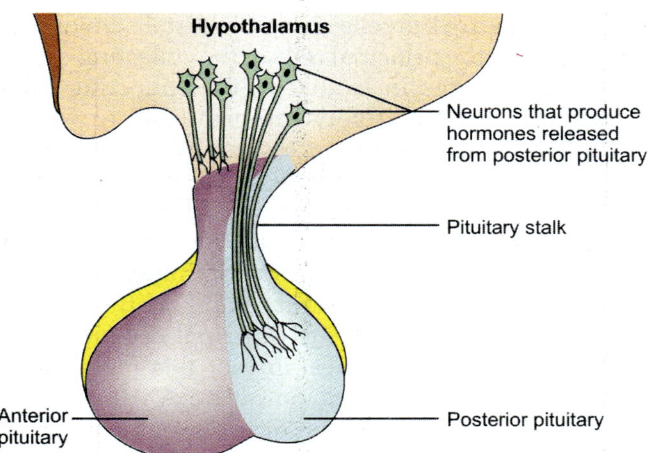

Fig. 9.29: Hypothalamohypophyseal tract

processed peptides are stored in the axonal termini of the posterior lobe.

Because the human hormone has an arginine in position 8 instead of the lysine found in the hormone that was originally isolated from pigs, it is called arginine vasopressin (AVP).

VASOPRESSIN

Transport

ADH circulates unbound.

Metabolism

Because of its small size, ADH is readily filtered at the glomerulus, but it is taken up by proximal tubule cells that degrade it to its constituent amino acids. It is also metabolized in the liver. The biologic half-life of ADH is approximately 15 to 20 minutes.

Vasopressin Receptors

There are three kinds of vasopressin receptors: V_{1A}, V_{1B} and V_2. All are G protein-coupled receptors (GPCR). V_2 is the receptor in the distal nephron and V_{1A} mediates the action of ADH on vascular smooth muscle. V_{1B} receptors (also called V_3 receptors) appear to be unique to the anterior pituitary, where they mediate increased ACTH secretion form the corticotropes.

Actions of ADH

The two actions of vasopressin are:

1. *Increased reabsorption of water in the kidney (antidiuretic effect):* This effect is of primary importance in the maintenance of normal water balance. The target cells are the cells lining the distal convoluted tubule and the principal cells of the collecting ducts. When vasopressin is absent, the collecting duct epithelium is relatively impermeable to water. ADH binds to the vasopressin 2 (V_2) receptor on the basolateral membranes of the renal cells. V_2 receptor is a G protein-coupled receptor (GPCR). Signaling from the V_2 receptor induces the rapid translocation of endosomes containing the water channel protein, called aquaporin 2, to the apical/luminal membrane of the principal cells, thereby increasing water permeability of this membrane. The effect is mediated via cyclic AMP, protein kinase A and a molecular motor, one of the dyneins. ADH also increases the gene expression and new synthesis of aquaporin 2. The overall effect is retention of water in excess of solute; consequently, the osmolarity of the body fluids is decreased. Therefore, in the absence of ADH, urine flow increases (diuresis).
2. *Contraction of arteriolar smooth muscle (pressor effect):* This effect only has a minor role in the normal regulation of blood pressure. In severe volume depletion, ADH levels increase to supra-physiological levels. At these levels, ADH binds to the V_{1A} receptor on vascular smooth muscle and increases vascular smooth muscle contraction.

Regulation of ADH Secretion (Fig. 9.30)

ADH secretion is stimulated by:

1. *Increased osmolarity of the ECF, which is detected by osmoreceptors in the anterior hypothalamus:* They are located in the circumventricular organs, primarily the organum vasculosum of the lamina terminalis, and are outside the blood-brain barrier. Osmoreceptive neurons innervate the magno-cellular neurons of the PVN and SON. When the plasma osmolarity rises, the osmoreceptor cells shrink. This serves as a signal for increased firing of nerve fibers running from the hypothalamic nuclei through the pituitary stalk to the posterior pituitary. This regulatory system is sensitive to serum osmolarity changes in the range between 280 and 295 mOsm/kg.
2. *Decreased circulating blood volume and pressure, as detected by low-pressure volume receptors, predominantly*

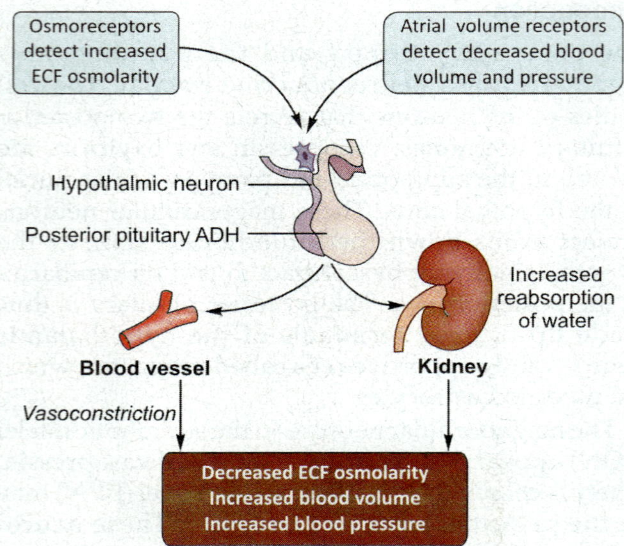

Fig. 9.30: Stimuli for ADH secretion and its actions

the atrial volume receptors: A fall in atrial pressure initiates a reflex release of ADH from the hypothalamus. The information is relayed via afferent neurons in the vagus to the nucleus of the tractus solitarius (NTS) and hence to the hypothalamus. ADH reduces fluid loss at the kidneys, which in-turn increases the blood volume. Haemorrhage is a potent stimulus for vasopressin secretion, when circulating blood volume decreases about 10% or more.

Other Factors Altering ADH Secretion

- Alcohol is an effective suppressor of ADH secretion. The hormones, atrial natriuretic peptide (ANP) and cortisol inhibit ADH secretion.
- Pain, surgical stress and some emotions increase vasopressin secretion.
- Nausea is associated with particularly large increases in ADH secretion.
- Angiotensin II increases vasopressin secretion by acting on the circumventricular organs.

Regulation of Thirst

Thirst is regulated by many of the same factors that regulate ADH secretion. Increased serum osmolarity, decreased vascular volume and ADH secretion are effective stimuli for thirst. Osmoreceptors are also located in the lateral preoptic hypothalamus near the SON. This area is referred to as the hypothalamic thirst center. Thirst and the associated drinking behavior come about when these osmoreceptors are stimulated by high plasma osmolarity. The receptors are stimulated most effectively by increases in the Na^+ concentration of plasma. Angiotensin II is also thought to play a major role in the regulation of thirst.

Applied Aspects

Diabetes Insipidus (DI)

DI is the syndrome that results when there is a vasopressin deficiency or when the kidneys fail to respond to the hormone. The word diabetes derives from the Greek meaning "passing through". It is used to describe the condition of passing large amounts of dilute urine (polyuria). The word insipidus refers to the fact that in this affliction the urine tastes bland or insipid. People with DI are unable to concentrate urine normally and therefore, excrete a large volume of urine. These individuals can have urinary flow rates as high as 25 liters/day. Thirst increases as a result of the dehydration caused by the high urinary flow and they drink large amounts of fluid (polydipsia).

Types of DI

- Neurogenic (pituitary-hypothalamic) diabetes insipidus. It is due to:
  - Destruction of the hypothalamus (e.g. by hypothalamic tumors)
  - Destruction of the pars nervosa (e.g. by metastatic disease, post-trauma)
  - Mutations in the preprovasophysin gene. People with neurogenic DI have a high urine volume and a low urinary osmolarity and high plasma osmolarity with inappropriately low ADH levels. If ADH is administered, they respond with a decrease in urinary volume and an increase in urinary osmolarity.
- Nephrogenic diabetes insipidus: Those with nephrogenic DI have normal ADH production but lack a normal renal ADH response. The two primary defects in congenital nephrogenic DI are:
  - Mutations in the V_2 receptor (an X-linked recessive condition because the V_2 gene is on the X chromosome)
  - Mutations in the autosomal gene for aquaporin 2, producing nonfunctional versions of this water channel.

  Blood ADH levels are normal or elevated in patients with nephrogenic DI and administration of exogenous ADH analogs does not decrease the urinary flow rate.
- *Psychogenic diabetes insipidus:* Those with this condition are compulsive water drinkers. If water is withheld, the ADH secretion increases and urinary flow decreases while osmolarity increases.
- *Syndrome of inappropriate hypersecretion of antidiuretic hormone (SIADH):* Many disorders can produce this syndrome: It is often an association with trauma, anesthesia and pain. Some neoplasms produce ADH. This is particularly common with pulmonary carcinomas.

In SIADH, falling serum osmolarity does not inhibit ADH secretion because control of ADH secretion is no longer linked to the normal regulatory mechanisms. With normal water consumption, water is retained because of the inappropriately high ADH levels. The resultant increase in blood volume and pressure increases renal glomerular filtration and therefore, increases the loss of sodium in urine. The hypervolemia stimulates release of ANP, which promotes renal sodium loss. The person consequently becomes hyponatremic and has a low serum osmolarity. The urine osmolarity is inappropriately high. If water is restricted in an individual with SIADH, serum sodium and osmolarity will return to normal. Patients with SIADH have been successfully treated with demeclocycline, an antibiotic that reduces the renal response to vasopressin.

Synthetic Agonists and Antagonists

- Desmopressin, a synthetic agonist, has very high antidiuretic activity with little pressor activity, making it valuable in the treatment of vasopressin deficiency.
- Antagonists that selectively block the V_2 receptors are used as diuretics.

OXYTOCIN

Metabolism

Like ADH, oxytocin circulates unbound. It has a relatively short $t_{1/2}$ of 3 to 5 minutes. Its degradation occurs primarily in the liver and kidney.

Actions of Oxytocin

The major actions of oxytocin are on:
- Uterine motility
- Milk release

Uterine motility: Oxytocin stimulates contraction of the myometrium. Estrogens increase the uterine response to oxytocin by stimulating the synthesis of oxytocin receptors while progestins decrease the response by direct action on the uterine oxytocin receptors. In late pregnancy, estrogen levels rise and oxytocin receptor synthesis increases, increasing uterine sensitivity to oxytocin. In early labor, the uterine contractions cause dilation of the cervix and descent of the fetus down the birth canal initiates impulses in the afferent nerves that are relayed to the SON and PVN causing oxytocin release, which enhances labor. This is a neuroendocrine reflex, which has a positive feedback nature: Increasing labor contractions stretch the cervix further, stimulating more oxytocin release, increasing labor contractions and so on. The positive feedback loop terminates on expulsion of the products of conception.

Oxytocin increases uterine contractions in two ways:
- It acts directly on uterine smooth muscle cells to make them contract.
- It stimulates the formation of prostaglandins in the decidua (the endometrium of pregnancy). The prostaglandins enhance the oxytocin-induced contractions (Fig. 9.31).

Milk "Let-Down" or milk ejection reflex: In this neuroendocrine reflex, suckling or tactile stimulation activates touch receptors located in the nipple and areola of the breast. Impulses generated in these receptors are relayed from the somatic touch pathways to the hypothalamic magnocellular neurons which results in release of a pulse of oxytocin from the posterior pituitary. Oxytocin stimulates contraction of the myoepithelial cells, smooth-muscle-like cells surrounding the mammary gland alveoli. Oxytocin receptors on these cells cause contraction through a Gq-phospholipase C signaling pathway that ultimately increases intracellular Ca^{2+}. Contraction of myoepithelial cells squeezes the milk out of the alveoli into the larger ducts and sinuses of the gland and hence out of

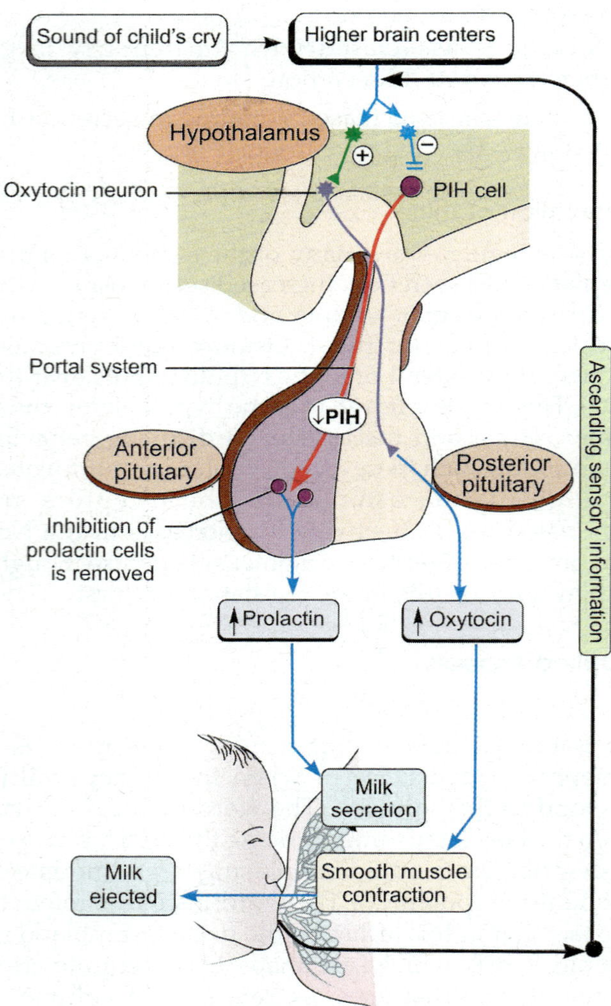

Fig. 9.31: Milk ejection reflex and reflex milk secretion

the nipple (milk ejection). Thus, the nursing infant does not gain milk by applying negative pressure to the breast from suckling. Rather, milk is actively ejected through a neuroendocrine reflex. In lactating women, psychogenic stimuli, such as the sound of a baby crying or thinking about the baby, also produce oxytocin secretion, sometimes causing milk to spurt from the breasts.

Milk must be removed regularly by suckling for continued lactation. Failure to empty the mammary alveoli causes lactation to stop within about a week and the lobuloalveolar structures to involute. Involution results partly from prolactin withdrawal. Thus, suckling triggers two neuroendocrine reflexes critical for the maintenance of lactation: the milk let-down reflex and surges of prolactin secretion.

Other Actions

Nonpregnant Women

Oxytocin may also act on the nonpregnant uterus to facilitate sperm transport.

The increased release of oxytocin during intercourse in women may aid the passage of sperm up the female genital tract to the uterine tubes, where fertilization normally takes place, by initiating specialized uterine contractions.

In Men

Circulating oxytocin increases at the time of ejaculation in males, and it is possible that this increase causes increased contraction of the smooth muscle of the vas deferens, propelling sperm toward the urethra.

Applied Aspects

Although a deficiency of oxytocin does not cause major problems, it can prolong labor and produce lactational difficulties as a result of poor milk ejection in some women. No pathologic problems associated with excess levels of oxytocin are known.

77. THYROID GLAND

Introduction

Thyroid hormones are indispensable for the growth and development of an individual and affect physiologic processes occurring in virtually every organ system.

They profoundly increase the metabolic rate of the body; complete lack of thyroid secretion causes the basal metabolic rate to fall about 50% below normal. They are not essential for life but act as modulators governing all the physiologic processes.

Anatomy of the Thyroid (Fig. 9.32)

The thyroid gland is a bilobed structure located at the base of the neck below the larynx and wraps around the trachea just below the cricoid cartilage. The two large lateral lobes that comprise the bulk of the gland lie on either side of the trachea and are connected by a thin bridge of tissue, the isthmus, which extends across the ventral surface of the trachea below the larynx. There is sometimes a third structure, the pyramidal lobe, arising from the isthmus in front of the larynx. The pyramidal lobe may be a remnant of the embryonic thyroglossal duct.

The thyroid gland in the normal human being weighs about 20 g but is capable of enormous growth when stimulated intensely over a long period of time.

Blood Supply and Lymphatics

The thyroid gland is well vascularized; the blood flow expressed as flow rate per gram of tissue exceeds that of the kidney. The gland is also endowed with a rich lymphatic system that may play an important role in delivery of hormone to the general circulation.

Innervation

The gland is innervated by adrenergic fibers from the cervical ganglia and by cholinergic fibers from the vagus. This autonomic innervation regulates blood flow: adrenergic fibers increase and cholinergic fibers decrease blood flow.

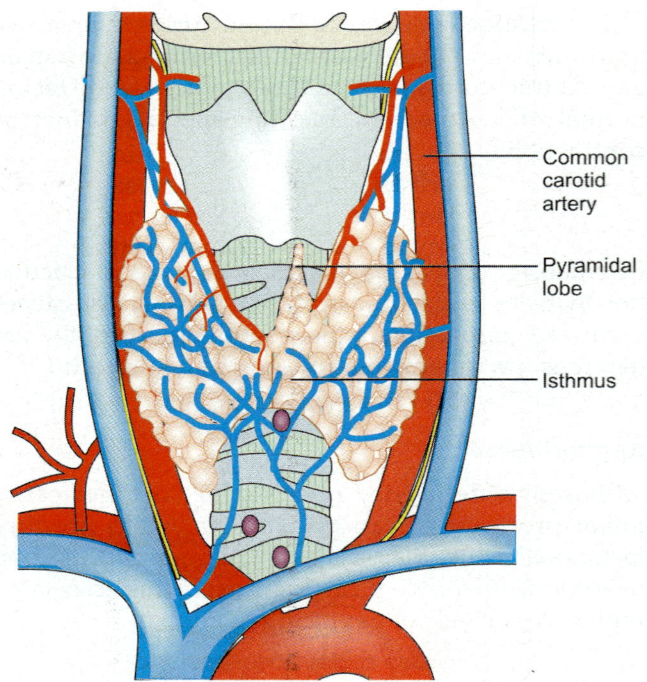

Fig. 9.32: Anatomy of the thyroid gland

Histology

The functional unit of the thyroid gland is the follicle (Fig. 9.33). The adult human thyroid gland has about 3 million follicles. Each follicle (acinus) is formed by a single layer of epithelial cells called follicular cells arranged as hollow vesicles. The height of the follicular cells is greatest when their activity is highest. These cells are squamous in an inactive gland, cuboidal in a normal gland and columnar in a highly stimulated gland.

9

A clear viscous material called colloid is found in the lumen. Colloid is the glycoprotein thyroglobulin (TG), which contains the molecular structure of the thyroid hormones. An inactive gland has large follicles and abundant colloid while an active gland has small follicles and the edge of the colloid is scalloped, forming many small "reabsorption lacunae". Microvilli project into the colloid from the apices of the follicular cells and canaliculi extend into them.

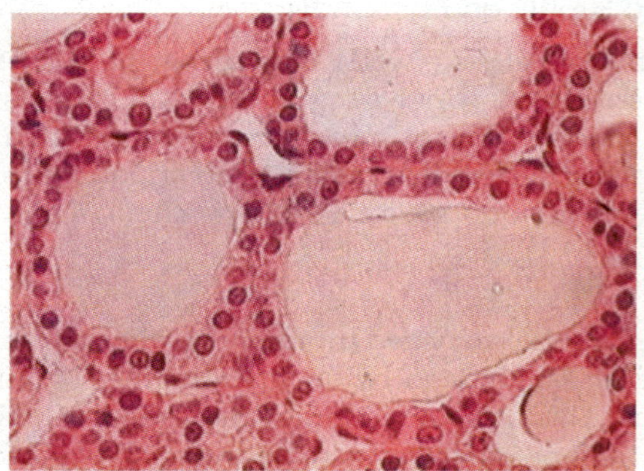

Fig. 9.33: Thyroid follicles (400 X)

In the stroma around the follicles are the parafollicular "light" or "C" cells that produce calcitonin.

Embryology

The thyroid originates from an evagination of the floor of the pharynx and a thyroglossal duct marking the path of the thyroid from the tongue to the neck sometimes persists in the adult. Follicular cells are derived from endoderm of the primitive pharynx.

Thyroid Hormones

Chemistry

The thyroid hormones are derivatives of tyrosine. Tyrosine is iodinated and two iodinated tyrosine molecules are coupled in an ether linkage.

The thyroid hormones include:

1. *Thyroxine (T_4 or 3, 5, 3′, 5′-tetraiodothyronine):* It constitutes 90% of the hormone secreted by the gland. The naturally occurring forms of T_4 are the L-isomers. Thyroxine is not the biologically active form of the hormone but serves as a prohormone. Most of it is eventually transformed to T_3 in the tissues.
2. *Triiodothyronine (T_3 or 3, 5, 3′-triiodothyronine):* T_3 constitutes only about 9% of the hormone secreted by the gland. It is also formed in the peripheral tissues by deiodination of T_4. T_3 is four times more potent than T_4.
3. *Reverse T_3 (rT_3 or 3, 3′, 5′-triiodothyronine):* This represents about 1% of the hormone secreted by the gland and is biologically inactive.

Synthesis of Thyroid Hormones (Fig. 9.34)

The steps in the biosynthesis of thyroid hormones are as follows:

1. Thyroglobulin synthesis and secretion into follicular lumen
2. Iodide trapping
3. Oxidation of iodide
4. Organification of thyroglobulin
5. Coupling reactions

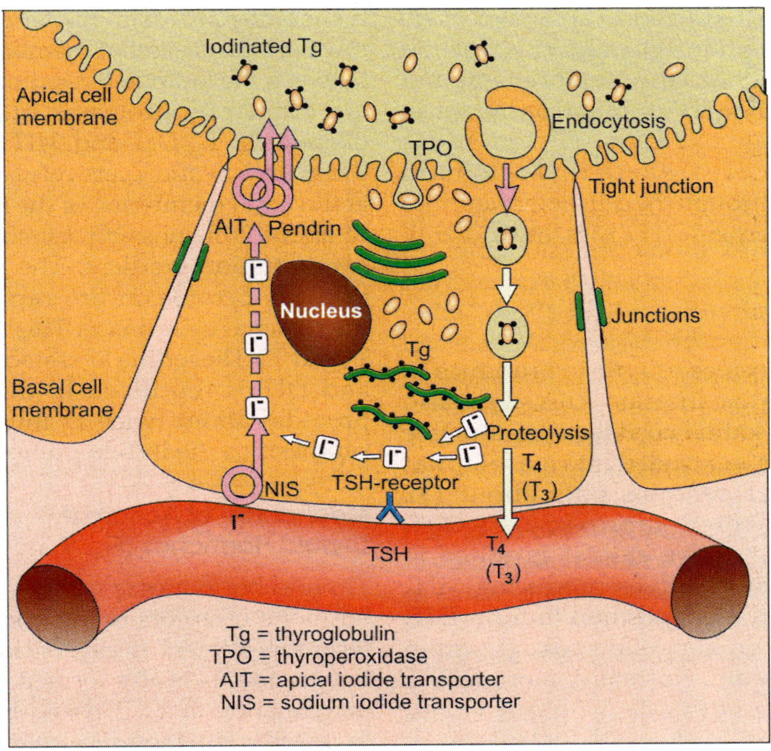

Fig. 9.34: Synthesis of thyroid hormone

6. Endocytosis and proteolysis of thyroglobulin to release free T_3 and T_4.

Thyroglobulin Synthesis and Secretion

TG is a large glycoprotein that serves as a matrix for thyroid hormone synthesis and is the form in which thyroid hormones are stored in the gland. It has a molecular mass of 660 kDa. Like other proteins in the cell, TG is synthesized on the rough endoplasmic reticulum of the follicular cell, glycosylated and translocated to the Golgi apparatus and then packaged in secretory vesicles that discharge it from the apical surface into the lumen of the follicle. The vesicles also contain thyroid peroxidase, the enzyme that catalyzes the steps in thyroid hormone synthesis.

Iodide Trapping

Iodine is a trace element essential for thyroid hormone synthesis. Ingested iodine is converted to iodide and absorbed into the bloodstream. The thyroid follicles have an efficient transport mechanism for selectively trapping iodide against its electrochemical gradient. The iodide pump is located in the basilar membrane of the follicular cell facing the capillaries. It is a Na^+/I^- symporter (NIS) that transports two Na^+ with each I^- into the cells. The secondary active transport of I^- is driven by the favorable electrochemical gradient for sodium. Energy is provided by the sodium potassium ATPase. Normally, the iodide pump concentrates the iodide to about 30 times its concentration in blood. When maximally active, it can raise this concentration ratio to even 250 times.

Iodide that enters at the basolateral surfaces of the follicular cell must be delivered to the follicular lumen where hormone biosynthesis takes place. Iodide diffuses throughout the follicular cell and exits from the apical membrane by way of a sodium-independent iodide transporter called pendrin.

The minimum daily iodine intake that will maintain normal thyroid function is 150 μg in adults. To prevent iodine deficiency, common table salt is iodized with about 1 part sodium iodide to every 100,000 parts sodium chloride.

Oxidation of Iodide

In order for iodination of the tyrosine residues of TG to occur, iodine must first be converted to some higher oxidized state. Iodide is oxidized to an active intermediate, either nascent iodine (IO) or I_3^-. This reaction is catalyzed by a thyroid-specific membrane-bound enzyme, thyroid peroxidase (TPO), found on the apical surface of the follicular cell. Thus, TPO provides oxidized iodine at the area where thyroglobulin molecule is exocytosed through the cell membrane into the colloid. Hydrogen peroxide (H_2O_2) is the oxidizing agent.

Organification (Iodination of Tyrosine)

Addition of iodine molecules to tyrosine residues in thyroglobulin is called organification. This step is also catalyzed by TPO. TG is iodinated at the apical surface of the follicular cells as it is extruded into the follicular lumen. Each TG dimer contains only about 132 tyrosine residues of which approximately 20% residues are iodinated. "Active iodide" is added to the 3 position of tyrosine residues producing MIT. MIT is next iodinated in the 5 position to form DIT. Both MIT and DIT remain in peptide linkage within the thyroglobulin molecule. Normally, more DIT is formed than MIT.

Coupling Reactions

This is the final stage of thyroxine biosynthesis. Only 20% of the iodinated tyrosine residues undergo coupling, with the rest remaining as MIT and DIT. Two DITs are coupled to form T_4 (an oxidative condensation) within the peptide chain. T_3 is formed by condensation of one MIT with one DIT. TPO also catalyzes the coupling reactions. After coupling is complete, there is about 10 times more T_4 than T_3 in TG, and only traces of rT_3, formed by condensation of DIT with MIT.

9

Endocytosis and Proteolysis of Thyroglobulin to Release Free T_3 and T_4

The thyroid hormones remain stored as part of the TG molecule in the lumen of the follicle until lysosomal enzymes set them free during the secretory process. In the normal individual, the thyroid gland stores about 2–3 months supply of hormone in the colloid.

On stimulation with TSH, pseudopodia reach out from the apical surfaces of follicular cells to surround the colloid in endocytic vesicles. This chewing away at the edge of the colloid produces the reabsorption lacunae seen in active follicles. In the cells, the membrane-bound endocytic vesicles merge with lysosomes to form lysoendosomes that migrate towards the basement membrane. The peptide bonds between the iodinated residues and the thyroglobulin are broken by proteases in the lysoendosomes to liberate T_4, T_3, DIT and MIT into the cytoplasm. Of these, only T_4 and T_3 are released into the bloodstream at the basal membrane of the follicular cells, in a ratio of about 20:1, possibly by simple diffusion down a concentration gradient. The DIT and MIT liberated into the cytoplasm are rapidly deiodinated by a microsomal deiodinase. This enzyme does not attack T_4 and T_3. The iodine liberated by deiodination of MIT and DIT is reutilized in the gland and normally provides about twice as much iodide for hormone synthesis as the iodide pump does.

Mechanism of Action of Thyroid Hormones (Fig. 9.35)

Thyroid hormones enter cells and T_3 binds to thyroid hormone receptors in the nuclei. T_4 also binds to the receptors but less avidly. Besides the T_3 taken up from the plasma, T_3 is also formed within the target cell by deiodination of T_4. Thyroid hormone receptors bind to specific nucleotide sequences (thyroid response elements or TREs) in the genes that they regulate.

Transport of Thyroid Hormones

More than 99% of thyroid hormone circulating in blood is firmly bound to three plasma proteins:

1. Thyroxine-binding globulin (TBG).
2. Transthyretin (TTR also called thyroxine-binding prealbumin).
- Albumin.

Of these, TBG accounts for more than 70% of the total protein-bound hormone (both T_4 and T_3), though

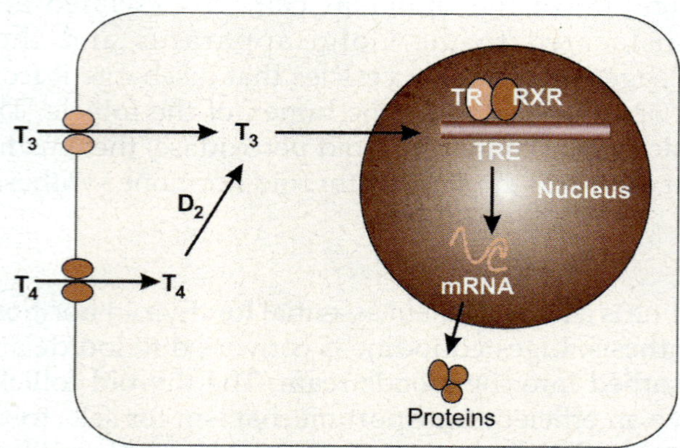

Fig. 9.35: Mechanism of action of thyroid hormone

its plasma concentration is lesser than that of the other proteins. This is so as its affinity for the thyroid hormones is much higher. About 10–15% of circulating T_4 and 10% of circulating T_3 is bound to TTR and nearly equal amounts are bound to albumin. All three binding proteins bind T_4 at least 10 times more avidly than T_3.

Metabolism of Thyroid Hormones

As T_4 is much more tightly bound to plasma proteins than T_3, the half-life of T_4 is six times that of T_3. However, because of the binding proteins, both the hormones have unusually long half-lives in plasma, measured in days: 6 days in the case of T_4 and 1 day in the case of T_3.

T_4 serves as a prohormone and is the precursor for extrathyroidal formation of T_3. 90% of thyroxine is metabolized by sequential deiodination catalyzed by enzymes called deiodinases. Less than 10% of thyroxine is metabolized to produce tetraiodothyroacetic acid (tetrac) and its subsequent deiodination products. The type I deiodinase is expressed mainly in the liver and kidney. It is located in the plasma membrane where it is thought to serve a major role in conversion of T_4 to T_3 before cellular entry. This enzyme is responsible for the majority of the T_4 to T_3 conversion that occurs in circulation. It can also form rT_3 from T_4.

The type II deiodinase is absent in liver but is found in many extrahepatic tissues including the brain, brown fat and pituitary gland where it is thought to produce T_3 to meet local tissue demands, although these tissues can also take up T_3 from the blood. Hormones that act via the cyclic AMP second messenger system, such as the sympathetic neurotransmitter norepinephrine, stimulate type II deiodinase expression.

The type III deiodinase forms only rT_3 and is solely degradative. It is located on the cell membrane and is widely expressed by many tissues throughout the body.

Thyroid hormones are also conjugated with glucuronic acid and excreted in the bile. Intestinal bacteria can split the glucuronide bond and some of the thyroxine liberated can be absorbed and returned to the general circulation. This cycle of excretion in bile and subsequent absorption form the intestine is called enterohepatic circulation. Thyroxine is one of the few naturally occurring hormones that is sufficiently resistant to intestinal and hepatic destruction that it can readily be given by mouth.

Actions of Thyroid Hormone

Effects of Thyroid Hormone on Growth and Maturation

Skeletal System

Although skeletal growth appears to be independent of the thyroid in the fetus, neonatal growth and attainment of normal adult stature require normal amounts of thyroid hormone. Thyroid hormones appear to act synergistically with growth hormone, IGFs and other growth factors that promote bone formation. Maturation of bone results in ossification and eventual fusion of the cartilaginous growth plates.

Central Nervous System

Thyroid hormones are required for normal fetal and neonatal brain development. They regulate neuronal proliferation and differentiation, myelinogenesis and synapse formation.

Effects of Thyroid Hormone on Organ Systems

Autonomic Nervous System

Many actions of excessive thyroid hormone levels resemble those of increased sympathetic nervous system activity. Thyroid hormones increase the number of receptors for epinephrine and norepinephrine (β-adrenergic receptors) in the myocardium and some other tissues.

Skeletal Muscle

- They increase both the content and activity of the electrogenic sodium potassium pump (calorigenic action) and increase the resting membrane potential.
- They increase the rate of calcium uptake in the sarcoplasmic reticulum, thereby increasing calcium availability on stimulation.
- Thyroid hormones also increase myosin ATPase activity.

Cardiovascular System

- Thyroid hormones act directly on the heart to increase the heart rate (chronotropic action), myocardial contractility (inotropic action) and consequently, the cardiac output. These actions can also be mediated by potentiating the effects of sympathetic stimulation. Hyperthyroidism produces myocardial hypertrophy. Peripheral resistance falls when thyroid hormones are in excess for two reasons:

1. Thyroid hormones act directly on vascular smooth muscle to cause vasodilatation.
2. The increased heat and metabolite production results in cutaneous vasodilatation.

- Because cardiac output increases and peripheral resistance decreases, the pulse pressure increases.

Respiratory System

The increase in metabolic rate increases the utilization of oxygen and formation of carbon dioxide increasing the rate and depth of respiration.

Gastrointestinal System

Thyroid hormone increases both the rate of secretion of digestive juices and the motility of the gastrointestinal tract. Therefore, hyperthyroidism often results in diarrhea.

Central Nervous System

Deficiency of thyroid hormone slows down cerebration; somnolence is a characteristic feature of hypothyroidism. Conversely, a hyperthyroid individual is extremely nervous, has difficulty in falling asleep and shows psychoneurotic tendencies, such as paranoia.

Other Endocrine Glands

As thyroxine increases the rate of glucose metabolism, there is a corresponding need for increased insulin secretion.

The acceleration of metabolic activities related to bone formation increases the need for parathormone. Thyroid hormone also increases the rate at which glucocorticoids are inactivated by the liver. This leads to a feedback increase in adrenocorticotropic hormone production by the anterior pituitary and therefore, increased rate of glucocorticoid secretion by the adrenal glands.

Reproductive System

Thyroid hormone is necessary for normal function of the reproductive system. Hypothyroidism is often associated with menorrhagia (excessive menstrual bleeding) and polymenorrhea (frequent menstrual bleeding) and decreased libido in both men and women. Excess thyroid hormone may cause impotence in men and oligomenorrhea (greatly reduced bleeding) in women.

Effect of Thyroid Hormones on Cellular Metabolic Activity

Thyroid hormones increase the metabolic activity of almost all the tissues in the body except brain, testes, uterus, lymph nodes, spleen and anterior pituitary. The rate of utilization of foods for energy is greatly accelerated. Thyroid hormones increase the number and activity of mitochondria in most cells.

Effect of Thyroid Hormones on Metabolic Pathways

Oxidative Metabolism

The basal metabolic rate (BMR), which is a measure of oxygen consumption under defined resting conditions, is highly sensitive to thyroid status: The BMR decreases in hypothyroidism and increases in hyperthyroidism.

Thermogenesis

Splitting of ATP not only energizes cellular processes but also results in heat production. Thyroid hormones are said to be calorigenic because they promote heat (thermogenesis in the newborn) production.

Brown fat is an important source of heat in the newborn. This form of adipose tissue is rich in mitochondria, which give it its unique brown color. Mitochondria in this tissue contain UCP 1 (uncoupling protein 1), sometimes called thermogenin, which allows them to produce heat by oxidation of large amounts of fatty acids. Both T_3 and the sympathetic neurotransmitter norepinephrine can induce the synthesis of UCP 1. In addition, T_3 increases the efficacy of norepinephrine to release fatty acids from stored triglycerides and thus provides fuel for heat production. Brown adipose tissue increases synthesis of the type II deiodinase in response to sympathetic stimulation, and produces abundant T_3 locally to meet its needs. Cold exposure increases TSH secretion from the pituitary and consequently, increases T_4 and T_3 secretion in the newborn but not in adults.

In adults, exposure to cold temperatures increases conversion of T_4 to T_3, probably as a result of increased sympathetic activity which leads to increased cyclic AMP production in various tissues. Cyclic AMP activates expression of the type II deiodinase which is involved in generation of T_3 from T_4 in extrahepatic tissues.

Link: One of the classical signs of hypothyroidism is decreased tolerance to cold, whereas excessive heat production and sweating are seen in hyperthyroidism.

Fuel Metabolism

In general, thyroid hormones stimulate all metabolic pathways, both anabolic and catabolic. This increases the requirement of vitamins to meet the metabolic needs of the body. Thus, a relative vitamin deficiency can occur when excess thyroid hormone is secreted.

Carbohydrate Metabolism

Thyroid hormones accelerate all aspects of carbohydrate metabolism:

- Thyroid hormones increase the rate of glucose absorption from the digestive tract. They increase glycogenolysis and gluconeogenesis in hepatocytes; with hyperthyroidism, glycogen concentration decreases.
- Thyroid hormones increase glycolysis in liver, fat and muscle cells.

Lipid Metabolism

- In general, thyroid hormones are lipolytic and increase hormone-sensitive lipase activity. This action increases the plasma FFA concentration and greatly accelerates the oxidation of FFA by the cells. In hypothyroidism, the percentage of body fat increases over time. Hyperthyroidism results in a decrease in total lipids.
- Thyroid hormones decrease the plasma concentrations of cholesterol, phospholipids and triglycerides. Cholesterol secretion in bile is significantly increased. A possible mechanism for the increased cholesterol secretion is that thyroid hormone induces an increase in the numbers of low-density lipoprotein (LDL) receptors and therefore, more cholesterol is cleared from serum. Serum cholesterol levels increase in hypothyroidism.

Protein Metabolism

Thyroid hormones increase cellular uptake of amino acids and incorporation of these amino acids into protein. In hypothyroidism, protein synthesis decreases and the percentage of body weight that is protein tends to decrease.

Regulation of Thyroid Function (Fig. 9.36)

The principal regulator of thyroid function is the thyroid-stimulating hormone (TSH) secreted by thyrotropes of the pituitary gland.

TSH binds to a G protein-coupled receptor in the basolateral surface membranes of thyroid follicular cells. Binding of the hormone to its receptor results in activation of both adenylyl cyclase through $G\alpha_s$ and phospholipase C through $G\alpha_q$ and leads to increases in both the cyclic AMP and diacylglycerol/IP_3 second messenger pathways.

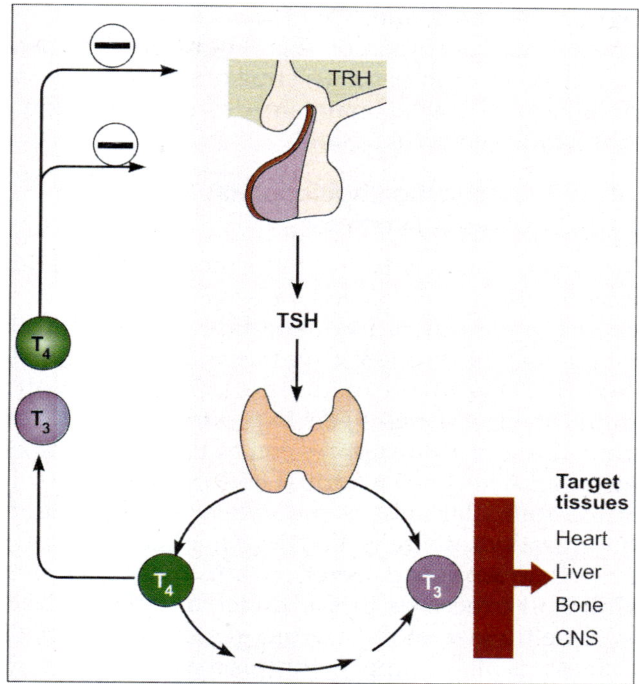

Fig. 9.36: Hypothalamic-pituitary-thyroid axis

Actions of TSH

- TSH regulates all aspects of hormone biosynthesis and secretion. It increases iodide uptake, oxidation of iodide, organification and coupling by increasing expression of the genes for NIS, thyroglobulin and thyroid peroxidase. Endocytosis of colloid and proteolysis of thyroglobulin also increases. Each step of hormone biosynthesis, storage and secretion appears to be accelerated independently of the preceding or following steps in the pathway.
- TSH increases blood flow to the thyroid gland.
- TSH also increases the height of the follicular epithelium (hypertrophy) and can stimulate division of follicular cells (hyperplasia). In the absence of TSH, thyroid cells are quiescent and atrophy.

Secretion of TSH by the pituitary gland is governed by positive input from the hypothalamic hormone thyrotropin-releasing hormone (TRH) and negative input from thyroid hormones. Maintaining constant levels of thyroid hormones in blood depends on the negative feedback effects of T_4 and T_3, which inhibit synthesis and secretion of TSH. High concentrations of thyroid hormones may shut off TSH secretion completely and, when maintained over time, produce atrophy of the thyroid gland.

Role of Iodide in the Regulation of Thyroid Hormone Synthesis

The production of thyroid hormones is severely impaired when too little iodide is available. However, when the concentration of iodide is high, iodide uptake and hormone biosynthesis are temporarily blocked. This effect of iodide, called the Wolff-Chaikoff effect, has been exploited clinically to produce short-term suppression of thyroid hormone secretion. As even the normal endocytosis of colloid by the follicular cells is paralyzed by high iodide concentrations, there is almost immediate shutdown of thyroid hormone secretion into blood. As they inhibit all processes in the follicular cells, iodides decrease the size of the thyroid gland and especially decrease its blood supply. For this reason, iodides are frequently administered to patients for 2 to 3 weeks before surgical removal of the thyroid gland to decrease the vascularity of the gland and thereby, reduce the amount of bleeding.

Applied Aspects

Hypothyroidism in Children

There are multiple causes of hypothyroidism in children. Dietary iodine deficiency beginning *in utero* impairs the biosynthesis of thyroid hormones and results in endemic cretinism (Fig. 9.37). For children whose hypothyroidism does not result from iodine deficiency, the term sporadic congenital hypothyroidism is used.

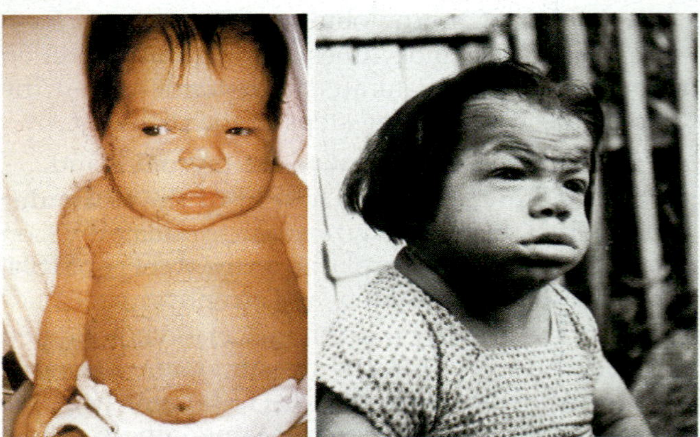

Fig. 9.37: Cretinism

Causes of Hypothyroidism in Children

- *Endemic cretinism:* Dietary iodine deficiency *in utero*
- *Sporadic congenital hypothyroidism*
  - Thyroid agenesis or dysgenesis
  - Thyroidal defects in hormone biosynthesis
  - Transfer of thyroid-blocking antibodies across the placenta from a mother with autoimmune thyroid disease
  - Hereditary thyroid hormone resistance.

The symptoms of hypothyroidism in children:

- Poor feeding
- Sluggish movements
- Hoarse cry
- Umbilical hernia
- Retarded bone age.
- Untreated hypothyroidism in children results in mental retardation and stunted growth. Skeletal growth is characteristically more affected than soft tissue growth giving the child an obese, stocky and short appearance.
- The tongue becomes so large in relation to the skeletal growth to obstruct swallowing and breathing, inducing a characteristic guttural breathing that sometimes chokes the child. These children may show delayed or absent sexual maturity.

Hypothyroidism in Adults

The common symptoms and signs of hypothyroidism in adults and their causative mechanisms are listed (*see* next page).

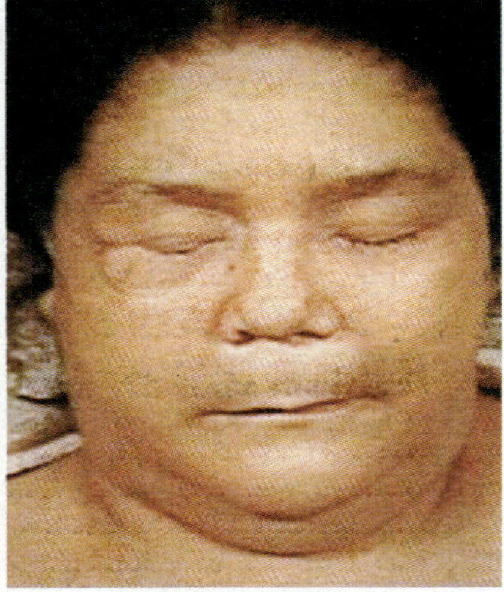

Fig. 9.38: Myxedema

9

Hypothyroidism in adults	
Symptom/Sign	*Causative mechanism*
Dullness, weakness, fatigue lethargy Mental slowness Slow speech Prolonged reflex times Somnolence Psychosis: Myxoedema madness	Effects of thyroid hormones on the central nervous system
Weight gain	Low BMR and caloric use despite decreased appetite and food consumption
Cold intolerance	Decreased thermogenesis
Dry, cold skin	Decreased sweating, decreased sebaceous gland secretion Cutaneous vasoconstriction
Decreased sweating	Lower heat production Insufficient ATP for normal sweat formation
Myxedema (Fig. 9.38)	Nonpitting edema that results from accumulation of glycosaminoglycans (mucopolysaccharides) in the interstitial spaces and fluid retention
Thick, coarse skin Thickened facial features Thick tongue Periorbital edema Husky voice	Myxoedema: Edema due to accumulation of a mucous material formed by certain proteins complexing with hyaluronic acid and chondroitin sulphate in extracellular matrices. Being osmotic, this complex draws water causing nonpitting edema in the skin
Thin, brittle, lustreless hair Loss of lateral one-third eyebrows Scaly skin	Effect of thyroid hormones on protein metabolism and hair follicle function
Goiter (Fig. 9.39)	Hypertrophy and hyperplasia of thyroid follicles stimulated by raised TSH levels, as there is no negative feedback by the thyroid hormones
Bradycardia	Loss of chronotropic action of thyroid hormones
Hypertension	Increased peripheral resistance at rest
Pericardial effusion	Interstitial edema
Muscle aches	Thyroid myopathy
Atherosclerosis leading to peripheral vascular disease, deafness and coronary artery disease	Elevated serum cholesterol and triglyceride levels
Constipation	Decreased gastrointestinal motility
Amenorrhea	Lack of the effects of thyroid hormones on gonads and gonadotropin secretion

Causes of Adult Hypothyroidism

a. *Destruction of Gland*

- Surgical
- Irradiation
- Autoimmune (Hashimoto's thyroiditis)
- Cancer
- Thyroiditis

b. *Inhibition of Thyroid Hormone Synthesis*

- Dietary iodine deficiency
- Enzyme defects in hormonogenesis
- Antithyroid drugs

c. *Hypothalamic or Pituitary Disorders*

d. *Resistance to Thyroid Hormone*

Hyperthyroidism

Hyperthyroidism occurs in various forms. The most prevalent form of hyperthyroidism is Graves' disease. Other forms of hyperthyroidism include toxic multinodular goiter, toxic adenoma and Hashimoto's thyroiditis.

Graves' Disease

This is an autoimmune disorder in which T lymphocytes become sensitized to antigens within the thyroid gland and stimulate B lymphocytes to produce antibodies to these antigens. In most cases, antibodies are produced to the TSH receptor, thyroglobulin and thyroid peroxidase. The antibodies produced to TSH receptor mimic the action of TSH on its thyroidal

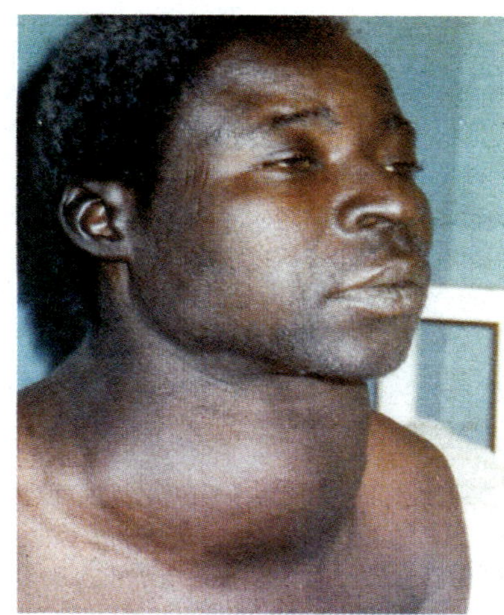

Fig. 9.39: Goiter

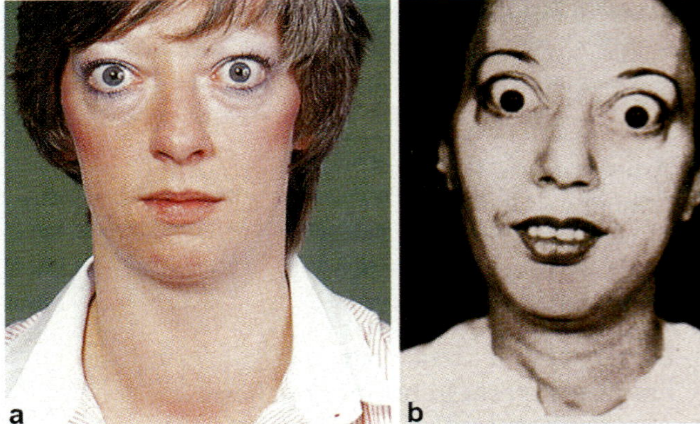

Figs 9.40a and b: Exophthalmos

receptors, serving as TSH agonists. They are called thyroid-stimulating immunoglobulins (TSIs). They bind to the follicular membrane and have a prolonged stimulating effect on the synthesis and secretion of thyroid hormones. Like TSH, these antibodies also stimulate the growth and vascularity of the thyroid gland.

There is strong familial predisposition for the disorder and women have 7 to 10 times the incidence in men. The hypothalamus-pituitary axis is no longer regulating the thyroid in this condition. The high circulating T_4 and T_3 levels inhibit pituitary TSH synthesis and secretion.

The symptoms and signs of hyperthyroidism and their causative mechanisms are listed below:

Symptoms of hyperthyroidism	*Causative mechanism*
Nervousness Tremor Inability to sleep	Thyroid hormones potentiate catecholamine action by increasing the number of β-adrenergic receptors
Heat intolerance increased BMR	Increased thermogenesis
Palpitations (symptom)/ Tachycardia (sign)	Potentiated catecholamine action
Muscle weakness fatigue	Thyroid myopathy
Increased appetite	Not known
Moist, warm skin	Increased sweating Cutaneous vasodilatation
Goiter bruit over thyroid (Fig. 9.39)	The antibodies stimulate thyroid growth and vascularity
Pretibial myxoedema in Graves' disease	The pathogenesis is thought to be an autoimmune disorder. T lymphocytes infiltrate the skin in the pretibial region, where fibroblasts have TSH receptors; these lymphocytes release cytokines that stimulate glycosaminoglycan production and subsequent edema
Eye problems	
Proptosis (Figs 9.40a and b) Lid lag Periorbital edema Extraocular muscle weakness Diplopia Eye irritation Lid retraction	Retro-orbital contents increase There is fibroblastic proliferation and glycosaminoglycans accumulate in the retro-orbital tissues. The retro-orbital fibroblasts and adipocytes are targets of the auto-immune attack. TSH receptors in these cells may promote the T lymphocytes activated against the TSH receptor to infiltrate the orbit and skin. These activated cells release cytokines such as interferon-γ, interleukin-I and transforming growth factor-β. The cytokines stimulate fibroblasts to produce glycosaminoglycans that accumulate and produce edema. Edema within the retro-orbital muscles and adipose tissue produces proptosis and extraocular muscle dysfunction (causing diplopia) Potentiated catecholamine action causes the lid retraction.
Varying degrees of diarrhea	Increased gastrointestinal motility

Dermopathy (pretibial myxoedema) may be associated with Graves' disease. The skin thickens in the pretibial area and/or feet and forms "pig-like" plaques. The edges of these plaques are well-defined. As with the myxoedema of hypothyroidism, glycosaminoglycans accumulate in the dermis. These regions itch and are sometimes painful.

Hashimoto's Thyroiditis

It is a common cause of acquired hypothyroidism. It is an autoimmune disorder characterized by the lymphocytic production of thyroid antibodies.

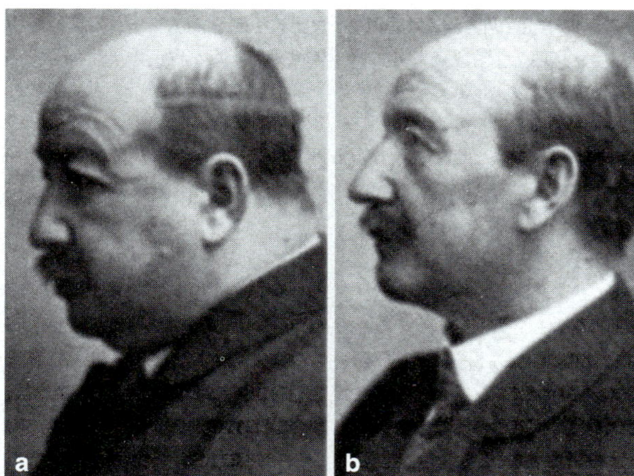

Figs 9.41a and b: Hypothyroidism: (a) Before treatment and (B) after treatment

Common thyroidal antigens are thyroid peroxidase and thyroglobulin. Lymphocytes infiltrate the gland and structural damage of the gland occurs with release of thyroglobulin into blood. Therefore, hyperthyroidism may be present early in the progression of Hashimoto's thyroiditis. However, as the disease progresses and the gland is destroyed, hypothyroidism develops, serum thyroid hormone levels fall and TSH levels rise. The patient usually has a goiter and most typically is either euthyroid or hypothyroid. High antibody titres to thyroid peroxidase or thyroglobulin are typical. Hashimoto's thyroiditis can sometimes be part of a syndrome involving multiple autoimmune endocrine disorders that can include the adrenals, pancreas, parathyroid and ovaries (Schmidt's syndrome).

Thyroid Function Tests

- *Serum TSH* represents the single best screening test for thyroid function.
- *Serum T_4 and T_3* are measured by radioimmunoassay. These tests do not distinguish bound from free hormone.
- *T_3 resin uptake* provides an index of thyroxine-binding globulin levels and therefore, is an index of the serum binding capacity. A tracer quantity of radioactive T_3 is mixed with serum. The radioactive T_3 should distribute itself between bound and free forms in accordance with the ratio of bound and free forms for the nonradioactive hormone. A synthetic resin that binds free T_3 is then added. The radioactive T_3 that was originally in the free form will now bind to the resin. The resin can be precipitated from the serum and the radioactivity measured. If the levels of free T_3 are high in the original serum, the percentage of resin ^{125}I–T_3 will be high.
- *Free T_4/T_3 index*
  Free T_4 index = $[T_4] \times [T_3$ resin uptake$]$
  Free T_3 index = $[T_3] \times [T_3$ resin uptake$]$
  These are nondimensional numbers that are an indirect approximation of the true free T_4 or T_3 levels.
- *Radioactive iodide uptake*
  It is increased in hyperthyroidism and iodine deficiency. It is decreased in hypothyroidism and after exogenous T_4, T_3 administration.
- *Thyroid antibodies*
  Anti-thyroid peroxidase or anti-thyroglobulin antibodies may be detected. Very high titers are common for Hashimoto's thyroiditis.
- *Serum thyroglobulin*
  These levels increase in disorders involving destruction of the thyroid, such as thyroid carcinoma and Hashimoto's thyroiditis. Serum thyroglobulin levels increase when thyroid hormone synthesis and secretion increase.
- *TRH challenge to TSH secretion*
  A bolus injection of TRH is given and the effects on TSH levels are measured. An increased TSH secretion is seen in primary hypothyroidism. There is no response in secondary hypothyroidism and hyperthyroid individuals.

CALCIUM AND PHOSPHATE METABOLISM

Calcium

Calcium is an integral structural component of the skeleton and plays a key role in many fundamental biological processes including muscle contraction, blood coagulation, enzyme activity, neural excitability, hormone release and membrane permeability. Therefore, special endocrine mechanisms are involved in the precise control of calcium concentration in the extracellular fluid.

The body of a young adult human contains about 1100 g of calcium. 99% of the total body calcium is in the skeleton. Bone can thus serve as a large reservoir of calcium, releasing it when plasma concentration decreases and storing calcium when it is in excess. The normal plasma calcium level is about 10 mg/dl, about 50% is bound to protein and cannot diffuse through the capillary membranes. Diffusible calcium is mostly in the free, ionized form, which is physiologically active and a small fraction (9%) is combined with anionic substances of the plasma and interstitial fluids (phosphate and citrate) (Fig. 9.42).

Calcium in the bone is of two types: A readily exchangeable form and a larger pool of stable calcium that is only slowly exchangeable. The two forms are regulated by two homeostatic systems; one is the system that regulates plasma Ca^{2+} and the other system is concerned with bone remodeling by the constant interplay between bone deposition and resorption.

Calcium is actively absorbed from the intestine and the process is regulated by 1, 25-dihydroxycholecalciferol. There is also some absorption by passive diffusion. When calcium intake is high, 1, 25-dihydroxycholecalciferol levels fall because of the increased plasma Ca^{2+}. Consequently, Ca^{2+} absorption is high when the calcium intake is low and decreased when the calcium intake is high. Calcium absorption is also decreased by substances that form insoluble salts with Ca^{2+}, (e.g. phosphates and oxalates) or by alkalis, which favor formation of insoluble calcium soaps.

A large amount of calcium is filtered in the kidneys but nearly 99% of the filtered calcium is reabsorbed. About 60% of the reabsorption occurs in the proximal tubules and the remainder in the ascending limb of the loop of Henle and the distal tubule. Parathyroid hormone regulates the distal tubular reabsorption of calcium.

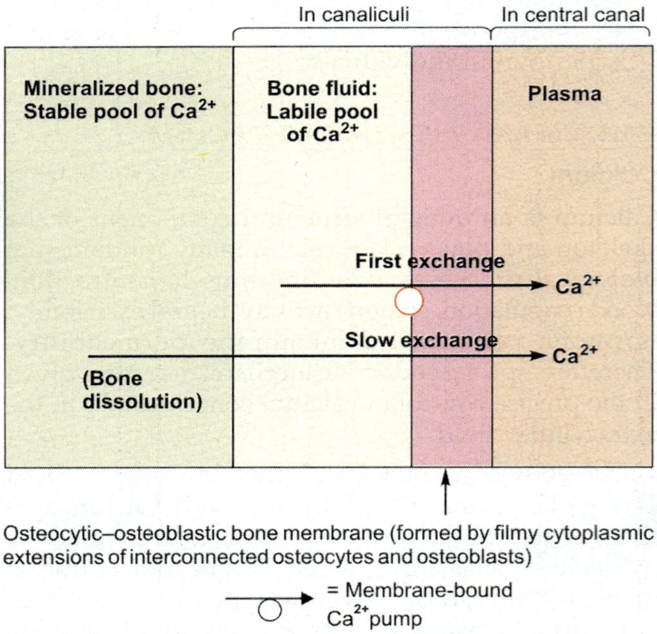

Fig. 9.42: Exchange of calcium between bone and plasma

Phosphorus

The total body phosphorus is 500–800 g, 85% of which is in the skeleton. Total plasma phosphorus is about 12 mg/dl, two-thirds of which is in organic compounds and the remaining inorganic phosphorus (Pi) in PO_4^{-3}, HPO_4^{-2} and $H_2PO_4^{-3}$. Organic phosphorus is a component of ATP, cAMP, 2, 3-diphosphoglycerate and many proteins. Phosphorylation and dephosphorylation of proteins are involved in the regulation of cell function. Therefore, phosphate metabolism is closely regulated.

The amount of phosphorus normally entering bone is about 3 mg/kg/day; an equal amount leaves via reabsorption.

Pi is absorbed in the duodenum and small intestine by both active transport and passive diffusion. The absorption of Pi is linearly proportionate to dietary intake.

Bone Physiology

Calcitropic Hormones

The primary hormones concerned with the regulation of calcium metabolism are parathyroid hormone (PTH), 1, 25-dihydroxycholecalciferol and calcitonin. PTH mobilizes calcium from bone and increases urinary phosphate excretion. 1, 25-dihydroxycholecalciferol is a steroid hormone whose primary action is to increase calcium absorption from the intestine. Calcitonin is a calcium-lowering hormone that inhibits bone resorption.

Parathyroid Glands and Parathyroid Hormone

Embryology of the Parathyroid Glands

The parathyroid glands develop from the endodermal lining of the third and fourth branchial pouches.

Anatomy of the Parathyroid Glands

There are typically four parathyroid glands in humans, two embedded in the superior poles of the thyroid gland and two in its inferior poles. However, the locations of the individual parathyroids and their number can vary considerably. More than 10% of humans harbor a fifth parathyroid gland.

Each gland is a flattened ellipsoid measuring about 6 mm in its longest diameter. The glands are well-vascularized and derive their blood supply mainly from the inferior thyroid arteries.

Parathyroid glands are composed of two types of cells: The chief or principal cells that secrete parathormone and the oxyphil cells that have no known function. The chief cells predominate and are arranged in clusters or cords. They have all of the cytological characteristics of cells that produce protein hormones: rough endoplasmic reticulum, prominent Golgi apparatus, and some membrane-bound storage granules. The larger eosinophilic oxyphil cells contain oxyphil granules and are rich in mitochondria.

Synthesis, Storage and Secretion of PTH

PTH is a simple straight-chain peptide of 84 amino acids with a molecular weight of 9500. It is synthesized as part of a larger 115-amino acid preproparathormone. Upon entry of preproparathormone into the endoplasmic reticulum, a leader sequence from the amino terminal is removed to form a 90-amino-acid proparathormone. In the Golgi apparatus, six additional amino acids are removed from the amino terminal of proparathormone to yield the mature hormone which is packaged in secretory granules.

Parathormone has a short half-life of only about 5 minutes. It is rapidly cleaved in the liver into fragments that are cleared from blood by filtration at the glomeruli.

PTHrP

A protein with PTH activity, parathyroid hormone related peptide (PTHrP), is synthesized by a wide range of tissues and acts primarily as a paracrine hormone to regulate a variety of processes unrelated to calcium homeostasis. It is found in the plasma of patients suffering from certain malignancies and accounts for the accompanying hypercalcemia. Little or no PTHrP is found in blood plasma of normal individuals.

PTHrP has a marked effect on the growth and development of cartilage *in utero*. In addition, there is evidence that it is involved in Ca^{2+} transport in the placenta. PTHrP is also found in keratinocytes in the skin, in smooth muscle and in the teeth, where it is present in the enamel epithelium that caps each tooth. In the absence of PTHrP, teeth cannot erupt.

Mechanism of Action of PTH

There are at least three different PTH receptors:

1. The hPTH/PTHrP receptor binds PTHrP as well. It is expressed on osteoblasts in bone and in the proximal and distal tubules of the kidney.
2. The hPTH-2 receptor does not bind PTHrP.
3. The third receptor, CPTH, reacts with the carboxyl terminal rather than the amino terminal of PTH.

The first two PTH receptors are G protein-coupled receptors that are linked to adenylyl cyclase via a stimulatory G protein (Gs). The hPTH/PTHrP receptor also activates phospholipase C through Gq. Thus binding of PTH to this receptor on the surfaces of target cells increases the formation of cyclic AMP and of inositol triphosphate (IP_3) and diacylglycerol (DAG). Consequently, protein kinases A and C are also activated and intracellular calcium is increased. Rapid responses to PTH result from protein phosphorylation while delayed responses are due to altered expression of genes regulated by cyclic AMP response element binding protein (CREB).

Actions of PTH

Parathormone is the principal regulator of the extracellular calcium pool. It increases the calcium concentration and decreases the phosphate concentration in blood. The direct targets of PTH are bone and kidney, while they act indirectly on the intestine to raise calcium levels. In its absence, plasma calcium concentration decreases dramatically while the concentration of phosphate increases.

Actions on Bone

PTH acts directly on bone to increase bone resorption and mobilize Ca^{2+} by increased osteoclastic activity; however, PTH receptors are expressed only on osteoblasts. Osteoclasts are thus not direct targets for PTH.

In bone remodeling, resorption is precisely coupled with bone formation. The signaling mechanisms that couple bone formation with bone resorption are not yet known but it appears that osteoblasts secrete a variety of autocrine and paracrine growth factors that are trapped and stored in the bone matrix during bone formation. Activated osteoclasts digest bone matrix and release previously sequestered growth factors that stimulate osteoblasts to lay down new bone. At this time PTH stimulates osteoblasts to synthesize and secrete growth factors including insulin-like growth factor I (IGF-I) and transforming growth factor beta

(TGF-β) that stimulate osteoblast progenitors to divide and differentiate. Intermittent stimulation with PTH leads to net formation of bone (anabolic); however, with prolonged continuous exposure to high concentrations of PTH, osteoclastic activity is greater than osteoblastic activity and bone resorption predominates, thereby reducing bone density.

Thus, PTH plays a critical role in maintaining blood calcium concentrations and in bone remodeling which continues throughout life.

Actions on Kidney

In the kidney, PTH produces three main effects:

1. PTH promotes calcium reabsorption in the distal tubule:
   - PTH receptors are present on the basolateral surface of cells in the distal convoluted tubule. In the basolateral membrane, PTH activates three transport proteins: Sodium-calcium antiporters (that exchange three ions of sodium for one ion of intracellular calcium), a calcium ATPase (that pumps calcium across the basolateral membrane) and the sodium-potassium ATPase (that maintains the electrochemical gradient across the membrane).

   About 90% of the filtered calcium is reabsorbed in the proximal tubule and the loop of Henle independently of PTH. In the proximal tubule, most of the Ca^{2+} is reabsorbed by a passive, paracellular pathway. In contrast to the proximal nephron, Ca^{2+} uptake in the thick ascending limb of the loop of Henle and the distal convoluted tubule occurs solely via the transcellular route.
2. In the proximal tubule, PTH inhibits phosphate reabsorption.
   - Phosphate is mostly reabsorbed in the proximal convoluted tubule via a hormonally-regulated transcellular route. It enters the tubular cells via a sodium-phosphate co-transporter in the luminal membrane. PTH decreases the abundance of these sodium-phosphate cotransporters in the proximal tubular cells by stimulating their translocation to intracellular vesicles. It powerfully inhibits tubular reabsorption of phosphate and thus increases the amount excreted in urine (phosphaturic action).
3. PTH promotes hydroxylation and activation of vitamin D.
   - PTH stimulates the renal enzyme 1-α hydroxylase that converts vitamin D_3 to its active form-1, 25-dihydroxycholecalciferol (1, 25-DHCC). This active metabolite of vitamin D_3 stimulates intestinal uptake of calcium. PTH has no direct effects on intestinal transport of either calcium or phosphate.

Regulation of PTH Secretion

The primary signal that stimulates PTH secretion is low circulating Ca^{2+} levels. Circulating ionized calcium acts directly on the chief cells in a negative feedback fashion to regulate the secretion of PTH. When the plasma Ca^{2+} level is high, PTH secretion is inhibited and Ca^{2+} is deposited in the bones. When it is low, secretion is increased and Ca^{2+} is mobilized from the bones. The key to this regulation is a cell membrane Ca^{2+}-sensing receptor (CaSR).

1, 25-dihyroxycholecalciferol, whose synthesis depends on PTH, is also a negative feedback inhibitor of PTH synthesis. There are two ways by which 1, $25(OH)_2D_3$ inhibits PTH secretion: Firstly, it acts directly on the parathyroid gland to inhibit the production of mRNA for PTH.

In a second negative feedback action, 1, $25(OH)_2D_3$ indirectly decreases PTH secretion by virtue of its actions to increase plasma calcium concentration.

Increased plasma phosphate stimulates PTH secretion by lowering plasma Ca^{2+} and inhibiting the formation of 1, 25-dihydroxycholecalciferol.

Magnesium is required to maintain normal parathyroid secretory responses.

Applied Aspects

Primary Hyperparathyroidism

Primary hyperparathyroidism is caused by excessive production of PTH by the parathyroid glands. It is usually caused by a parathyroid adenoma confined to one of the parathyroid glands.

Patients with primary hyperparathyroidism are usually asymptomatic. They have high serum calcium levels and low serum phosphate levels. The hypercalcemia is a result of bone resorption, increased gastrointestinal calcium absorption (mediated by 1, 25-dihydroxyvitamin D_3) and increased renal calcium reabsorption. High serum calcium levels decrease neuromuscular excitability. Minor personality changes, particularly depression, may be associated with increased serum calcium levels. Renal stones (nephrolithiasis) are common because the high urinary calcium and phosphate concentrations increase the tendency for precipitation of calcium-phosphate salts in the soft tissues of the kidney. Hypercalcemia can result in peptic ulcer because calcium increases gastrin secretion and it can also cause cardiac arrest.

Secondary Hyperparathyroidism

Chronically, low plasma Ca^{2+} levels, seen in rickets and chronic renal disease, cause stimulation of the parathyroid glands resulting in compensatory parathyroid hypertrophy and secondary hyperparathyroidism.

Hypoparathyroidism

PTH is essential for life. In humans, hypoparathyroidism is most often due to inadvertent parathyroidectomy during thyroid surgery. There is a steady decline in the plasma Ca^{2+} level after parathyroidectomy resulting in hypocalcemic tetany. The most prominent feature is increased neuromuscular excitability. Low serum calcium levels decrease the neuromuscular threshold. This is manifested as spontaneous neuromuscular discharge or as repetitive responses to a single stimulus. The increased neuromuscular excitability can result in tingling in the fingers, toes and perioral area (paraesthesia) and extensive spasms of skeletal muscle, especially the muscles of the extremities and the larynx. Laryngospasm can be so severe that the airway is obstructed and fatal asphyxia is produced. The low serum calcium level decreases myocardial contractility and can produce a first-degree heart block.

The signs of tetany are (Fig. 9.43):

Chvostek's sign: There is a quick contraction of the ipsilateral facial muscles elicited by tapping over the facial nerve at the angle of the jaw.

Trousseau's sign or Carpopedal spasm: This is a spasm of the muscles of the upper extremity that causes flexion of the wrist and thumb with extension of the fingers.

Erb's sign: Sometimes the serum calcium level is not low enough to produce overt tetany; latent tetany can be demonstrated by occluding the circulation in the upper limb for a few minutes with a blood pressure cuff. The resultant oxygen deficiency precipitates overt tetany.

Pseudohypoparathyroidism

It is a rare familial disorder characterized by tissue resistance to PTH. Individuals with pseudohypoparathyroidism demonstrate increased PTH secretion and low serum calcium levels. Congenital skeletal defects are sometimes associated, including shortened metacarpal and metatarsal bones.

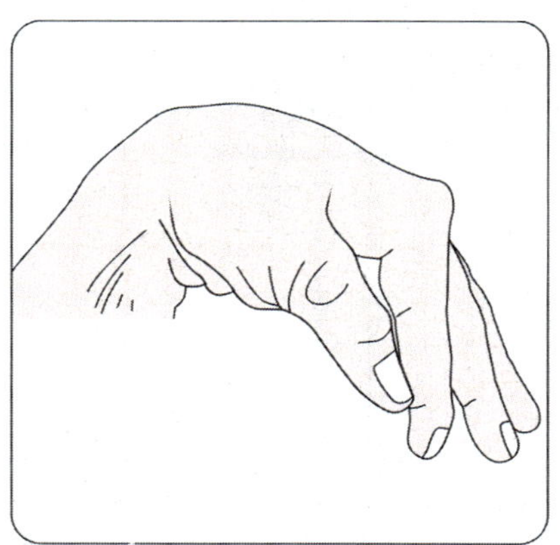

Recognizing carpopedal spasm: In the hand, carpal carpopedal spasm involves adduction of the thumb over the palm, followed by flexion of the metacarpophalangeal joints, extension of the interphalangeal joints (fingers together), adduction of the hyperextended fingers, and flexion of the wrist and elbow joints. Similar effects occur in the joints of the feet.

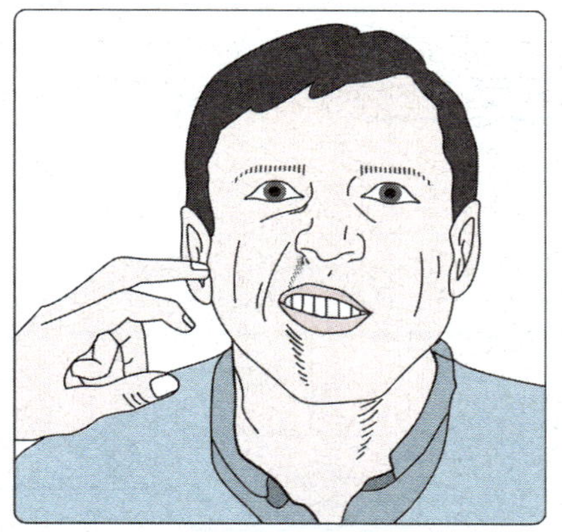

Eliciting Chvostek's sign: Begin by telling the patient to relax his facial muscles. Then stand directly in front of him, and tap the facial nerve either just anterior to the ear-lobe and below the zygomatic arch and the corner of his mouth. A positive response varies from twitching of lip at the corner of the mouth to spasm of all facial muscles, depending on the severity of hypocalcemia

Fig. 9.43: Hypocalcemic features: Trousseau's sign and Chvostek's sign

VITAMIN D

The term "vitamin D" is used to refer to a group of closely related sterols produced by the action of ultraviolet light on certain provitamins. Vitamin D_3, also called cholecalciferol, is produced in the skin of mammals from 7-dehydrocholesterol by the action of sunlight; hence the name sunshine vitamin. Vitamin D_3 is also ingested in the diet.

Vitamin D_3 and its derivatives are secosteroids, i.e. they are steroids in which one of the rings has been opened.

Vitamin D_3 is actually a prohormone, which must be converted to an active form, 1, 25-dihydroxy-cholecalciferol (1, 25 $(OH)_2D_3$).

Synthesis and Transport (Fig. 9.44)

The immediate precursor of vitamin D_3, 7-dehydro-cholesterol, is synthesized from acetyl coenzyme A (CoA) and is stored in the basal layers of the skin. Ultraviolet radiation converts cholesterol into vitamin D_3. The vitamin is biologically inert but has a high affinity for a vitamin D-binding protein in plasma. The

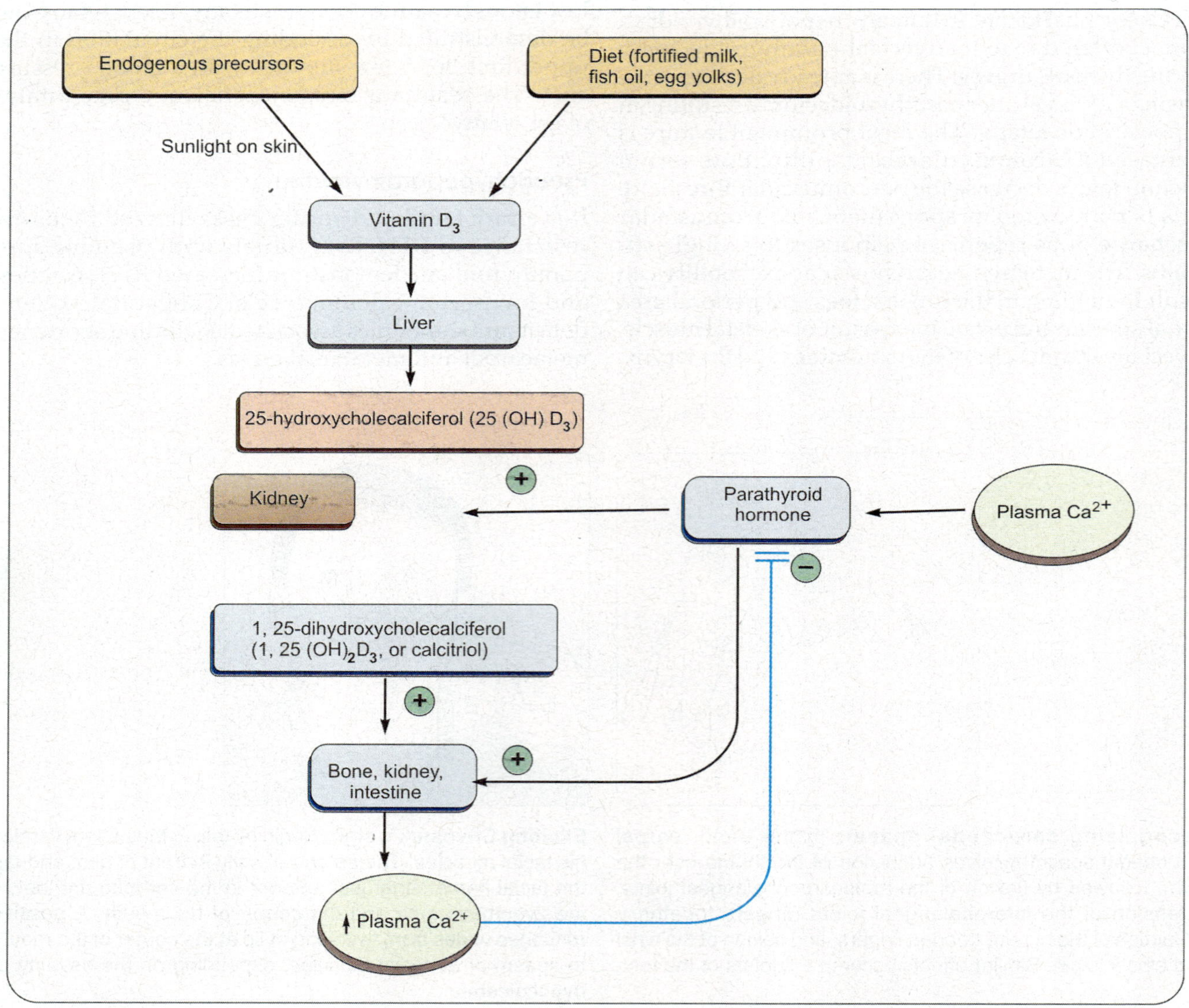

Fig. 9.44: Synthesis and action of active vitamin D_3

bound vitamin D_3 is transported to the liver, where it is converted to 25-hydroxycholecalciferol (25-OH-D_3, calcidiol) by enzymes that are members of the cytochrome P450 superfamily.

Mechanism of Action

Since 1, 25 $(OH)_2D_3$ is a steroid, it binds to a specific nuclear receptor that is a member of the same superfamily as the receptors for steroid and thyroid hormones. Binding of the hormone to the receptor exposes a DNA-binding region and gene expression is regulated in its target tissues.

Role of 1, 25 $(OH)_2D_3$ in Calcium Homeostasis

The principal actions of 1, 25 $(OH)_2D_3$ is to increase calcium and phosphate concentrations in extracellular fluid. These effects are exerted, primarily on intestine and bone and, to a lesser extent, on kidney.

Actions on Intestine

Calcium absorption from the small intestine is stimulated by 1, 25 $(OH)_2D_3$. Dietary calcium is absorbed by epithelial cells lining the duodenum and jejunum through an active transcellular route as well as a passive, bulk-flow paracellular route.

Calcium enters the duodenal epithelial cells passively down its electrochemical gradient through two channels: the epithelial calcium channel (ECaC) and calcium transporter 1 (CaT1). Once inside the cell, calcium is bound by abundant calcium binding proteins called calbindin-Ds and carried through the cytosol to the basolateral membrane where it is extruded into the interstitium against an electrochemical gradient by calcium ATPase and sodium/calcium antiporters.

Phosphate absorption in the jejunum is proportional to the amount of phosphate in the diet and is only under minor hormonal control by 1, 25 $(OH)_2D_3$ which regulates expression of sodium-phosphate cotransporters in the luminal membrane.

Actions on Bone

Mineralization of bone occurs spontaneously when adequate amounts of calcium and phosphate ions are available. 1, 25 $(OH)_2D_3$ brings about increased bone mineralization by increased intestinal absorption of calcium and phosphate, it does not directly increase bone formation.

Actions on Kidney

In the kidney, 1, 25 $(OH)_2D_3$ increases reabsorption of both calcium and phosphate in vitamin D-deficient subjects.

1, 25 $(OH)_2D_3$ acts in a permissive way to support the actions of PTH on calcium reabsorption.

Regulation of 1, 25 $(OH)_2D_3$ Production

The most important regulatory step is the production of 1, 25 $(OH)_2D_3$ by cells in the proximal tubules of the kidney. PTH facilitates formation of 1, 25 $(OH)_2D_3$ by regulating transcription of the gene that codes for 1-α-hydroxylase.

Formation of 1, 25 $(OH)_2D_3$ is subject to feedback regulation by plasma Ca^{2+} and PO_4^{-3}. When the plasma Ca^{2+} level is low, PTH secretion is increased and production of 1, 25 $(OH)_2D_3$ is enhanced. When the plasma Ca^{2+} is high, PTH secretion is inhibited.

Prolactin increases the activity of 1-α-hydroxylase and circulating 1, 25 $(OH)_2D_3$ is increased during lactation.

Growth hormone, hCS and calcitonin also stimulate 1, 25 $(OH)_2D_3$ formation.

Applied Aspects

Rickets and Osteomalacia

Vitamin D deficiency causes rickets in children and osteomalacia in adults. The main defect in this condition is impaired mineralization of bone (Fig. 9.45). Osteoid is formed, but it does not mineralize adequately. As there is decreased gastrointestinal absorption of calcium and phosphate when vitamin D is deficient, the serum calcium level drops. This

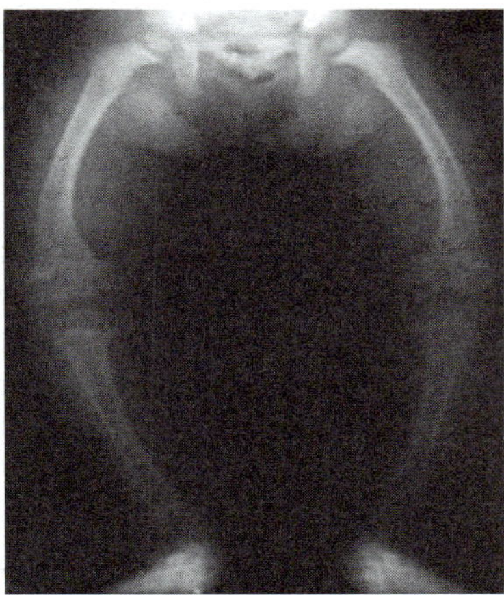

Fig. 9.45: X-ray showing ricketic "bow legs"

9

stimulates PTH secretion, which increases phosphate excretion, thereby aggravating the phosphate loss. The secondary elevation in PTH can produce osteoporosis.

Rickets is caused by vitamin D deficiency before skeletal maturation. It is characterized by weakness and bowing of weight-bearing bones, dental defects and hypocalcemia. It may result from inadequate exposure to the sun or inadequate intake of the provitamins on which the sun acts in the skin. These cases respond to vitamin D.

The condition can also be caused by inactivating mutations of the gene for 1-α-hydroxylase, in which case there is no response to vitamin D but a normal response to 1, 25 $(OH)_2D_3$ (type I vitamin D-resistant rickets). In rare instances, it can be due to inactivating mutations of the gene for the 1, 25 $(OH)_2D_3$ receptor (type II vitamin D-resistant rickets), in which there is a deficient response to both vitamin D and 1, 25 $(OH)_2D_3$.

Osteomalacia results when vitamin D deficiency occurs after skeletal growth is complete and the epiphyses have closed. It is characterized by poorly calcified osteoid associated with pain, increased risk of fracture and vertebral collapse.

CALCITONIN

Calcitonin is a Ca^{2+}-lowering hormone secreted by the parafollicular cells (clear or C cells) distributed around the follicles in the thyroid gland. These cells are neuroectodermal in origin and are derived from the ultimobranchial bodies that are a pair of glands derived embryologically from the fifth branchial arches (Fig. 9.46).

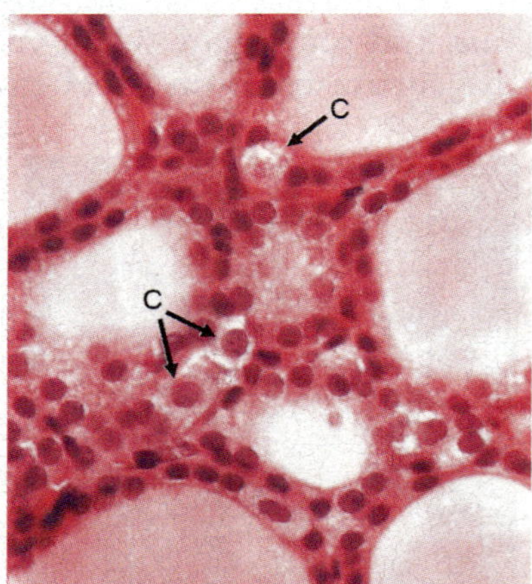

C = Parafollicular cell

Fig. 9.46: Thyroid gland showing parafollicular cells

Chemistry

Human calcitonin contains 32 amino acid residues and has a molecular weight of 3500. In the nervous system, the calcitonin gene is processed differently to form the neuropeptide, calcitonin gene-related peptide (CGRP).

Secretion and Metabolism

Parafollicular cells respond directly to ionized calcium in blood and the secretion of calcitonin is primarily regulated by the same CaSR that regulates PTH secretion. Increase in plasma Ca^{2+} levels stimulate the synthesis and secretion of calcitonin.

Calcitonin secretion may also increase after eating. Gastrin, a hormone produced by gastric mucosal cells, stimulates parafollicular cells to secrete calcitonin. Cholecystokinin, glucagon and secretin have all been reported to stimulate calcitonin secretion but gastrin is the most potent stimulus among them.

The half-life of calcitonin in circulation is less than 10 minutes. It is primarily inactivated in the kidney.

The Calcitonin Receptor

The calcitonin receptor is a G protein-coupled receptor that acts primarily through cAMP-dependent signaling pathways and is closely related to the PTH/PTHrP receptor. In contrast to the PTH/PTHrP receptor, the calcitonin receptor is expressed in osteoclasts.

Actions of Calcitonin

Calcitonin lowers the circulating calcium and phosphate levels. The calcium-lowering effect is due to its inhibition of bone resorption by direct inhibition of osteoclastic activity. It also increases Ca^{2+} excretion in the urine.

Calcitonin may protect against postprandial hypercalcemia.

More calcitonin is secreted in young individuals, and it may play a role in skeletal development.

During pregnancy, it may protect the bones of the mother from excess calcium loss.

Calcitonin is useful in the treatment of Paget's disease, a condition in which there is increased osteoclastic activity, which triggers compensatory formation of disorganized new bone.

78. ADRENAL GLANDS

Overview

The adrenal glands are complex endocrine structures that produce two structurally distinct classes of hormones: steroids and catecholamines. The outer adrenal cortex secretes steroid hormones that act at the level of the genome to regulate gene expression in virtually all cells. The inner adrenal medulla is actually a component of the sympathetic nervous system and secretes catecholamines. The three major categories of adrenal steroid hormones are:

- Mineralocorticoids, essential for the maintenance of sodium balance and ECF volume
- Glucocorticoids, whose actions affect body fuel metabolism, immunity and responses to injury and inflammation
- Androgens that exert minor effects on reproductive function.

The secretion of mineralocorticoids is primarily controlled by the renin-angiotensin system in the kidney while the secretion of glucocorticoids and androgens is controlled by ACTH from the anterior pituitary.

The mineralocorticoids and glucocorticoids are necessary for survival while adrenal medullary hormones are not essential for life.

Morphology and Histology

The adrenal or suprarenal glands are bilateral structures situated on the superior pole of each kidney, weighing about 4 grams each. The outer cortex makes up more than three-quarters of the adrenal mass. The inner medulla is a modified sympathetic ganglion that is innervated by cholinergic, preganglionic sympathetic neurons (Fig. 9.47).

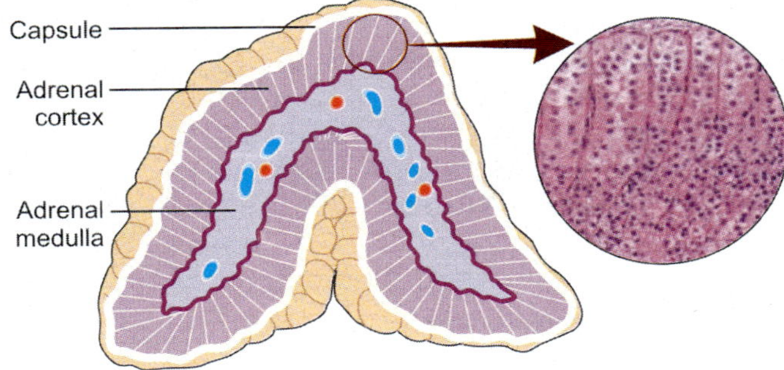

Fig. 9.47: Zone of the adrenal cortex

The cortex is subdivided histologically into three zones:

- The zona glomerulosa (makes up 15% of the mass of the adrenal gland)
- The zona fasciculata (50%)
- The zona reticularis (7%).

Cells in the outer zona glomerulosa are arranged in clusters (glomeruli) and produce the hormone aldosterone. In addition to aldosterone biosynthesis, another function performed by this zone is the formation of new cortical cells. In the zona fasciculata, which comprises the bulk of the cortex, columns of lipid-laden cells are arranged radially in bundles of parallel cords (fasces). These columns are separated by venous sinuses. The lipid droplets represent stored cholesterol esters. The inner region of the cortex consists of a tangled network of cells and is called the zona reticularis. Zona fasciculata and zona reticularis possess the enzymes for producing both glucocorticoids and androgens. The cells of the adrenal cortex contain large amounts of smooth endoplasmic reticulum, which is involved in the steroid-forming process.

The adrenal medulla is made up of interlacing cords of densely innervated granule-containing cells that abut on venous sinuses. The two cell types that can be distinguished morphologically are an epinephrine-secreting type that has larger, less dense granules and a norepinephrine-secreting type in which smaller, very dense granules are present. In humans, 90% of the cells are the epinephrine-secreting type and the rest are norepinephrine-secreting.

Embryology

The adrenal glands are derived from both neuronal and epithelial tissue. The adrenal cortex arises from mesodermal cells in the vicinity of the superior pole of the developing kidney. These cells form cords of epithelial endocrine cells. Soon after the cortex forms, neural crest-derived cells that are associated with the sympathetic ganglia–called chromaffin cells migrate into the cortical cells and become encapsulated by them. Thus, the chromaffin cells establish the inner adrenal medulla.

During fetal life, the human adrenal is large and under pituitary control but the three zones of the

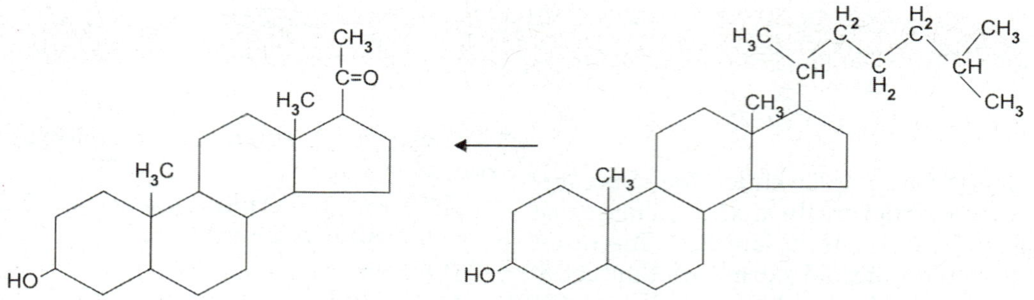

Fig. 9.48: Pregnane (21 carbons), cholesterol (27 carbons)

permanent cortex represent only 20% of the gland. The remaining 80% is the large fetal adrenal cortex, which undergoes rapid degeneration at the time of birth.

Blood Supply

The adrenal glands receive a rich arterial supply. These arteries penetrate the adrenal capsule and divide to form the subcapsular plexus from which small arterial branches pass centripetally toward the medulla. These vessels supply oxygen and nutrients to the adrenal medullary cells. The cortical cells secrete steroid hormones into these vessels. Sinusoidal blood collects through venules into a single large central vein in each adrenal gland. Thus, adrenal cortical secretions percolate through the medullary cells, bathing them in high concentrations of cortisol.

ADRENOCORTICAL HORMONES

All adrenal steroids are derivatives of cholesterol. They contain the cyclopentanoperhydrophenanthrene nucleus, which is also present in bile acids, vitamin D and gonadal steroids.

Synthesis of Adrenocortical Hormones

The adrenal cortex secretes primarily C21 and C19 steroids. Most of the C19 steroids have a keto group at carbon 17 and are therefore called 17-ketosteroids. The C21 steroids that have a side chain in addition to the hydroxyl group at carbon 17 are called 17-hydroxycorticosteroids (Fig. 9.48).

The C19 steroids have androgenic activity. The C21 steroids are classified, using Hans Selye's terminology, as mineralocorticoids or glucocorticoids. The C21 steroids secreted by adrenocortical tissue in humans are aldosterone, cortisol and corticosterone.

The starting material for steroid hormone biosynthesis is cholesterol. Most of the cholesterol is taken up from low-density lipoproteins (LDL) in the circulation. Adrenal cortical cells avidly capture LDL by receptor-mediated endocytosis. The cells also synthesize some cholesterol *de novo* from acetate. Free cholesterol is then esterified and stored in lipid droplets. When hormone synthesis is to occur, the stored cholesterol is released from its esterified storage by a cholesterol ester hydrolase. This step is stimulated by ACTH (Figs 9.49 and 9.50).

Free cholesterol must enter the mitochondria to gain access to the first enzyme in the steroidogenic pathway, CYP11A1, located on the matrix space side of the inner mitochondrial membrane. Thus, the rate-limiting reaction in steroidogenesis is the transfer of cholesterol from the outer mitochondrial membrane to the inner mitochondrial membrane. A sterol carrier protein called steroidogenic acute regulatory protein (StAR protein) is indispensable for this process.

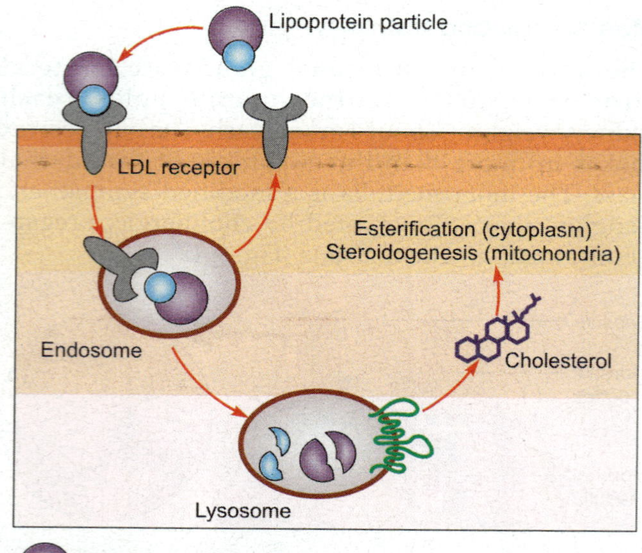

Fig. 9.49: Cholesterol uptake in the adrenocortical cell

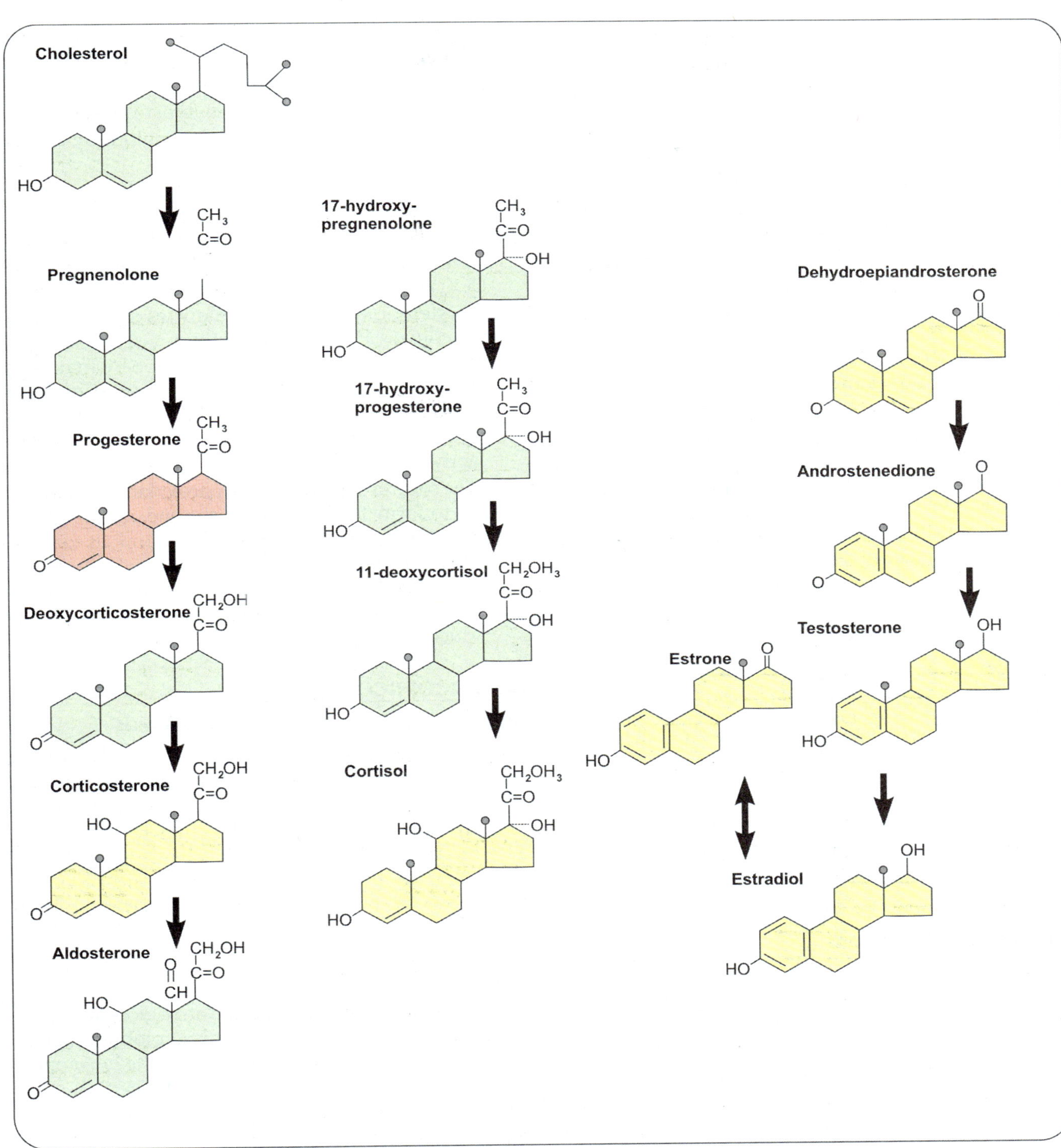

Fig. 9.50: Synthesis of steroid hormones in adrenal cortex

Biosynthesis of adrenocortical steroids is catalyzed by a particular class of oxidizing enzymes called the cytochrome P450 monoxygenases that are referred to as CYPs. They contain a heme group and absorb light in the visible range. The name P450 derives from the property of these pigments to absorb light at 450 nm when reduced by carbon monoxide.

Formation of Cortisol

Cortisol is a C21 steroid that is the principal hormone secreted by zona fasciculata. It is the most potent of the naturally occurring glucocorticoids. Free cholesterol is modified to cortisol in five steps (Fig. 9.50).

1. The side chain of cholesterol (carbon 22 to 27) is removed by side chain cleavage enzyme (CYP11A1 or cholesterol desmolase) in the mitochondria to generate a C21 steroid intermediate, pregnenolone. Pregnenolone is the common precursor of all steroid hormones produced by the adrenals or the gonads.
2. Pregnenolone moves to the smooth endoplasmic reticulum where it is converted to progesterone by the action of the enzyme, 3β-hydroxysteroid dehydrogenase (3β-HSD). This enzyme converts the hydroxyl group on carbon 3 to a ketone (-one) and converts the Δ5 steroid to a Δ4 steroid. All active steroid hormones must be converted to Δ4 structures.
3. Progesterone is then hydroxylated to 17-hydroxy-progesterone in the smooth endoplasmic reticulum by 17α-hydroxylase (CYP17).
4. 17-hydroxyprogesterone is hydroxylated on the 21 carbon by 21β-hydroxylase (CYP21B2), producing 11-deoxycortisol. This reaction also occurs in the smooth endoplasmic reticulum.
5. 11-deoxycortisol moves back to the mitochondria and is then efficiently hydroxylated on the 11 carbon by 11β-hydroxylase (CYP11B1), producing cortisol.

9

Formation of Androgens

Adrenal androgens are the main product of the zona reticularis. The zona reticularis begins to appear at about 5 years of age and androgens are detectable in the circulation at about 6 years of age. The onset of adrenal androgen production is called adrenarche and contributes to the appearance of axillary and pubic hair at about 8 years of age.

Formation of Aldosterone

Aldosterone is secreted only by cells in the zona glomerulosa as the enzyme that catalyzes its formation, CYP11B2 (aldosterone synthase), is expressed only in them. Another important feature of zona glomerulosa is that it does not express CYP17. Therefore, these cells never make cortisol or androgens.

The steps in the biosynthesis of aldosterone are:

1. Cholesterol is converted to pregnenolone by CYP11 A1.
2. Pregnenolone is converted to progesterone by 3β-HSD.
3. Progesterone is acted upon by CYP21B2 and hydroxylated at carbon 21 to form 11-deoxycorticosterone (DOC) which has some mineralocorticoid activity.
4. Aldosterone synthase then catalyzes the three steps that convert DOC to aldosterone:
   i. DOC is converted to corticosterone by hydroxylation at carbon 11. This hydroxylation step reduces the mineralocorticoid activity of DOC and confers corticosterone with glucocorticoid activity.
   ii. The second step involves hydroxylation of carbon 18 to form 18 (OH)-corticosterone.
   iii. The final step is oxidation of carbon 18 to form aldosterone. The oxygen at carbon 18 increases the mineralocorticoid activity of corticosterone by a factor of 200 and only slightly decreases glucocorticoid activity.

GLUCOCORTICOIDS

Mechanism of Action of Glucocorticoids

The glucocorticoid receptor resides in the cytoplasm in a stable complex with several molecular chaperones. The glucocorticoid hormones bind to their receptors and promote dissociation of the chaperone proteins. The hormone-receptor complex migrates to the nucleus where it binds to glucocorticoid-response elements in the target genes and acts as a transcription factor.

Transport of Glucocorticoids

Cortisol is bound in circulation to an α-globulin called transcortin or corticosteroid-binding globulin (CBG) and albumin. CBG binds about 90% of the hormone. Bound steroids are physiologically inactive. There is an equilibrium between the bound and free forms of cortisol and the bound form functions as a circulating reservoir that keeps a supply of free hormone available to the tissues.

CBG is synthesized in the liver and its production is increased by estrogen. CBG levels are increased in pregnancy (high estrogen levels) and depressed in cirrhosis (decreased production) and nephrosis (increased renal clearance).

Metabolism of Glucocorticoids

The liver is the principal site of glucocorticoid catabolism. Cortisol is reduced to dihydrocortisol and then to tetrahydrocortisol, which is conjugated with glucuronic acid.

Cortisol is also reversibly inactivated by conversion to cortisone. This is catalyzed by the enzyme, 11β-hydroxysteroid dehydrogenase type II. The inactivation is reversible in that another enzyme 11β-hydroxysteroid dehydrogenase type I, converts cortisone back to cortisol. This occurs in the liver, adipose tissue, central nervous system and skin.

Hepatic Metabolism of Glucocorticoids

Cortisone formed in the liver is promptly reduced and conjugated to tetrahydrocortisone glucuronide. The conjugates of cortisol and corticosterone are freely soluble. They enter the circulation, where they remain unbound and are rapidly excreted in the urine.

About 10% of the secreted cortisol is converted in the liver to the 17-ketosteroid derivatives of cortisol and cortisone. The ketosteroids are conjugated to sulfate and excreted in the urine.

There is an enterohepatic circulation of glucocorticoids and about 15% of the secreted cortisol is excreted in the stool.

Physiologic Effects of Glucocorticoids

Resistance to "Stress"

Glucocorticoids prepare the individual for the "fight" response or the "flight" response during stress. When an individual is exposed to noxious or potentially noxious stimuli, there is an increased secretion of ACTH. The increase in ACTH secretion raises circulating glucocorticoid level. This rise is essential for survival. In the 1930s, Hans-Selye defined noxious stimuli that increase ACTH secretion as "stressors" and cortisol is often characterized as a "stress hormone".

Most of the stressful stimuli that increase ACTH secretion also cause release of catecholamines from the sympathetic nervous system. Glucocorticoids are necessary for the catecholamines to exert their effects.

The term "permissive action" is used for those actions of glucocorticoids that require their presence to occur but are not produced by the hormones themselves.

Permissive actions of glucocorticoids
Calorigenic effects of catecholamines and glucagon
Lipolytic effects of catecholamines
Glucocorticoids are essential for the mobilization of free fatty acids by catecholamines
Pressor responses of catecholamines
In adrenal insufficiency, vascular smooth muscle becomes unresponsive to catecholamines. Capillaries dilate and their permeablility increases leading to vascular collapse. Glucocorticoids restore vascular reactivity
Bronchodilation produced by catecholamines

Effects on Intermediary Metabolism

Carbohydrate Metabolism

Glucocorticoids have major diabetogenic effects. They increase blood glucose by stimulating gluconeogenesis. Glucose-6-phosphatase activity is increased, glucose phosphate formed in the liver is converted to glucose which enters circulation and consequently, plasma glucose level rises.

Cortisol also decreases peripheral glucose utilization; this effect may be due to inhibition of glucose phosphorylation or due to a reduction in GLUT-4-mediated glucose uptake in skeletal muscle and adipose tissue (anti-insulin effect). The brain and the heart are spared, so the increase in plasma glucose provides extra glucose to these vital organs.

Lipid Metabolism

Glucocorticoids potentiate the effects of catecholamines on lipolysis and increase the activity of hormone-sensitive lipase.

Protein Metabolism

Cortisol inhibits protein synthesis and increases proteolysis, especially in skeletal muscle, thereby providing a rich source of carbon for hepatic gluconeogenesis.

Cardiovascular System

Cortisol is permissive on the actions of catecholamines and thereby contributes to a rise in cardiac output and blood pressure.

Blood Cells and Lymphatic Organs

Cortisol stimulates erythropoietin synthesis and hence, increases red blood cell production.

Glucocorticoids also increase the number of neutrophils and platelets. They decrease the number of circulating eosinophils by increasing their sequestration in the spleen and lungs. Glucocorticoids also lower the number of basophils in the circulation.

Glucocorticoids decrease the circulating lymphocyte count and the size of the lymph nodes and thymus by inhibiting lymphocyte mitotic activity.

Fetal Development

Cortisol is required for normal development of the CNS, retina, lungs, skin and gastrointestinal tract. The best-studied effect is that of cortisol on the differentiation and maturation of type II alveolar cells in the lungs. These cells produce surfactant during late gestation that reduces surface tension in the lungs and thus allows for the onset of respiration at birth.

Effects of Glucocorticoids

Gastrointestinal Tract

Glucocorticoids exert a trophic effect on the gastrointestinal mucosa. Cortisol-mediated stimulation of gastric acid and pepsin secretion increases the risk of peptic ulcer development. As cortisol stimulates appetite, hypercortisolism is frequently associated with weight gain.

Anti-inflammatory, antiallergic and immunosuppressive effects of glucocorticoids.

Inflammation and immune responses are often part of a response to stress. However, they have the potential to do significant harm if not held in homeostatic balance.

9

Inflammation is a complex localized response to foreign substances such as bacteria or tissue injury. It includes a sequence of reactions initially involving cytokines, neutrophils, complement and IgG. Prostaglandins, leukotrienes and thromboxanes are mediators of inflammation. Later, monocytes and lymphocytes are involved. Arterioles in the inflamed area dilate and capillary permeability is increased. When the inflammation occurs in or just under the skin, it is characterized by redness, swelling, tenderness and pain.

As a stress hormone, cortisol plays an important role in inflammation response. It brings about its effects through various mechanisms:

- Cortisol inhibits phospholipase A_2, a key enzyme in prostaglandin, leukotriene and thromboxane synthesis.
- Cortisol also stabilizes lysosomal membranes, thereby decreasing the release of proteolytic enzymes that augment local edema.
- The migration of neutrophils to the site of injury and their phagocytic activity is inhibited by cortisol.
- Proliferation of fibroblasts is involved in inflammation. This response is important for the formation of barriers to the spread of infectious agents. Cortisol inhibits this response.

Cortisol inhibits the immune response; hence, glucocorticoid analogs have been used as immunosuppressants in organ transplants. High cortisol levels decrease the number of circulating T lymphocytes and decrease their ability to migrate to the site of antigenic stimulation.

Kidney

Cortisol inhibits ADH secretion and action; it is an ADH antagonist.

The mineralocorticoid activity is manifested at high levels of the hormone. Cortisol increases the glomerular filtration rate by direct action on the kidney and by increasing the cardiac output.

Reproductive System

Cortisol decreases the function of the reproductive axis at the hypothalamic, pituitary and gonadal levels.

Effects on Other Hormones

Large doses of glucocorticoids decrease growth hormone and TSH secretion. They induce phenylethanolamine-N-methyltransferase (PNMT), the enzyme that catalyzes the conversion of norepinephrine to epinephrine.

Regulation of Glucocorticoid Secretion

Cortisol synthesis and secretion is stimulated primarily by ACTH from the anterior pituitary. Cortisol inhibits further secretion of ACTH in a typical negative feedback arrangement.

Chemistry and Metabolism of ACTH

ACTH is a single-chain polypeptide containing 39 amino acids. Its half-life in circulation is about 10 minutes. The site of its inactivation is not known.

Mechanism of Action of ACTH

ACTH binds to high-affinity receptors on the plasma membrane of adrenocortical cells. This activates adenylyl cyclase via Gs and results in an increase in intracellular cAMP that activates protein kinase A.

Stimulation of cortisol synthesis results from the following actions of ACTH:

- Accelerated conversion of cholesteryl esters to free cholesterol by increasing the activity of cholesteryl ester hydrolase
- Increased synthesis and activity of StAR protein.

Thus the immediate actions of ACTH accelerate the delivery of cholesterol to the mitochondria to form pregnenolone.

Regulation of ACTH Secretion

The rate of ACTH secretion is determined by CRH (corticotrophin) from hypothalamus. Figures 9.51a to c illustrates the hypothalamus-pituitary-adrenal axis involving CRH, ACTH and cortisol.

This polypeptide is produced by neurons in the paraventricular nuclei. It is secreted in the median eminence and transported by the portal hypophyseal vessels to the anterior pituitary where it stimulates ACTH secretion.

Stimuli for CRH secretion

Emotional stresses: Fibers from the amygdaloid nuclei mediate responses to emotional stresses. Fear and anxiety markedly increase ACTH secretion

Input from the suprachiasmatic nucleus: This provides the drive for the diurnal rhythm

Hypoglycemia

Haemorrhage

Proinflammatory cytokines

Pain: Impulses ascending to the hypothalamus via the nociceptive pathways and the reticular formation trigger ACTH secretion in response to injury

Mechanism of Action of CRH

CRH binds to G protein-coupled receptors in the corticotrope membrane and activates adenylyl cyclase resulting in increase in cyclic AMP.

Diurnal Rhythm of Cortisol Secretion

ACTH is secreted in irregular bursts throughout the day and plasma cortisol levels rise and fall with a 24-hour periodicity in response to these bursts. The bursts are more frequent in the early morning and cortisol levels are highest in the early morning hours. This diurnal (circadian) rhythm is sensitive to the daily pattern of physical activity. The biologic clock responsible for the diurnal ACTH rhythm is located in the suprachiasmatic nucleus of the hypothalamus (Figs 9.39, 9.47 to 9.49).

MINERALOCORTICOIDS

Mechanism of Action

Like cortisol, aldosterone also acts by binding to a specific intracellular receptor, i.e. mineralocorticoid receptor. After dissociation of chaperone proteins, nuclear translocation and binding to mineralocorticoid-response element, the hormone-receptor complex alters the transcription of mRNAs which increases the production of certain proteins.

Transport and Metabolism of Aldosterone

Aldosterone has low affinity for the corticosteroid-binding globulin and albumin; therefore, it has a short half-life of about 20 minutes. Most of the aldosterone is inactivated in the liver to the tetrahydroglucuronide derivative and excreted by the kidney.

Actions of Aldosterone

Kidney

The principal action of aldosterone is to increase the reabsorption of Na^+, followed by water, in the distal nephron. Thus, mineralocorticoids cause retention of Na^+ in the ECF. This expands ECF volume. Sodium reabsorption is brought about primarily by the increase in activity of the ENaC channels in the apical membrane. Na^+ diffuses into the cell through these channels along its electrochemical gradient. The primary site of action is the principal cell (P cell) of the renal collecting ducts.

Aldosterone also stimulates K^+ and H^+ secretion. Increased amounts of Na^+ are exchanged for K^+ or H^+ in the renal tubules, producing a K^+ diuresis and an increase in urine acidity.

9

Actions on Other Epithelia

As in the distal nephron, aldosterone increases sodium and water reabsorption and increases K^+ excretion in the colon. Aldosterone has similar effects on epithelia of salivary glands, sweat glands and gastric glands.

Aldosterone Escape

With prolonged exposure to excess mineralocorticoids, Na^+ excretion is increased in spite of the continued action of the hormone on renal tubules. This phenomenon is called aldosterone escape. Initially, there is sodium retention and volume expansion. Plasma Na^+ is elevated only slightly if at all, because water is retained with the osmotically active sodium ions. When the ECF expansion passes a certain point, the escape phenomenon occurs. As ECF volume is expanded, the glomerular filtration rate increases. This increases the rate of sodium delivery to the nephron and therefore the rate of renal sodium excretion, which limits the ability of aldosterone to expand extracellular volume. Increased atrial natriuretic peptide (ANP) secretion may contribute to the escape phenomenon. The increase in vascular volume will stimulate the release of ANP which promotes renal Na^+ excretion. However, "escape" from the effects of aldosterone on potassium and hydrogen ion secretion does not occur and potassium depletion and metabolic alkalosis can persist.

Regulation of Aldosterone Secretion

- Angiotensin II is a potent stimulus for aldosterone production. The early action is on the conversion of cholesterol to pregnenolone and the late action is on the conversion of corticosterone to 18-hydroxycorticosterone, which in-turn facilitates the production of aldosterone.
- Like angiotensin II, plasma K^+ stimulates the conversion of cholesterol to pregnenolone and the conversion of corticosterone to aldosterone.
- ACTH from the anterior pituitary is not required for basal aldosterone secretion but is responsible for the normal increase in rate of secretion produced by surgery and other stresses.
- ANP acts directly on the zona glomerulosa to inhibit aldosterone secretion. It also acts indirectly by inhibiting renin secretion and plays an important role in aldosterone escape.

Stimuli that increase aldosterone secretion
Surgery
Anxiety
Physical trauma
Hemorrhage
High potassium intake
Low sodium intake
Standing

ADRENAL ANDROGENS

Transport and Metabolism of Adrenal Androgen

DHEAS binds to albumin and other transport globulins with low affinity and has a half-life of 15 to 30 minutes. It is excreted by the kidney. In contrast, DHEAS binds to albumin with very high affinity and has a half-life of 7 to 10 hours.

Physiological Actions of Adrenal Androgens

Androgens are the hormones that exert masculinizing effects and they promote protein anabolism and growth. Adrenal androgens do not have a significant role in men; in women, however, they constitute 50% of the circulating active androgens. They are required for the appearance of axillary and pubic hair as well as libido.

The adrenal androgen androstenedione is converted to testosterone and to estrogen (aromatized) in fat and other peripheral tissues. This is an important source of estrogens in men and postmenopausal women.

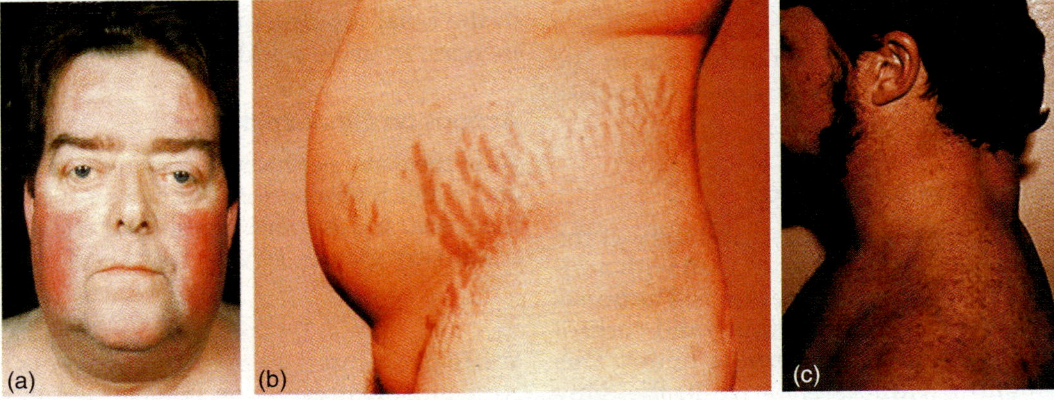

Figs 9.51a to c: (a) Cushing syndrome; (b) abdominal striae and (c) buffalo hump

Regulation of Adrenal Androgens

ACTH stimulates production of adrenal androgens but neither adrenal androgens nor their potent metabolites (i.e. testosterone, dihydrotestosterone, estradiol-17β) negatively feedback on ACTH or CRH.

Applied Aspects

Adrenocortical Excess

Cushing's Syndrome

The clinical picture produced by prolonged increases in plasma glucocorticoids was described by Harvey Cushing and is called Cushing's syndrome (Fig. 9.51a). It may be ACTH-independent or ACTH-dependent.

Causes

Pharmacologic use of exogenous corticosteroids is now the most common cause of this condition (ACTH-independent Cushing's syndrome).

The next most prevalent cause is ACTH-secreting tumors, such as functional tumors of the anterior pituitary gland and lung cancers that produce ACTH (ectopic ACTH syndrome). Cushing's syndrome due to anterior pituitary tumors is often called Cushing's disease because these tumors were the cause of the cases described by Cushing.

Other causes of ACTH-independent Cushing's syndrome include glucocorticoid-secreting adrenal tumors and adrenal hyperplasia.

Clinical features and causes	
Clinical feature	*Cause*
Centripetal fat distribution: Truncal obesity with thin limbs	For reasons not fully understood, adipose tissue accumulates in the abdomen. The limbs are thin as a result of increased muscle proteolysis
Protruding abdomen with purple striae (Fig. 9.51b)	Accumulation of abdominal fat with poor abdominal muscle tone due to proteolysis; increased proteolysis causes thinning of skin that is rapidly stretched by the increased intra-abdominal fat
Buffalo hump (Fig. 9.51c)	Increase in the size of sub-clavicular fat pads
Moon face	Fat deposition; salt and water retention
Flushed face	Polycythemia
Bruises and ecchymoses	Increased capillary fragility as a result of damage to the connective tissue supporting the capillaries
Muscle weakness	Increased muscle proteolysis
Poor wound healing	Inhibit fibroblastic proliferation and collagen synthesis
Osteoporosis	Inhibit osteoblastic activity; Decrease intestinal absorption of calcium which lowers plasma calcium levels and increases PTH secretion
Increased susceptibility to infection	Immunosuppression by glucocorticoids
Hypertension	Mineralocorticoid activity seen with excessive glucocorticoids or increased aldosterone secretion causes salt and water retention; direct glucocorticoid effect on blood vessels
Hirsutism, male pattern of baldness and enlargement of the clitoris in women (adrenogenital syndrome) and precocious pseudo-puberty in boys	Excessive adrenal androgen secretion
Personality changes	Effect on the CNS
Metabolic effects:	
Hyperglycemia, glucose intolerance and Insulin resistance	Increased gluconeogenesis and decreased peripheral utilization of glucose
Increase in total body fat	Increase in appetite due to action on the CNS resulting in increased caloric consumption; Increase in plasma glucose levels increases insulin secretion. Insulin is a strong lipogenic hormone and cortisol is a weak lipolytic hormone

Conn's Syndrome

Hyperaldosteronism of adrenal origin (primary hyperaldosteronism) is called Conn's syndrome. It is seen with adenoma of the zona glomerulosa, adrenal hyperplasia and adrenal carcinoma. Excess mineralocorticoid secretion leads to K^+ depletion and Na^+ retention. Edema is not an accompanying feature due to the phenomenon of aldosterone escape. Other clinical features are:

- Muscle weakness
- Hypertension
- Tetany
- Polyuria
- Hypokalemic alkalosis

Secondary Hyperaldosteronism

The causes of secondary hyperaldosteronism are:

- Cirrhosis
- Cardiac failure
- Nephrosis
- Renal arterial constriction

Adrenocortical Insufficiency

Addison's Disease

Primary adrenal insufficiency due to disease processes that destroy the adrenal cortex is called Addison's disease. Usually, both mineralocorticoids and glucocorticoids are deficient. It used to be a common complication of tuberculosis but the common cause of this condition now is autoimmune destruction of the adrenal cortex.

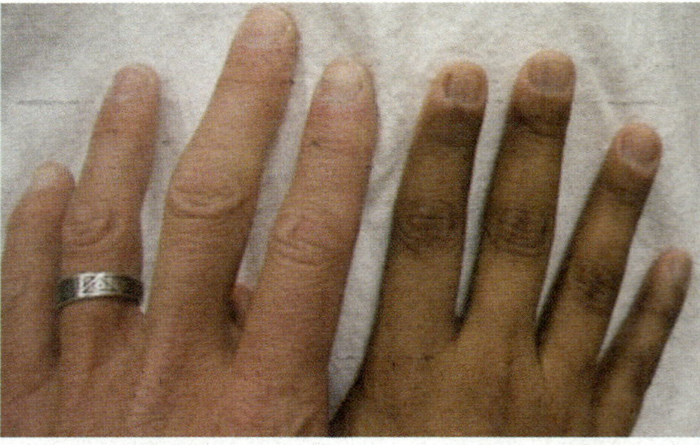

Fig. 9.52: Hyperpigmentation in Addison's diseases

Clinical Features

Clinical manifestation	*Cause*
Orthostatic hypotension: Inability to maintain normal mean arterial pressure with postural change to a standing position	Decreased baroreceptor mediated vasoconstriction (loss of the permissive action of glucocorticoids for pressor effects of catecholamines) causes a drop in peripheral resistance
Circulatory shock	Deficiency of mineralocorticoids results in contraction of ECF volume, producing circulatory hypovolemia and therefore, a decrease in blood pressure and cardiac output
Muscle weakness	Glucocorticoids are important for muscle function
Hypoglycemia when fasting or in stress	Impaired gluconeogenesis and increasd insulin sensitivity; hyperglycemic actions of other hormones, namely, glucagon, epinephrine and growth hormone, generally prevent hypoglycemia
Water intoxication	Though hypovolemia occurs, water intoxication can develop if a water load is given as the loss of glucocorticoids impairs the ability to excrete a water load
Increased pigmentation of skin, particularly in creases, scars and gums and spotty pigmentation (Fig. 9.52)	Elevated levels of ACTH have MSH activity and compete the melanotropin-1 receptor (MC1R) in melanocytes
Weight loss	Decreased appetite and decreased gastrointestinal secretion due to glucocorticoid deficiency
Hyperkalemia metabolic acidosis	Impaired renal excretion of potassium and hydrogen ions
Anemia	Decreased erythropoiesis due to cortisol deficiency; decreased iron and vitamin B_{12} absorption
Depression, psychosis	Cortisol deficiency

Secondary adrenocortical insufficiency is caused by pituitary disorders that decrease ACTH secretion and tertiary adrenocortical insufficiency is caused by hypothalamic disorders disrupting CRH secretion. Both are usually milder than primary adrenal insufficiency because electrolyte metabolism is affected to a lesser degree. In these conditions, there is no increase in pigmentation because plasma ACTH is low.

ADRENAL MEDULLARY HORMONES

Norepinephrine, epinephrine and dopamine are the catecholamines secreted by the adrenal medulla. Circulating epinephrine is derived entirely from the adrenals; in contrast, only 30% of the circulating norepinephrine comes from the medulla. The remaining 70% is released from the terminals of postganglionic sympathetic fibers and diffuses into the circulation. Though medullary hormones affect virtually every tissue of the body and play a crucial role in the acute response to stress, the adrenal medulla is not essential for life as long as the rest of the sympathetic nervous system is intact.

Chemistry and Synthesis of Catecholamines

The structure of catecholamines is illustrated in Fig. 9.53.

Catecholamine synthesis begins with the transport of the amino acid, tyrosine, into the chromaffin cell cytoplasm. Most tyrosine is of dietary origin. Tyrosine is hydroxylated and decarboxylated to form norepinephrine; norepinephrine is methylated to form epinephrine.

The biosynthetic steps are illustrated in Fig. 9.54.

Tyrosine is hydroxylated by the rate-limiting enzyme, tyrosine hydroxylase, to produce dihydroxyphenylalanine (DOPA). The enzyme is subject to feedback inhibition by dopamine and norepinephrine, thus providing internal control of the synthetic process.

DOPA is converted to dopamine by the cytoplasmic enzyme, aromatic amino acid decarboxylase (DOPA decarboxylase) and is then transported into the secretory vesicle.

Within the vesicle, dopamine is converted to norepinephrine by the enzyme, dopamine-β-hydroxylase. Essentially, all of the dopamine is converted to norepinephrine and remains in the vesicle in norepinephrine-secreting neurons until secreted.

In epinephrine-secreting cells, norepinephrine diffuses out of the vesicle by facilitated transport and is methylated by the cytoplasmic enzyme, phenylethanolamine-N-methyltransferase (PNMT), to form epinephrine. Epinephrine is then transported back into the secretory vesicle.

Norepinephrine and epinephrine are stored in the secretory vesicles with ATP and a protein called chromogranin A. This protein may play a general role in hormone storage or secretion.

Secretion is initiated by acetylcholine released from the preganglionic sympathetic neurons that innervate the medulla. Acetylcholine binds to nicotinic receptors and opens cation channels; the Ca^{2+} that enters the cells from the ECF triggers exocytosis and causes

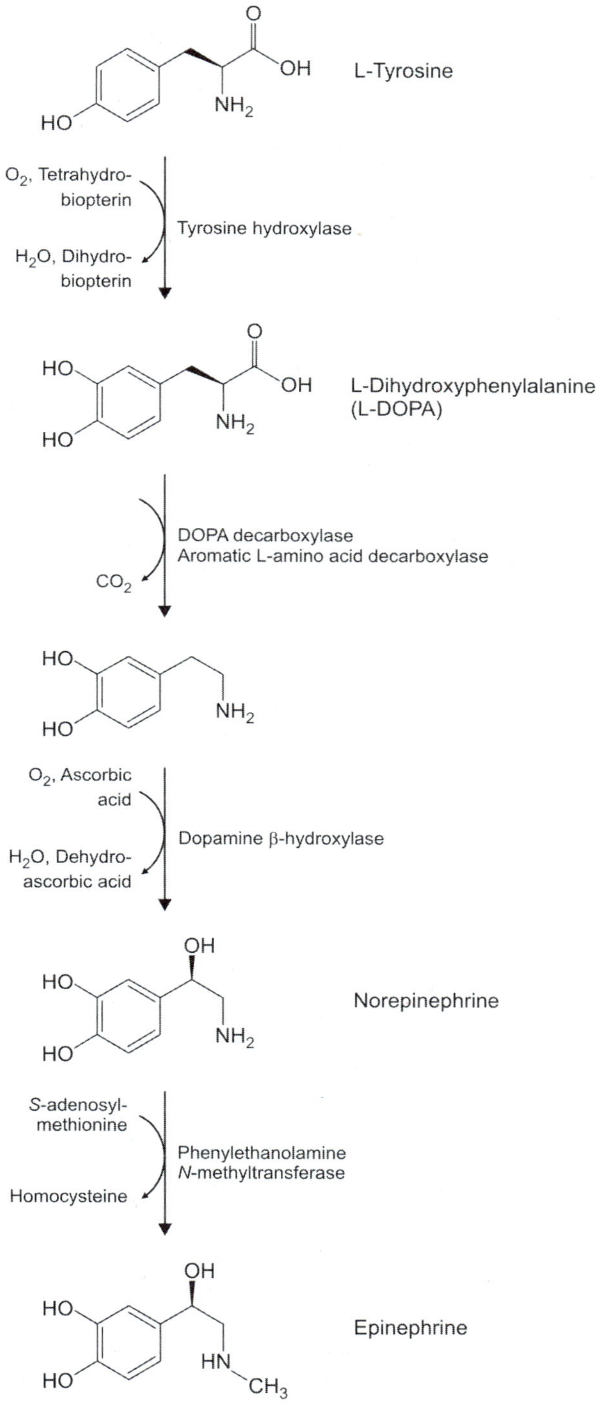

L-Tyrosine

O_2, Tetrahydrobiopterin → H_2O, Dihydrobiopterin — Tyrosine hydroxylase

L-Dihydroxyphenylalanine (L-DOPA)

DOPA decarboxylase / Aromatic L-amino acid decarboxylase — CO_2

O_2, Ascorbic acid → H_2O, Dehydroascorbic acid — Dopamine β-hydroxylase

Norepinephrine

S-adenosylmethionine → Homocysteine — Phenylethanolamine N-methyltransferase

Epinephrine

Fig. 9.53: Structure of catecholamines

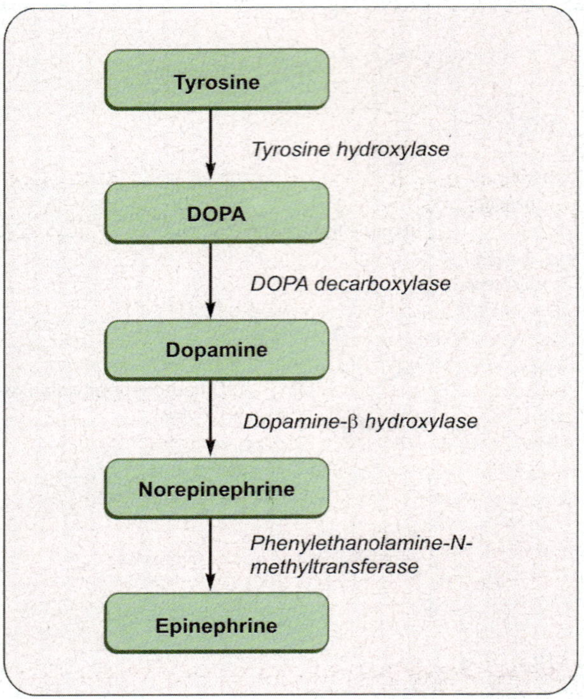

Fig. 9.54: Synthesis of epinephrine in adrenal medulus

release of the catecholamines, ATP, chromogranin A and the enzyme, dopamine β-hydroxylase contained in the vesicles.

Circulating levels of chromogranin A appear to be an index of sympathetic activity.

Adrenomedullin is a polypeptide found in adrenal medullary cells that causes vasodilatation. It appears to act by increasing the production of nitric oxide. It is found in many other tissues, including the kidney and the brain.

9

Transport and Metabolism of Catecholamines

In plasma, about 70% of the norepinephrine and epinephrine are conjugated to sulfate. Sulfate conjugates are inactive. Catecholamines have a half-life of about 2 minutes in the circulation.

Epinephrine and norepinephrine are metabolized to biologically inactive compounds by oxidation and methylation. Oxidation is catalyzed by monoamine oxidase (MAO) located in the outer surface of the mitochondria. It is widely distributed and particularly plentiful in the nerve endings at which catecholamines are secreted (Fig. 9.55).

The methylation of catecholamines is catalyzed by the enzyme, catechol-O-methyltransferase (COMT)

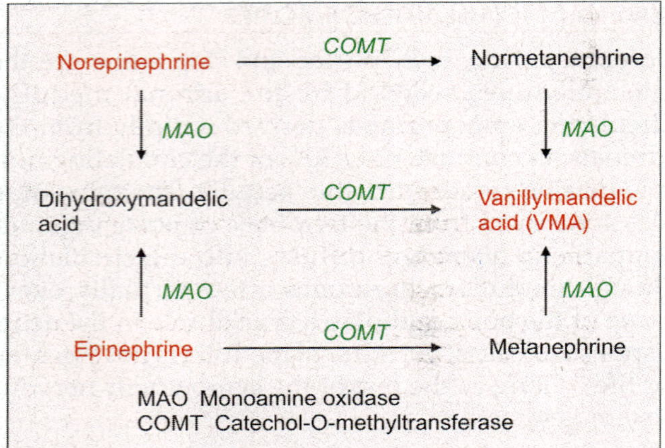

Fig. 9.55: Metabolism of catecholamines

which acts primarily on secreted catecholamines. It is particularly abundant in the liver, kidneys and smooth muscle and is not found in presynaptic noradrenergic neurons.

The O-methylated derivatives that are not excreted are largely oxidized to vanillylmandelic acid (VMA), the most abundant catecholamine metabolite in the urine.

Mechanism of Action of Catecholamines

Catecholamines act via G protein-coupled receptors in the cell membrane. The individual types of adrenergic receptors were first classified based on their pharmacology. Adrenergic receptors are generally classified as α-adrenergic and β-adrenergic receptors. α-adrenergic receptors are further divided into α_1 and α_2 receptors; β-adrenergic receptors are divided into β_1, β_2 and β_3 receptors.

Regulation of Adrenal Medullary Hormones

Secretion of epinephrine and norepinephrine from the adrenal medulla is primarily under sympathetic neural control. The primary autonomic centers that initiate sympathetic responses are in the hypothalamus and brainstem. Autonomic signals descend in the preganglionic sympathetic neurons that directly innervate the adrenal medulla. Thus, stimuli that activate the sympathetic nervous system almost always stimulate adrenal medullary secretion. This association of the sympathetic nervous system with the adrenal medulla is referred to as the 'sympatho-adrenal' system.

Actions of Catecholamines

Metabolic Effects

Norepinephrine and epinephrine promote glycogenolysis in liver and skeletal muscle and lipolysis in adipose tissue. These actions increase circulating levels of lactate and glycerol which can be used by the liver as gluconeogenic substrates to increase glucose. Lactate oxidation in the liver may be responsible for the calorigenic effect of epinephrine.

Catecholamines stimulate glucagon secretion through β_2 receptors and inhibit insulin secretion (α_2 receptors).

They produce a rise in the basal metabolic rate.

Cardiovascular Effects

Norepinephrine and epinephrine increase both the rate (chronotropic action) and force of contraction (inotropic action) of the isolated heart through their action on β_1 receptors.

Norepinephrine produces vasoconstriction in most organs via α_1 receptors and increases the systolic and diastolic pressure. The hypertension stimulates the carotid and aortic baroreceptors, producing reflex bradycardia that overrides the direct cardioacceleratory effect of norepinephrine.

Epinephrine dilates the blood vessels in skeletal muscle and the liver via α_2 receptors. This overbalances the vasoconstriction produced by epinephrine elsewhere and the total peripheral resistance drops. Epinephrine, thus, causes a widening of the pulse pressure because baroreceptor stimulation is insufficient to obscure the direct effect of the hormone on the heart, cardiac rate and output increase (Fig. 9.56).

Circulating Epinephrine Causes

- Increased heart rate and inotropy (β_1-adrenoceptor mediated)
- Vasoconstriction in most systemic arteries and veins (postjunctional α_1 and α_2 adrenoceptors)
- Vasodilation in muscle and liver vasculatures at low concentrations (β_2-adrenoceptor)
- The overall cardiovascular response epinephrine is increased cardiac output with only a small change in mean arterial pressure.

Circulating Norepinephrine Causes

- Increased heart rate (although only transiently) and increased inotropy (β_1-adrenoceptor mediated) are the direct effects of norepinephrine on the heart.
- Vasoconstriction occurs in most systemic arteries and veins (postjunctional α_1- and α_2- adrenoceptors)
- The overall cardiovascular response is increased cardiac output and systemic vascular resistance, which results in an elevation in arterial blood pressure. Heart rate, although initially stimulated by norepinephrine, decreases due to activation of baroreceptors and vagal-mediated slowing of the heart rate.

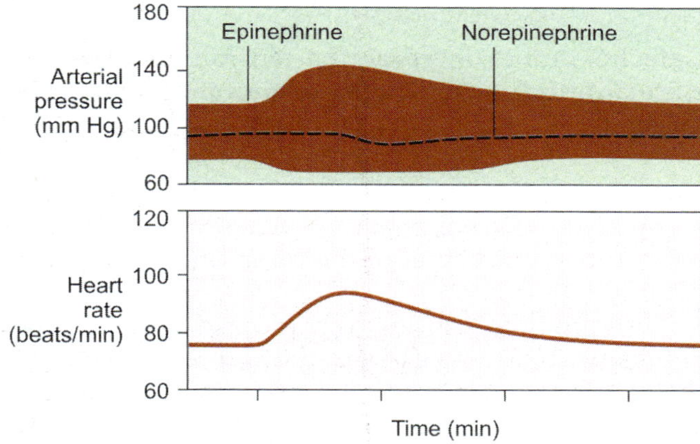

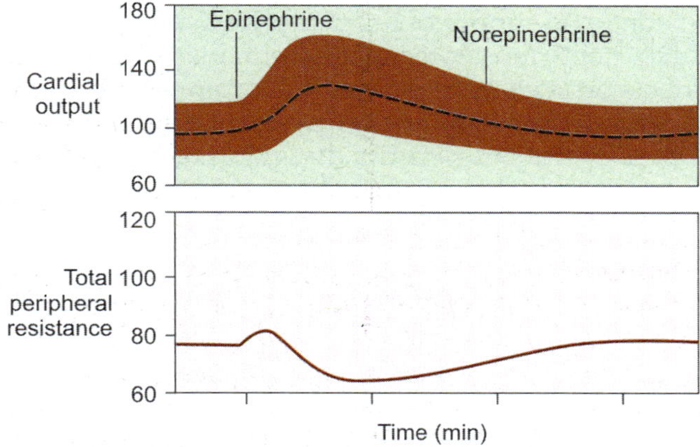

Fig. 9.56: Circulatory changes produces after administration of epinephrine and norepinephrine

Effect on Bronchial Smooth Muscle

Epinephrine promotes relaxation of bronchiolar smooth muscle through β_2 receptors.

Effect on Visceral Smooth Muscle

A sympathoadrenal response decreases gastrointestinal motility and decreases the energy demand of visceral smooth muscle.

9

Effects on Skeletal Muscle

Catecholamines increase the tension generated in skeletal muscles and increase neuromuscular transmission.

Ocular Effects

Sympathetic discharge causes dilatation of the pupil by causing contraction of the radial muscle fibers of the iris.

Thus, the effects of catecholamines on various tissues are coordinated to help the individual cope with the challenges to survival. Cardiovascular effects maximize cardiac output and ensure perfusion of the brain and working muscles. Metabolic effects ensure an adequate supply of nutrients. Relaxation of bronchial smooth muscle facilitates pulmonary ventilation. Effects on skeletal muscle and neuromuscular transmission increase muscular performance and quiescence of the gut permits diversion of blood flow, oxygen and fuel to reinforce these effect (Fig. 9.57).

Applied Aspects

A pheochromocytoma is a tumor of the chromaffin tissue that produces excessive catecholamines. Pheochromocytomas are the most common source of hyperadrenal medullary function. The catecholamine most frequently elevated in pheocromocytoma is norepinephrine.

Clinical Features

The symptoms of excessive catecholamine secretion are often sporadic. These include hypertension, headaches (from hypertension), sweating, anxiety, palpitations and chest pain. Patients may experience orthostatic hypotension (despite the tendency for hypertension. This occurs because hypersecretion of catecholamines decreases the postsynaptic response to norepinephrine as a result of down-regulation of the receptors. Consequently, the baroreceptor response to the volume shifts that occur on standing is blunted.

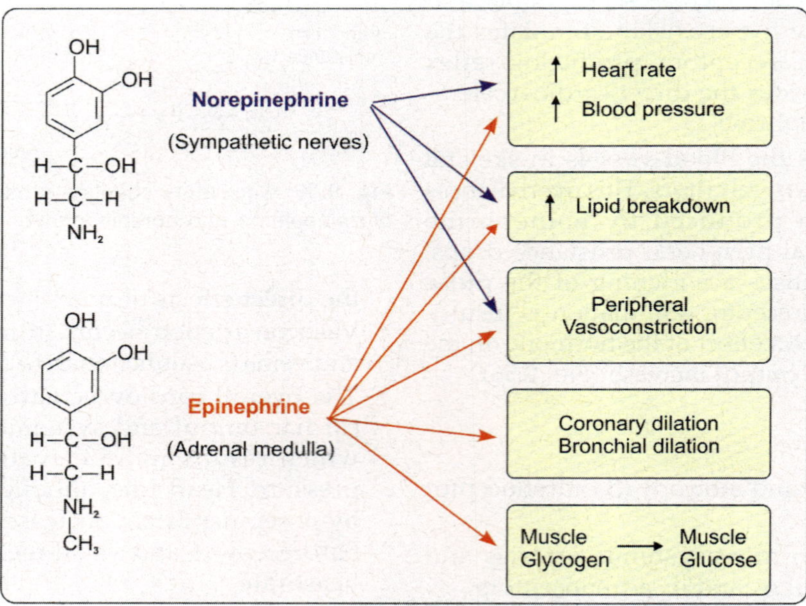

Fig. 9.57

9

79. MISCELLANEOUS HORMONES

Besides the classical endocrine glands, there are additional organs with endocrine functions.

- The kidneys produce two hormones: 1, 25-dihydroxycholecalciferol, a calcitropic hormone and erythropoietin.
- The heart secretes natriuretic peptides
- The adipocytes secrete at least three established protein hormones that have an effect on insulin sensitivity.
- The pineal gland secretes melatonin.

Renin, produced by juxtaglomerular cells in the kidney, is an acid protease secreted into the bloodstream. Its only known function is to form angiotensin I from the plasma protein, angiotensinogen. As it does not require receptors to mediate its action and there is no signal transduction involved, renin should not be considered a hormone.

PINEAL GLAND

The pineal gland (epiphysis) secretes melatonin, which may function as a timing device to keep internal events synchronized with the light-dark cycle in the environment (Fig. 9.58).

Anatomy

The pineal gland arises from the roof of the third ventricle under the posterior end of the corpus callosum. The pineal stroma contains neuroglia and parenchymal cells with features suggesting that they have a secretory function. Like other endocrine glands, the pineal has highly permeable fenestrated capillaries. In infants, the pineal is large; it begins to involute before puberty, and small concretions of calcium phosphate and carbonate (pineal sand) appear in the tissue. Because the concretions are radiopaque, the normal pineal is often visible on X-ray films of the skull in adults.

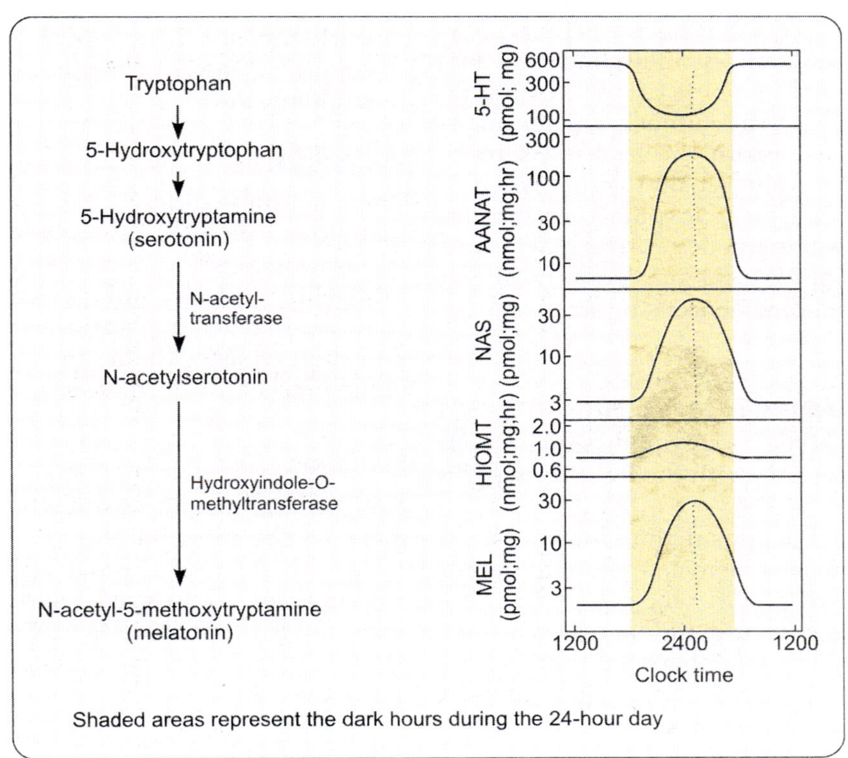

Fig. 9.58: Diurnal rhythms of various compounds in the pineal and melatonin in blood

Displacement of a calcified pineal from its normal position indicates the presence of a space-occupying lesion such as a brain tumor.

Melatonin

Synthesis and Secretion

Melatonin is synthesized from serotonin by N-acetylation and O-methylation and secreted into the blood and the cerebrospinal fluid.

Receptors

The melatonin receptors are of many types and they are all coupled to G proteins; However, the functions of each remain to be determined.

Regulation of Secretion

Melatonin synthesis and secretion is increased during the dark period of the day and maintained at a low level during daylight hours. This diurnal variation is brought about by norepinephrine secreted by the postganglionic sympathetic nerves (nervi conarii) that innervate the pineal. The norepinephrine acts via β-adrenergic receptors in the pineal to increase intracellular cAmP and the cAMP in turn produces a marked increase in N-acetyltransferase activity. This results in increased melatonin synthesis and secretion.

The retinohypothalamic fibers carry information about the light-dark cycle to the suprachiasmatic nuclei in the hypothalamus. From the hypothalamus, descending pathways converge on the inter-medio-lateral gray column of the thoracic spinal cord and end on the preganglionic sympathetic neurons that in-turn innervate the superior cervical ganglion, the site of origin of the postganglionic neurons to the pineal.

9

Function of the Pineal

It is hypothesized that the diurnal change in melatonin secretion functions as some sort of timing signal which coordinates internal events with the light-dark cycle in the environment.

There is a leading proposal that focuses on a potential role for the hormone melatonin in initiating the onset of puberty. Melatonin, whose secretion decreases during exposure to light and increases during exposure to the dark, has an antigonadotropic effect in many species. Some researchers suggest that an observed reduction in the overall rate of melatonin secretion at puberty in humans–particularly during the night, when the peaks of GnRH secretion first occur–is the trigger for the onset of puberty.

HORMONES OF THE HEART

Two natriuretic hormones are secreted by the heart. The first natriuretic hormone isolated from the heart was atrial natriuretic peptide (ANP). The second was first isolated from brain and named brain natriuretic peptide (BNP); subsequently more BNP was found in the human heart, including the ventricles.

Actions

- ANP and BNP in the circulation act on the kidneys to increase Na^+ excretion. They appear to produce this effect by dilating afferent arterioles and relaxing mesangial cells. Both the actions increase glomerular filtration rate.
- They act on the renal tubules to inhibit Na^+ reabsorption.
- They also increase capillary permeability, leading to extravasation of fluid and a decline in blood pressure.
- These peptides relax vascular smooth muscle in arterioles and venules.
- Both the peptides inhibit renin secretion and counteract the pressor effects of catecholamines and angiotensin II.

Receptors

There are three different types of natriuretic peptide receptors. Two of them have intracellular guanylyl cyclase domains; the third receptor does not trigger any intracellular activity and is a clearance receptor which removes natriuretic peptides from the bloodstream and then releases them later, maintaining a steady blood level of the hormones.

Secretion

ANP secretion is increased when the ECF volume is increased by infusion of isotonic saline or ingestion of a high-sodium diet. It appears that the atria respond directly to stretch and that the rate of ANP secretion is proportionate to the degree to which the atria are stretched by increases in central venous pressure.

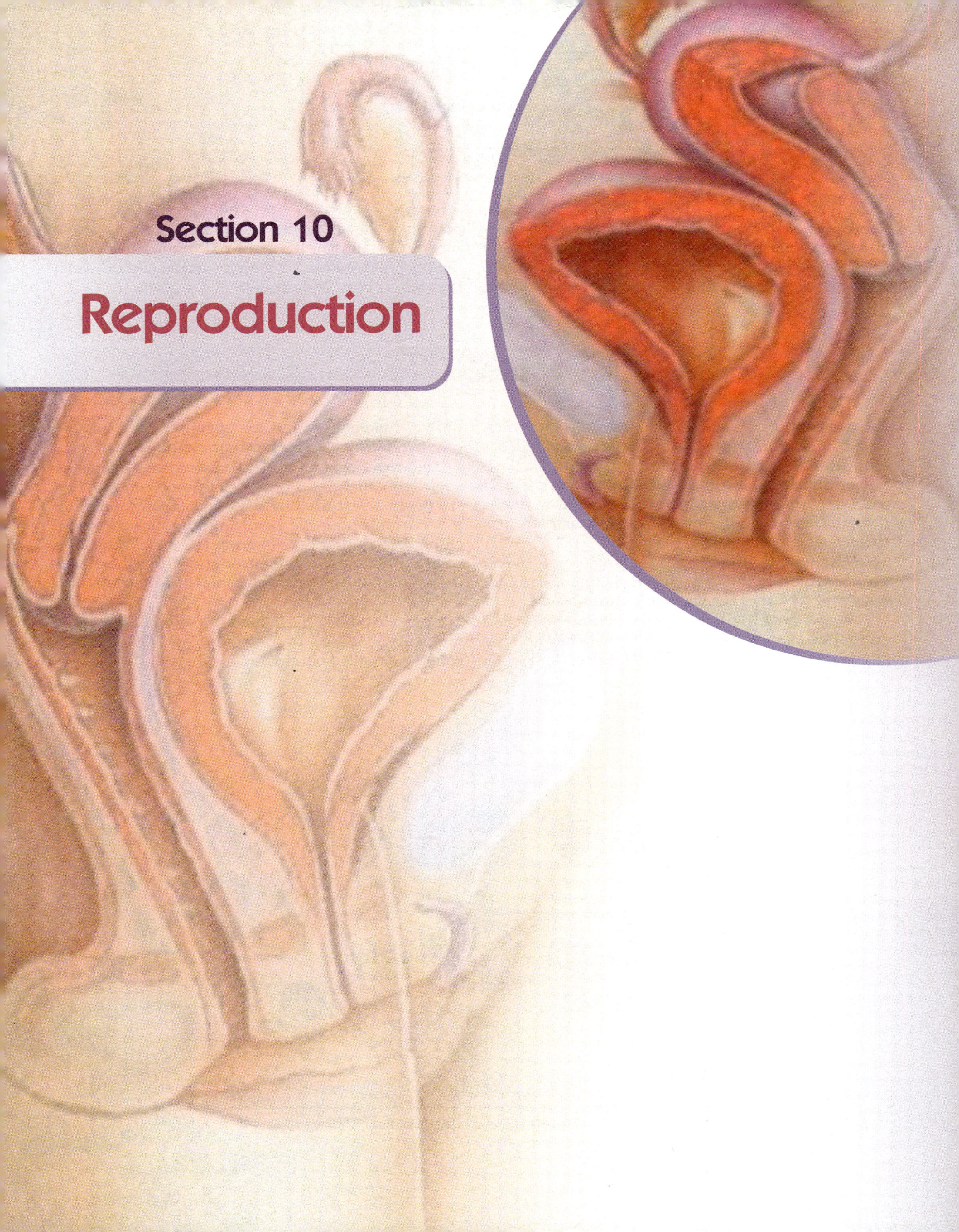

Section 10

Reproduction

80. INTRODUCTION

Reproduction is the process by which new members of a species are produced. It ensures the survival of the species. Sexual reproduction is by union of two sex cells or gametes, one male and one female. In mammals, development occurs in the uterus of the mother. In human, the fertilized ovum develops in the uterus for ten lunar months, at the end of which the child is born and cared by the mother.

81. DETERMINATION OF SEX

Sex is determined genetically by two chromosomes, called the sex chromosomes but the sex characteristics are influenced by sex hormones (Fig. 10.1). Each human somatic cell contain 46 chromosomes (i.e. 23 pairs of chromosomes) of these 22 pairs are somatic chromosomes or autosomes and one pair is the sex chromosome.

In the female, the sex chromosomes are two X chromosomes. In the male, one is a large X chromosome and the other is a smaller Y chromosome.

During gametogenesis, meiotic division (reduction division) occurs, by which each gamete has half the number of chromosomes (haploid number) and when union of gametes occur, the zygote formed has the original number of chromosomes (diploid number).

The ovum contains 22 + X chromosomes and the sperm contains 22 + X or 22 + Y chromosomes. When the ovum is fertilized by a spermatozoan containing a Y chromosome the resulting zygote has 44 XY chromosomes and the offspring is a male. When the sperm containing X chromosome fertilizes the ovum, the zygote has 44 XX chromosomes and develops into a female.

Each chromosome is made up of a large DNA molecule, covered by protein. The DNA-protein complex is called chromatin.

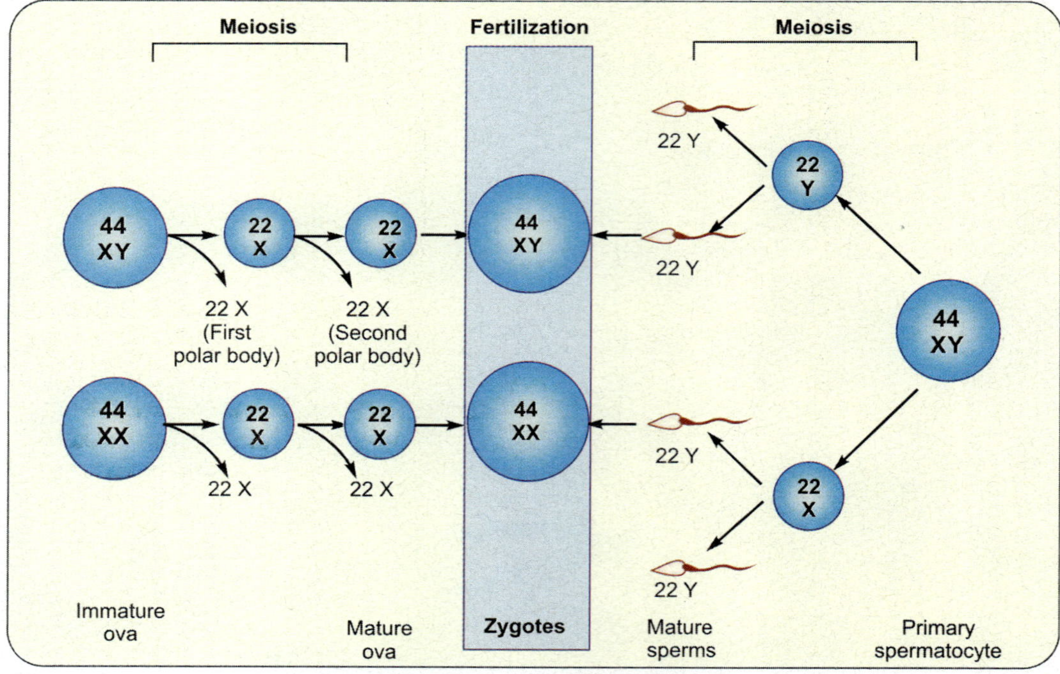

Fig. 10.1: Determination of sex

10

82. SEX CHROMATIN (BARR BODY)

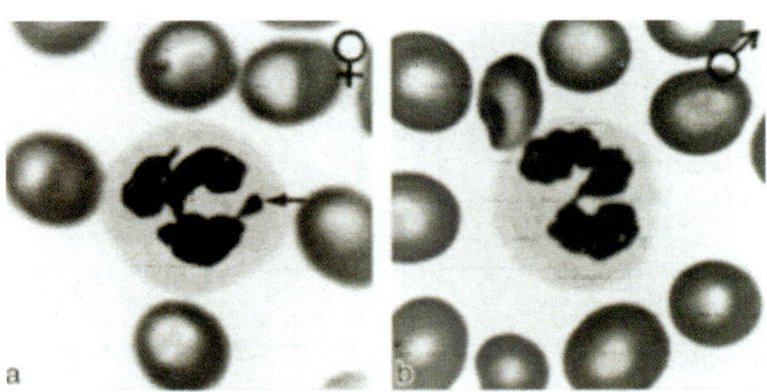

Figs 10.2a and b: Sex chromatin (Barr body) *Left:* An-arrow depicts the drumstick pattern of Barr body in the white blood cells of female

The somatic cells of a woman show chromatin mass called sex chromatin or Barr body (Figs 10.2a and b).

This is an inactivated X chromosome of the female cell.

One of the X chromosomes of each somatic cell of the female fetus becomes inactive in early embryonic life.

The DNA becomes tightly coiled and this prevents the release of messenger RNA rendering it non-functional. This inactivation is random, about half the cells carry an active maternal X chromosome and inactive paternal X chromosome and the other half has an active paternal chromosome and inactive maternal chromosome. The number of Barr bodies is one less than the number of X chromosomes.

Hence, a normal female with 46 XX chromosomes has one Barr body, while a normal male with 46 XY chromosomes has no Barr body.

83. DEVELOPMENT OF REPRODUCTIVE SYSTEM

GONADS

On each side of the embryo, a primitive gonad arises from the genital ridge by condensation of tissue near the adrenal gland. The gonad develops a cortex and a medulla. Until the 6th week of development, the structures are identical in both sexes.

In genetic males, the medulla develops during the 7th and 8th week into a testis and the cortex regresses. Leydig and Sertoli cells appear. Testosterone and Müllerian inhibiting substance are secreted.

In genetic females, the cortex develops into an ovary and the medulla regresses. The embryonic ovary does not secrete hormones (Fig. 10.3)

GENITALIA

In the 7th week of gestation, the embryo has both male and female primordial genital ducts. In a normal female fetus, the Müllerian duct system then develops into uterine tubes (oviducts) and a uterus. In the normal male fetus, the Wolffian duct system on each side develops into the epididymis and vas deferens. The external genitalia are similarly bipotential until the 8th week. Thereafter, the urogenital slit disappears and male genitalia forms or alternatively, it remains open and female genitalia forms.

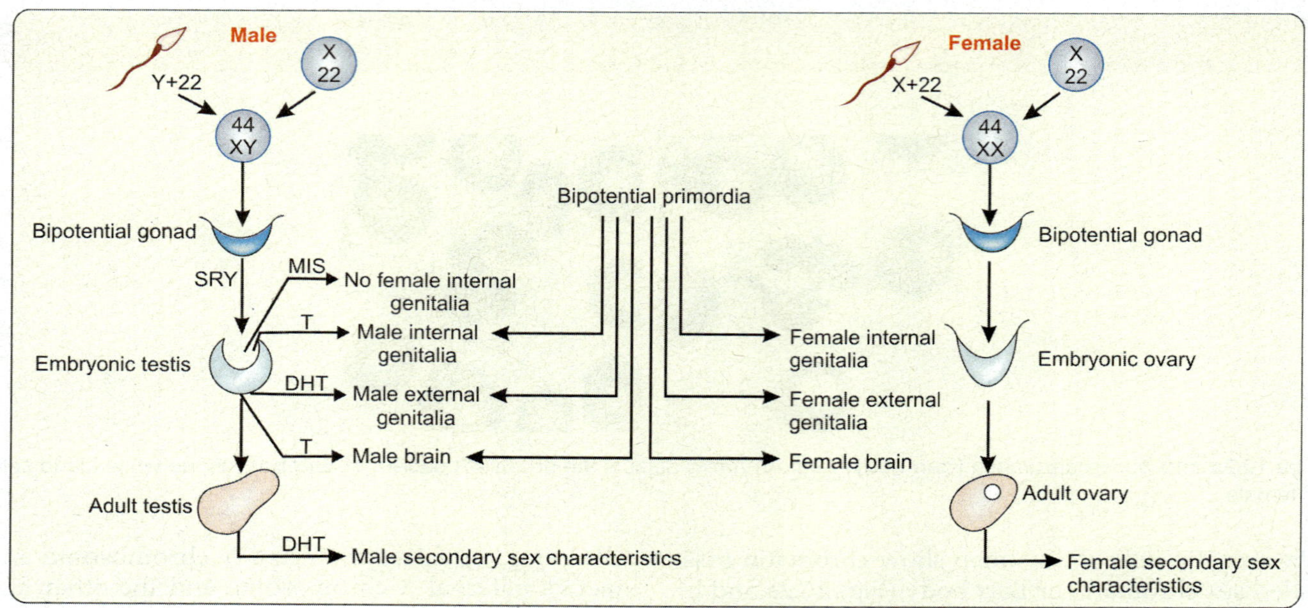

Fig. 10.3: Normal sex determination, differentiation and development in humans

84. ABERRANT SEXUAL DIFFERENTIATION

10

CHROMOSOMAL ABNORMALITIES (Fig. 10.4)

Turner's Syndrome
(Gonadal Dysgenesis, Ovarian Agenesis)

In individuals with the XO chromosomal pattern (45 XO), the gonads are rudimentary or absent, so that female external genitalia develop.

- Stature is short.
- Webbing of neck and primary amenorrhea are present
- Congenital abnormalities are often present
- No sexual maturation occurs at puberty.

Klinefelter's Syndrome
(Seminiferous Tubule Dysgenesis)

Individuals with the 47 XXY pattern, the most common sex chromosome disorder have the genitalia of normal male. Testosterone secretion at puberty is enough for the development of male characteristics.

- They are usually tall with bilateral gynecomastia.
- The seminiferous tubules are abnormal.
- Incidence of mental retardation is higher than normal.

Down's Syndrome (Trisomy 21, Mongolism)

- Nondisjunction of chromosome 21 produces trisomy 21.

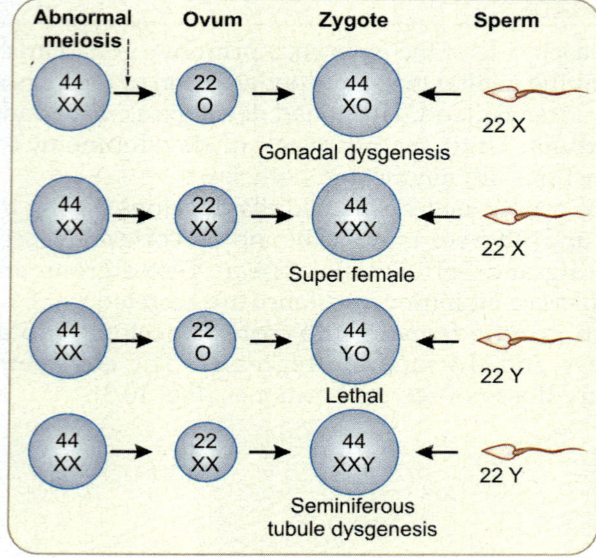

Fig. 10.4: Aberrant sexual differentiation

- Features are small head, slanting eyes and mental retardation.

Super Female (XXX)

- True hermaphroditism
- In this condition, the individual has both ovaries and testes
- Due to XX/XY mosaicism

These chromosomal abnormalities can be diagnosed *in utero* by analysis of fetal cells in a sample of amniotic fluid collected by inserting a needle through the abdominal wall (aminocentesis) or early in pregnancy by examining fetal cells obtained by a needle biopsy of chorionic villi (chorionic villus sampling).

HORMONAL ABNORMALITIES

Female Pseudohermaphroditism

Male genital development occur in genetic females exposed to androgens secreted by the embryonic testes causing hypertrophy of the clitoris.

A pseudohermaphrodite is an individual with the genetic constitution and gonads of one sex and the genitalia of the other.

It may be due to congenital virilizing adrenal hyperplasia.

Male Pseudohermaphroditism

The development of female external genitalia in genetic males is due to defective testicular development.

The testes also secrete Müllerian inhibiting substance (MIS) hence, genetic males with defective testes have female internal genitalia.

Another cause is due to androgen resistance: One form is 5 α-reductase deficiency.

It also occurs when there is congenital deficiency of 17 α-hydroxylase.

Testicular Feminizing Syndrome or Complete Androgen Resistance Syndrome

- When the loss of receptor function is complete, this syndrome results.
- MIS is present and testosterone is secreted in normal or elevated rate.
- The external genitalia is female, but the vagina ends blindly because there is no female internal genitalia.
- There is enlarged breasts at puberty.
- Diagnosed only by lack of menstruation.

85. PUBERTY

It is the period or time when gametogenic and endocrine functions of the gonads develop to the point where reproduction becomes possible. The accessory sex organs enlarge and the characteristic secondary sex characters appear.

In girls, the first event is thelarche, the development of breast, followed by pubarche, the development of axillary and pubic hair and then by menarche, the first menstrual period. This occurs between the ages of 11–15 years. Another event that occurs is an increase in the secretion of adrenal androgens–adrenarche. The interval between thelarche and menarche is about two years.

Puberty is due to the secretion of pituitary gonadotropic hormones, which are released by the hypothalamic gonadotropin releasing hormone. The gonadotropic hormones stimulate the production of gametes and secretion of gonadal hormones. These sex hormones stimulate the growth of accessory sex organs and cause the appearance of secondary sex characters. This period is also called adolescence.

The factors that bring about puberty may be due to:

Stimulation of hypothalamus by some area in the brain or withdrawal of some inhibitory influence on the hypothalamus. The brain region involved may be the amygdala of the limbic system.

There may be a mechanism in the hypothalamus itself which may keep the pituitary gonadotropin secretion in check.

Another factor may be that before puberty the hypothalamus is highly sensitive to the negative feedback inhibitory effects of small amounts of gonadal hormones. At puberty, the sensitivity is decreased and gonadotropins are released. The pineal gland may be involved in puberty control.

CLASSIFICATION OF PUBERTY

Precocious Puberty

a. True precocious puberty
   - Constitutional (cause not known, common in girls)
   - *Gonadotropin:* Independent precocity
   - *Cerebral:* Disorders involving posterior hypothalamus
   - Tumors
   - Infections
   - Developmental abnormalities

b. Precocious pseudopuberty (no spermatogenesis or ovarian development)
   - Adrenal
   - Congenital virilizing adrenal hyperplasia
   - *Androgen:* Secreting tumors (in males)
   - *Estrogen:* Secreting tumors (in females)
   - Gonadal
   - Leydig cell tumors of testis
   - Granulosa cell tumors of ovary
   - Miscellaneous

Delayed or Absent Puberty

- Failure of menarche by the age of 17 years (or) testicular development by the age of 20 years
- Enuchoidism (males)
- Primary amenorrhea (females).

86. MENOPAUSE

With advancing age, the human ovaries become unresponsive to gonadotropins and their functions decline, so that sexual cycles disappear. This results in the decline in the number of primordial follicles.

Menopause is the final cessation of menstruation which usually occurs from the ages of 45–55 years.

Changes during Menopause

Some women about 75% show emotional instability, palpitations, insomnia, irritability, depression or vasomotor disturbances called "hot flushes" or "hot flashes", i.e. flushing of skin of face and neck with a feeling of warmth followed by night sweating. Some estrogen sensitive event in the hypothalamus initiates both the release of LH and the episode of flushing.

There is gradual progressive atrophy of gonads and accessory sex organs. Sex hormone secretions (estrogen and progesterone) are reduced, gonadotropins (FSH and LH) are increased, breasts shrink and become pendulous due to atrophy of glandular tissue. Serum lipids increase, osteoporosis and atheroscleosis also occur.

Treatment

Hormone replacement therapy (HRT): Combination of estrogen and progesterone.

In males, there is no actual menopause (andropause).

CLIMACTERIC

It is a gradual period of transition over a period of 1 to 5 years during which involution of genitalia occurs following diminished gonadal function.

87. STRUCTURE OF MALE REPRODUCTIVE SYSTEM

The testes are the primary male sex organ, which are ovoid bodies lying in the scrotum (Fig. 10.5). The testes are made up of loops of convoluted seminiferous tubules, in the walls of which the spermatozoa are formed from the primitive cells (spermatogenesis). Both ends of each loop drain into a network of ducts in the head of the epididymis. From there, spermatozoa pass through the tail of the epididymis into the vas deferens. They enter through the ejaculatory ducts into the urethra in the body of the prostate at the time of ejaculation.

Between the tubules in the testes are nests of cells containing lipid granules, the interstitial cells of Leydig, which secrete testosterone into the blood-stream. The seminal vesicles are two coiled tubes situated between the lower parts of the urinary bladder and rectum.

The spermatic arteries to the testes are tortuous and blood in them runs parallel but in the opposite direction to blood in the pampiniform plexus of spermatic veins. This anatomic arrangement may permit countercurrent exchange of heat and testosterone.

SPERMATOGENESIS (Figs 10.6 and 10.7)

Spermatogenesis is the process by which the male gametes—spermatozoa (sperms) are formed from the primitive germ cells (spermatogonia) in the testis. The spermatogonia begin to undergo mitotic division, beginning at puberty, continue to proliferate and differentiate through definite stages of development to form sperm.

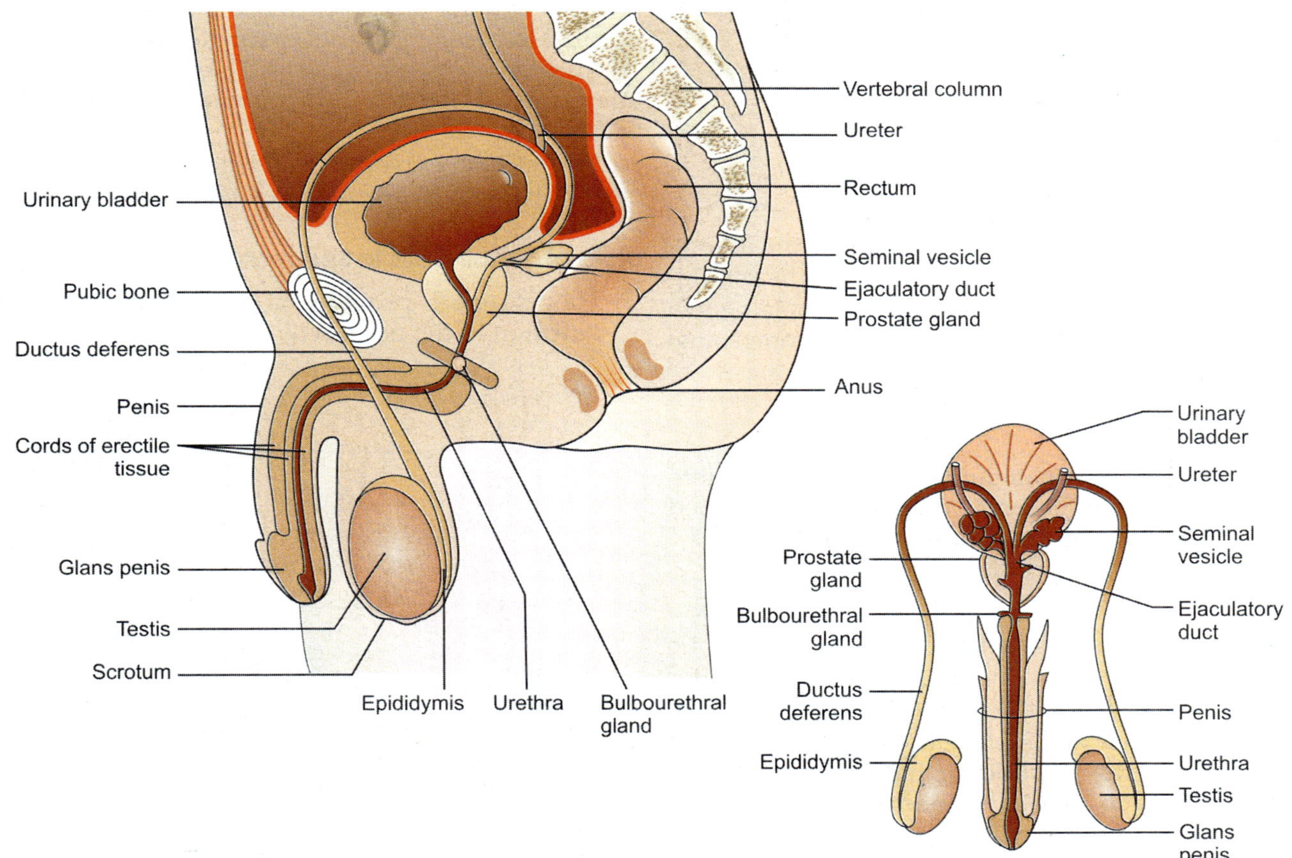

Fig. 10.5: Male reproductive system

10

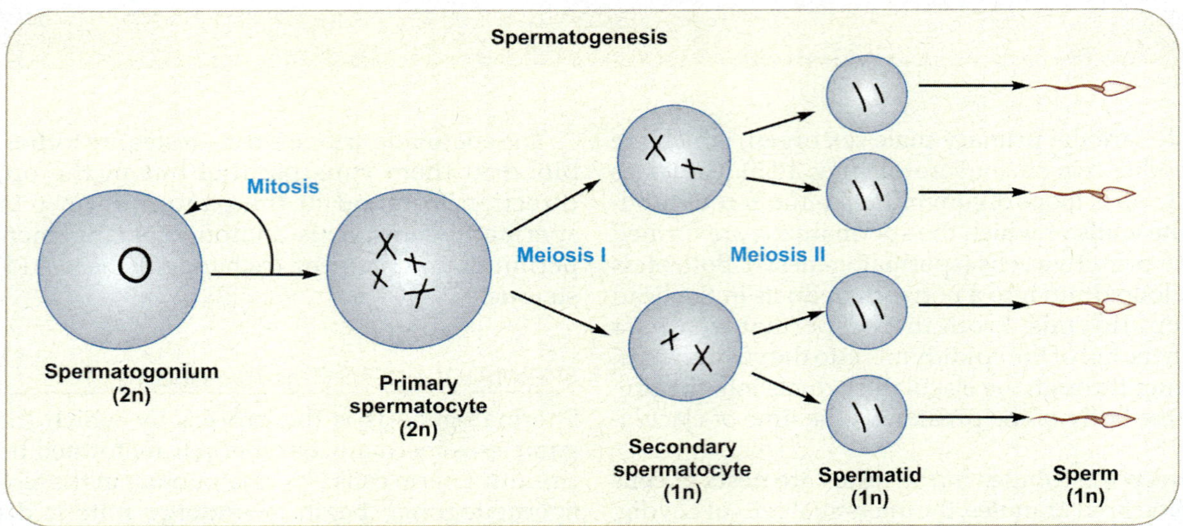

Fig. 10.6: Spermatogenesis

Stages of Spermatogenesis

Stages in the development of sperm from spermatogonia

1. Stage of proliferation
2. Stage of growth
3. Stage of maturation
4. Stage of transformation

Stage of Proliferation

In the first stage, the spermatogonia migrate among Sertoli cells toward the central lumen of the seminiferous tubules. During this stage, the spermatogonia divide by mitosis without change in the chromosomal number.

Stage of Growth

In this stage, the spermatogonia cross the barrier into the Sertoli cell layer, becomes progressively modified and enlarged to form large primary spermatocytes.

10

Stage of Maturation

Each of the primary spermatocyte undergo meiotic division to form two secondary spermatocytes. After another few days, these too divide to form spermatids.

The importance of this stage is that each spermatid receives only the haploid or half the number of chromosomes, so that only one-half of the genetic characteristics of the eventual fetus are provided by the father, while the other half are derived from the oocyte provided by the mother.

Stage of Transformation

The spermatids are eventually modified or transformed to become mature spermatozoa (sperm) by a process called spermiogenesis. The estimated number of spermatids formed from a single spermatogonium is 512.

The entire period of spermatogenesis—from spermatogonia to spermatozoa takes about 74 days.

Role of Sertoli Cells in Spermatogenesis

1. They support, provide suitable temperature and nutrition to the germ cells

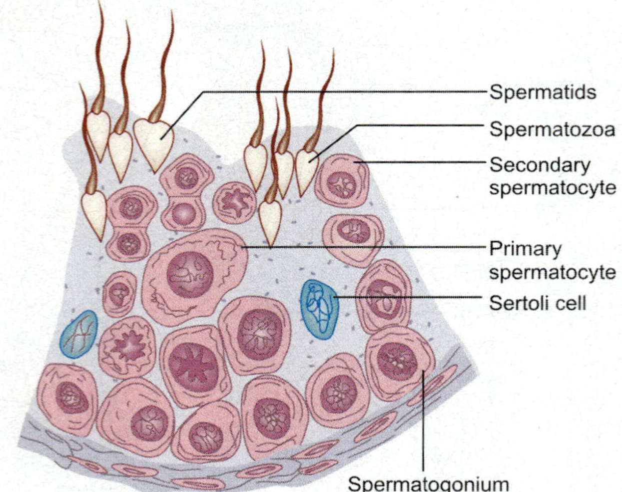

Fig. 10.7: Spermatogenesis

2. Provide hormones necessary for spermatogenesis
3. Secrete ABP (androgen binding protein) which is essential for testosterone activity
4. Release the sperms into lumen of seminiferous tubules (spermination).

Role of Hormones in Spermatogenesis

1. *Testosterone:* Secreted by the Leydig cells is essential for the growth and division of the testicular germinal cells which is the first stage in forming sperm.
2. *Luteinizing hormone (LH):* Secreted by the anterior pituitary gland, stimulates the Leydig cells to secrete testosterone.
3. *Follicle-stimulating hormone (FSH):* Also secreted by the anterior pituitary gland, stimulates the Sertoli cells for the conversion of spermatids to sperms (the process of spermiogenesis).
4. *Estrogens:* Formed from testosterone by the Sertoli cells when they are stimulated by FSH are also essential for spermiogenesis.

Growth hormone (GH): It is necessary for controlling background metabolic functions of the testes. It specifically promotes early division of the spermatogonia. In the absence of GH as in pituitary dwarfs, spermatogenesis is deficient or absent resulting in infertility.

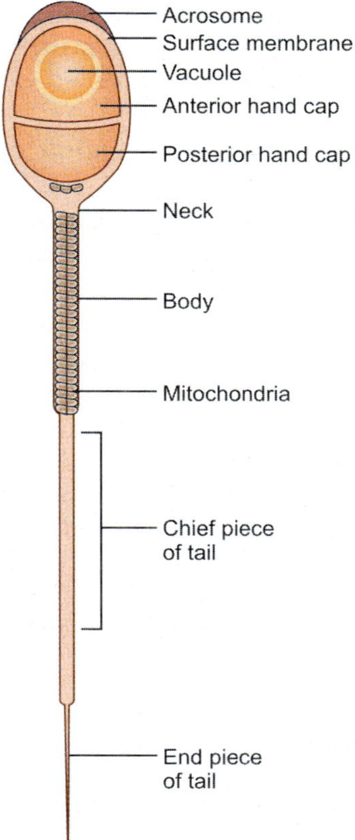

Fig. 10.8: Structure of human sperm

HUMAN SPERM (Fig. 10.8)

Formation of Sperm

Each spermatozoan is an intricate motile cell, rich in DNA which is composed of a head and a tail.

The head comprises the condensed nucleus of the cell with only a thin cytoplasmic cell membrane layer around its surface. On the outside of the anterior two-thirds of the head, is a thick cap called the acrosome that is formed mainly from the Golgi apparatus. This contains a number of enzymes—hyaluronidase (which can digest proteoglycan filaments of tissues) and powerful proteolytic enzymes (which can digest proteins). These enzymes play important role in allowing the sperm to enter the ovum and fertilize it. The membranes of late spermatids and spermatozoa contain a special small form of angiotensin-converting enzyme called germinal angiotensin-converting enzyme (the function of this enzyme in sperm is unknown).

The tail of the sperm called the flagellum has three major components:

1. A central skeleton constructed of 11 microtubules–axoneme
2. A thin cell membrane covering the axoneme
3. A collection of mitochondria surrounding the axoneme in the proximal portion of the tail.

Back and forth movement of the tail (flagellar movement) provides motility for the sperm. This movement results from a rhythmical longitudinal sliding motion between the anterior and posterior tubules that make up the axoneme. The energy for this process is supplied in the form of ATP that is synthesized by the mitochondria in the body of the tail.

The normal motile, fertile sperm move in a fluid medium at a velocity of 1–4 mm/min. This allows them to move through the female genital tract in quest of the ovum. The activity of sperm is greatly enhanced in a neutral and slightly alkaline medium but it is greatly depressed in a mildly acidic medium.

After the formation in the seminiferous tubules, the sperm require several days to pass through the 6 meter long tubule of the epididymis, where they attain maturation and also acquire motility. The ability to move forward (progressive motility) involves activation of a unique protein called Catsper present in the tail.

The two testes of the human adult form up to 120 million sperm each day.

The matured sperms are released from the Sertoli cells into the lumen of seminiferous tubules.

Effect of Temperature

Spermatogenesis requires a temperature lower than that of the interior of the body. The testes are normally maintained at a temperature of about 32°C. They are kept cool by air circulating around the scrotum and probably by heat exchange in a countercurrent fashion between the spermatic arteries and veins.

When the testes are retained in the abdomen, degeneration of tubular walls and sterility result. Hot baths (43–45°C for 30 min/day) reduce the sperm count.

BLOOD–TESTIS BARRIER

Seminiferous epithelium: The mature germ cells remain connected by cytoplasmic bridges from the early spermatid stage, closely invested by Sertoli cell from the basal lamina to the lumen.

The walls of the seminiferous tubules are lined by primitive germ cells and Sertoli cells (large, complex glycoprotein containing cells) that stretch from the basal lamina of the seminiferous tubules to the lumen.

Germ cells must stay in contact with Sertoli cells to survive and this contact is maintained by cytoplasmic bridges (Fig. 10.9).

Tight junctions between adjacent Sertoli cells near the basal lamina form a blood–testis barrier that prevents many large molecules from passing from the interstitial tissue and the part of the tubule near the basal lamina (basal compartment) to the region near the tubular lumen (adluminal compartment) and the lumen. Steroids and some proteins penetrate this barrier from the Sertoli cells to the Leydig cells and vice versa in a paracrine fashion.

In addition, maturing germ cells must pass through the barrier as they move to the lumen. This occurs without disruption of the barrier by progressive breakdown of the tight junctions above the germ cells with concomitant formation of new tight junctions below them.

The fluid in the lumen contains very little protein and glucose but is rich in androgens, estrogens, potassium, inositol, glutamic and aspartic acids. The barrier also protects the germ cells from blood borne noxious agents, prevents antigenic products of germ cells entering circulation, generating an autoimmune response and may help establish an osmotic gradient that facilitates movement of fluid into the tubular lumen.

SEMEN

Semen is a milky, opalescent mucoid fluid which contains sperms and the secretions of the seminal vesicles, prostate, Cowper's and bulbourethral glands. Testes contribute sperms and the prostatic secretions give milky appearance to semen. Semen clots in a few minutes after ejaculation and then liquefies due to fibrinolysin within 1/2 hour.

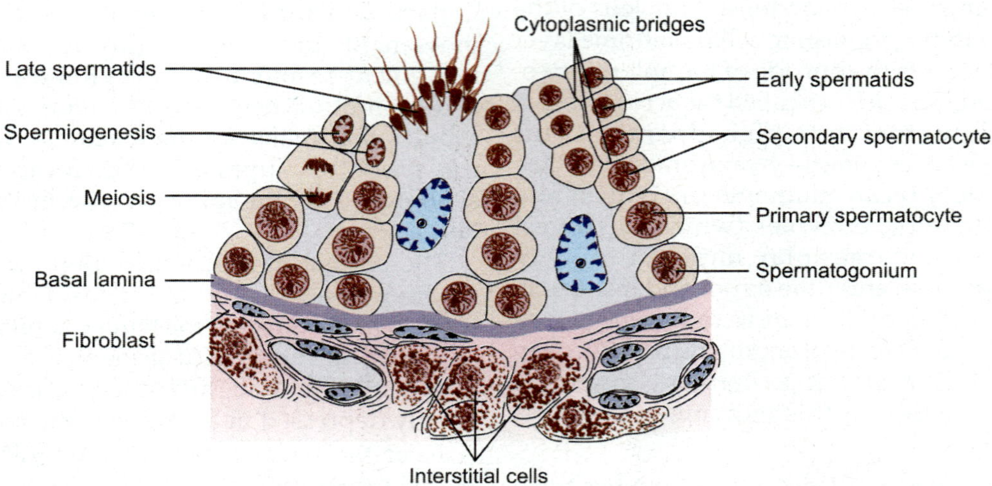

Fig. 10.9: Blood–testis barrier

Specific gravity: 1.028
pH: 7.35–7.50
Volume per ejaculate: 2.5 to 3.5 ml

Each ml of semen contains about 100 million sperms, 50% of men have 20–40 million sperms.
Rate of motility of sperm: 3 mm/min.

Contributions

From seminal vesicles: 60%, alkaline, contains fructose, prostaglandins.

From prostate: 20%, acidic, contains citric acid, cholesterol, fibrinolysin.

Buffers: Phosphate and bicarbonate.

Enzymes: Hyaluronidase.

For fertility

- Volume of semen should be at least 2 ml
- Sperm count should be more than 40 million/ml
- More than 60% of sperms should be normal
- Atleast 50% of sperms should be motile for 1 hour after incubation at 37°.

Oligozoospermia: Reduction in the sperm count between 10 and 25 million/ejaculate.

Azoospermia: Absence of sperms.

Oligospermia: Reduction in the volume of seminal fluid.

ERECTION

Erection is initiated by dilation of the arterioles of the penis. As the erectile tissue of the penis fills with blood, the veins are compressed, blocking outflow and adding to the turgor of the organ.

The integrating centers in the lumbar segments of the spinal cord are activated by impulses in afferents form the genitalia and descending tracts that mediate erection in response to erotic psychological stimuli.

The efferent parasympathetic fibers are in the pelvic splanchnic nerves (nervi erigentes). The fibers release acetylcholine and the vasodilator vasoactive intestinal peptide as cotransmitters.

Nonadrenergic noncholinergic fibers are also present in the nervi erigentes and these contain large amounts of NO synthase, the enzyme that catalyzes the formation of NO.

NO activates guanylyl cyclase resulting in increased production of cGMP which is a potent vasodilator.

This plays a prominent role in the production of erection.

EJACULATION

Ejaculation is a two-part spinal reflex that involves

a. *Emission:* Movement of the semen into the urethra.
b. *Ejaculation proper:* Propulsion of the semen out of the urethra at the time of orgasm.

The afferent pathways are fibers from the touch receptors in the glans penis that reach the spinal cord through the internal pudendal nerves.

Emission is a sympathetic response, integrated in the upper lumbar segment of the spinal cord and effected by the contraction of the smooth muscle of the vasa deferentia and the seminal vesicles in response to stimuli in the hypogastric nerves.

The semen is propelled out of the urethra by the contraction of the bulbocavernosus muscle, a skeletal muscle.

The spinal reflex center are in the upper sacral and lowest lumbar segment of the spinal cord, and the motor pathways traverse the first to the third sacral roots and the internal pudendal nerves.

Carbon monoxide may be involved in the control of the ejaculation.

ENDOCRINE FUNCTION OF THE TESTES

The testes secrete several male sex hormones which are collectively called androgens. They are:

1. Testosterone
2. Dihydrotestosterone
3. Androstenedione.

Testosterone is more abundant than the others.

Chemistry and Biosynthesis of Testosterone

The prinicipal hormone of the testes is testosterone (C 19). It is a 19-carbon steroid which has a hydroxyl (OH) group at 17 position. It is synthesized from cholesterol in the Leydig cells and is also formed from androstenedione secreted by the adrenal cortex.

Leydig cells are numerous in the newborn male infant for the first few months of life and in the adult male after puberty and hence, the testes secrete large quantities of testosterone (Fig. 10.10). During childhood, Leydig cells are absent and so no testosterone is secreted.

Biosynthesis of Testosterone (Fig. 10.11)

Cholesterol (Leydig cells) is converted to pregnenolone, which in-turn is converted by 17 α-hydroxylase to 17-hydroxypregnenolone. This is converted to dehydroepiandrosterone which is further converted to androstenedione.

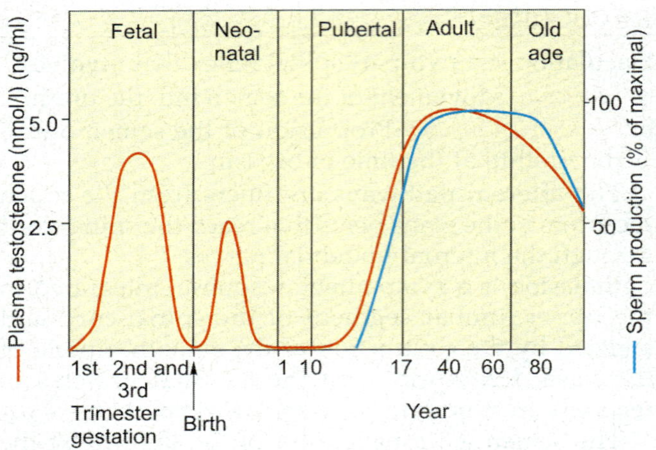

Fig. 10.10: Testosterone concentration and sperm production

Pregnenolone is also converted to progesterone which in-turn is converted by 17 α-hydroxylase to 17-hydroxyprogesterone. This is converted to androstenedione.

From androstenedione, testosterone is formed.

Secretion

The secretion of testosterone is under the control of LH, and the mechanism by which LH stimulates the Leydig cells involves increased formation of cAMP.

The testosterone secretion rate is 4–9 mg/dl in normal adult males.

Small amount is also secreted in females (ovary + adrenal).

Transport and Metabolism

98% of testosterone in plasma is bound to protein (65% bound to β-globulin called gonadal steroid-binding globulin (GBG) or sex steroid-binding globulin, 33% to albumin).

Most of the testosterone is converted to 17-keto-steroids—principally androsterone and excreted in urine.

Functions of Testosterone

1. During fetal development.
2. Development of adult primary and secondary sexual characteristics.

During Fetal Development

- Sex differentiation and development of sexual organs.
- Descent of testes.

Testosterone is secreted by the male fetal testes, genital ridge at about the 7th week of embryonic life. This is responsible for the development of the male body characteristics, including the formation of a penis, scrotum, prostate gland, seminal vesicles and male genital ducts while at the same time suppressing the formation of female genital organs.

Secondly, the stimulus for the descent of the testes is testosterone. The testes usually descend into the scrotum during the last 2–3 months of gestation when the testes begins to secrete testosterone.

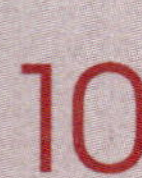

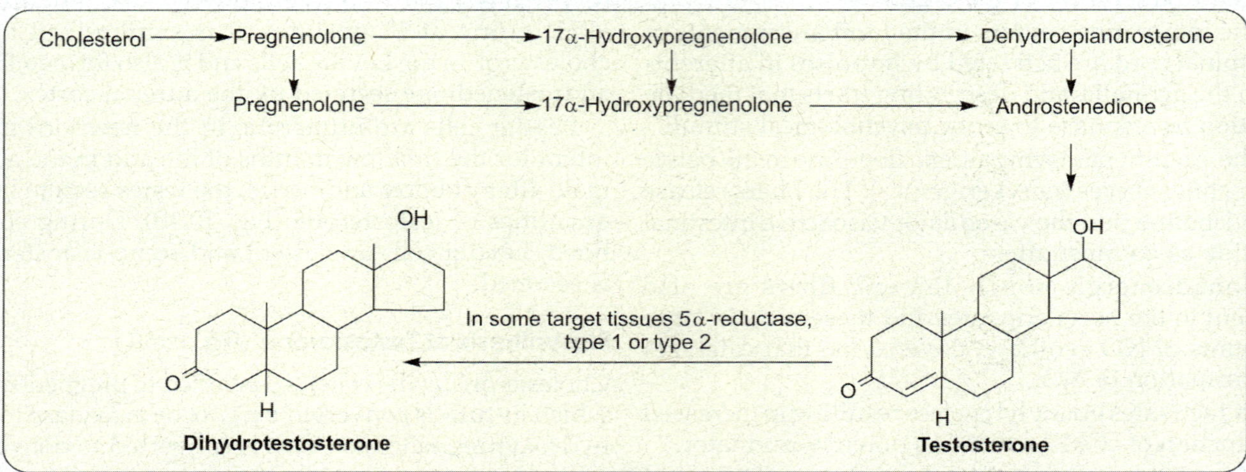

Fig. 10.11: Biosynthesis of testosterone

Development of Adult Primary and Secondary Sexual Characteristics

After puberty, the increasing amounts of testosterone secretion cause the penis, scrotum and testes to enlarge about eightfold before the age of 20 years.

Secondary Characteristics

1. *Effect on the distribution of body hair:* The distribution of hair is of male type–testosterone causes hair growth over the pubis, along linea alba up to umbilicus, face, chest and back. The pubic hair in males has the base of the triangle downwards.
2. *Baldness:* It decreases the growth of hair on the top of the head and cause baldness, which may occur if there is genetic background for the development of baldness and also when there is large secretion of androgenic hormones.
3. *Effect on the voice:* Testosterone causes hypertrophy of laryngeal mucosa, enlargement of larynx, which causes cracking of voice at the time of adolescence. But, this gradually changes into the typical adult masculine voice.
4. *Increases thickness of the skin/development of acne:* It increases the thickness of the skin over the entire body and increases the ruggedness of the sub-cutaneous tissues. Testosterone also causes excessive secretion by the sebaceous glands which results in acne.
5. *Increases protein formation/muscle development:* One of the most important male sexual characters is the development of musculature after puberty, about 50% increase in muscle mass. This is associated with anabolic activity of testosterone on proteins.
6. *Increases bone matrix/calcium retention:* At puberty, the bones grow thicker and deposit additional calcium. Testosterone increases the total quantity of bone matrix and causes calcium retention. The increase in bone matrix is due to protein anabolic function of testosterone plus deposition of calcium salts in response to the increased protein. Testosterone has a specific effect on the pelvis to:
   i. Narrow the pelvic outlet
   ii. Lengthen it
   iii. Funnel like shape of the pelvis
   iv. Greatly increase the strength of the entire pelvis for load-bearing.

   In addition, it also causes the epiphysis of the long bones to unite with the shafts of the bone at an early date. So, if testes are removed before puberty, the fusion of epiphyses is delayed and the height of the person increases.
7. *Increases basal metabolism:* During adolescence and early adult life, testosterone increases the rate of metabolism to 5–10%. It is due to anabolic effect of testosterone on protein metabolism.
8. *Effect on red blood cells:* There is a 15–20% increase in red blood cells following injection of normal quantities of testosterone into a castrated adult, partly due to increased metabolic rate.
9. *Effect on electrolyte and water balance:* Testosterone increases the reabsorption of sodium to minor extent. After puberty, the blood and extracellular fluid volumes increase 5–10% in relation to body weight.

Mode of Action of Testosterone (Fig. 10.12)

Figure 10.12 depicts the action of testosterone and DHT via the same receptor but DHT binds more effectively testosterone is converted to dihydro-testosterone (DHT) under the influence of intracellular enzyme 5α-reductase in the target cells of accessory sex organs—prostate, seminal vesicles, epididymis, penis and other organs. The dihydrotestosterone combines with intracellular receptor proteins. The hormone-receptor complex binds to DNA in the nucleus facilitating transcription process of various genes.

Testosterone is responsible for the formation of male internal genitalia, increase in muscle mass, development of male sex drive and libido but DHT-receptor complexes are needed to form male external genitalia, facial hair, acne and temporal recession of the hairline.

Control of Testicular Function

1. *GnRH:* GnRH secreted by the hypothalamus, reaches the pituitary via the hypophyseal portal vessels and causes the release of FSH and LH.
2. *FSH:* It acts on the germinal epithelial cells of the seminiferous tubules and promotes sperma-togenesis. It also stimulates Sertoli cell activity and inhibin secretion.
3. *LH:* It acts on Leydig cells and causes testosterone secretion.
4. *Inhibin:* It reduces FSH secretion by a negative feed-back mechanism acting on the pituitary.
5. *Testosterone:* It inhibits LH secretion by a negative feedback mechanism acting at the level of hypothalamus and reducing GnRH secretion. This

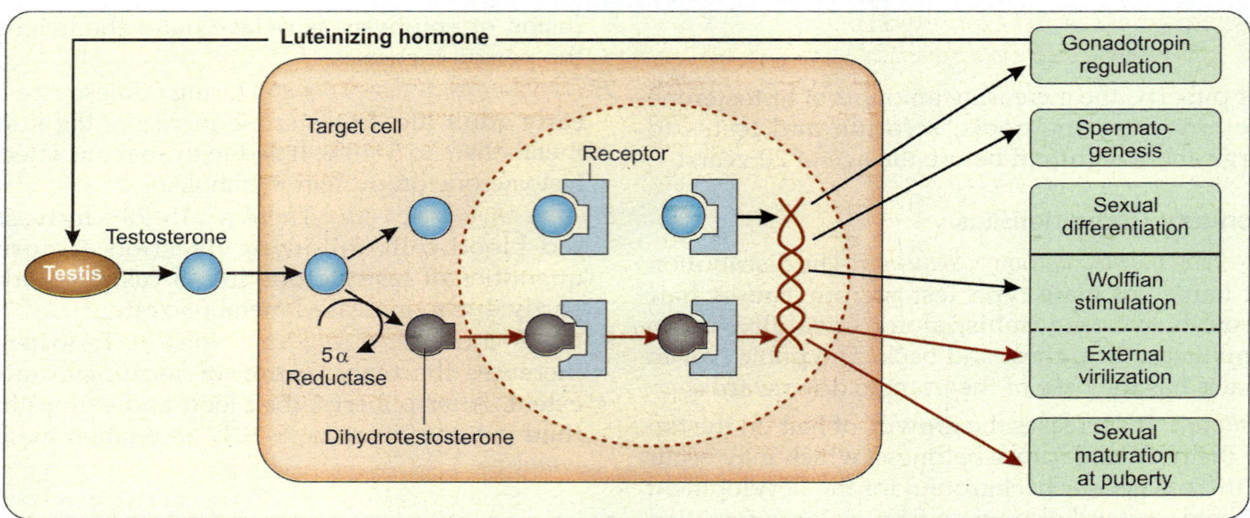

Fig. 10.12: Action of testosterone

negative feedback mechanism maintains optimal testosterone level.

6. Optimal thyroid and adrenal cortical hormones are also necessary for normal sex function.

Applied Aspects

Congenital 5α-reductase deficiency results in male pseudohermaphroditism:

- Features are male internal genitalia including testes but with female external genitalia and are usually raised as girls.
- Following puberty, LH secretion and testosterone levels are increased and consequently develop into male body contours and become boys.

Castration (Removal of Testes)

Before Puberty

- Pubertal changes are absent
- Secondary male sex characters do not appear
- Female type of deposition of fat
- Delay in union of epiphysis and the individual is tall.

There is impotence (inability to perform the sexual act), sterility (inability to procreate) and absence of libido (sex desire and drive).

After Puberty

- Atrophy of accessory sex organs and secondary sex characters.
- There is sterility but libido is present, though reduced.

Abnormalities of Testicular Function

1. *Male hypogonadism:* Similar to castration before and after puberty.
2. *Undescended testes (cryptorchidism):* Failure of descent of testes into the scrotum in the last few months of fetal life. In a few children, it remains in the abdominal cavity or inguinal canal at birth and descends in the first year. Sometimes, it continues to remain undescended. Gametogenic function does not occur and there is also a higher incidence of malignancy in cryptorchidism.

88. STRUCTURE OF FEMALE REPRODUCTIVE SYSTEM

OVARY

Ovary is the primary female sex organ. A pair of ovaries are situated one on either side of the lateral pelvic wall in the peritoneal cavity. It is shelled, almond shaped and is of varying sizes. The ovary has gametogenic and endocrine functions (Fig. 10.13).

FALLOPIAN TUBE (UTERINE TUBE, OVIDUCT)

They are two in number, one on each side, about 10 cm long, and 1 cm wide. Each tube has an outer peritoneal coat, a middle muscular coat containing outer longitudinal and inner mucous membrane lined by ciliated columnar epithelium. The cilia beat towards the uterus. The lateral portion, the ampullla has a wide lateral half and the expanded end is fimbriated, funnel shaped which lies in close relation to the ovary and receives the ovum.

UTERUS

Uterus or womb is a hollow pear shaped organ lying in the pelvic cavity between the rectum and bladder. It has:

i. An outer serous coat
ii. A thick middle muscular coat (myometrium), made up of longitudinal, circular, oblique and transverse smooth muscle fibers
iii. Inner mucus coat (endometrium) of varying thickness containing tubular glands.

A slight constriction divides the uterus into an upper body about 5 cm in length, and a lower cervix about 2.5 cm long which projects into the vagina. The portion of the body above the attachment of the fallopian tube is called the fundus (Fig. 10.14).

VAGINA

It is a narrow but distensible musculomembranous canal which leads from the uterus to the vulva outside. In the virgin, the outlet is covered by membrane called the hymen which has a small opening.

MENSTRUAL CYCLE

Definition

The monthly cyclic events that take place in a rhythmic fashion in the rates of secretion of the female hormones

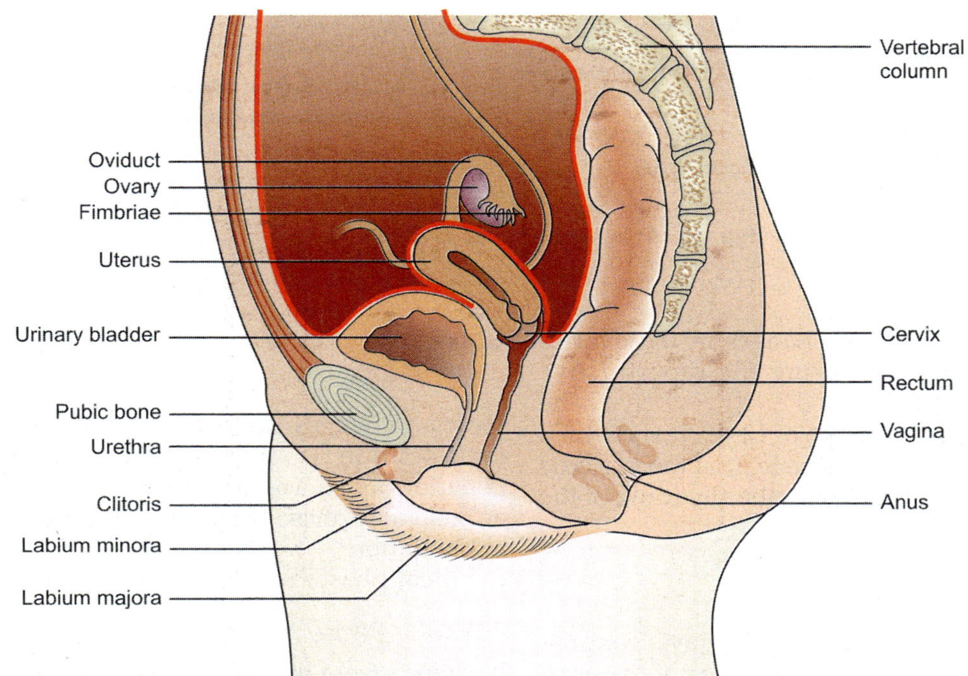

Fig. 10.13: Female reproductive system

10

Uterine tube (sectioned)
Uterine cavity
Uterine tube
Ovary
Fimbriae
Entrance to uterine tube
Cervix
Vagina

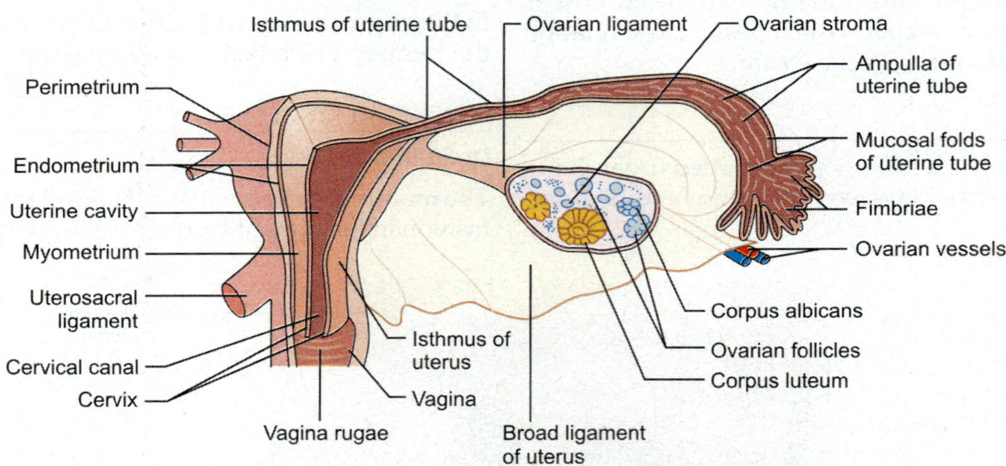

Fig. 10.14: Internal structures of the uterus

and corresponding physical changes in the ovaries and other sexual organs during the reproductive period of a woman's life is called menstrual cycle. The menstrual cycle starts at the age of 12–15 years, which marks the onset of menstrual cycle. It is the periodic vaginal bleeding that occurs with the shedding of the uterine mucosa.

Duration of Menstrual Cycle

The duration of menstrual cycle is 28 days from the start of one menstrual period to the start of the next. It may vary between 20 and 40 days.

Changes

Ovarian Changes

Ovarian changes that occur during each menstrual cycle occur in two phases and depend completely on gonadotropic hormones (FSH and LH).

a. Follicular phase/Proliferative phase
b. Ovulation
c. Luteal phase/Secretory phase

Follicular Phase

It extends from the 5th day of the cycle until the time of ovulation. There is maturation of ovum with development of ovarian follicles through different stages:

1. Primordial follicle
2. Primary follicle
3. Vesicular follicle
4. Matured follicle or graafian follicle.

Primordial Follicle

During fetal development, the ovaries contain over 7 million primordial follicles. Before birth, many follicles undergo atresia. At the time of birth, there are 2 million ova but 50% of these atretic. The million that are normal undergo the first part of 1st meiotic division enter a stage of arrest in prophase, in which those that survive persist until adulthood. At the time of puberty, both the ovaries contain about 3,00,000 primordial follicles.

Each contains an immature ovum which is surrounded by the granulosa cells. These cells provide nutrition to the ovum throughout childhood. They also secrete the oocyte maturation inhibiting factor which keeps the ovum in the immature stage.

Primary Follicle

The primordial follicle becomes the primary follicle, when the ovum is surrounded by additional layers of granulosa cells.

Vesicular Follicle

Under the influence of FSH, about 6–12 primary follicles start growing and develop into vesicular follicles. There is rapid proliferation of granulosa cells giving rise to many more layers of these cells. In addition, spindle cells develop outside the granulosa cells giving rise to a second mass of cells called the theca. This is divided into two layers—theca interna which secrete estrogen and progesterone and theca externa (outer layer) which forms the capsule of the developing follicle. The granulosa cells also secretes a follicular fluid and accumulation of this fluid causes an antrum.

The accelerated growth of follicles occur leading to larger follicles called vesicular follicles. This is due to increasing estrogen, FSH and LH receptors.

Graafian Follicle

After 1 week or more, one of the follicles begins to outgrow all the others and the remaining 5 to 11 follicles undergo atresia. This is due to increasing estrogen from the largest follicle acting on hypothalamus suppressing FSH secretion from the anterior pituitary. The single, matured graafian follicle reaches a diameter of 1–1.5 cm.

Ovulation

Ovulation is the process in which there is rupture of distended mature graafian follicle with consequent discharge of ovum into the abdominal cavity, which is influenced by LH. It occurs on the 14th day of menstrual cycle in a normal cycle of 28 days. The ovum is picked up by the fimbriated ends of the fallopian tube.

Process of Ovulation

Before ovulation, the protruding outer wall of the follicle swells rapidly and a small area in the center of the follicular capsule, called the stigma, protrudes like a nipple. After ½ hour, fluid begins to ooze through the stigma and the stigma ruptures. The ovum is expelled surrounded by several thousand granulosa cells called the corona radiata.

Without the initial preovulatory surge of LH, ovulation will not take place. Just 2 days before ovulation, LH rises to 10-fold and FSH rises to 2–3-fold. Both FSH and LH act synergistically to cause rapid swelling of the follicle and converting the granulosa and theca cells to secrete progesterone.

Luteal Phase

This phase extends between 15th and 28th day of menstrual cycle. The follicle that ruptures at the time of ovulation fills with blood, forms "corpus hemorrhagicum". Minor bleeding from the follicle into the abdominal cavity may cause peritoneal irritation and fleeting abdominal pain called "mittelschmerz". The granulosa and theca cells of the follicle begins to proliferate and the clotted blood is rapidly replaced with yellowish, lipid rich luteal cells, forming the corpus luteum. This initiates the luteal phase which is dependent on LH secretion and hence the name "lutenizing" for "yellowing". The corpus luteum is a highly secretory organ, secreting large amounts of both estrogen and progesterone. The corpus luteum grows to 1.5 cm in diameter.

Functions of Corpus Luteum

1. Secretion of hormones (estrogen and progesterone)
2. Maintenance of pregnancy: Corpus luteum is active until placenta starts secreting estrogen and progesterone for a period of 3 months of pregnancy.

Fate of Corpus Luteum

If fertilization occurs, the corpus luteum persists for 3–4 months, secreting large amounts of estrogen and progesterone, which is essential for maintenance of pregnancy.

If fertilization does not occur, inhibin secreted by the corpus luteum inhibits FSH and LH secretion. This causes the corpus luteum to degenerate completely and replaced by scar tissue, forming corpus albicans.

Uterine Changes

These changes in uterus takes place in three phases (Fig. 10.15):

1. Proliferative phase
2. Secretory phase
3. Menstrual phase

Proliferative Phase (Preovulatory Phase, Postmenstrual Phase or Follicular Phase)

This phase begins on the 5th day after the beginning of menstruation and ends with ovulation on the 14th day in 28 day cycle. At the beginning of this phase, the endometrium increases rapidly in thickness, uterine glands lengthen and show proliferative changes and hence called proliferative phase. The mucosa is 3–4 mm thick. This phase represents restoration of the epithelium from the preceding menstruation.

Secretory Phase (Postovulatory Phase, Pre-menstrual, Luteal Phase or Progestational Phase)

This phase starts from the 15th to 28th day of the cycle—14 days which is constant. The endometrium shows marked hypertrophy and is about 5–6 mm thick. The uterine glands become elongated, coiled and tortuous and begin to secrete fluid. Consequently, this phase is called secretory phase.

The endometrium is supplied by two type of arteries:
The superficial 2/3—stratum functionale which is shed during menstruation is supplied by long, coiled spiral arteries. The deep layer—stratum basale, that is not shed, is supplied by short, straight basilar arteries.

There is increase in the number of spiral arteries, blood flow is increased, vessels are congested as increased coiling impedes blood flow. The stromal cells proliferate, cytoplasm increases due to deposition of glycogen and lipids and size of the uterus is increased.

At the end of this phase, the mucosa resembles the decidua of pregnancy, which represents preparation of the uterus for implantation of the fertilized ovum. If fertilization does not occur, next phase—menstrual phase results.

Menstrual Phase (Phase of Bleeding, Destructive Phase)

At the end of the secretory phase, when the corpus luteum regresses, hormone support for the endo-metrium is withdrawn. The endometrium becomes thinner, which adds to the coiling of the spiral arteries. Vasoconstriction of the spiral arteries of the mucosa occurs causing ischemia, leading to necrosis of endometrium and these coalesce. In addition, spasm and degeneration of the walls of the spiral arteries take place, leading to spotty hemorrhages and that become confluent and produce the menstrual flow. The vasospasm is produced by the locally released prostaglandins.

About 75% of the blood is arterial and 25% is venous. It contains tissue debris, prostaglandins and

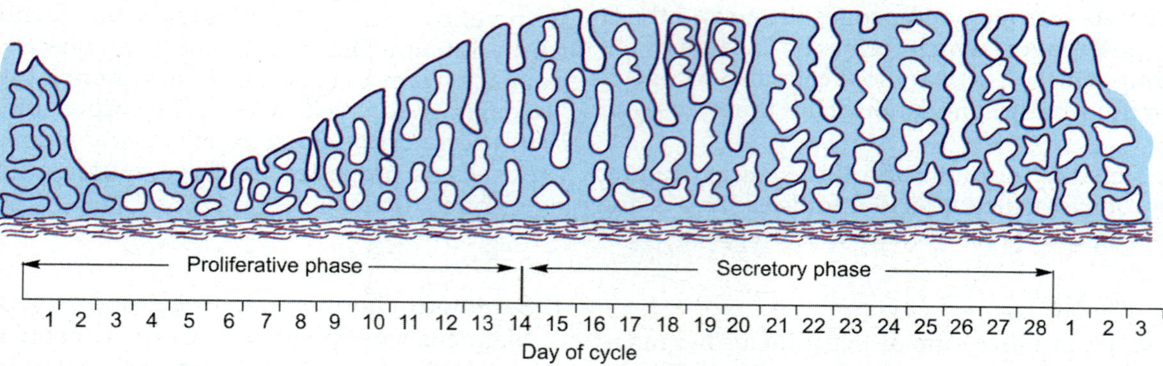

Fig. 10.15: Endometrial changes during menstrual cycle

10

fibrinolysins. The fibrinolysin lyses clot, so that menstrual blood does not clot normally unless the flow is excessive. The usual duration of menstrual flow is 3–5 days but may be short as 1 day or long as 8 days in normal women. The average amount of blood loss is about 30 ml but may range normally between slight spotting to 80 ml.

Vaginal Changes

1. *Proliferative phase:* Under the influence of estrogens, the vaginal epithelium becomes cornified.
2. *Secretory phase:* Under the influence of progesterone, a thick mucus is secreted, and the epithelium proliferates and becomes infiltrated with leukocytes.

Cervical Changes

1. *Proliferative phase:* Estrogen makes the mucus of cervix thinner and more alkaline. It helps in the survival and motility of spermatozoa.
2. *Ovulation:* The mucus is thinnest at the time of ovulation and its elasticity (spinnbarkeit) increases so that a drop can be stretched into a long, thin thread that may be 8–12 cm or more in length. In addition, it dries in an arborizing, fern-like pattern when a thin layer is spread on a slide.
3. *Secretory phase:* Progesterone makes the cervical mucus thick, tenacious and cellular.

Indicators of Ovulation

1. A rise in the basal body temperature. The rise starts 1–2 days after ovulation. Temperature is recorded in the morning by using a thermometer (oral or rectal) before getting out of bed. The rise is due to thermogenic effect of progesterone.
2. The cervical mucus shows fern pattern.
3. Hormone detection in plasma and urine. There is an increase in the urinary excretion of estrogen and progesterone metabolic end-products.
4. Ultrasound scan.
5. *Endometrial biopsy:* Significance of determining ovulation time is essential for family planning by adopting "rhythm method".

Hormonal Contol of Menstrual Cycle (Figs 10.16 and 10.17)

The regulatory system functions through hypo-thalamo-pituitary-ovarian axis. Hormones involved are:

1. Hypothalamic hormones—GnRH
2. Anterior pituitary hormones—FSH and LH
3. Ovarian hormones—estrogen and progesterone.

Hypothalamic Hormones—GnRH

It releases FSH and LH from the anterior pituitary. The secretion of GnRH depends on psychosocial events as well as feedback effects of ovarian changes via ovarian hormones.

Anterior Pituitary Hormones—FSH and LH

FSH and LH secreted from anterior pituitary modulate the ovarian and uterine changes by acting directly and/or indirectly via ovarian hormones.

FSH: It induces the development of graafian follicle and secretion of estrogen, which is responsible for the proliferative phase of menstrual cycle.

LH: LH is essential for the formation and maintenance of corpus luteum.

Ovarian Hormones—Estrogen and Progesterone

Both the ovarian hormones are under the influence of GnRH which acts via FSH and LH.

Estrogen: The high level of estrogen is responsible for the LH burst which is essential for ovulation.

Progesterone: It is responsible for the endometrial changes of the secretory phase.

Applied Physiology

Menstrual Abnormalities

1. Premenstrual Syndrome (PMS)

It is the symptoms of stress that appears 4–5 days before the onset of menstruation. It is also called pre-menstrual stress or tension. The symptoms occur due to salt and water retention caused by estrogens and the features are:

Mood swings, anxiety, irritability, emotional instability, headache, depression, constipation, abdominal cramping and bloating.

Treatment: Antidepressant–Fluoxetine
Benzodiazepine–Alprazolam

2. Amenorrhea

Absence of menstruation during reproductive period.

Primary amenorrhea: If menarche does not occur beyond 18 years, it is called primary amenorrhea.

10

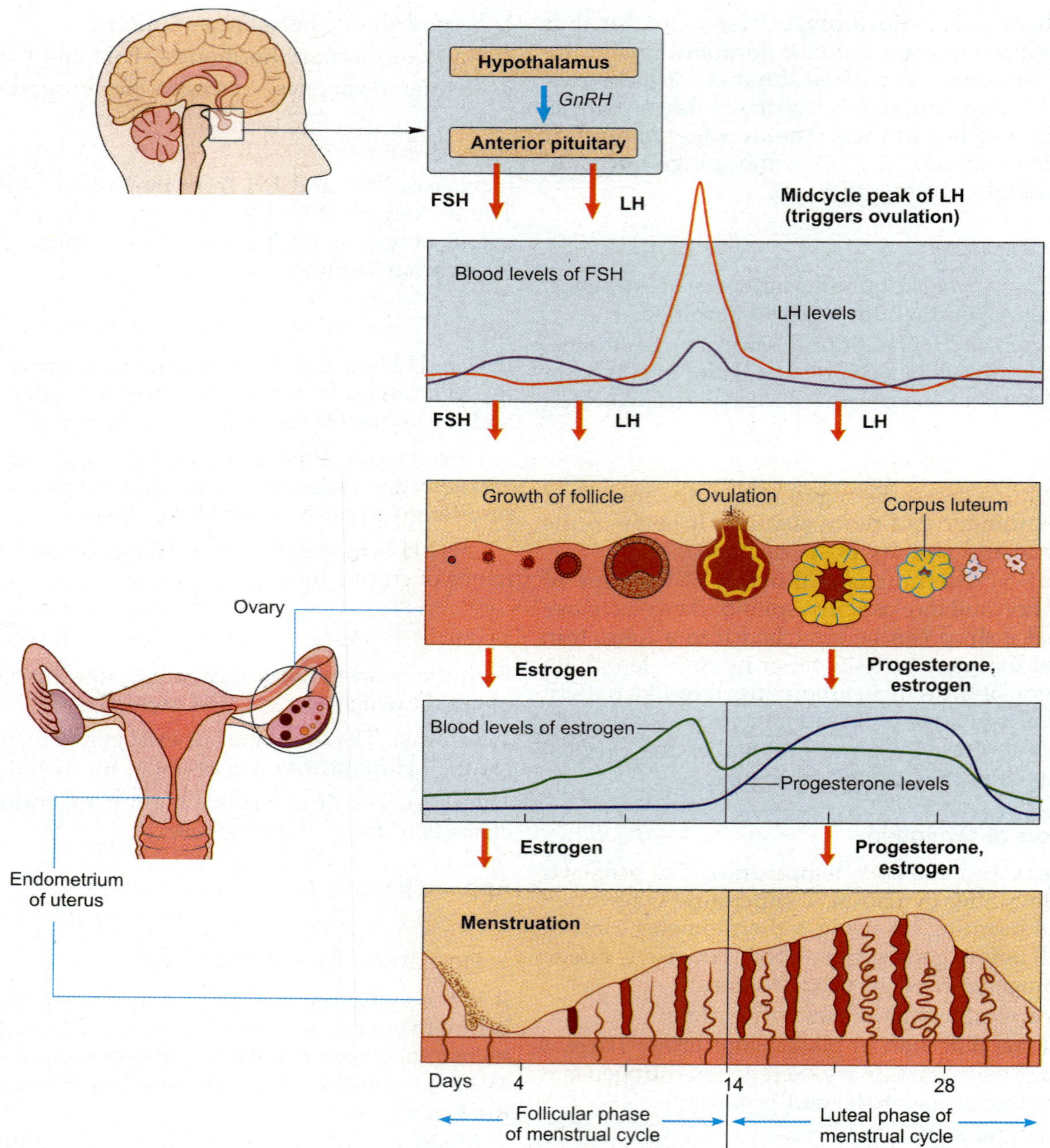

Fig. 10.16: Hormonal control of menstrual cycle

10

Secondary amenorrhea: Absence of menstruation for over 3 months, at any time, after menstruation has set in, is secondary amenorrhea.

The commonest cause of amenorrhea in young women is pregnancy.

Physiological cause of amenorrhea: Occurs during lactation.

Pathological cause: Abnormalities of hypothalamic-pituitary-ovarian axis, ovarian and uterine disorders, endocrine disorders or systemic diseases.

3. *Menorrhagia*

Excessive bleeding during a menstrual period.

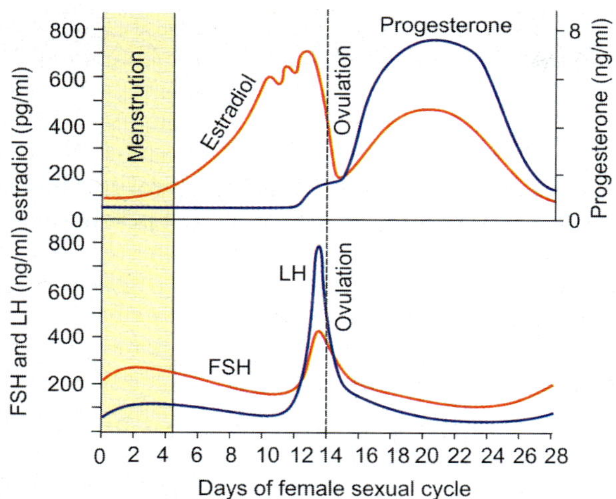

Fig. 10.17: Hormonal changes during normal female sexual cycle

4. *Metrorrhagia*

Uterine bleeding in between menstruations

5. *Hypomenorrhea*

Scanty menstruation

6. *Oligomenorrhea*

Decreased frequency of menstrual bleeding

7. *Polymenorrhea*

Increased frequency of menstrual bleeding

8. *Dysmenorrhea*

Painful menstruation

9. *Anovulatory Cycle*

If ovulation does not occur in a menstrual cycle, it is called anovulatory cycle. It is common during puberty and a few years before menopause.

Common Causes

1. Hormonal imbalance
2. Prolonged strenuous exercise
3. Hypothalamic dysfunctions
4. Tumors in pituitary, adrenal gland or ovary
5. Long use of oral contraceptives.

89. GENETIC DEFECTS

A number of single-gene mutations cause reproductive abnormalities in women.

Loss of Function Mutations

1. *Kallmann's syndrome:* Hypogonadotropic hypogonadism
2. *GnRH resistance, FSH resistance, LH resistance:* Defects in GnRH, FSH and LH receptors.
3. *Aromatase deficiency:* Prevents the formation of estrogens.

Gain of Function Mutations

McCune-Albright syndrome:

Associated with multiple endocrine abnormalities, including precocious puberty, amenorrhea and galactorrhea.

90. OVARIAN HORMONES

The hormones produced by the ovaries are:

a. Steroid hormones
   1. Estrogens
   2. Progestins

b. Nonsteroidal hormones
   1. Relaxin
   2. Inhibin
   3. Activin

STEROID HORMONES

Chemistry of Steroid Hormones

Biosynthesis and metabolism of estrogens (Fig. 10.18).

1. *Estrogen*

The ovarian estrogens are 18 carbon steroids. They are:

1. β-estradiol is the principal and most potent ovarian estrogen
2. Estrone
3. Estriol (least potent estrogen).

Estradiol Synthesis and Secretion

In normal nonpregnant female, major quantity of estrogens are secreted by the granulosa cells of ovarian follicles, the corpus luteum and minute amounts by the adrenal cortex (Fig. 10.19).

During pregnancy, estrogens are also secreted by the placenta.

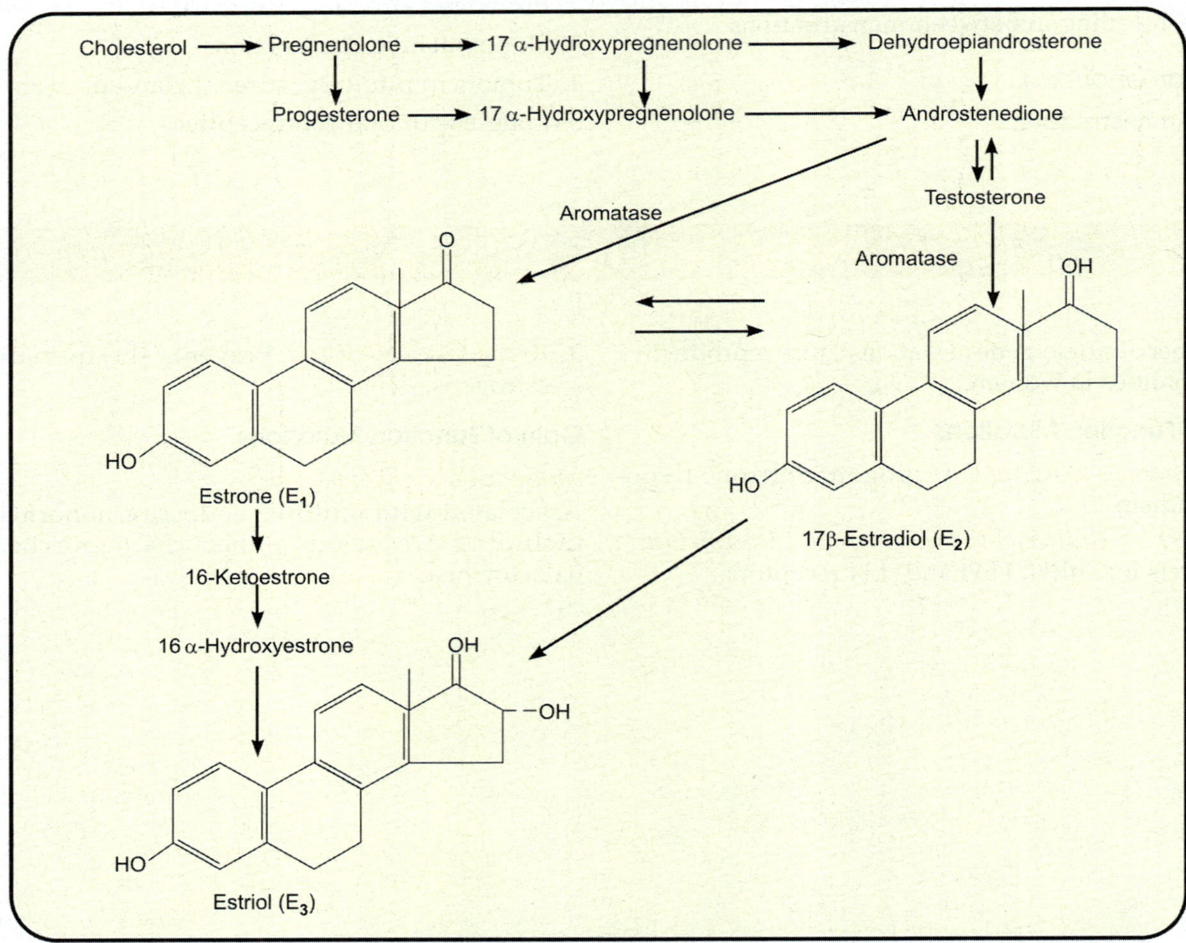

Fig. 10.18

10

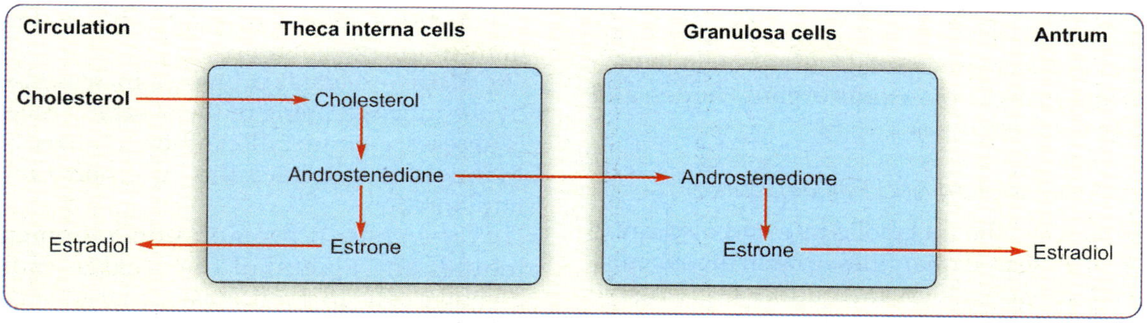

Fig. 10.19: Estradiol synthesis and secretion

2. Progestins

The most important progestins is progesterone. Another progestins is 17α-hydroxyprogesterone.

In normal nonpregnant female, progesterone is secreted by the corpus luteum.

Duing pregnancy, large amounts of progesterone are also secreted by the placenta after the 4th month of gestation.

Biosynthesis

They are synthesized from cholesterol derived from blood and acetyl coenzyme A.

Mainly progesterone and male hormone testosterone are synthesized first. Then, enzyme aromatase converts testosterone to estradiol.

Transport and Metabolism

Both estrogens and progesterone are transported in the blood bound mainly with plasma albumin and with globulins.

In the liver, the estrogens are converted to glucuronide and sulfate conjugates. Most of estrogens and metabolites are excreted in the urine and small amounts in the bile, which is reabsorbed into the blood stream (enterohepatic circulation).

Progesterone is also degraded in the liver to pregnenediol and 10% of original progesterone is excreted in urine.

Functions of Estrogens

Effects on Primary and Secondary Female Sex Organs

1. On Female Genitalia

The ovaries, fallopian tubes, uterus and vagina all increase several times in size along with enlargement of external genitalia, labia minora and deposition of fat in the mons pubis and labia majora.

Estrogens change the vaginal epithelium from a cuboidal into a stratified type, which is more resistant to trauma and infection.

Uterus increases in size along with marked proliferation of the endometrial, glands. It also increases the uterine blood flow, musculature and contractile proteins which makes the muscle more active, excitable and action potentials become more frequent. The estrogen dominated uterus is also more sensitive to oxytocin.

Estrogens increase the number of cilated epithelial cells lining the fallopian tube and their activity (motility).

2. On Breasts

Estrogen causes:

a. Developmental of the stromal tissues of the breasts
b. Growth of an extensive ductile system
c. Deposition of fat

It is called the growth hormone of the breast as it is largely responsible for breast enlargement at puberty in girls.

3. On the Skeleton

a. Estrogens inhibit osteoclastic activity in the bones and therefore stimulate bone growth.
b. It causes uniting of the epiphysis with the shafts of the long bones.

Women have narrow shoulders, broad hips and thighs that converge and arms that diverge (wide carrying angle).

After menopause, estrogen deficiency causes increased osteoclastic activity, decreased bone matrix and decreased deposition of bone calcium and phosphate which becomes more severe in some women leading to osteoporosis.

4. On Protein Deposition

There is a slight increase in total body protein, which promotes the growth of sexual organs, bones and other tissues of the body.

5. On Body Metabolism and Fat Deposition

Estrogens increase the metabolic rate and also cause deposition of increased quantities of fat in the subcutaneous tissues (breasts, thigh and buttocks– giving the feminine figure).

6. On Hair Distribution

Women have less body hair and more scalp hair. Pubic hair has a characteristic flat-topped pattern. Androgens from female adrenal gland are mainly responsible for this.

7. On Skin

Estrogen causes the skin texture to be soft, smooth and more vascular.

8. On Electrolyte Balance

Estrogen causes salt and water retention by the kidney tubules.

Other effects: Estrogens inhibit the formation of comedones (black heads) and acne.

They have a significant plasma cholesterol lowering action. Also, produce vasodilation by increasing the local production of NO (prevent heart attacks and strokes).

Mechanism of Action

Most of the effects of estrogens are due to the actions on the nucleus. There are two nuclear estrogen receptors–estrogen receptor α (ER α – found in uterus) and estrogen receptor β (ER β – found in ovaries).

10

Synthetic Estrogens

1. Digoxins
2. Tamoxifene and raloxifene
3. SERMs (selective estrogen receptor modulators).

Functions of Progesterone

1. *On uterus:* Progesterone promotes secretory changes in the endometrium during the latter half of the monthly female sexual cycle, thus preparing the uterus for implantation of the fertilized ovum. It also decreases the frequency and intensity of uterine contractions thereby helping to prevent expulsion of the implanted ovum.
2. *On fallopian tubes:* It promotes increased secretion by the mucosal lining of the fallopian tubes, which is necessary for nutrition of the fertilized, dividing ovum as it traverses the fallopian tube before implantation.
3. *On the breasts:* It promotes development of the lobules and alveoli of the breasts, causing the alveolar cells to proliferate, enlarge and become secretory in nature.

NONSTEROID HORMONES

Relaxin

It is a polypeptide hormone, molecular weight 6000, produced by the corpus luteum of the ovary, cytotrophoblast cells of the placenta, decidua and the secretory uterine endometrium.

It has two polypeptide chains linked by disulfide bridges (resembling insulin) but alpha chain contains 24 amnio acids and beta chain contains 32 amino acids. Its concentration reaches a peak during the 36th week of pregnancy, remains high till delivery and then falls.

Actions

a. Loosening of the pubis symphysis and sacroiliac joints and softening of cervix during pregnancy, thereby facilitating delivery.
b. Inhibition of uterine contractions during pregnancy.
c. It also promotes tubuloalveolar growth of mammary glands.

Inhibin

Inhibin is of testicular origin and it inhibits the secretion of FSH.

- It belongs to TGF β family of growth factors
- It is found both in females and males.

Chemical Structure

Made up of three polypeptide subunits: α, βA, βB

α–Glycosylated, molecular weight of 18,000

β–Nonglycosylated, molecular weight of 14,000

There are two types:
Inhibin A – α combines with βA
Inhibin B – α combines with βB

They are linked by S-S bridges. Both inhibin A and B inhibit FSH secretion by direct action on pituitary but inhibin B is the one that regulates FSH in adult men and women.

Source

- In males—Sertoli cells
- In females—Granulosa cells

Other sites: Brainstem

Activins

Are found when the β subunits link, with each other by S-S bridges. Three types are formed βA βA, βB βB, βA βB.

It belongs to TGF β superfamily of growth factors.

Action

Stimulates FSH secretion

Other sites: Brain and bone marrow

Functions

In bone marrow:

1. Helps in the development of WBC.
2. In embryonic life, it is involved in the formation of mesoderm.

91. PREGNANCY, PARTURITION AND LACTATION

MATURATION AND FERTILIZATION OF THE OVUM

While in the ovary, the ovum is in the primary oocyte stage.

Shortly before it is released from the ovarian follicle, its nucleus divides by meiosis and a secondary oocyte is formed with the expulsion of the I polar body.

The secondary oocyte has only 23 chromosomes and it is extruded out of the ovary into the abdominal cavity during ovulation. It then enters the fimbriated end of the fallopian tube.

In the fallopian tube, the secondary oocyte is extruded into 100 or more granulosa cells on its surface which forms the corona radiata. The fimbrial ends of the fallopian tube contains cilia which are activated by the estrogens from the ovaries, causing the cilia to beat towards the opening or OSTIA of the fallopian tube. 98% of the ova are drawn into the fallopian tube by the movement of the cilia.

FERTILIZATION OF THE OVUM

Once the semen is released into the vagina, a few sperms are transported within 5–10 min upwards from the vagina through the uterus and the fallopian tube to the ampullae of the fallopian tube.

The transport of the sperm is aided by:

1. Prostaglandins in the male seminal gland.
2. Oxytocin released from the posterior pituitary gland of the female during orgasm.

Fertilization of the ovum normally takes place in the ampulla of the fallopian tube soon after both the sperm and ovum enter it.

Fertilization Involves (Fig. 10.20)

1. Chemoattraction of the sperm to the ovum by substances produced by the ovum.
2. Adherence to the zona pellucida (ZP), the membranous structure surrounding the ovum.
3. Penetration of the ZP and the acrosome reaction.
4. Adherence of the sperm head to the cell membrane of the ovum, with the breakdown of the area of fusion and the release of the sperm nucleus into the cytoplasm of the ovum.

Millions of sperms are deposited in the vagina but eventually 50–100 sperms reach the ovum. Sperms

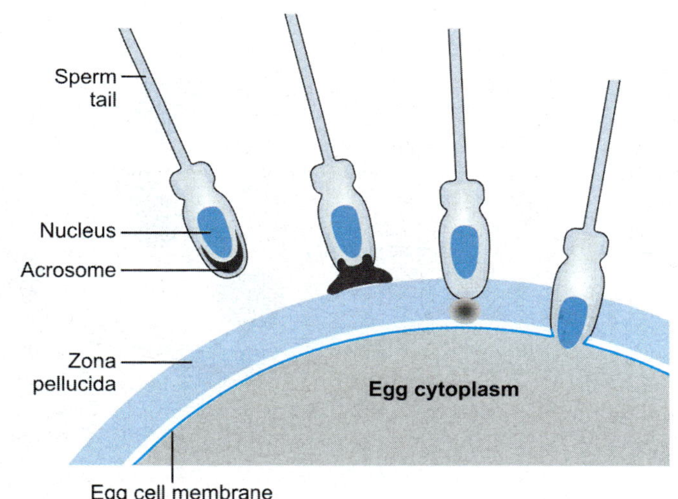

Fig. 10.20: Fertilization of the ovum

10

bind to the sperm receptor in the ZP and is followed by the acrosomal reaction, i.e. the acrosome (lysosomal liker organelle) in the head of the sperm releases various enzymes including trypsin-like-protease-acrosin.

Acrosin facilitates the penetration of the sperm through the ZP.

When one sperm reaches the membrane of the ovum, fusion to the ovum membrane is facilitated by fertilin, a protein on the surface of the sperm head (which resembles viral fusion proteins).

The fusion provides the signal for further development.

In addition, fusion sets off a reduction in the membrane potential of the ovum that prevents polyspermy—the fertilization of the ovum by more than one sperm.

There is a diffusion of calcium into through the oocyte membrane and this causes multiple cortical granules to be released by exocytosis from the oocyte into the perivitelline space.

These granules contain substances that permeate all functions of the ZP and prevent binding of additional sperm and cause any sperm that have already begin to bind to fall off.

Fertilization (Fig. 10.21)

Once a sperm has entered the ovum (which is in the secondary oocyte stage of development) the oocyte divides again to form the mature ovum and the second polar body that is expelled.

The mature ovum is called the female pronucleus and it contains 23 chromosomes.

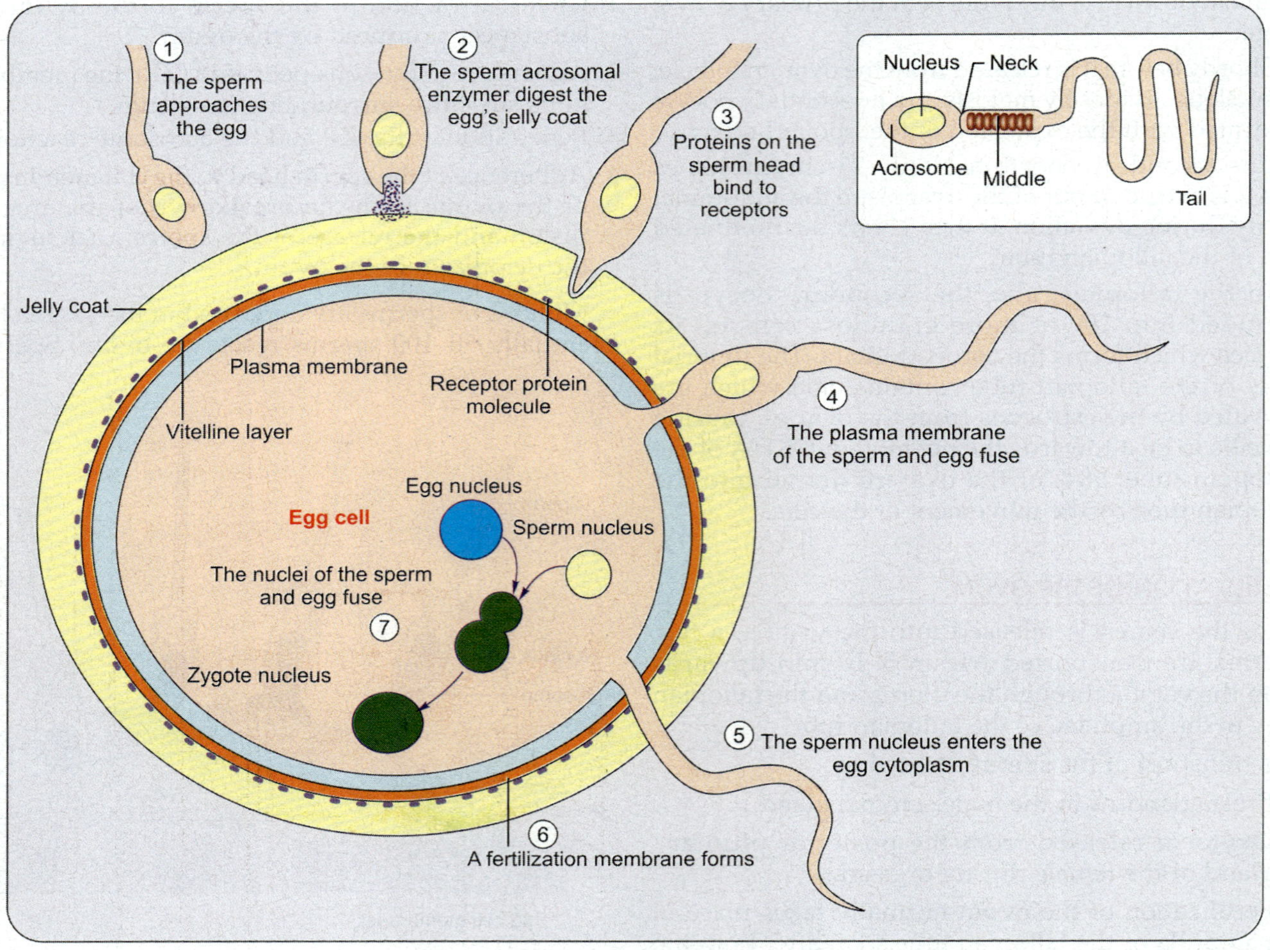

Fig. 10.21: Process of fertilization

10

The fertilizing sperm has also changed. On entering the ovum, its head swells to form the male pronucleus. Later the 23 unpaired chromosomes of the male and female pronucleus align themselves to reform the complete complement of 46 chromosomes (23 pairs) in the fertilized ovum.

Transport of the Fertilized Ovum in the Fallopian Tube

After fertilization, it takes 3–5 days for the transport of the fertilized ovum through the remainder of the fallopian tube into the uterus. This transport is affected mainly by:

1. Feeble fluid current in the tube resulting from epithelial secretions.
2. Action of ciliated epithelium towards the uterus.
3. Weak contractions of the fallopian tube.

Factors which impede movement through fallopian tube:

1. Fallopian tube are lined with rugged, cryptoid surface that impedes passage of the ovum despite the fluid current.
2. The isthmus of the fallopian tube remains spastically contracted for the first 3 days after ovulation.

After this the increased progesterone secreted by corpus luteum, exerts a tubular relaxing effect by increasing the progesterone receptors in fallopian tube and allows entry of sperm into the uterus.

IMPLANTATION

The site of implantation is usually on the dorsal wall of the uterus (Fig. 10.22).

At the site of implantation, the placenta develops and the trophoblast remains associated with it.

Till the 8th week, the fertilized ovum is called embryo and thereafter it is called fetus.

As the trophoblast cells invade the decidua, it digests it and imbibes the stored nutrients for growth and development.

The decidua provides nutrition up to 8 weeks and later the placenta takes up this function.

FAILURE TO REJECT THE FETAL GRAFT

The fetus and the mother are two genetically distinct individuals and the fetus is a foreign tissue in the mother. The transplant is tolerated and the rejection reaction when foreign tissue is transplanted does not occur.

This is because the placental trophoblast which separates the fetal and maternal tissues does not express class I and II MHC genes and instead express HLA-G, a nonpolymorphic gene. Therefore, antibodies against fetus do not develop.

(Also, a Fas ligand on the surface of the placenta binds to T cells, causing them to undergo apoptosis). The developing embryo is called the blastocyst and it undergoes rapid cell division and reaches the 8–16 cell stage when it reaches the uterus. It obtains nutrition from the uterine endometrial secretions "uterine milk".

Once in contact with the endometrium, the blastocyst becomes surrounded by:

a. An outer layer of syncytiotrophoblast, a multinucleate layer with no cell boundaries.
b. An inner cellular layer called cytotrophoblast.

The syncytiotrophoblast erodes the endometrium and the blastocyst burrows into it. This is called implantation.

Development of Placenta

While the trophoblastic cords from the blastocyst are attaching to the uterus, blood capillaries grow into the cords from the vascular system of the embryo.

By the 16th day after fertilization, blood is pumped by the heart of the embryo. Simultaneosuly, blood sinuses supplied with blood from the mother develop around the outside of the trophoblastic cords.

The trophoblastic cells send out more and more projections which become placental villi into which fetal capillaries grow.

Thus the villi carry fetal blood and are surrounded by sinuses that contain maternal blood.

On cross-section, the fetus blood flows through the two umbilical arteries and then into the capillaries of the villi and finally back through the single umbilical vein into the fetus.

The mother's blood flows from the uterine arteries into large maternal sinuses that surround the villi and then back into the uterine veins.

Structure of Placenta

Placenta is formed by the union of the maternal decidua and the fetal chorionic villi.

It lies embedded on the uterine wall and is connected to the fetus by the umbilical cord. It is formed during 6th to 12th week of pregnancy.

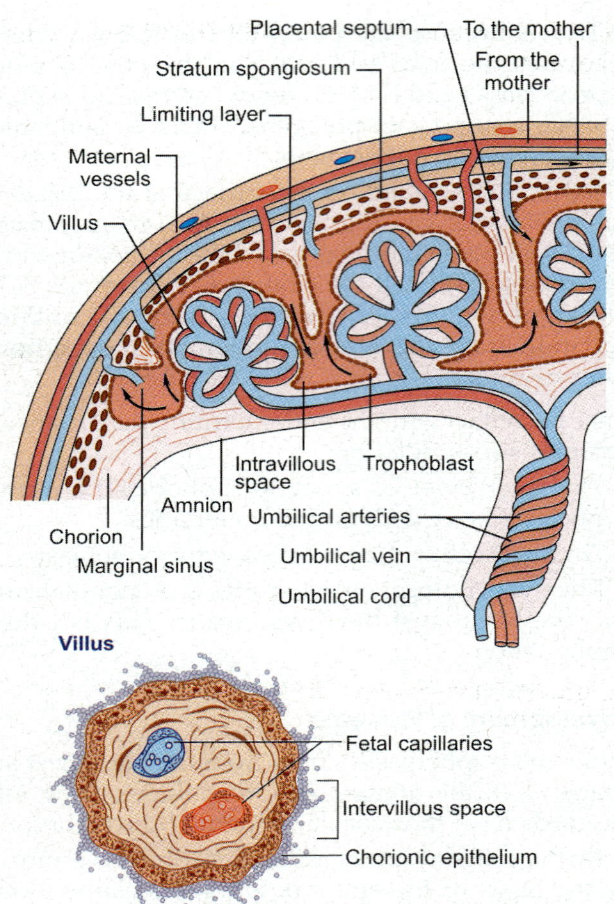

Fig. 10.22: Structure of placenta

Diameter: 15–20 cm
Thickness: 2–5 cm
Weight: 500 gm
Fetal surface: Smooth and glistening and covered by amnion.
Maternal surface: Has 15–20 lobes called cotyledons.

There are numerous fetal chorionic villi lined by trophoblast cells with large stem villi extending from the fetal side to the spongy layer of the decidua. They branch and rebranch to form secondary and tertiary villi.

Function

The major function of the placenta is to provide diffusion of nutrients and oxygen from the mother's blood into the fetus blood and diffusion of excretory products from the fetus back into the mother.

Diffusion of Oxygen through the Placental Membrane

Dissolved oxygen in the blood of the maternal sinuses passes into the fetal blood by simple diffusion, driven by an oxygen pressure gradient from the mother's blood to the fetus blood.

The PO_2 in the mother's blood in placental sinuses is around 50 mm Hg and the mean PO_2 in the fetal blood after oxygenation in placenta is 30 mm Hg.

The mean pressure gradient for diffusion of O_2 through placental membrane is 20 mm Hg.

Even at this low PO_2, adequate oxygenation of fetal tissue occurs because:

1. Hb is of the HbF type: The O_2 dissociation curve of HbF is shifted to the left of the maternal curve showing that at low PO_2 in fetal blood, the HbF is able to carry 20–50% more O_2 than maternal Hb can carry.
2. The Hb concentration of fetal blood is 50% greater than that of the mother. Therefore, it increases O_2 transport to tissues.
3. Bohr effect: The Hb can carry more O_2 at a low PCO_2 than it can at high PCO_2. The fetal blood entering the placenta carries large amount of CO_2, but most of it diffuses into the maternal blood.

Loss of CO_2 makes the blood more alkaline, whereas increase in CO_2 in maternal blood makes it acidic.

The capacity of the fetal blood to combine with oxygen increase and that of maternal blood decrease. This causes more oxygen from the maternal blood to flow into the fetal blood.

Thus the Bohr shift operates in one direction in the maternal blood and in the other direction in the fetal blood.

Then, 2 effects make the Bohr shift twice as important in the placenta as it is for O_2 exchange in the lungs. Therefore, it is called double Bohr effect.

By these three means, the fetus is capable of receiving more than adequate oxygen through the placental membrane.

The total diffusing capacity of the entire placenta for O_2 at term is 1.2 ml of O_2/minute/mm of Hg O_2 pressure difference across the membrane.

Diffusion of CO_2 through the Placental Membrane

CO_2 is being continuously formed in the tissues of the fetus and the only means for excreting the CO_2 from the fetus is through the placenta into the mother's blood.

The PCO_2 of fetal blood is 2–3 mm Hg higher than that of the maternal blood. This pressue gradient across the placental membrane allows adequate diffusion of CO_2 because of the extreme solubility of CO_2 in the placental membrane and allows CO_2 to diffuse about 20 times as rapidly as oxygen.

Diffusion of Food Stuffs through the Placental Membrane

In the late stages of pregnancy, the fetus uses as much glucose as the mother does. The trophoblast cells lining the placental villi provide facilitated diffusion of glucose through the placental membrane with the help of carrier proteins. Even then concentration of glucose is 20–30% lower in fetal blood than maternal blood.

Fatty acids have high solubility in cell membrane and they diffuse easily, but more slower than glucose.

Glucose is more easily used by fetus for nutrition. Ketone bodies, K^+, Na, Cl^- also diffuse easily from maternal blood to fetal blood.

Excretion of Waste Products through the Placental Membrane

Urea, uric acid, nonprotein nitrogenous substances and creatinine diffuse out of the fetus blood in a similar fashion to that of CO_2 because of its higher concentration in fetal blood than in maternal blood.

Hormones

Placenta is the temporary endocrine organ of pregnancy and synthesizes many hormones:

a. Protein hormones
b. Steroid hormones

Protein Hormones

- hCG
- Relaxin
- LHRH: Involved in regulation of hCG secretion
- A substance with TSH activity
- POMC, endorphins, prorenin, inhibin and substances with ACTH and TRH activity.
- hCG: Human chorionic gonadotropin.

hCG is a glycoprotein that contains galactose and hexosamine:

- It is produced by the syncytiotrophoblast.
- It is made up of α and β subunits.
- hCG α is identical to the α subunit of FSH, LH and TSH with molecular weight of 18,000.
- Molecular weight of hCG is 28,000.
- hCG is primarily luteinizing, luteotropic and has little FSH activity.

It can be measured by RIA (radioimmunoassay) and detected in the blood as early as 6 days after conception.

Its presence in the urine as early as 14 days after conception is the basis of laboratory test for pregnancy.

Small amounts are secreted by fetal liver, kidney and a variety of gastrointestinal and other tumors in both sexes and hence used as 'tumor marker'.

hCS: Human chorionic somatomammotropin.

The syncytiotrophoblast also secretes large amounts of a protein hormone that is lactogenic and has a small amount of growth-stimulating activity. Initially, it was called as chorionic growth hormone prolactin (CGP) and human placental lactogen (hPL).

Structure is similar to human growth hormone. Most of the actions of hCS are similar to growth hormone and functions as "maternal growth hormone of pregnancy" to bring about the nitrogen, potassium and calcium retention, lipolysis and decreased glucose utilization. The last two functions divert glucose to the fetus.

Amount secreted is proportionate to the size of the placenta.

Low hCS level is a sign of placental insufficiency.

Steroid Hormones

1. Estrogen
2. Progesterone

Estrogen

Placenta forms estradiol and estrone. The most abundant is estriol. Its concentration increases towards the end of pregnancy.

It is synthesized in the syncytiotrophoblast and are responsible for the enormous growth of the uterus and increased vascularity.

Progesterone

It is synthesized in the syncytiotrophoblast from maternal cholesterol.

Its concentration greatly increases and reaches a peak towards the end of pregnancy.

It is the hormone of pregnancy and it suppresses ovulation and menstruation, inhibits uterine motility, maintains pregnancy and causes great increase in the development of the alveolar system of the mammary gland.

TESTS FOR PREGNANCY

These tests are based on the detection of hCG in urine of pregnant women. hCG appears in urine as early as the 14th day after conception.

Immunoassay

i. Without isotopes
ii. With radioisotopes

hCG has both α and β subunits. Antigen-antibody reactions are used to detect its presence in the serum and urine.

The tests using hCG antibodies for α subunits are not specific. Cross reaction with LH occurs as the α subunit is identical for both.

Antibody against β subunit of hCG are highly specific and do not cross react with LH.

Latex particles coated with hCG or RBC are used as indicators of angiten-antibody (Ag-Ab) reaction. Levels of 1.5–3 IU/ml of hCG can be detected.

Without Isotopes

1. *ELISA test:* The enzyme-linked immunosorbent assay uses a monoclonal antibody, which binds the hCG in the test sample. A second antibody is added to sandwich test sample hCG. An enzyme is lined to the second antibody. When substrate for this enzyme is added, a blue color develops. A clear blue color means positive for pregnancy. Absence of it, means negative.
2. *Immunofluorometric assay (IFMA):* In this test, photon emission from a fluorescent label is used.

With Radioisotopes

10

1. *Radioimmunoassay (RIA):* In this test, Iodine 125 hCG is used as the radiolabeled ligand for antibody against hCG.
2. *Immunoradiometric assay (IRMA):* This test uses excessive antibody as the radiolabeled material rather than the ligand hCG.
3. *Radiological diagnosis:* The fetal skeleton can be seen in X-ray as early as 16–18 weeks and is confirmative of pregnancy.

It is not possible to detect by X-ray earlier than 16 weeks as there is hazards of radiation.

Ultrasound

Ultrasonics by the pulse echo sonar method is widely applied for diagnostic purposes in obstetrics and gynecology.

The gestational sac is detected as a well-defined white ring by the fourth to fifth week.

Fetal echo within the sac appears by the 7th week. Fetal heart reaction detected by the end of 7th week.

At 8–14 weeks, CRL of embryo allows accurate estimation of gestational age.

Biological Tests

1. *Ascheim-Zondek test:* This was the first test introduced in 1927. 2 ml of urine from the woman suspected for pregnancy is injected subcutaneously into immature female mice twice a day for 3 days. The animal is killed and examined on the 5th day. The presence of corpora lutea or hemorrhagic follicle in ovary indicates pregnancy.
2. *Friedman's test:* In this test, 10–15 ml of urine is injected intravenously in virgin or isolated female rabbit. The presence of ovulated or hemorrhagic follicles in 24–48 hours is positive for pregnancy.
3. *Kupperman test:* This test is the modification of Ascheim-Zondek test. In this, 2 ml of urine is injected in an immature female rat and the presence of hyperemia or ovarian hemorrhage indicates pregnancy.
4. *Hogben test:* In this test, about 20–30 ml of urine is injected in female frog and toad. The extrusion of ova in 12 hours is positive.
5. *Galli-Manini test:* In this test, 2 ml of urine is injected in male frog or toad. The presence of spermatozoa in the cloaca within 4 hours is positive.

Immunological Tests

The presence of hCG is also determined by the basis of antigen-antibody reaction. The most commonly performed immunological test is known as Gravindex test.

Requirements

First, the antiserum for hCG is prepared by injecting hCG which is isolated from urine of pregnant woman into rabbits. Antibodies for hCG are formed in the rabbit's blood.

or

Sheep's RBCs or latex particles are coated with hCG obtained from pregnant woman urine.

These two preparations are commercially available. Secondly, urine of the woman who needs to confirm pregnancy.

Procedure: One drop of the above prepared hCG antiserum is taken on a glass slide. One drop of urine from the woman who wants to confirm pregnancy is added to this and both are mixed well. If urine contains all the antibodies of antiserum, the agglutination of hCG molecules by the antiserum is not visible because it is colorless. Now, one drop of latex particles is added to this and mixed. The particles are not agglutinated because, the free antibody is not available. Thus, the absence of agglutination of latex particles confirms pregnancy.

If the urine without hCG is mixed with antiserum, the antibodies are freely available. When the latex particles are added, the antibodies cause agglutination of these latex particles which can be seen clearly even with naked eye. Thus, the presence of agglutination of latex particles indicates the woman is not pregnant.

Advantages

1. More sensitive and accurate.
2. Result is quickly obtained within a few minutes.
3. Tests are done easily.
4. The tests can be performed on the 5th day of conception.

These tests may be positive in some uterine tumors like choriocarcinoma and hydatidiform mole.

Duration of Pregnancy

280 ± 20 days from the first day of the last menstrual period.

1–12 weeks: First trimester
13–28 weeks: Second trimester
29–40 weeks: Third trimester

RESPONSE OF MOTHER'S BODY TO PREGNANCY

1. Menstruation ceases and ovulation does not occur.
2. Corpus luteum persists and reaches maximum size (2–3 cm) by the second month and then regresses after the third month and remains small till the end of pregnancy.
3. *Uterus enlarges:* Muscle fibers increase in length and width. Size of lumen increase from 2–5 to 5000–7000 ml. Weight increase from 50 to 1000 gm. This growth is due to placental estrogens which also increases the oxytocin receptors. Cervix is softened, mucosa is thickened.
4. Abdominal wall distends: Rupture of subcutaneous elastic fibers cause the appearance of irregular depressed lines called striae gravidarum. They heal after delivery leaving typical whitish lines called linea albicans.
5. *Weight gain:* Total weight gain: 10–12 kg
   3–4 kg: Fetal weight
   2 kg: Amnotic fluid, placenta and fetal membranes
   1 kg: Uterus
   3 kg: Increase blood volume and ECF volume
   1–2 kg: Fat accumulation
   Increase appetite causes increase in weight gain.

Metabolism

Increase secretion of many hormones during pregnancy namely thyroxine, adrenocortical hormones and sex hormones. The BMR increases by 15% during the latter half of pregnancy. Because of the increase load, extra energy should be expended for muscular activity.

Nutrition during Pregnancy

Greatest growth of the fetus occurs during the last trimester of pregnancy—weight of fetus doubles in the last 2 months of pregnancy.

Adequate amount of nutrition should be supplemented in the mother's diet.

Iron: Fetal requirement–375 mg
Maternal: 600 mg
Normal stores: 100 mg—not more than 700 mg

If not supplemented, leads to hypochromic anemia. Vit D to be supplemented to enhance calcium absorption.

Vit K in last trimester to prevent brain hemorrhage during delivery.

Changes in CVS of Mother

Cardiac output: Increases by 30% in third trimester. The blood flow through the placenta is 625 ml/min and increase in the metabolism of the mother increase the cardiac output.

Blood volume: Increases by 30% above normal especially in the last trimester.

This is due to the action of hormones especially aldosterone and estrogen which increases in pregnancy and cause fluid retention by the kidney.

The bone marrow becomes active and produces increase RBC to compensate the increase fluid volume. Therefore, at term the mother has 1–2 liters of blood extra in her CVS.

Only ¼ of this amount is lost by the mother during delivery of the baby, thereby allowing a considerable safety factor for the mother.

Maternal Respiration

Due to increase in BMR and weight gain, amount of oxygen consumed increases to 20% above normal and equal amount of CO_2 is also expelled. Therefore, the minute ventilation also increases, as progesterone increases the sensitivity of the respiratory center to CO_2.

This results in increase in minute volume >50% of normal and ↓ in PCO_2 several mm of Hg below that of normal woman.

Due to increase in uterus height, it presses upward against the diaphragm thereby the movement of diaphragm is reduced and the respiratory rate is increased to maintain extra ventilation.

Urinary System

- Increased urinary output due to increased fluid intake
- Increase in BMR increases the load of excretory products.
- The renal tubular reabsorptive capacity for Na^+, Cl^- and water increases by 50% due to increased production of steroid hormones by placenta and adrenal cortex.
- GFR increases by 50%
- Increased rate of water and electrolyte excretion in urine.

Gastrointestinal Tract

Nausea and vomiting may occur in the morning in first trimester called morning sickness.

Excessive and persistent vomiting (hyperemesis gravidarum) may affect health.

10

Endocrine Glands

The activity of various endocrine glands—pituitary, thyroid, parathyroid, adrenal cortex and pancreatic islets is increased.

The pituitary becomes nearly twice its normal size due to increased number of lactotrophs but LH, FSH and GH secretions are reduced.

AMNIOTIC FLUID AND ITS FORMATION

The volume of amniotic fluid is between 500 ml and 1 liter. The water in the amniotic fluid is replaced once in every 3 hours. Na^+ and K^+ are replaced once every 15 hours. Most of the amniotic fluid is obtained from renal excretion by the fetus. Some amount of absorption occurs by way of GI tract and lungs of fetus. Some amount is directly formed and absorbed through the amniotic membrane.

Functions

1. Provides medium for movement of fetus
2. Protection from trauma
3. Growth and development of lungs and GI tract
4. Maintains temperature.

Clinical importance: It helps in detection of:

1. Sex-linked disease
2. Chromosomal abnormalities
3. Metabolic disease
4. Rh isoimmunization
5. Acute fetal distress
6. Placental insufficiency
7. Fetal maturity
8. Antenatal fetal surveillance.

FETOPLACENTAL UNIT

Interactions between the placenta and the fetal adrenal cortex in the production of steroids are shown in Fig. 10.23.

The fetus and the placenta interact in the formation of steroid hormones. The placenta synthesizes pregnenolone and progesterone from cholesterol in the maternal blood. Some of the progesterone enters

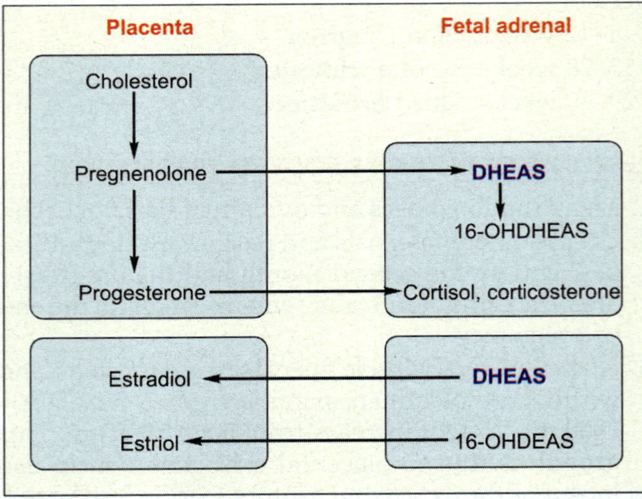

Fig. 10.23: Fetoplacental unit

the fetal circulation and provides the substrate for the formation of cortisol and corticosterone in the fetal adrenal glands.

Some of the pregnenolone enters the fetus and along with pregnenolone synthesized in the fetal liver is the substrate for the formation of dehydroepiandrosterone sulfate (DHEAS) and 16-hydroxydehydroepiandrosterone sulfate (16-OHDHEAS) in the fetal adrenal. Some 16-hydroxylation also occurs in the fetal liver. DHEAS and 16-OHDHEAS are transported back to the placenta, where DHEAS forms estradiol and 16-OHDHEAS forms estriol.

The principal estrogen formed is estriol and since fetal 16-OHDHEAS is the principal substrate for the estrogens, the urinary estriol excretion of the mother can be monitored as an index of the state of the fetus.

PARTURITION

Parturition means birth of the baby. Towards the end of pregnancy, uterus becomes progressively more and more excitable until it develops strong rhythmical contractions and the baby is expelled. Caused by two factors:

1. Hormonal changes
2. Mechanical changes.

Hormonal Changes

Increase in Ratio of Estrogen to Progesterone

Progesterone inhibits uterine contractility during pregnancy, thereby preventing expulsion of the fetus. Estrogen has the tendency to increase the degree of uterine contractility.

Towards end of pregnancy, the placental secretion of estrogen increases while that of progesterone remains constant. This causes increased contractility of uterus.

Effect of Oxytocin on Uterus (Fig. 10.24)

Oxytocin secreted by neurohypophysis causes uterine contraction.

There is increase in oxytocin receptors in the uterine muscle nearer term and the sensitivity of the receptors is increased by estrogen.

The rate of oxytocin secretion greatly increases at the time of labor.

Stretching of the cervix by the descent of the head causes a neurogenic reflex through the para-ventricular and supraoptic nuclei of the hypothalamus that causes the posterior pituitary to increase the secretion of oxytocin.

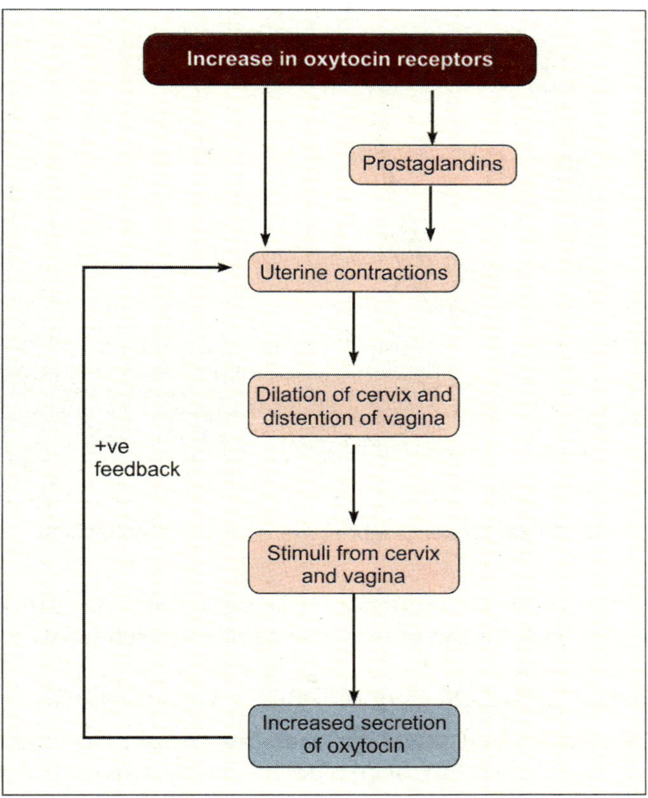

Fig. 10.24: Role of oxytocin in parturition

Effect of Fetal Hormones on Uterus

Fetal pituitary gland secretes increased quantity of oxytocin.

Fetal adrenal glands also secrete large quantities of cortisol which is also a uterine stimulant.

Fetal membranes release prostaglandins (PGs) in high concentration which increase the intensity of uterine contractions.

Mechanical Changes (Fig. 10.25)

Stretch of Uterine Muscles

Stretching of smooth muscles usually causes their contraction . So, intermittent stretching of uterus due to fetal movements can cause smooth muscle contraction.

Stretch and Irritation of Cervix

Stretching or irritation of nerves in the cervix initiates reflexes that go to the body of the uterus.

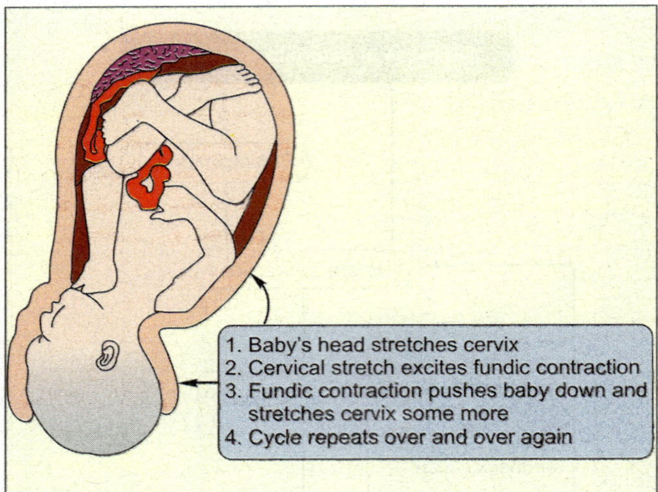

Fig. 10.25: Onset of labor (+ve feedback mechanism)

Myogenic transmission of signals from the cervix to the body of the uterus also causes contractions.

ONSET OF LABOR (+VE FEEDBACK MECHANISM)

Braxton Hicks contractions are slow, weak, rhythmic contractions that occur periodically throughout pregnancy.

They become stronger towards the end of pregnancy, stronger contractions causing stretching of cervix, followed by pushing of the baby through the birth canal.

This process is called labor and the strong contraction which results in final parturition is called labor contraction.

This occurs through a positive feedback mechanism. The stretching of the cervix by the baby's head further increases the force of contractions in the body of uterus which pushes the baby out through the outlet.

Stretching of Cervix

10

1. Increases the force of uterine contractions
2. Increases oxytocin secretion which in-turn increases the uterine contractions.

Mechanics of Parturition

Uterine contractions begin at the top of uterine fundus and spread downwards to the body of uterus.

The intensity of contraction is great at the top and body of uterus but weak in the lower segment of uterus close to cervix. This pushes the baby downwards towards the cervix.

Initially contractions occur once in every 30 minutes.

- Increase to 1 in 3 minutes with short periods of relaxation.
- Head of baby is delivered first—95%
- Intermittent contractions enable the fetus to receive adequate oxygen in between.

Stages of Labor

First stage: Onset of pains to full cervical dilatation (8–24 hours).

Second stage: Rupture of membranes to birth of baby (30 minutes).

Third stage: Delivery of placenta (10–45 minutes after delivery of baby).

Bleeding: 350–500 ml of blood lost.

Smooth muscles of uterine musculature are arranged in figure of eight around the blood vessel. Therefore, contraction of uterus after delivery of the baby constricts the blood vessel and decreases the bleeding.

Prostaglandins secreted at the site of placental separation cause additional vasospasm.

Involution of Uterus after Parturition

In 4–5 weeks after parturition, uterus becomes less than half of postpartum weight in 1 week.

In 4 weeks, it assumes the original size.

Lochia: Early postpartal discharge from the site of placental detachment due to autolysis on the endometrial surface.

Initially bloody and then later serous which last for 10 days.

Later endometrial surface become re-epithelialized to continue normal nongravid sexual life.

Mammary Glands and Lactation

Structure of Breast

The breast arises from the surface epithelium as solid columns of cells which gradually is hollowed out to become ducts. These ducts branch to give rise to terminal ductules which in-turn, leads to alveoli.

At birth, the breast is rudimentary. Further development occurs at the time of puberty.

At Puberty

There is considerable growth and branching of duct system, which undergoes further proliferative changes with the recurrence of each menstrual cycle followed by regression. There is progressive enlargement due to deposition of fat.

Between each menstrual period, there is hyperemia of the breasts, increase in interalveolar stroma with formation of new alveoli. However, these changes are transient.

During Pregnancy

The breasts enlarge greatly with marked change in structure (Fig. 10.26).

1. During the first half of pregnancy, there is further duct development accompanied by the appearance of many alveoli which form lobules. No milk is secreted by the breast gland at this stage.
2. During the second half of pregnancy, there is initiation of secretory activity and slow accumulation of milk in the alveolar lumen. The further enlargement takes place due to distension of the breast with its secretion.

Role of Hormones in the Breast Development

1. *Estrogen:* It causes ductal development—marked growth and branching of the ducts and thickening of the nipple.
2. *Progesterone:* It is responsible for the lobular development.
3. *Prolactin:* It increases steadily until term and levels of estrogen and progesterone are also elevated as well producing full lobuloalveolar development. This action is increased by growth hormone, corticosteroids and thyroxine.
4. *Placental lactogen:* During pregnancy, in addition to estrogen and progesterone, the placenta also produces a prolactin growth hormone-like factor, called placental lactogen.

All these hormones promote the growth and development of the breast during pregnancy.

LACTATION

Lactation consists of two processes:

1. Milk secretion
2. Milk ejection

Milk Secretion

It is the synthesis of milk by the alveolar epithelium and its passage into the lumen of the gland. It occurs in two phases—initiation and maintenance of secretion. Initiation of milk secretion is called lactogenesis.

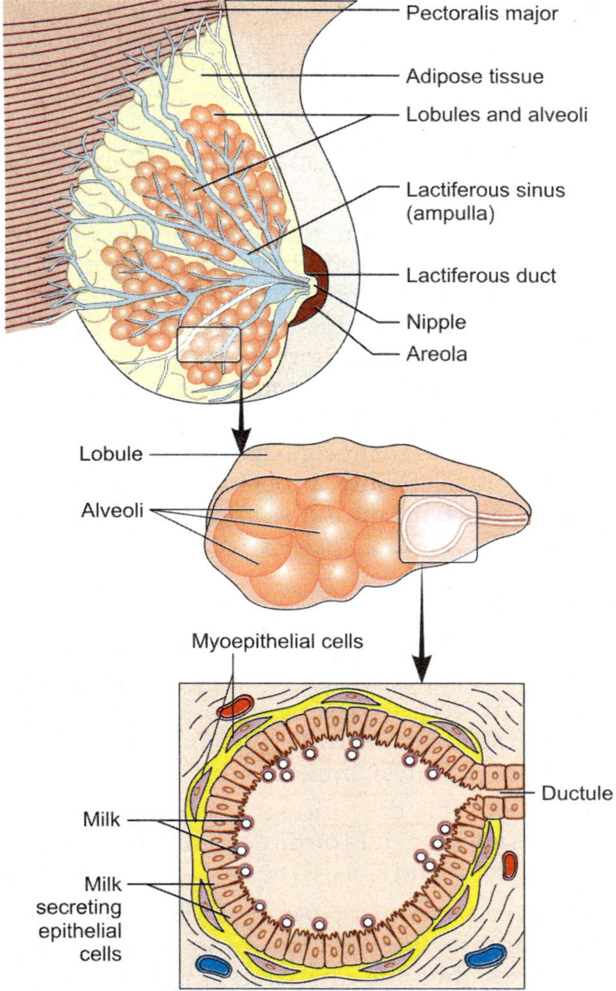

Fig. 10.26: Structure of breast

i. Though some secretion is present in the breasts during the second half of pregnancy, a free flow of milk occurs only 1–3 days after the child birth. The initiation of milk secretion is controlled by low circulating levels of estrogen which activate the lactogenic function of the anterior pituitary mediated by prolactin. This effect is due to reduced secretion of prolactin inhibiting factor (PIF) by the hypothalamus.
ii. During pregnancy, the lactogenic action of estrogen is inhibited by progesterone. After child birth, the rate of progesterone secretion decreases markedly before the decrease in estrogen occurs, thus allowing the estrogen to perform its lactogenic action.

Maintenance of milk secretion is called galactopoiesis. This is also controlled by prolactin along with other hormones like growth hormone, thyroid hormone, insulin and adrenal cortical hormones.

Milk Ejection Reflex (Neuroendocrine Reflex)

Suckling by fetus stimulates the tactile (touch) receptors in the areolar region of the breast, which activates somasthetic neural pathways which transmit signal to the paraventricular nuclei of hypothalamus which causes reflex stimulation of oxytocin into blood stream. This oxytocin is responsible for the milk ejection following 30–60 seconds. This is called neuroendocrine reflex.

Lactation amenorrhea: Stoppage of menstrual periods and temporary sterility, probably due to inhibitory action of prolactin on the secretion of the gonadotropins FSH and LH.

Human Milk

Milk is a natural balanced food and requires only the minimum of supplements to form a perfect diet. It contains protein (caseinogens and lactalbumin), carbohydrates (disaccharide—glucose and galactose), fat (minute globules), mineral salts, vitamins.

Colostrum: It is the fluid secreted during the first three days after the child birth, deep yellow in color and rich in proteins and salts.

Difference between human and cow milk

1. Human milk contains less protein, less salt and more carbohydrate compared to the cow milk.
2. Cow milk contains about six times as much caseinogen as human milk.
3. Cow milk contains more fatty acids and calcium than human milk.

Applied Aspects

10

1. *Gynecomastia:* Breast development in the male is called gynecomastia. It may be unilateral or bilateral. It is common in 75% newborns because of transplacental passage of maternal estrogen. It is a complication of estrogen therapy and is seen in patients with estrogen–secreting tumors. It is found in hyperthyroidism, cirrhosis of liver, eunuchoidism.
2. *Chiari-Frommel syndrome:* It is a rare condition, in which there is persistence of lactation (galactorrhea) and amenorrhea in woman who do not nurse after delivery. It may be associated with some genital atrophy and is due to persistent prolactin secretion without the secretion of the FSH and LH necessary to produce maturation of new follicles and ovulation.

INFERTILITY

It is the inability to conceive. The defect may be in the male or female. Hence, both partners must be investigated.

In the Male

Semen is collected by masturbation or coitus interruptus after abstinence for 5 days. It is analyzed within 2 hours for volume, sperm count and motility, etc.

In the Female

a. To determine if ovulation is occurring by an endometrial biopsy or by other methods described earlier under indicators for ovulation.
b. Patency of the fallopian tube by injection of radio-opaque material via cervix (hysterosalpingography).

Artificial Insemination

- It is introduction of semen into the vagina or into the uterus.
- It is widely used in veterinary practice.
- It is also done in couples where wife is fertile, and husband's semen analysis is normal but has problems of ejaculation.
- It is done at the time of ovulation.

In Vitro Fertilization (IVF) and Embryo Transfer Technique (ETT) Test Tube Baby

This is the latest technique by which infertile women with tubal block or some defects can still bear a child. Basic principles are:

1. Woman is given ovulation inducing agent such as clomiphene and when the graafian follicles have matured, oocytes are recovered by laparoscopy.
2. Each oocyte is placed in a separate petri dish containing a suitable culture medium along with sperms obtained from the husband 1½–2 hrs earlier.
3. This is incubated at 37°C and monitored to see if fertilization has occurred.
4. The presence of 2 pronuclei in the oocyte indicates successful fertilization.
5. It is allowed to grow in the incubation till embryo reaches 4 to 8 cell stage.

6. Now, the embryo is passed into the uterine cavity via the cervix through a fine Teflon catheter and implanted into the uterus (embryotransfer). Thereafter, the pregnant woman needs to be well cared for.

Gamete Intrafallopian Transfer (GIFT)

In this new method, the fertilized ova are introduced into the fallopian tube from where they naturally pass to the uterus for implantation. This method is considered to have a higher success rate than IVF.

CONTRACEPTION

A method or a system which allows intercourse and yet prevents conception is called a contraceptive method. At its present rate, the population of the world will double in 54 years and that of many poorer countries in the world will double in about 20 years.

For the individual and for the planet, reproductive health requires careful use of effective means to prevent both pregnancy and sexually transmitted diseases.

The practice of contraception is as old as human existence. Although medical history has documented the desire to control fertility since ancient times, safe and effective contraception did not exist until the beginning of the 20th century.

Need for Contraception

Individual level: Limiting family size, arises due to increased cost of living, scarcity of accommodation desire for better education of children in competitive world and desire for improved standard of living.

National level: Control of population, socio-economic problems of overpopulation.

Medical Grounds

1. Pregnancy in women <20 yrs, high-risk case, low birth weight.
2. Spacing birth (3 yrs) beneficial for both mother and child.
3. Multiparous woman from lower socioeconomic group suffers from malnutrition which predisposes to prolapse, stress incontinence, chronic cervicitis and carcinoma of cervix.
4. Previous cesarean section—surgical risks advised sterilization after second delivery.
5. Mentally retarded woman and serious psychiatric disorders.
6. Woman who has a child with genetic disorder needs genetic counseling and advised against further pregnancy.

Classification

- Spacing (temporary)
  1. Barrier
     a. Physical
     b. Chemical
     c. Combination
  2. Intrauterine device
  3. Hormonal
  4. Postconceptional
- Terminal (permanent)
  1. Male sterilization
  2. Female sterilization.

Temporary Methods

The effect of preventing pregnancy lasts while the couple uses the method, but the fertility returns immediately or within a few months of its discontinuation.

Older Methods

Natural and Behavioral Methods

The predominant methods of preventing births in most parts of the world were based on sexual behavior and required the cooperation of men.

- Abstinence
- Withdrawal technique
- Predicting fertility
- Breastfeeding was used to prevent unintended pregnancy.

Methods	*Advantages*	*Disadvantages*	*Noncontraceptives benefits*	*Risks*
Coitus interruptus	Available free	Depends on male control	Decreased HIV risk	Pregnancy
Lactation free	Available free	Unreliable duration of effect	Decreased breast cancer	Pregnancy
Periodic abstinence	Available free	Complex methodology motivation is necessary	None	Pregnancy

Breastfeeding

Ovulation is suppressed during lactation. Breastfeeding elevates prolactin levels and reduces gonadotropin releasing hormone (GnRH) from the hypothalamus reducing luteinizing hormone (LH) release and thus inhibiting follicular maturation.

The duration of this suppression is variable and is influenced by the frequency and duration of nursing, length of time since birth and mother's nutritional status.

Efficacy of Contraceptive Methods

Pearl formula – Pregnancy rate per 100 women/year

$$= \frac{\text{No. of pregnancies}}{\text{Total no. of months contributed by all couples}} \times 1200$$

Fertility Awareness

Periodic abstinence, also described as "natural contraception" or "fertility awareness" requires avoiding intercourse during the fertile period around the time of ovulation.

A variety of methods are used:

1. Calendar method (rhythm method)
2. The mucous method (Billings or ovulation method)
3. Symptothermal method is a combination of the first two methods.

In symptothermal method, the first day of abstinence is predicted either from the calendar by subtracting 21 from the length of the shortest menstrual cycle in the preceding 6 months or the first day mucus is detected, whichever comes first. The end of the fertile period is predicted by use of basal body temperature, i.e. 3 days after the rise in temperature signaling corpus luteum producing progesterone and ovulation has occurred. Because sperm may survive 5–7 days in the female genital tract, even a week's abstinence around the time of actual ovulation offers no guarantee against pregnancy.

10

Barrier Methods

- Male condom
- Female
  - Condom
  - Diaphragm
  - Cap
  - Sponge

Male Condom

The condom is the oldest and most widely used form of birth control in the world.

Advantages of Condom

1. Easily available
2. Cheap
3. Easy to carry
4. Free from side effects
5. Prevents sperm allergy
6. No adverse effects on pregnancy
7. Prevents transmission of sexually transmitted diseases
8. Occurrence of carcinoma of cervix low in partners.

Female Barrier Methods

Vaginal barriers are following types:

- Vaginal diaphragm
- Cervical cap
- Vault cap
- Vimule
- Sponge
- Condom

When used consistently, vaginal barriers are highly effective. They are safe, have contraceptive benefit and protection from sexually transmitted diseases.

Diaphragm

The diaphragm consists of a circular spring covered with fine latex rubber.

Risks: Prolonged use increases the risk of bladder infections.

Cervical Cap

FEM cap is a new version of cervical cap made of silicon rubber. It looks like a sailor's hat with the dome covering the cervix and the brim fitting into the vaginal fornices. The brim serves to form a seal against the vaginal wall, thereby acting as a funnel to direct the ejaculate fluid into the groove facing the vaginal opening, which is filled with spermicides.

Lea's shield: It is another vaginal barrier device made of silicon rubber and recently approved by FDA.

The Sponge

The today sponge contains nonoxynol-9. It is moistened with water and then inserted high in the vagina to cover the cervix. It combines the advantages of a disposable barrier with spermicide and provides protection for 24 hours.

IUCD

Intrauterine contraceptive device (Fig. 10.27)

Classification

First generation: Nonmedicated IUCD. Biological inert, e.g. Lippe's loop, Saf. *T. coil.*

Second generation: Cu IUCDs-Cu T 200, 220 (3 years)

Paraguard: Cu T 380 A (10 years), Multiload Cu 250, Nova T-Ag^+ Cu (5 years)

Third generation: Hormone releasing IUCD

- Progestasert
- Mirena

Mechanism of Action

1. Presence of foreign body in uterine cavity renders the migration of spermatozoa difficult.
2. Foreign body within the uterus provokes uterine contractility and increased tubal peristalsis, so that fertilized egg is moved down fallopian tube more rapidly and reaches the uterine cavity before development of chorionic villi and hence implantation does not occur.
3. Leucocytic infiltration: Macrophages engulf the fertilized egg in endometrial tissue.

IUCDs cause the formation of "biologic foam" within the uterine cavity that contains strands of fibrin, phagocytic cells and proteolytic enzymes.

Copper IUCDs continuously release a small amount of the metal, producing an inflammatory response. All IUCDs stimulate the formation of prostaglandins within the uterus, consistent with both smooth muscle contraction and inflammation.

Electron microscopy studies show alternations in the surface morphology of cells, especially of the microvilli of ciliated cells.

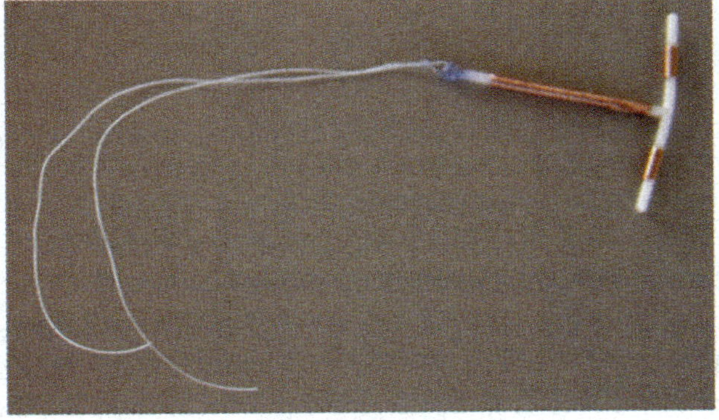

Fig. 10.27: IUCD

The altered intrauterine environment interferes with sperm passage through the uterus, preventing fertilization.

IUCD with Hormone

Progestasert: 38 mgm of progesterone releases 65 mcg/day. Its mechanism of action is similar to Copper-T.

Benefits of IUCDs

Both provide safe, long-term contraception with effectiveness equivalent to tubal pregnancy. It does not require continued effort by the user. It has low pregnancy rate.

The Levonorgestrol T acts by releasing Levonorgesterol which reduces menstrual bleeding and cramping. Additional noncontraceptive benefits include a reduced risk of endometrial cancer and improvement in symptoms of endometriosis.

Risks

1. Infection

Exposure to sexually transmitted pathogens is a more important determinant of pelvic inflammatory disease than wearing an IUCD. The only pelvic infection that is related to IUCD use is actinomycosis.

2. Ectopic Pregnancy

Occurs in 5% of cases. This is because the fallopian tubes are less well-protected from pregnancy than is the uterus.

3. Bleeding

Contraindications

a. Pregnancy
b. Puerperal sepsis
c. Pelvic inflammatory disease
d. Sexually transmitted disease
e. Endometrial or cervical cancer
f. Uterine anomalies

Hormonal Contraception

Hormonal contraceptives are:

1. Female sex steroids
2. Synthetic estrogen and progesterone (progestin)
3. Progestin only

They can be administered in the form of oral contraception, patches, implants and injectables. The most widely used hormonal contraceptive is the combination oral contraceptives.

Combination oral contraceptives can be monophasic with the same dose of estrogen and progestin administered each day or multiphasic in which varying doses are given through a 21-day cycle.

Typically they are administered for 21 days beginning on the fifth day of a menstrual period, then discontinued for 7 days to allow for withdrawal bleeding that mimics normal menstrual cycle.

The 28 day version provides placebo tablets for the last seven days of the cycle so the user simply takes one pill a day and starts a new pack as soon as the first pack is completed.

Steroid Hormone

Estrogens

Oral contraceptive (OC) contain either mestranol or ethinyl estradiol (EE).

Mestranol is EE with an extra methyl group. It requires bioactivation in the liver, where the methyl group is cleaved releasing the active agent EE.

Combination Estrogen Progestin Contraceptives

Ovulation can be inhibited by estrogen or by progestin alone. Synergism is exhibited when the 2 hormones are combined and ovulation is suppressed at a much lower dose of each agent. Combination OCs patches and the Nuva Ring suppress basal FSH and LH. They diminish the ability of the pituitary gland to synthesize gonadotropins when it is stimulated by the hypothalamic GnRH.

Ovulation does not occur, the corpus luteum does not form and progesterone is not produced. This blockade of ovulation is dose related.

Progestin only Preparation

As synthetic compounds that mimic the effect of natural progesterone but differ from it structurally. With the progestin—only "mini-pill" which supplies 0.3 mgm of norethindrone.

Transdermal Hormonal Contraception

The patch (Orthoevra) which is affixed to the user's skin and the vaginal Nuva Ring both contain combinations of ethinyl estradiol and a potent progestin. Both provide sustained release of the steroids and result in relatively constant serum levels that are less than peak levels seen with OCs but sufficient to prevent ovulation.

Hormonal Implants

With the subdermal implant that releases Levonorgesterel there is some follicular maturation and estrogen production but LH peak levels are low and ovulation is often inhibited.

The scant, dry cervical mucus that occurs in women using these preparations inhibit sperm migration into the upper tract.

Progestins decrease nuclear estrogen receptor level, decrease progesterone receptors and induce activity of the enzyme 17 OH steroid dehydrogenase which metabolizes natural estradiol 17 β.

Mifepristone

It is an antiprogesterone. Progesterone is essential for ovulation, and if the antiprogesterone is given before ovulation, this can be delayed for several days.

Mini Pills

Low progestogen only pill

1. Norethisterone—350 µg
2. Norgestrel—75 µg
3. Levonorgestrel—30 µg

Daily same dose starting 5–7 days after periods.

Depot Injections

1. Depot medroxyprogesterone acetate (DMPA) in aqueous suspension
2. Norethisterone enanthrate (NETO) in castor oil suspension.

Failure Rate

Progestin only OCs are less effective than combination E-P preparations.

Subdermal Implants

- Norplant-I
- Norplant-II

Implants inserted on the I day of menstrual cycle or 5 days after abortion or 3 weeks after delivery.

Site: Medial aspect of upper arm or forearm.

Hormonal Suppression of Spermatogenesis

Gossypol: Yellow pigment, isolated from cotton seed oil.

Dose: 10–20 mg, orally for 3 months, then 20 mg twice weekly.

Acts directly on seminiferous tubules inhibiting spermatogenesis without altering FSH and LH levels.

Side Effects

- Weakness, hypokalemia
- Permanent sterility—20%

Spermicidal agents: Contain surfactants that kill sperm before entry into cervical canal.

They may be in the form of foam tablets, soluble pessaries, creams and jelly.

Effective for 1–2 hours after application.

Postcoital Contraception (Emergency Contraception)

1. 2 tablets of high dose of combined pills containing
   i. 100 µg EE + 1 mg norethisterone
   ii. 500 µg LNG
   Taken within 72 hours of intercourse followed by 2 tablets after 12 hours.
2. *EE:* 1 mg daily × 5 days within 72 hours of exposure.
3. *RU 486:* Mifepristone is a steroid with affinity for progesterone receptors.
4. *Cu T IUCD:* Inserted within 5 days of intercourse prevents implantation of fertilized ovum.

Silastic Vaginal Rings (Nuva Ring)

Contents: LNG—releases 20 µg/day.

Effects cervical mucous

Permanent Methods of Sterilization

Female: Tubectomy (Fig. 10.28)

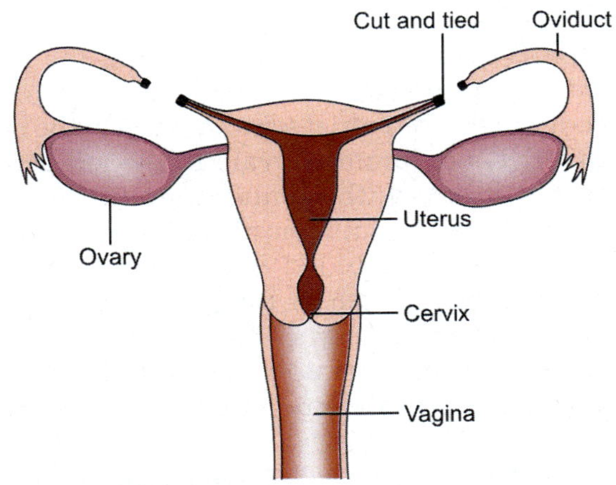

Fig. 10.28: Tubectomy

Postpartum

1. *Puerperal sterilization:* Done within 24–48 hours of childbirth.
2. *Cesarean ligation:* Combined with cesarean section.
3. *Internal ligation:* 6 weeks after delivery or any time in nonpregnant women. It should be done within 7–10 days of onset of menstruation.

Tubectomy consists of two steps routes:

1. Abdominal route
   a. Laparotomy (LSCS) 5–10 cm incision
   b. Mini laparotomy (puerperal) 5 cm.
   c. Laparoscopy (single puncture or incision technique) 1 cm (double puncture).
2. Vaginal route
   i. Colpotomy
   ii. Culdoscopy

Methods of Occluding Fallopian Tubes

1. Pomeroy's technique
2. *Laproscopic technique:* Occlusion of the fallopian tube using Fallope's ring/band: Avascular necrosis of the loop of the tube results in tubal occlusion
3. Occlusion of tubes using clips.

Male Sterilization (Permanent)

Vasectomy: Nonscalpel vasectomy(Fig. 10.29).

This is simple open patient department procedure under LA. The vas is grasped extracutaneously using a ringed clamp. The scrotal skin is punctured with

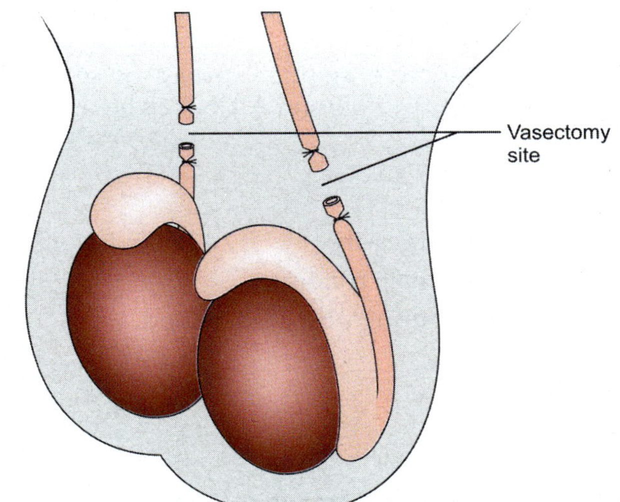

Fig. 10.29: Vasectomy

10

dissecting forceps to make a skin opening twice the diameter of the vas.

The wall of the vas is pierced with a dissecting forceps, vas is elevated outside and grasped with the ringed clamp. The vas is occluded by ligation or cautery.

Procedure repeated on other side. The vas is reinserted back and no sutures required.

Male Sterilization with Sclerosing Agents

Injection of 90% ethanol, 36% formaldehyde or acetic acid cause sclerosis of vas.

Contraceptive Vaccines

Contraceptive vaccines (CV) may provide viable and valuable alternative to presently available methods of contraception. The molecules that are being developed for CV target either:

1. Gamete production (LHRH/GnRH, FSH)
2. Gamete function (sperm antigens and oocyte ZP)
3. Gamete outcome (HCG).

Vaccines in Males

Blocking the production of sperms by mobilizing a selective inbuilt autoreaction approach against partners emerging with spermatogenesis in adulthood.

Female Condom—Femshield

- It has combined features of diaphragm and condom.
- It covers the entire vagina, cervix and external genitalia partially.

Highly protective against spread of sexually transmitted disease (STD) and AIDS. Can be removed after intercourse.

Advantages

1. Does not slip off easily
2. Stronger than male condom
3. Can be worn during puerperal period.

Disadvantage

Expensive.

Organization of Fetal Circulation (Fig. 10.30)

Fetal circulation differs from adult circulation because:

a. Fetal heart pumps blood to the fetal body as well as the placenta.
b. Since fetal lungs are not functioning, blood from the right heart is shunted into left heart, via the foramen ovale and ductus arteriosus, bypassing the lungs. Hence, the two ventricles in the fetus pump in parallel, unlike in the adult in whom they pump in series.
c. As gas exchange occurs in the placenta, outside the body of the fetus, in blood vessels carry a mixture of oxygenated and deoxygenated blood.

The foramen ovale is an oblique valvular opening through which the right and left atria communicate. The valve allows blood to flow from the right to left atrium.

Ductus arteriosus is a short channel communicating the arch of aorta beyond the origin of the left subclavian artery to the beginning of the left branch of the pulmonary artery.

Ductus venosus connects the umbilical vein to the inferior vena cava.

Deoxygenated (venous) blood from the fetus passes via two umbilical arteries to the placenta, while oxygenated (arterial) blood reaches the fetus from the placenta through the umbilical vein. These vessels are coiled round one another and covered by a jelly-like material and form the umbilical cord.

1. The umbilical vein carrying oxygenated blood (80%) from the placenta enters the fetus and passes to the liver. Most of the blood is diverted through a large branch, the ductus venosus to the inferior vena cava (IVC). A smaller branch joins the portal vein which supplies the liver and drains into the IVC via hepatic veins. The blood in the IVC is better oxygenated.
2. As the IVC reaches the right atrium, the blood divides into two streams at the crista dividens at the edge of the interatrial septum. Most of the blood is diverted via foramen ovale to the left atrium, where it mixes with a small amount of blood received from the pulmonary veins and enters the left ventricle. This blood is pumped by the left ventricle into the arch or the aorta, and supplies the heart, head and upper part of the body. This arrangement ensures adequate supply of better oxygenated blood to the two vital organs, brain and heart.
3. The smaller stream from IVC which enters the right atrium is joined by the deoxygenated blood from

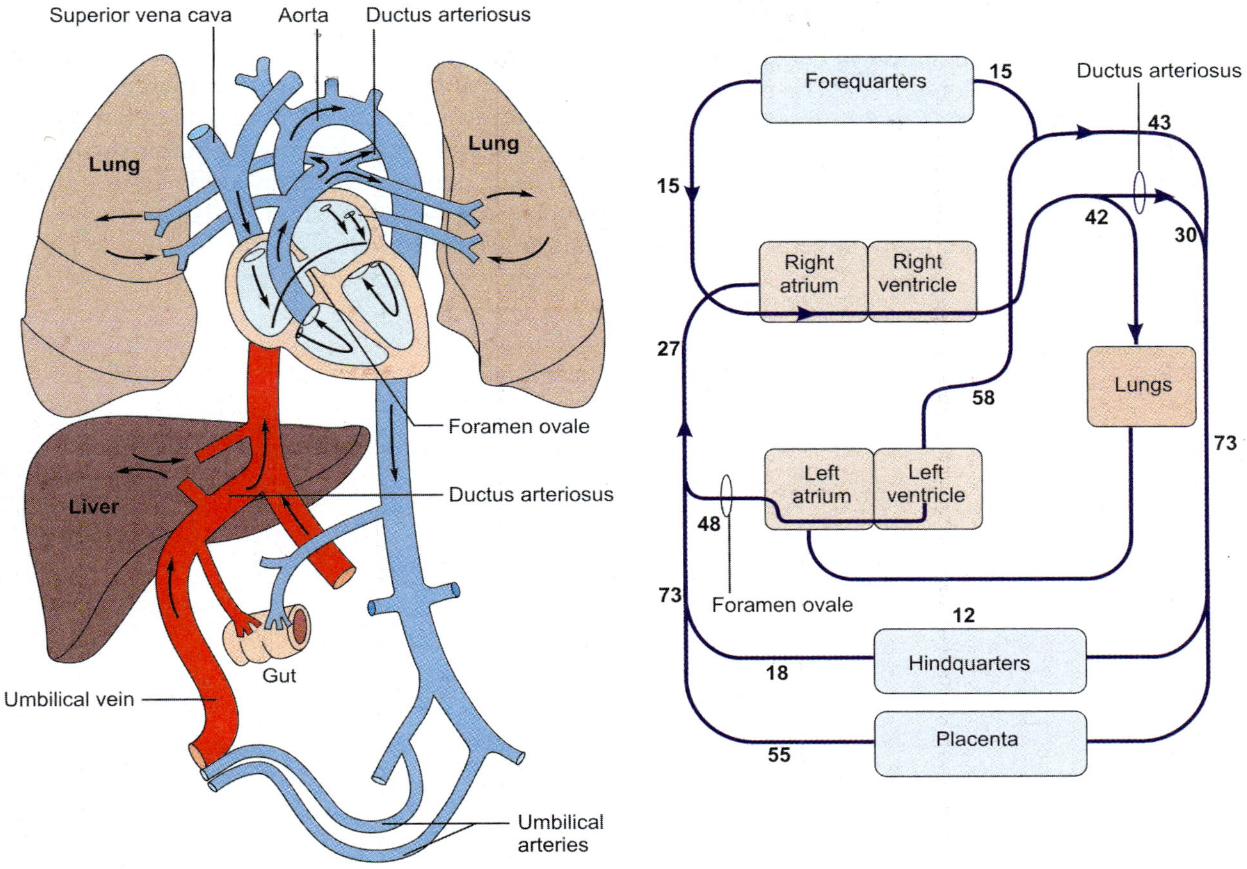

Fig. 10.30: Fetal circulation

the superior vena cava and coronary sinus and passes into the right ventricle and pulmonary trunk. Since, the lungs are collapsed and resistance is high, very little blood (10%) enters the lungs; most of the blood from the pulmonary trunk passes via ductus arteriosus into the aorta. This blood is less well oxygenated as the propotion of oxygenated to deoxygenated blood is only 2 to 1. Some of this blood goes to the lower half of the body and rests return to the placenta via two hypogastric arteries which become the umbilical arteries. The umbilical arteries carries deoxygenated blood to the placenta.

The cardiac output is high, the minute output per kg body weight is estimated to be about three times the adult value, and is due to rapid fetal heart rate and low peripheral resistance. About 40% of cardiac output goes to the placenta and rests to fetal tissues. The fetal heart and brain receive about 5% of the blood each.

Fetal Respiration

The placenta is the "fetal lung". Its maternal portion is in effect a large blood sinus. Into this "lake" project the villi of the fetal portion containing the small branches of the fetal umbilical arteries and vein. O_2 is taken up by the fetal blood and CO_2 is discharged into the maternal circulation across the walls of the villi.

The fetal tissues have a remarkable resistant to hypoxia. The O_2 saturation of the maternal blood in the placenta is so low that the fetus might suffer hypoxic damage if fetal red cells did not have a greater O_2 affinity than adult red cells. The fetal red cells contain fetal hemoglobin (hemoglobin F) whereas the adult cells contain adult hemoglobin (hemoglobin A. The cause of the difference in O_2 affinity between the two is that hemoglobin F binds 2, 3-DPG less effectively than hemoglobin A does.

Changes in Fetal Circulation and Respiration at Birth

At birth, the placental circulation is cut off and the peripheral resistance suddenly rises. The pressure in the aorta rises until it exceeds that in the pulmonary artery.

Meanwhile, because the placental circulation has been cut off, the infant becomes increasingly asphyxial. Finally, the infant gasps several times and the lungs expand.

Once the lungs are expanded, the pulmonary vascular resistance falls to less than 20% of the in utero value and pulmonary blood flow increases markedly. Blood returning from the lungs raises the pressure in the left atrium, closing the foramen ovale. Ductus arteriosus constricts within a few hours afterbirth, producing functional closure and permanent anatomic closure follows in the next 24–48 hours due to extensive intimal thickening.

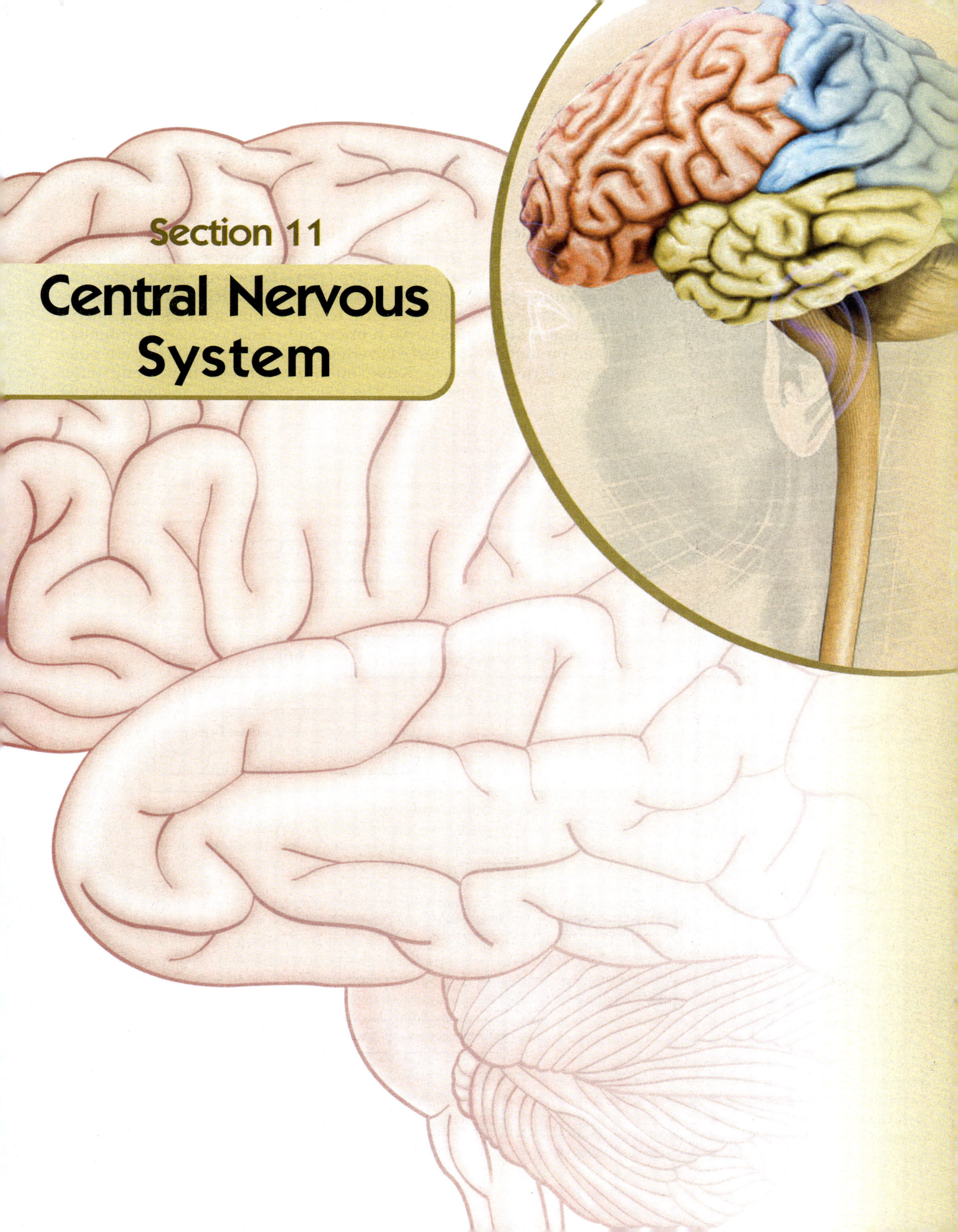

Section 11

Central Nervous System

92. INTRODUCTION TO NERVOUS SYSTEM

Our body is mainly under the control of two systems:

1. The chemical system
2. The nervous system

The chemical system includes the endocrinal system which regulates the functions of the body through various hormones. The nervous system controls all the activities of the body and provides a rapid means of communication between different parts of the body (Fig. 11.1a).

CENTRAL NERVOUS SYSTEM

The structure of the brain and the spinal cord are arranged in two layers, namely the gray matter and the white matter. The gray matter is formed by nerve cell bodies whereas the white matter contains nerve fibers. Both brain and spinal cord are surrounded by three coverings called meninges. They are outer dura mater, middle arachnoid mater and inner piamater. The space between the arachnoid mater

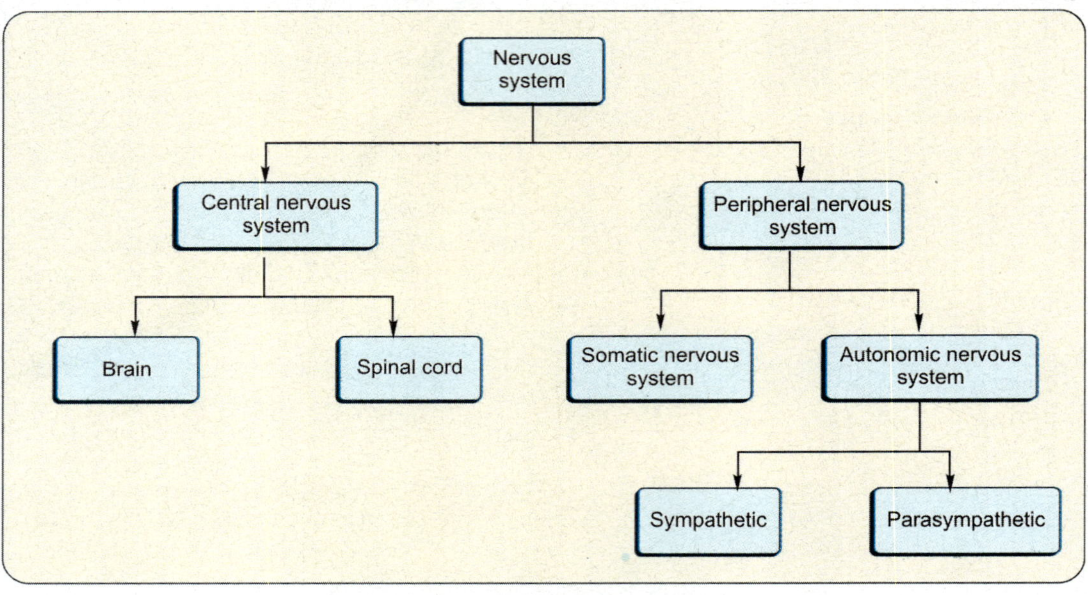

(a)

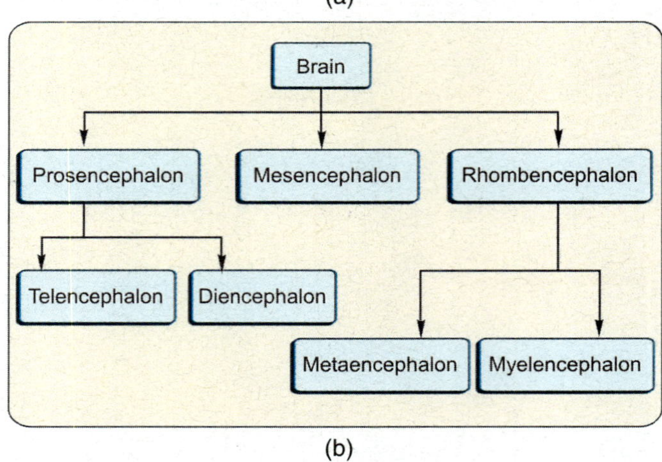

(b)

Figs 11.1a and b: Nervous system

11

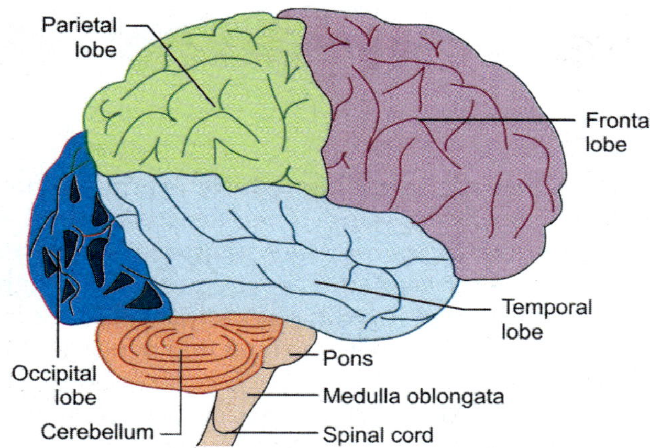

Fig. 11.2: Brain

and the pia mater is known as the subarachnoid space. This space is filled with cerebrospinal fluid (CSF) (Fig. 11.2).

Brain (Encephalon)

The brain is situated inside the skull. It has three divisions (Fig. 11.1b).

I. Prosencephalon (Forebrain)

It is further divided into two parts:

1. *Telencephalon:* It includes cerebral hemisphere, basal ganglia, hippocampus, amygdala and corpus callosum.
2. *Diencephalon:* It consists of thalamus, hypothalamus, metathalamus and subthalamus.

II. Mesencephalon (Midbrain)

It includes corpora quadrigemina and cerebral peduncles.

III. Rhombencephalon (Hindbrain)

It is divided into two parts:

1. *Metaencephalon:* Consists of the pons and the cerebellum.
2. *Myelencephalon:* Includes medulla oblongata. Midbrain, pons and medulla oblongata constitute the brainstem.

DIVISIONS OF THE BRAIN

Peripheral Nervous System (PNS)

It consists of various nerve fibers in the limbs, trunk, head and neck. It is divided into two systems:

1. Somatic nervous system
2. Autonomic nervous system.

Somatic Nervous System

It includes the nerves supplying skeletal muscles, 31 pairs of spinal nerves and 12 pairs of cranial nerves. It is concerned with somatic functions of the body.

Autonomic Nervous System

It is concerned with vegetative functions of the body. It is further divided into two systems:

1. Sympathetic system
2. Parasympathetic system.

93. NEURON

INTRODUCTION

Neuron is defined as the structure and functional unit of the nervous system. It is also known as the nerve cell. There are about 100 billion neurons in our body. During one's lifetime, the number of neurons remains constant. But the size increases as the organism grows. Neuron does not have centrosome, so it cannot undergo division. If there is death of the neuron due to any cause, it cannot be replaced by a new one. Recently it has been shown that in humans, neurons in hippocampus and olfactory bulb have the capacity to divide and proliferate.

STRUCTURE OF A NEURON (Fig. 11.3)

Neuron consists of:

1. Nerve cell body
2. Dendrite
3. Axon

Nerve Cell Body (Fig. 11.4)

It is also known as soma or perikaryon. It consists of cytoplasm which has nucleus, Nissl bodies, neurofibrils, mitochondria and Golgi apparatus.

Nucleus

Nucleus occupies the central part of the soma. It has usually one nucleolus. There is no centrosome, so the nerve cell cannot multiply.

Nissl Bodies (Nissl Granules)

Nissl bodies are small basophilic granules, first described by Franz Nissl. They are also called as 'tigroid substances' as they produce a spotted appearance when stained. They are present throughout the soma except in axon hillock (part of the soma where axon emerges). They extend into dendrites but not into axon.

Nissl bodies contain ribosomes and are concerned with protein systhesis in neurons. The proteins formed in soma are transported to axon by axonal flow. When there is a greater demand for proteins, Nissl granules overwork and disappear. This process is called 'chromatolysis'. It occurs when there is injury or fatigue of the neurons. They reappear after recovery from fatigue or regeneration of nerve fibers.

Mitochondria

They are present in the soma and in axon. ATP is produced here by Kreb's cycle.

Golgi Apparatus

It is similar to that of other cells. It is concerned with processing and package of proteins into granules.

Neurofibrils

They are thread-like structures present in soma and nerve processes. They consist of microfilaments and microtubules.

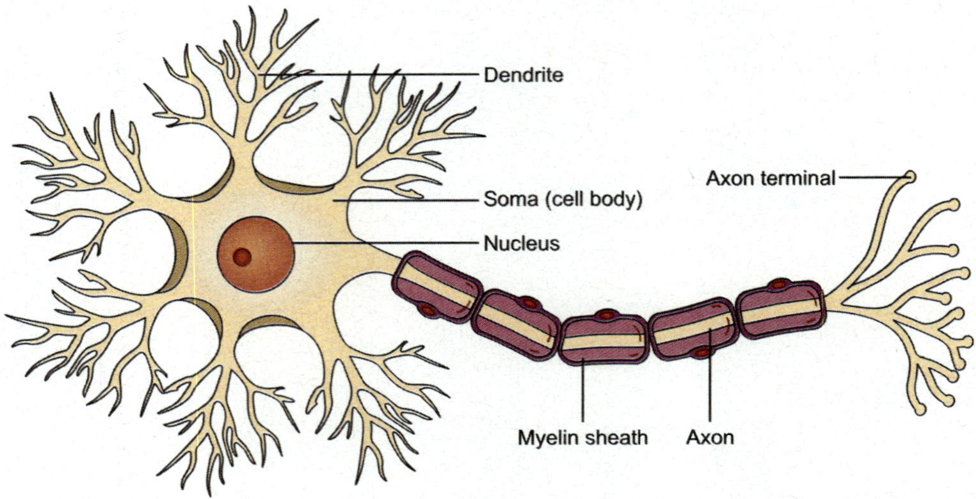

Fig. 11.3

11

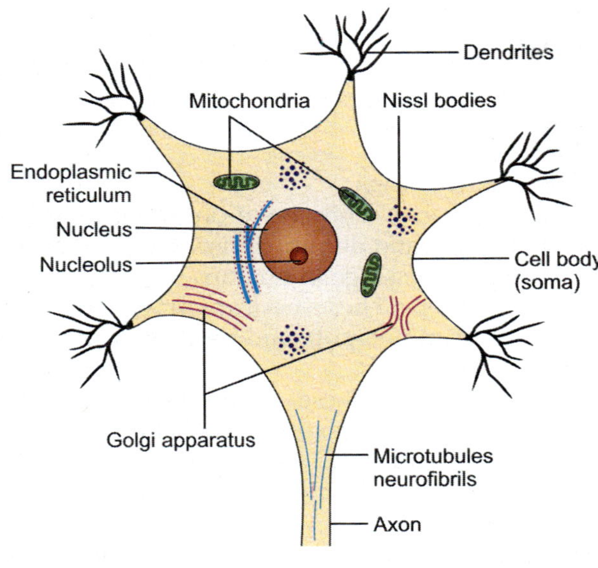

Fig. 11.4

PROCESSES OF NEURON (Fig. 11.5)

Dendrite

It is a short process of neuron which branches repeatedly. It has Nissl granules and neurofibrils. It transmits impulses towards the nerve cell body.

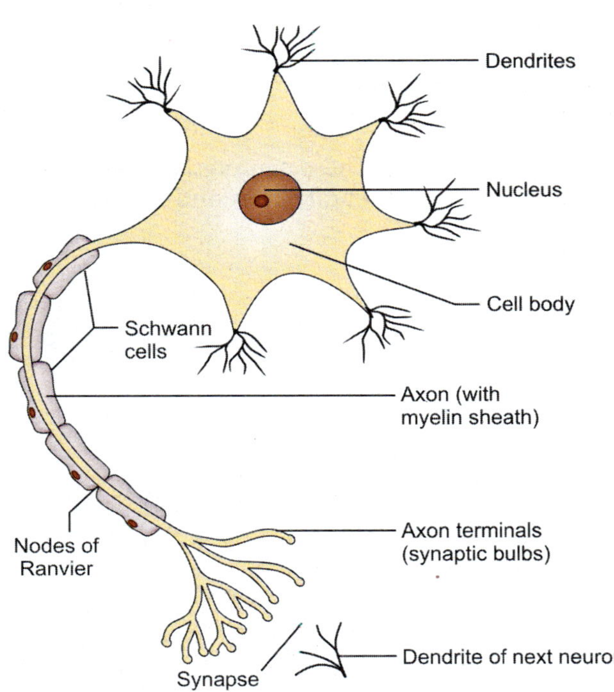

Fig. 11.5: Nerve cell (neuron)

Axon

It is a longer process of neuron. Each neuron has only one axon. It arises from an elevated portion of the cell body called the axon hillock. The first part of the axon is called initial segment which is more excitable than other parts of the neuron due to the presence of more number of ionic channels.

Structure of Axon

Many axons together form a bundle called fasciculus. Many fasciculi together form a nerve trunk. Each nerve fiber is covered by endoneurium. Each fasciculus is covered by perineurium. Entire nerve trunk is covered by epineurium.

The axon has a long central core of cytoplasm called axoplasm. This is covered by a tubular sheath called axolemma. The axoplasm along with the axolemma is called axon cylinder of the nerve fiber. This axon cylinder is covered by a membrane called neurilemma.

Types of Axons (Nerve Fibers)

There are two types of axons:

1. Myelinated (Fig. 11.6)
2. Nonmyelinated

Myelinated axons: These axons are covered by myelin sheath which acts as an insulator. Myelin sheath is a lipoprotein complex (lipids are sphingomyelin, cerebroside and cholesterol), which is absent at regular intervals. The area where the myelin sheath is absent is called node of Ranvier. The segment of nerve fiber between two nodes is called internode. Myelin gives white color to the nerves (Fig. 11.6).

Myelinogenesis: The formation of myelin sheath around the axon is called myelinogenesis. It is formed by Schwann cells in the peripheral nervous system

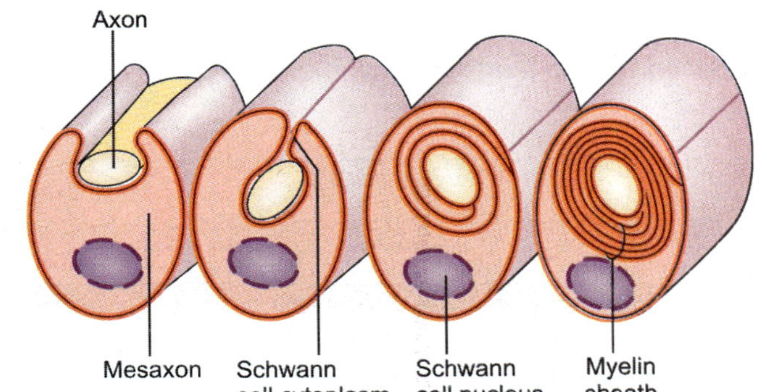

Fig. 11.6

11

and by oligodendroglia in the central nervous system. In the PNS, myelinogenesis starts at 4th month of intrauterine life and is completed only in the second year of life afterbirth.

Before myelinogenesis, Schwann cells of the neurilemma are applied close to the axolemma as in nonmyelinated nerve fibers. The membrane of the Schwan cells is double layered. The Schwann cells wrap up and rotate around the axis cylinder in many concentric layers. Eventually these concentric layers fuse to produce a heavily lipid rich membrane called myelin sheath. The neurilemma is the outermost cell membrane of the Schwann cell. The nuclei of the Schwann cell resides between the neurilemma and the myelin sheath.

Functions of Myelin

- Faster conduction
- Insulator

Faster conduction: In myelinated nerve fibers, the impulses jump from one node to the another node of Ranvier aiding in faster conduction of impulses (Fig. 11.7). This type of conduction is called saltatory conduction.

Insulator: Myelin sheath acts as an insulator and restricts the nerve impulse within stimulated nerve fibers.

Nonmyelinated Nerves

As there is no myelin sheath, these nerve fibers are small. The neurilemma and axis cylinder are present.

Classification of Neurons

The neurons are classified by three methods:

1. Based on the number of poles
2. Based on the function
3. Based on the length of the axon.

11

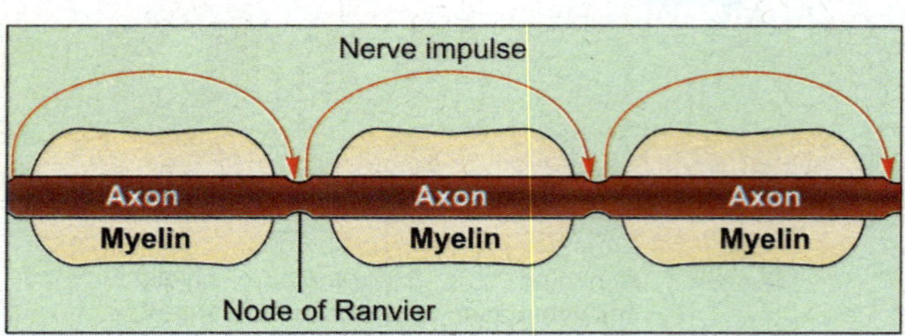

Fig. 11.7

Based on the Number of Poles

There are three types of neurons based on the number of poles (Fig. 11.8):
1. Unipolar neurons
2. Bipolar neurons
3. Multipolar neurons

Unipolar neurons: They have only one pole from which both axon and dendrite arise. They are present only in embryonic stage in humans.

Bipolar neurons: These neurons have two poles, axon arises from one pole and dendrites arise from the other pole.

Multipolar neurons: These neurons have many poles. one pole gives rise to axon and all the other poles gives rise to dendrites.

Based on the Function

There are two types of neurons based on their function:
a. Motor neuron, b. Sensory neuron

Motor neuron: They carry the motor impulses from central nervous system to the effector organs like the muscles and glands.

Sensory neuron: They carry the sensory impulses from the periphery to the central nervous system.

Based on the Length of the Axon

Based on the length of the axon, neurons are divided into two types:
1. Golgi type I neurons
2. Golgi type II neurons

Golgi type I neurons: These have long axons.

Golgi type II neurons: These neurons have short axons. They are present in cerebral cortex and spinal cord.

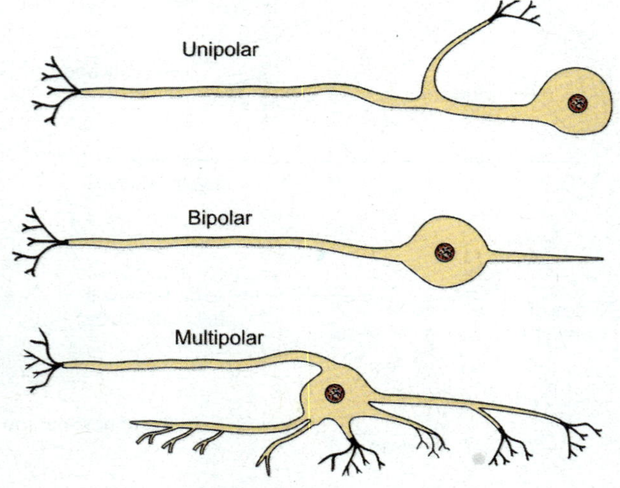

Fig. 11.8: Types of neurons

94. NEUROGLIA

Definition

Neuroglia are the cells which support the neurons (glia=glue). They are nonexcitable and do not transmit impulses. There are 10 times as many glial cells as neurons. They are capable of multiplying by mitosis.

Classification

There are three main types of neuroglia (Fig. 11.9).

1. Microglia
2. Astrocytes
3. Oligodendrocytes.

Apart from these Schwann cells, satellite cells and ependymal cells are also glial cells.

Microglia

- The smallest glial cells
- Mesodermal in origin
- Belong to reticuloendothelial system.

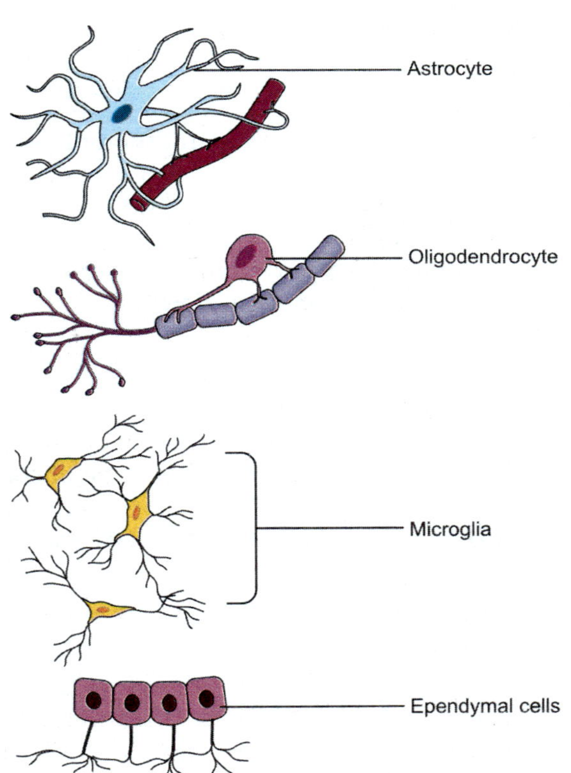

Fig. 11.9: Neuroglial cells of the CNS

Function

Phagocytosis of microorganisms and cellular debris in CNS and hence called macrophages of CNS.

Astrocytes

Star shaped neuroglial cells.

There are two types:

1. Fibrous astrocytes—found in white matter.
2. Protoplasmic astrocytes—found in gray matter.

Functions

- Their processes surround the blood vessels and capillaries forming tight junctions which are responsible for blood–brain barrier.
- Also surround the synapses and neurons and segregate and insulate them.
- Produce substances that are trophic to neurons.
- Help in maintaining proper ionic and neurotransmitter concentrations.

Oligodendrocytes

- Also called as oligodendroglia.
- Have fewer dendrites.

Function

Provide myelination around the nerve fibers in CNS.

Schwann Cells

Present in the peripheral nervous system.

Functions

- Provide myelination around the peripheral nerves.
- Play a role in nerve regeneration.

Satellite Cells

Present on the external surface of dorsal root and cranial nerve ganglion cells.

Function

Help in regulation of chemical environment around the neuron.

Ependymal Cells

Line the surface of the ventricles in the brain and the central canal of the spinal cord.

Functions

- Produce CSF along with choroidal cells.
- Also participate in blood-CSF barrier.

95. NERVE FIBERS

CLASSIFICATION OF NERVE FIBERS

Nerve fibers are classified based on different methods:

1. Based on diameter and conduction velocity. (Erlanger–Gasser classification)
2. Sensory nerve classification
3. Based on function
4. Based on origin
5. Based on type of neurotransmitter released.

Based on Diameter and Conduction Velocity: (Erlanger–Gasser Classification)

Erlanger and Gasser classified the nerve fibers into three major types:

a. Type-A
b. Type-B
c. Type-C

Type: A fibers are subdivided into α, β, γ and δ.

Erlanger–Gasser classification of nerve fibers

Type	Diameter (μm)	Conduction velocity (m/sec)	Location
Aα	12–22	70–120	Proprioceptive and motor nerves
Aβ	6–12	30–70	Afferents for touch
Aγ	3–6	15–30	Motor nerves to intrafusal fibers of muscle spindle
Aδ	2–5	12–15	Afferents for thermal senses and fast pain
B	1–2	3–10	Preganglionic fibers of ANS
C	1.5–0.3	0.5–2	Afferents for pain, post-ganglionic sympathetic fibers

Sensory Nerve Classification

This is the alternative classification used by sensory physiologists. The nerve fibers are divided into four groups.

Group of nerve fiber	Corresponds to	Function
IA	Aα	Fibers from annulospiral endings of muscle spindles.
IB	Aα	Fibers from Golgi tendon organs.
II	Aβ and Aγ	Fibers from flower-spray endings of muscle spindle and cutaneous tactile receptors.
III	Aδ	Fibers carrying temperature, crude touch and pricking pain sensation
IV	C	Unmyelinated fibers carrying slow pain, itch and temperature

Based on Function

There are two types

1. Sensory nerve fibers
   a. Carry sensory impulses from different parts of the body to CNS.
   b. Also called as afferent nerve fibers.
2. Motor nerve fibers
   a. Carry motor impulses from CNS to periphery.
   b. Also called as efferent nerve fibers.

Based on Origin

There are two types of nerve fibers

1. Cranial nerves which originate from brain.
2. Spinal nerves which originate from spinal cord.

Based on Type of Neurotransmitter Released

There are two types

1. Adrenergic fibers which secrete adrenaline.
2. Cholinergic fibers which secrete acetylcholine.

PROPERTIES OF NERVE FIBERS

Following are the properties of nerve fibers

- Excitability
- Conductivity

- Refractory period
- Infatiguability
- All-or-none law
- Adaptation
- Summation

Excitability

Excitability is defined as the physiochemical change that occurs in a tissue when a stimulus is applied. A stimulus is defined as an external agent which produces excitability in the tissues. When a threshold stimulus is applied, the nerve fibers get excited. The process of eliciting an action potential can also be called as excitation.

Excitability of the nerve fiber is measured using the strength duration curves. Chronaxie indicates the excitability of nerve fibers. There is an inverse relation between chronaxie and excitability.

Factors Affecting Excitability

- *Temperature:* Increase in temperature increases excitability by increasing the activity of ionic pump.
- *Ions:* An increase in K^+ decreases excitability. Ca^{++} and Mg^{++} have an inverse relation with excitability.
- *Oxygen supply:* Severe hypoxia decreases the excitability.
- *pH:* Alkaline pH increases and acidic pH decreases excitability.
- *Toxins:* Tetanus and rabies increase the excitability.
- *Drugs:* Anesthetics abolish excitability.

Conductivity

The ability of nerve fibers to transmit the impulse from the area of stimulation to other areas is called conductivity. Nerve fibers can conduct impulses in both directions but normally, in the body, the action potential is transmitted through the nerve fiber in only one direction.

Mechanism of Conduction of Action Potential

The depolarization occurs first at the site of stimulation in the nerve fibers. This causes depolarization of the neighboring areas. Depolarization is followed by repolarization.

Conduction in Myelinated Nerve Fibers

Conduction of impulses through a myelinated nerve fiber is 50 times faster than that through a non myelinated fiber (Fig. 11.7). This is because the myelin sheath is impermeable to ions. So, the entry of Na^+ from ECF into the nerve fiber occurs only in the node of Ranvier, where the myelin sheath is absent. It causes depolarization in the node only. Thus, the depolarization occurs at successive nodes. So, the action potential jumps from one node to another. Hence, it is called saltatory conduction.

Factors that Affect Conduction Velocity

1. *Temperature*

Rise in temperature increases the conduction velocity as the rate of conductance of Na^+ increases at higher temperature.

2. *Diameter of the Nerve Fiber*

Conduction is directly proportional to the diameter.

3. *Myelination*

Conduction velocity of nerve impulses is faster in myelinated, nerve fibers.

Hypoxia: Hypoxia decreases the conduction velocity of nerve impulses as it is energy dependent.

Drugs

- Tetradotoxin blocks voltage-gated Na^+ channels.
- Tetraethyl ammonium (TEA) blocks voltage-gated K^+ channels. These drugs block the conduction of impulses in the nerve fibers.

Orthodromic and Antidromic Conduction

Normally, impulses travel in one direction only, i.e. from the synaptic junctions or receptors along axons to their terminations. Such conduction is called orthodromic conduction.

Conduction in the opposite direction is called antidromic conduction.

Refractory Period

It is the period during which the nerve does not respond to a stimulus. It is of two types:

1. Absolute refractory period
2. Relative refractory period.

Absolute Refractory Period

It is the period during which the nerve does not respond at all, however, strong the stimulus may be.

Relative Refractory Period

It is the period during which the nerve fiber shows a response, if a stronger stimulus is given.

Absolute refractory period corresponds to the period from the time when firing level is reached till the time when 1/3rd of repolarization is completed. The relative refractory period extends through rest of the repolarization period.

Infatiguability

A nerve fiber cannot be fatigued, even if it is stimulated continuously for a long-time. This is because the nerve fiber can conduct only one action potential at a time. At that time, it is completely refractory and does not conduct another action potential.

All-or-None Law

This states that when a nerve is stimulated by a stimulus, it gives maximum response or does not respond at all.

Adaptation (Accommodation)

When a nerve fiber is stimulated continuously the excitability of the nerve fiber is greater in the beginning. But later, the response decreases slowly and finally the nerve does not show any response at all. This is because continuous depolarization inactivates the sodium pump and increases efflux of K^+.

Summation

When a subliminal stimulus is applied, it does not produce any response in the nerve fiber because the subliminal stimulus is very weak. However, if two or more subliminal stimuli are applied within a short interval of about 0.5 second, response is produced. This is due to summation of all the subliminal stimuli.

DEGENERATION AND REGENERATION OF NERVE FIBER

Introduction

11

When there is a nerve injury many changes occur in the nerve fiber and nerve cell body. All these changes are collectively known as degenerative changes. Nerve injury may be due to trauma, obstruction of blood flow or local injection of toxic substances.

Degrees of Injury

Sunderland had classified nerve injuries into five degrees based on the severity of the injury.

First Degree Injury

This is the most common type of injury to the nerves. It is caused by compression of the nerve for a short period leading to ischemia and hypoxia. There is mild demyelination but axon is not destroyed. Axon loses its function temporarily for a short-time which is called conduction block. The function returns within a short-time. This is also called as Seddons neuropraxia.

Second Degree Injury

This is due to prolonged severe pressure causing Wallerian degeneration. But the endoneurium is intact. Repair and restoration of function takes about 18 months. This is also called as axonotmesis.

Third Degree Injury

The endoneurium is injured but epineurium and perineurium are intact. The recovery is slow, poor or incomplete.

Fourth Degree Injury

The injury is severe, so epineurium and perineurium are also injured. Regeneration is poor or incomplete.

Fifth Degree Injury

This involves complete transection of the nerve trunk. Regeneration is possible only if the cut ends are sutured surgically. Third, fourth and fifth degree of nerve injuries of Sunderland are together known as neurotmesis.

DEGENERATION OF NERVE

When a nerve fiber is cut, it undergoes degenerative changes, which are seen in distal end, proximal end and soma.

Changes in the Distal End

This was first described by Augustus Waller in 1862 and hence it is called Wallerian degeneration. It is also known as orthograde degeneration.

1. The axis cylinder swells up and breaks into small rodlets. After a few days the broken pieces appear as debris.
2. The myelin sheath disintegrates. Hydrolysis of lipids occurs and the products of hydrolysis (cerebrosides, sphingomyelin, cholesterol and fatty acids) appear as droplets. Ultimately the myelin sheath is replaced by fatty droplets. Myelin degeneration occurs from 8th day to 32nd day.

3. The neurilemma remains intact. Schwann cells multiply rapidly. The macrophages invade from outside and phagocytose the broken down pieces of axis cylinder. Finally, a hollow tube of neurilemma containing large number of phagocytes is seen. This was described as 'ghost tube' by Edward Sharpey-Schafer.

Changes in the Proximal Part

This is also known as retrograde degeneration.

1. The same degenerative changes are seen in the proximal stump, but only up to the node of Ranvier nearest to the injury.
2. Changes in the soma
   a. Nissl granules disintegrate into fragments,a process called chromatolysis.
   b. The cell body swells due to accumulation of fluid.
   c. Golgi apparatus, mitochondria and neurofibrils disappear.
   d. The nucleus is pushed to one side or extruded out.

CRANIAL NERVES

Name	*Type nerve*	*Function*
Olfactory nerve	Sensory	Olfaction (smell)
Optic nerve	Sensory	Vision
Oculomotor nerve	Motor	Innervates extrinsic muscle of eyeball like inferior oblique, medial rectus, superior rectus, inferior rectus and intrinsic muscles of eye and participate in accomodation and light reflex. Carry proprioception from eye muscles
Trochlear nerve	Motor	Innervates superior oblique muscle of eyeball. Carry proprioception from superior oblique
Trigeminal nerve	Mixed nerve a. Motor b. Sensory	Innervates the muscles of mastication, tensor tympani, tensor veli palatine, myolohyoid and the anterior belly of digastric muscle Bring general senation from face, scalp, teeth, periodontal tissues, oral cavity, nasal cavity and cranial dura mater They carry proprioception from muscles of mastication, facial muscles and extrinsic ocular muscles
Abducent nerve	Motor	Innervates the lateral rectus of the eyeball, it carries proprioception from the same muscle
Facial nerve	Mixed	
	a. Motor	Innervates the skeletal muscles that participate in facial expressions Supply secretomotor fibers to nasal, palatine, lacrimal and salivary glands
	b. Sensory	Carries taste sensation from anterior 2/3rds of the tongue
Vestibulocochlear	Sensory	Concerned with hearing and equilibrium
Glossopharyngeal nerve	Mixed	
	a. Motor	Innervates skeletal muscles involved in swallowing. Supply secretomotor fibers to parotid gland
	b. Sensory	Carries taste sensation from posterior 1/3rd of the tongue Aids in reflex control of blood pressure and respiration
Vagus nerve	Mixed	
	a. Motor	Innervates the heart and GIT, and skeletal muscles of pharynx and larynx Provide secretomotor fibers to thoracic and abdominal glands
	b. Sensory	Carries information from visceral receptors from thorax and abdomen Participate in reflex control of heart rate, BP and respiration
Accessory nerve	Motor	Innervates sternocleidomastoid and trapezius muscles. Controls movements of head
Hypoglossal nerve	Motor	Innervates muscles of tongue and bring about its movements

11

96. SYNAPSE

Definition

Synapse is a physiological junction between two neurons without anatomical continuation.

Classification

Synapse is classified by two methods:
1. Anatomical classification.
2. Functional classification.

Anatomical Classification

There are three types of synapses:

Axodendritic

It is the synapse between axon of one neuron and dendrite of another neuron.

Axosomatic

It is the synapse between axon of one neuron and soma of another neuron.

Axoaxonic

Here synapse is between two axons.

Functional Classification

Synapses are classified into two types based on the mode of impulse transmission:
1. Chemical synapse
2. Electrical synapse

Chemical Synapse

Almost all the synapses used for signal transmission in CNS are chemical synapses. The first neuron or presynaptic neuron secretes a chemical substance called neurotransmitter. This transmitter acts on receptor proteins in the membrane of the next neuron to excite or inhibit it.

Electrical Synapse

In this type of synapse there are direct open fluid channels that conduct electricity from one cell to the next. Most of these consist of small protein tubular structures called gap junctions that allow free movement of ions from the interior of one cell to the interior of the next.

Physiologic Anatomy of Synapse

Synapse is composed of three major parts:
1. Soma, the main body of the neuron.
2. A single axon, which extends from soma into a peripheral nerve.
3. Dendrites which are branching processes of the soma.

The neuron from which the axon arises is called presynaptic neuron and the neuron on which the axon ends is called postsynaptic neuron.

Presynaptic terminals: About 10,000 to 2,00,000 minute synaptic knobs called presynaptic terminals lie on the surfaces of the dendrites and soma of the neuron. About 80 to 95 percent of them lie on the dendrites and only 5 to 20 percent lie on the soma. These are the ends of nerve fibrils that originate from many other neurons. They resemble small round or oval knobs and hence called as terminal knobs, boutons, end-feet or synaptic knobs (Fig. 11.10a)

The presynaptic terminal is separated from the post- synaptic neuronal soma by a synaptic cleft having a width of 200 to 300 angstroms. There are transmitter vesicles and mitochondria inside the presynaptic terminal. The transmitter vesicles contain the neurotransmitter. The mitochondria provide ATP which supplies the energy for synthesizing new

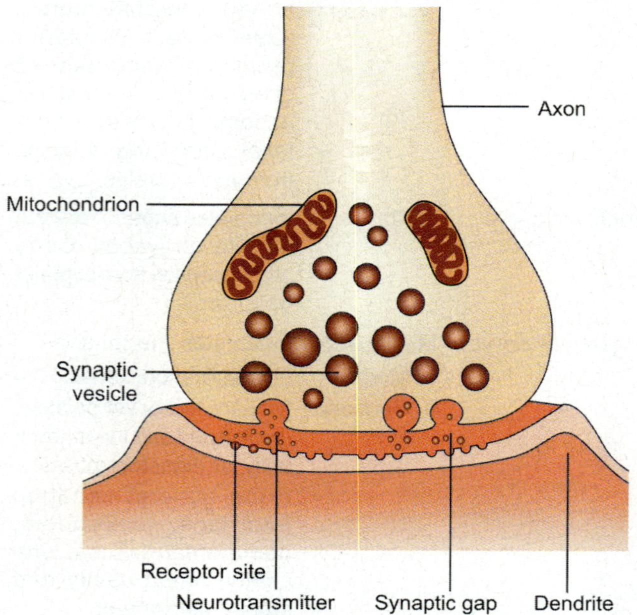

Fig. 11.10a

neurotransmitter. The postsynaptic neuronal membrane has receptor proteins to which the neurotransmitter binds.

Mechanism of Transmission of Impulses at Synapse

The presynaptic membrane contains large numbers of voltage-gated calcium channels. When an action potential depolarizes the presynaptic membrane, these calcium channels open and allow large numbers of calcium ions into the terminal and bind special protein molecules on the inner surface called release sites. This binding causes the release sites to open through the membrane, allowing transmitter vesicles to release the neurotransmitter into the cleft. In case of acetylcholine vesicles about 2000 to 10,000 molecules of acetylcholine are present in each vesicle. The membrane of the postsynaptic neuron contains receptor proteins which have two components:

1. A binding component that protrudes outward.
2. An ionophore component that passes through the membrane into the postsynaptic neuron. The ionophore is of two types:
   i. An ion channel
   ii. A second messenger activator.

Ion Channels

They are of 2 types:

1. Cation channels
   a. Allow mostly sodium ions and also potassium and calcium ions.
   b. Lined with negative charges, so repel anions.
   c. Any transmitter that opens cation channels is called an excitatory transmitter.
2. Anion channels
   a. Allow mainly chloride ions.
   b. Any transmitter that opens anion channels is called an inhibitory transmitter.

Second Messenger System in Postsynaptic Neuron

This system is essential for prolonged postsynaptic neuronal changes as the ionic channels close within milliseconds after the transmitter is no longer present (Fig. 11.10b).

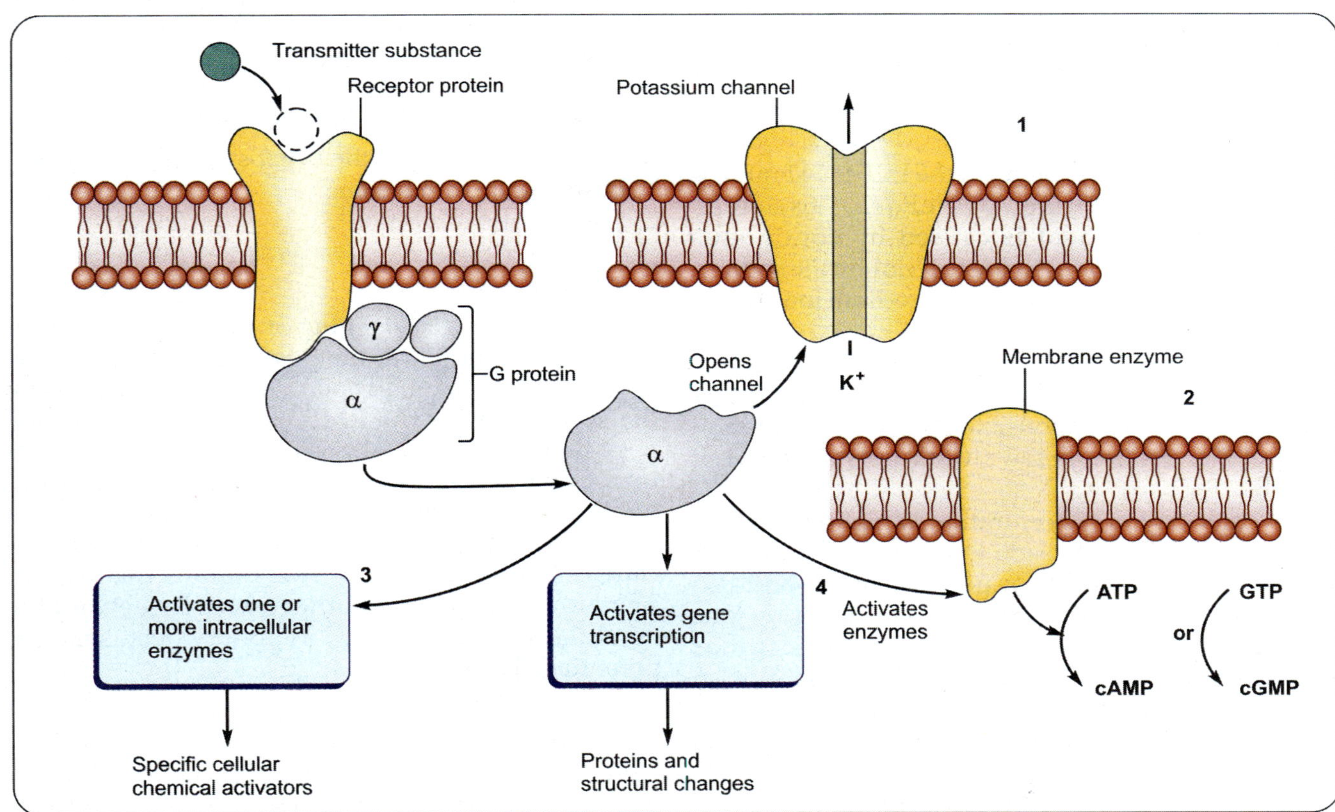

Fig. 11.10b

ACTION OF G PROTEIN

G-proteins are used by the second messenger systems to produce postsynaptic neuronal changes. A G-protein is attached to the portion of the receptor that protrudes into the interior of the cell. It has three components (Fig. 11.10b).

1. Alpha
2. Beta
3. Gamma

On activation by a nerve impulse the alpha portion of the G protein seperates from the beta and gamma portions, moves inside the cell and brings about the following changes:

1. Opening specific ion channels through postsynaptic cell membrane which stay open for a prolonged time
2. Activation of cAMP or cGMP
3. Activation of intracellular enzymes
4. Activation of gene transcription to form new proteins.

Electrical Events during Neuronal Excitation

Resting membrane potential (RMP) of neuronal soma: Consider the soma of a spinal motor neuron which has an RMP of about –65 mV.

Nernst Potential

The sodium ion concentration in the ECF is 142 mEq/L but inside the neuron it is only 14 mEq/L. This sodium concentration gradient is caused by continuous pumping of sodium ions to the exterior by the sodium pump on the somal membrane. So, sodium ion always tries to enter the cell.

The potassium ion concentration is high inside soma (120 mEq/L) but low in ECF (4.5 mEq/L). A potassium pump is responsible for this concentration gradient. So, potassium ion always tries to go out of the cell.

The chloride ion concentration is high in the ECF (107 mEq/L) but low inside the soma (8 mEq/L). A weak chloride pump may be involved in this and also the negative voltage of RMP repels the chloride ions forcing them out of the soma. An intracellular potential that exactly opposes the movement of an ion across the cell membrane is called Nernst potential for that ion. It can be calculated by the following equation:

Nernst potential = ± 61 log [concentration inside/ concentration outside]

Ions	*Nernst potential mV*
Sodium	+61
Potassium	–86
Chloride	–70

Excitatory Postsynaptic Potential (EPSP)

The RMP of the neuronal soma is –65 mV. The presynaptic terminal secretes an excitatory neurotransmitter into the cleft. This transmitter acts on the excitatory receptor to increase the membrane permeability to Na^+. Because of the large concentration and electrical gradient, sodium ions diffuse rapidly into the soma. Now, this increases the RMP in the positive direction from –65 to –45 mV. This positive increase in voltage above the normal RMP is called excitatory postsynaptic potential (EPSP). This can increase further to elicit an action potential in the postsynaptic neuron. This is achieved by simultaneous discharge of many terminals. The action potential originates in the initial segment of the axon because the membrane of this portion of axon has seven times as great a concentration of voltage–gated sodium channels as does the soma. Once the action potential begins, it travels peripherally along the axon but also backward over the soma and dendrites too.

Inhibitory Postsynaptic Potential (IPSP)

Inhibition occurring at the synapse is of two types:

1. Postsynaptic inhibition.
2. Presynaptic inhibition.

Postsynaptic Inhibition

Inhibition occurs by opening of chloride channels or potassium channels at the postsynaptic membrane. When chloride channels open, chloride ions move into the soma making the RMP more negative. When potassium channels open, positively charged potassium ions move to the exterior making the RMP more negative. Thus, both chloride influx and potassium efflux increase the intracellular negativity, which is called hyperpolarization. This inhibits the neuron. Therefore, an increase in the negativity beyond the normal RMP level is called inhibitory post- synaptic potential (IPSP).

Presynaptic Inhibition

Here, inhibition occurs at the presynaptic terminal before the signal ever reaches the synapse. This is caused by release of an inhibitory substance onto the outsides of presynaptic nerve fibrils before their own endings terminate on the postsynaptic neuron. The inhibitory neurotransmitter is gamma-aminobutyric acid (GABA) which opens the anion channels. Chloride influx into the terminal fibril inhibits synaptic transmission by neutralizing the excitatory effect of sodium ions that also enter the terminal fibrils when an action potential arrives.

Presynaptic inhibition occurs in sensory pathways in the nervous system.

Properties of Synapse

1. One Way Conduction

Synapse conducts impulses in one direction only. This is due to the presence of receptors only on the postsynaptic membrane to the neurotransmitters released from presynaptic terminal.

2. Synaptic Delay

- It is the delay that occurs during the transmission of impulses through the synapse. It is due to the time taken for the following:
  - Release of neurotransmitter.
  - Passage of neurotransmitter from axon terminal to postsynaptic membrane.
  - Opening the ion channels.

The normal duration of synaptic delay is 0.5 millisecond.

3. Summation

It is the fusion of effects of stimulation of presynaptic terminals. It is of two types:

1. *Spatial summation:* Occurs when many presynaptic terminals are stimulated simultaneously.
2. *Temporal summation:* Occurs when one presynaptic terminal is stimulated repeatedly.

4. Fatigue

On repeated stimulation of presynaptic terminal, the synapse goes into fatigue due to exhaustion of the neurotransmitter, acetylcholine.

5. Occlusion

This is the decline in the response obtained when two afferent nerves are stimulated together. This is because the presynaptic fibers share the postsynaptic neurons.

6. Facilitation

Sometimes, the summated postsynaptic potential has not risen high enough to reach the threshold for firing by the postsynaptic neuron. When this happens, the neuron is said to be facilitated. That is, its membrane potential is nearer the threshold for firing than normal, but not yet at the firing level. When another excitatory signal enters the neuron, it can excite the neuron very easily.

7. Subliminal Fringe

This means partial state of excitation. Neurons in the sublimal fringe have a few active knobs ending on them. Neurons which have many active knobs ending on them are in the discharge zone.

8. Convergence

Several neurons can converge on one neuron. This is called convergence, e.g. anterior horn cells in gray matter of spinal cord receive impulses from several descending tracts and interneurons (Fig. 11.10c).

9. Divergence

When one neuron connects with several neurons it is called divergence, e.g. reticular activating system sending nerve impulses to many parts of central nervous system for wide spread activation of brain.

10. Synaptic Plasticity

The changes that may occur in synaptic function after repeated stimulation is called plasticity. The effects may be either facilitation or inhibition of conduction and may be of short duration or long duration. This plays an important role in memory. The changes produced are the following.

Post Tetanic Potentiation or Facilitation

If an excitatory presynaptic neuron is stimulated for a short time by a tetanizing current, the synapse becomes a more excitable after cessation of stimulus. This is a short-term effect lasting for a few seconds or a minute. This is due to accumulation of Ca^{++} in the presynaptic endings caused by the tetanizing stimuli. The Ca^{++} facilitates transmission by increasing transmitter release.

Long-term Potentiation (LTP)

This is a prolonged increase in excitability of the synapse following brief tetanic stimulation of pre- synaptic neuron. This is due to Ca^{++} increase in the postsynaptic neuron. Glutamate released from pre- synaptic terminal

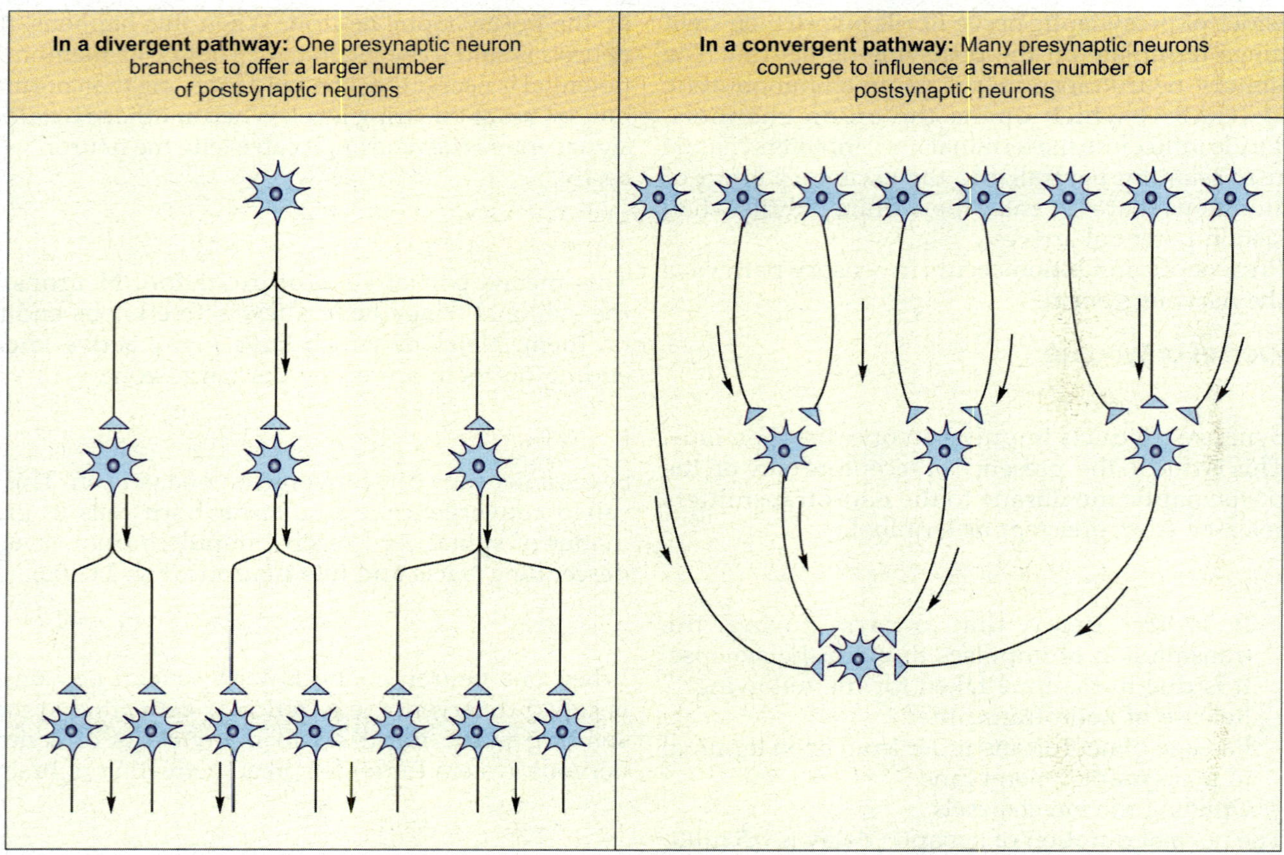

Fig. 11.10c

facilitates entry of Ca^{++} and Na^{++} into the postsynaptic neuron. The retrograde signals from postsynaptic neuron to presynaptic neuron through nitric oxide favors long-term release of glutamate from the presynaptic neuron.

Habituation and Sensitization

Repeated application of a benign stimulus causes the response to disappear. This is called habituation. This is brought about by gradual inactivation of Ca^{++} channels and reduction in the release of a neurotransmitter. When a habituated stimulus is coupled with a noxious stimulus, there is an increase in the postsynaptic response. This is refered to as sensitization. This is due to increased level of cAMP via an increase in Ca^{++} levels in the postsynaptic neuron. The long-term effects result from growth of presynaptic and postsynaptic neurons and increase in their connections.

Inhibition or Depression

Short-term depression may appear with repeated stimulation of inhibitory afferent inputs. Long-term depression (LTD) is just opposite of LTP. This may be due to either partial or total inactivation of the Ca^{++} channels. Nitric oxide appears to cause LTD in cerebellum and LTP in hippocampus.

Importance of Synaptic Plasticity

1. Helps in short-term and long-term memory.
2. Imparts individuality in learning, memory and other behavior.
3. Forms the basis for elimination of unwanted matter.

97. NEUROTRANSMITTERS

Definition

Neurotransmitter is a chemical substance that acts as a mediator for the transmission of nerve impulse from one neuron to another through synapse.

Amino Acids

The neurotransmitters of this group are involved in fast synaptic transmission. Glutamate, Aspartate, Glycine and GABA belong to this group.

Amines

These are modified amino acids. Noradrenaline, adrenaline, serotonin and histamine belong to this group.

Others

Acetylcholine is formed from choline and acetyl CoA in the presence of the enzyme choline acetyl transferase. Nitric oxide also belongs to this group.

Based on the Function

Neurotransmitters are classified into two types based on the function:

1. Excitatory neurotransmitters
2. Inhibitory neurotransmitters.

Excitatory Neurotransmitters

These neurotransmitters, after released from presynaptic terminal, produce EPSP in the post-synaptic neuron by opening sodium channels, e.g. acetylcholine, noradrenaline.

Inhibitory Neurotransmitters

These substances inhibit the conduction of impulse from presynaptic neuron to postsynaptic neuron by opening potassium channel causing potassium efflux or by opening chloride channels causing chloride influx, e.g. GABA, dopamine.

Based on the Molecular Size

- Small molecule, rapidly acting neurotransmitters
- Neuropeptides

Small Molecule, Rapidly Acting Neurotransmitters

- Rapidly acting neurotransmitters
- Cause most acute responses of the nervous system like transmission of sensory signals to the brain and of motor signals back to the muscles.
- Synthesized in the cytosol of presynaptic terminals.

Classified into Four Classes

Class	*Neurotransmitters*
I	Acetylcholine
II	The amines Norepinephrine, epinehrine, dopamine, serotonin, histamine
III	Aminoacids GABA, glycine, glutamate, aspartate
IV	Nitric oxide

Neuropeptides

- Slow in action
- Synthesized by ribosomes in the neuronal cell body by a laborious method
- More potent than small molecule transmitters
- Cause prolonged actions, lasting for even months or years; examples are as follows.

Hypothalamic Releasing Hormones

- TRH
- LHRH
- Somatostatin

Pituitary Peptides

- ACTH
- Beta endorphin
- Alpha MSH
- Prolactin
- LH
- Thyrotropin
- GH
- Vasopressin
- Oxytocin

Peptides that Act on Gut and Brain

- Leucin
- Methionine enkephalin

- Substance P
- Gastrin
- Cholecystokinin
- VIP
- Nerve growth factor
- Brain derived neurotropic factor
- Neurotensin
- Insulin
- Glucagon

From other Tissues

- Bradykinin
- Carnosine
- Sleep peptides
- Calcitonin

Fate of Neurotransmitters

The neurotransmitter is produced in the cell body of the neuron and transported through the axon. It is stored in vesicles in the axon terminal. It is released into the synaptic cleft when a stimulus arrives. Once released it can undergo any of the following:

1. It may bind to the specific receptors on the surface of the postsynaptic neuron
2. It may be destroyed by enzymes
3. It may be removed by means of reuptake into the axon terminal.

Name	*Site of secretion*	*Action*
GABA	Cerebral cortex, cerebellum, basal ganglia, spinal cord, retina	Inhibitory
Glycine	Spinal cord, retina	Inhibitory
Glutamate	Cerebral cortex, cerebellum, sensory pathway	Excitatory
Aspartate	Spinal cord, cerebellum, retina	Excitatory
Noradrenaline	Brainstem, hypothalamus, locus ceruleus, spinal cord, basal ganglia, postganglionic sympathetic nerve endings	Excitatory and inhibitory
Adrenaline	Hypothalamus, spinal cord, thalamus	Excitatory and inhibitory
Dopamine	Basal ganglia, hypothalamus, limbic system, retina, sympathetic ganglia	Inhibitory
Serotonin	Hypothalamus, limbic system, cerebellum, spinal cord, retina, lungs, platelets	Inhibitory
Histamine	Hypothalamus, cerebral cortex, GIT and mast cells	Excitatory
Nitric oxide	GIT, NMJ many parts of CNS	Excitatory
Acetylcholine	Parasympathetic postganglionic nerve endings, NMJ, hypothalamus, basal ganglia, thalamus, hippocampus, retina	Excitatory

11

98. REFLEX ACTION

Definition

Reflex action is the involuntary response resulting from stimulation of a receptor. For example: Withdrawal of the hand when placed on a hot object.

Reflex Arc (Fig. 11.11)

Reflex arc is the anatomical nervous pathway for a reflex action. A simple reflex arc consists of five components:

1. *Receptor or sense organ:* It is the peripheral part of the afferent neuron that responds to a stimulus.
2. *Afferent nerve:* Afferent or sensory nerve transmits sensory impulses from the receptor to the center.
3. *Center:* This is the junction between afferent and efferent neurons. It is located either in the spinal cord or brain.
4. *Efferent nerve:* Efferent or motor nerve transmits motor impulses from the center to the effector organ.
5. *Effector organ:* It can be a muscle or a gland where the activity occurs in response to the stimulus.

CLASSIFICATION OF REFLEXES

Reflexes are classified by five methods:

1. Anatomical classification
2. Based on the number of synapses involved
3. Functional classification
4. Whether inborn or acquired.
5. Clinical classification

Anatomical Classification

This is based on the region of the spinal cord involved.

Segmental Reflexes

These reflexes are those whose arcs pass through only one anatomical segment, e.g. knee jerk.

Intersegmental Reflexes

These reflexes involve more than one segment, e.g. withdrawal reflex.

Suprasegmental Reflexes

These reflexes involve interactions between the nuclei above the spinal cord and the segments of the spinal cord itself.

Based on the Number of Synapses

Monosynaptic reflexes: Have only one synapse in the reflex arc, e.g. stretch reflex.

Polysynaptic reflexes: Involve more than one synapse in the reflex arc, e.g. flexor reflexes.

Functional Classification

- Flexor reflexes
- Extensor reflexes

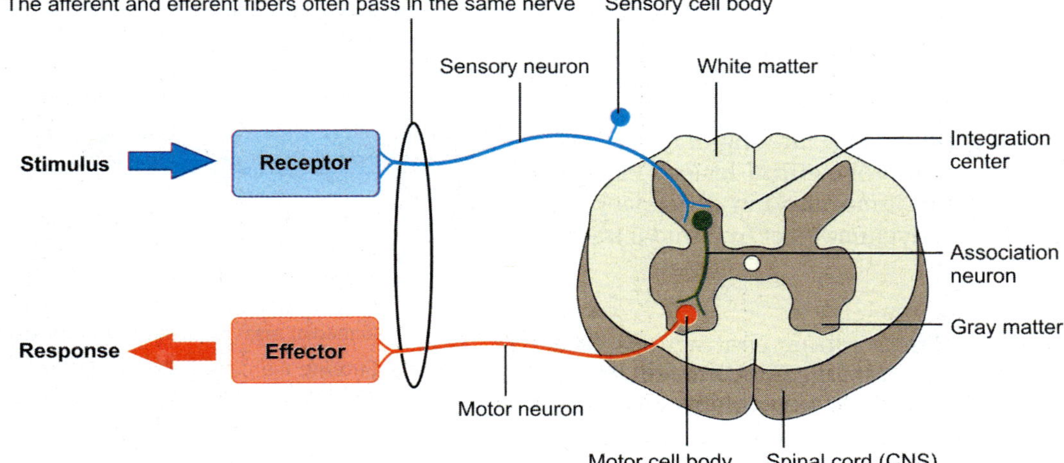

Fig. 11.11

- Righting reflexes
- Postural reflexes

Whether Inborn or Acquired

Unconditioned Reflexes

- Present since the time of birth
- Do not require previous learning, e.g. secretion of saliva when food is placed in the mouth.

Conditioned Reflexes

- Develop after training
- Secretion of saliva by the thought, smell or sight of a known food.

Clinical Classification

The reflexes are classified into four types:

1. *Superficial reflexes:* These reflexes can be obtained by stimulating the skin or mucous membrane.
2. *Deep reflexes:* These reflexes can be elicited by stimulating deep structures like tendon. They are also known as tendon reflexes.
3. *Visceral reflexes:* These are the reflexes arising from the viscera, e.g. baroreceptor and chemoreceptor reflex.
4. *Pathological reflexes:* They are elicited only in pathological condition. Three pathological reflexes are well known:
   1. Babinski sign
   2. Clonus
   3. Pendular movements

Babinski Sign

This is an abnormal plantar reflex first described by Joseph Babinski. In the normal plantar reflex, a gentle stroke over the sole of the foot causes plantar flexion and adduction of all toes. But in Babinski's sign, there is dorsiflexion of great toe and fanning of other toes. This is seen in upper motor neuron lesion. Physiologically, it is present in infants and in deep sleep. In infants, it is due to nonmyelination of pyramidal tracts.

Clonus

It is a series of regular rhythmic contractions of a muscle subjected to sudden maintained stretch. When deep reflex is elicited in a normal person the contractions of the muscle are smooth and continuous. But clonus occurs when the deep reflexes are exaggerated due to hypertonicity of muscles in pyramidal tract lesion. Clonus is seen in calf muscles producing ankle clonus and quadriceps producing patellar clonus.

Patellar Clonus

It is the rhythmic regular movements of the patella produced by grasping it between the thumb and index finger of the examiner and pushing it down forcibly towards the foot. It is caused by clonic contractions of quadriceps muscle.

Ankle Clonus

It is the rhythmic contractions of calf muscles on sudden dorsiflexion of foot and sustaining it.

Pendular Movements

These are slow oscillatory movements like a pendulum that are seen while eliciting a tendon jerk. A tap on the patellar tendon where the leg is hanging freely causes a brisk extension of the leg due to the contraction of the quadriceps muscle in knee jerk. Normally, the leg returns back to the resting position immediately. In cerebellar lesion the leg swings forwards and backwards several times before coming to rest. This is due to the hypotonia of the muscles caused by cerebellar lesion.

Superficial reflexes

Reflex	*Stimulus*	*Response*	*Center*
Corneal	Touching the cornea with a wisp of cotton wool	Closure of the eyelids	5th and 7th nerve nuclei in pons
Conjunctival	Touching the conjunctiva with a wisp of cotton wool	Closure of the eyelids	5th and 7th nerve nuclei in pons
Anal	Stroking skin near anus	Contraction of anal sphincter	S3 and S4
Cremastric	Stroking the inner side of the thigh	Drawing up of testicles	L1 and L2
Abdominal			
Upper	Stroking the abdominal wall below, the costal margin from lateral to medial side	Contraction of abdominal muscles, movement of umbilicus towards the site of stroke	T8–T10
Lower	Stroking the abdominal wall at umbilical and iliac level	Contraction of lower abdominal wall	T10 and T12

Contd.

Superficial reflexes *(Contd.)*			
Reflex	*Stimulus*	*Response*	*Center*
Plantar	Stroking the sole of the foot on the lateral side from heel to toes	Plantar flexion of toes and adduction	L5 and S1
Pupillary	Flashing light into the eye	Constriction of the pupil	3rd nerve nucleus

Deep reflexes			
Reflex	*Stimulus*	*Response*	*Center*
Biceps jerk	Tapping the biceps tendon in the front of elbow	Flexion of forearm, contraction of biceps	C5, C6
Triceps jerk	Tapping the triceps tendon above olecranon process	Extension of elbow due to contraction of triceps	C6, C7
Supinator jerk	Tapping the tendon over the styloid process	Flexion of elbow (Contraction of supinator and flexors of the elbow)	C5, C6
Jaw jerk	Striking the chin with the mouth slightly open	Closure of the mouth by contraction of the masseter	V nerve and pons
Knee jerk	Tapping the patellar tendon	Forward extension of leg	L2, L3, L4
Ankle jerk	Tapping the tendo achilles	Plantar flexion of the foot due to contraction of the calf muscles	S1, S2

Properties of Reflexes

1. One Way Conduction

During any reflex activity the impulses are transmitted in only one direction, i.e. towards the center in afferent nerve and away from the center in the efferent nerve.

2. Delay (Reaction Time)

This is the time interval between application of stimulus and the onset of reflex.

3. Summation

It is of two types:

Spatial Summation

When subthreshold stimulus is applied, no response is obtained but it produces a local EPSP. When sub threshold stimuli are applied at several points simultaneously, then a response is obtained. This is called spatial summation.

Temporal Summation

When one nerve fiber is stimulated repeatedly with subliminal stimuli, these stimuli are summed up to give response in the muscle. It is called temporal summation.

4. Occlusion

This is the decline in the response obtained when two afferent nerves are stimulated together.

5. Subliminal Fringe

The reflex response that is obtained by stimulating two afferent nerves together is more than the response obtained when they are stimulated separately

6. Recruitment

The reflex response can be obtained by applying a threshold stimulus to an afferent fiber and by increasing the strength of the stimulus, the magnitude of response can be increased. This is called recruitment and is due to activation of more number of motor units.

7. After Discharge

This is the persistence or continuation of response for some more time even after the cessation of the stimulus. This is due to the discharge of the impulses through the reverberatory circuits.

8. Rebound Phenomenon

A reflex response becomes more forceful when the inhibition is suddenly removed. This is called rebound phenomenon.

9. Fatigue

On continued stimulation the reflex response obtained gradually gets lessened. This type of failure to give response to a stimulus is called fatigue. Synapse is the seat of fatigue.

10. Reciprocal Innervation and Reciprocal Inhibition

Reciprocal Inhibition (Figs 11.12a and b)

Usually, excitation of one group of muscles is associated with inhibition of another, i.e. antagonist group of muscles to bring about a smooth motor act, e.g. when a flexor reflex is elicited, flexor muscles are excited and the extensor muscles are inhibited on that side. This is called reciprocal inhibition.

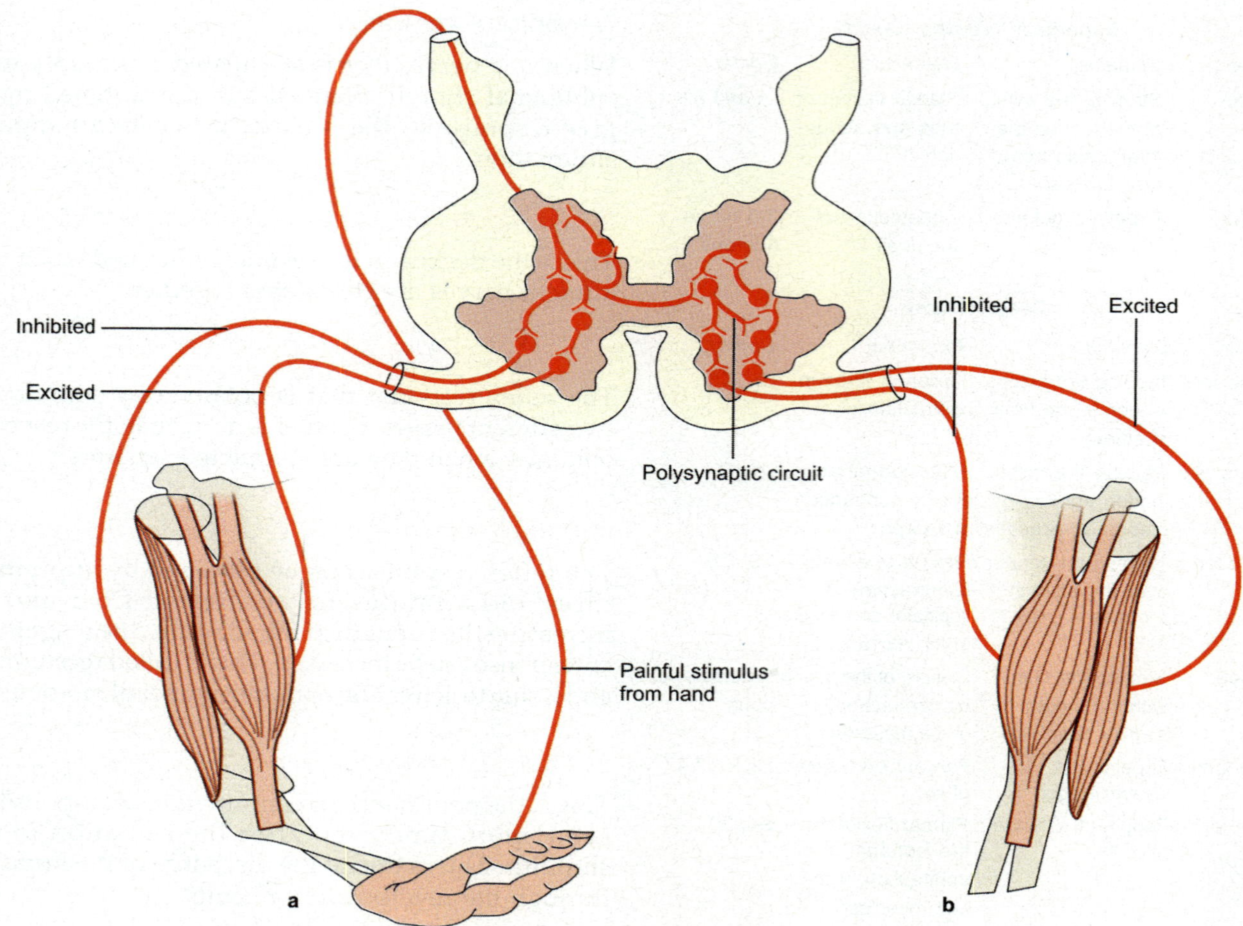

Figs 11.12a and b: (a) Flexor reflex; (b) crossed extensor reflex

Reciprocal Innervation

Reciprocal inhibition occurs because of reciprocal innervation. This mechanism was explained by Sherrington.

Hence, it is called Sherrington law of reciprocal innervation. According to this, the afferent nerve fibers which produce a flexor reflex in a limb have connections with motor neurons supplying not only the flexors but also the extensors. When they excite the motor neurons supplying the flexors, the motor neurons supplying the extensors are inhibited simultaneously. The inhibition is brought about through inhibitory internuncial neurons. This is referred to as reciprocal innervations.

99. RECEPTORS

Definition

Receptors are specialized afferent nerve endings which produce a nerve impulse in response to an adequate stimulus. They act as transducers that convert various forms of energy in to electrical energy.

Classification

Receptors are of two types:
1. Exteroceptors
2. Interoceptors.

Exteroceptors

- Respond to stimuli from external environment.
- It is divided into three types.

a. *Cutaneous Receptors* (Fig. 11.13)

- Receptors located in the skin.
- Also called as mechanoreceptors as they respond to mechanical stimuli like touch, pressure, etc.

Cutaneous receptors	
Sensory modality	*Receptor*
• Touch	Meissner's corpuscles and Merkel's disc
• Pressure	Pacinian corpuscle
• Warmth	Ruffini's end organ
• Cold	Krause's end bulb
• Pain	Free nerve endings (nociceptor)

b. *Chemoreceptors*

1. Respond to chemical stimuli like taste and smell.
   - Taste : Taste buds
   - Smell : Olfactory receptors

c. *Telereceptors*

1. Excited by stimuli—vision and hearing.
   - Vision : Rods and cones
   - Hearing : Hair cells in organ of Corti.

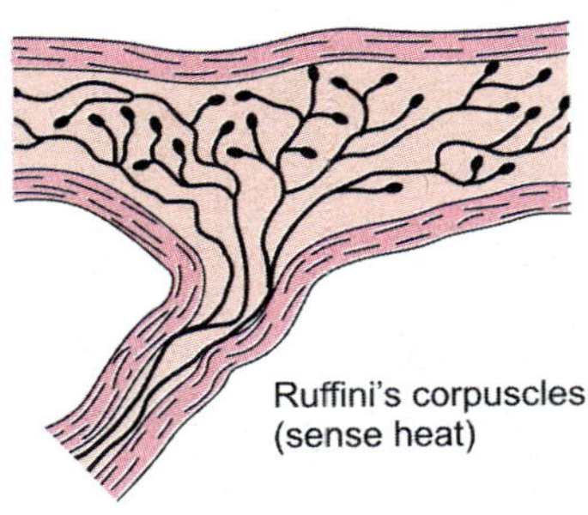

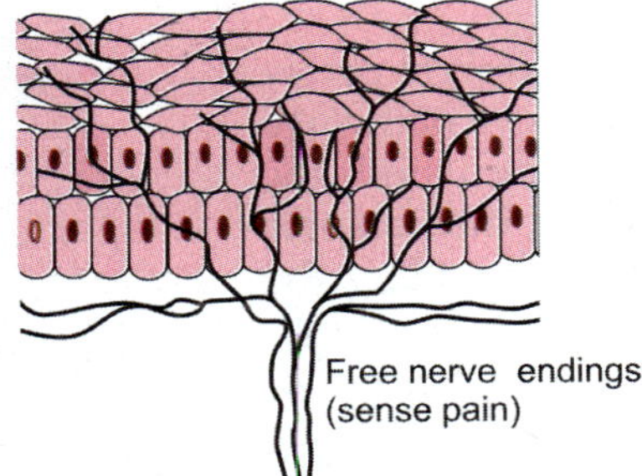

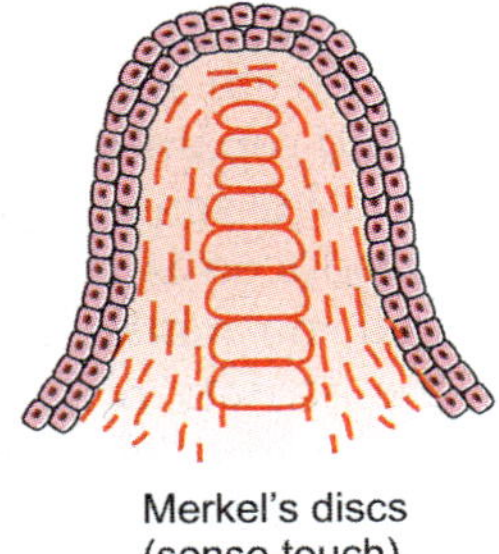

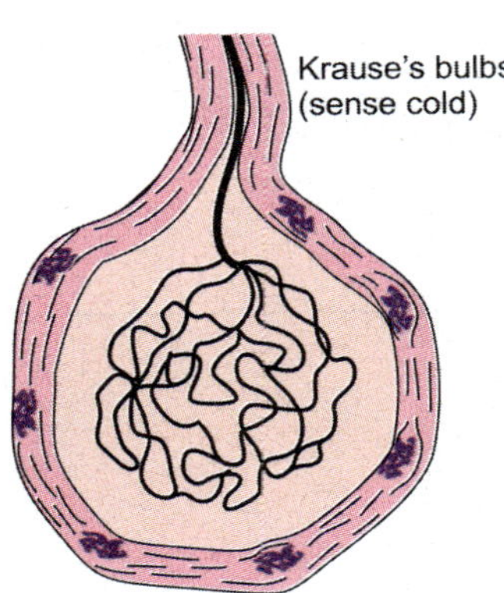

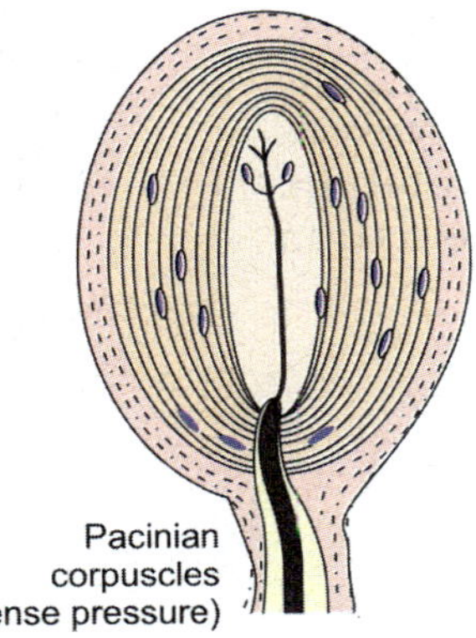

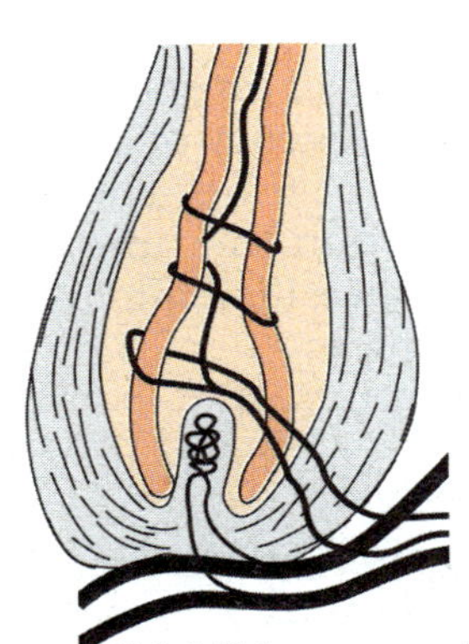

Fig. 11.13

11

Interoceptors

- Excited by stimuli arising within the body.
- Interoceptors are of 2 types.
  a. Visceroceptors.
  b. Proprioceptors.

Visceroceptors: Situated in the viscera	
Receptors	*Location*
Stretch receptors	Alveoli of lungs, heart
Chemoreceptors	Aortic and carotid bodies
Baroreceptors	Carotid sinus and aortic arch
Osmoreceptors	Hypothalamus

Proprioceptors: Respond to changes in position of different parts of the body	
Receptors	*Location*
Muscle spindle	Muscle
Golgi tendon organ	Tendon

Properties of Receptors

1. Specificity of Response (Müller's Law)

- Refers to the response given by a particular type of receptor to a specific sensation.
- For example, pain receptors respond only to pain sensation.
- The pathways from sense organs to cerebral cortex are specific and separate. When the nerve pathways from a particular sense organ are stimulated, the sensation produced is that for which the receptor is specialized, no matter how or where along the pathway the activity originates. This was established by Müller and is called Müller's doctrine of specific nerve energies. The specificity of nerve fibers for transmitting only one modality of sensation is called the labeled live principle.

2. Adaptation

When a stimulus of constant strength is applied to the receptor the frequency of action potential decreases over a period of time. This is called adaptation. Depending upon the time taken for adaptation receptors are classified into two types:

- Tonic receptors
- Phasic receptors.

11

Tonic Receptors

- Slowly adapting receptors.
- For example, muscle spindle, Golgi tendon organ, pain receptors, baroreceptors, chemoreceptors, receptors of the macula in vestibular apparatus.

Phasic Receptors

- Adapt rapidly
- Also called as movement receptors or rate receptors as they react strongly while a change is actually taking place
- For example, pacinian corpuscle.

Mechanism of Adaptation (Fig. 11.14)

This can be explained in Pacinian corpuscle in which extensive studies have been made. Adaptation occurs in two ways:

1. Pacinian corpuscle is a viscoelastic structure. When a distorting force is suddenly applied to one side of the corpuscle, this force is instantly transmitted by the viscous component of the corpuscle directly to the same side of the central nerve fiber, this producing a receptor potential. However, with a few hundredth of a second, the fluid within the corpuscle redistributes, so that the receptor potential is no longer elicited. Thus, the receptor potential appears at the beginning of the compression but

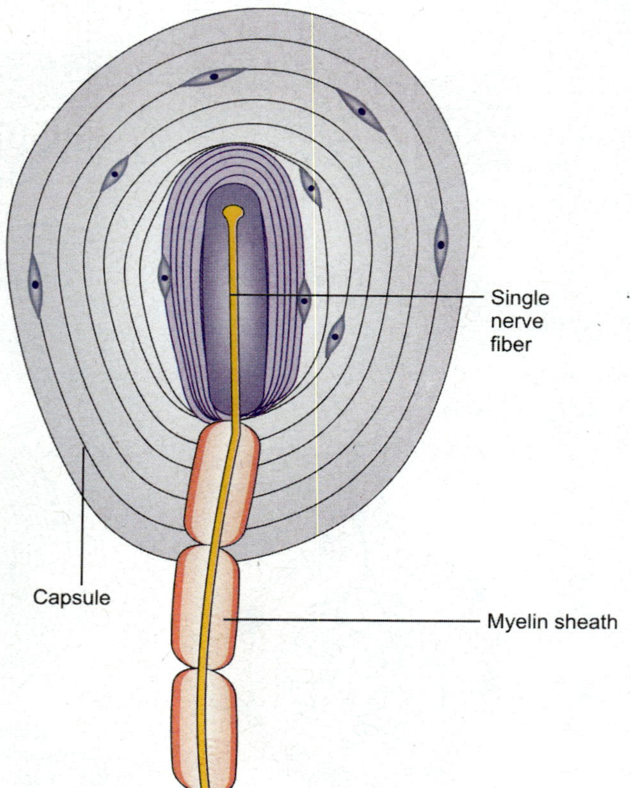

Fig. 11.14: Pacinian corpuscle

disappears within a fraction of second even though the compression continues.

2. The second mechanism of adaptation occurs from a process called accommodation which occurs in the nerve fiber itself. That is, even if the central core fiber continues to be distorted, the tip of the fiber gradually becomes accommodated to the stimulus. This results from the progressive inactivation of sodium channel in the nerve fiber membrane.
3. *Law of projection:* No matter where a particular sensory pathway is stimulated along its course to the cortex, the conscious sensation produced is referred to the location of the receptor. This is called the law of projection.

   Phantom limb: A person whose limb is amputated often complains of pain in the limb which is not present. This phenomenon of pain in an absent limb is referred to as phantom limb and the pain is called phantom pain. This pain is due to the irritation of the damaged nociceptive and proprioceptive afferents at the amputated stump. This generates impulses in nerve fibers that previously came from the receptors in the removed limb and the sensations produced are projected to where the receptors used to be located.
4. Intensity discrimination

   Weber-Fechner law: The magnitude of sensation felt is proportionate to the log of the intensity of the stimulus.
5. *Receptor potential:* This is the nonpropagated transmembrane potential difference that occurs in a receptor when stimulated. It is also called as generator potential. It is not action potential and it does not obey all-or-none law.

Mechanism of Development of Receptor Potential (Fig. 11.15)

Pacinian corpuscles have been extensively used to study the receptor potential because of their large size and accessibility in the mesentery of experimental animals.

Each capsule consists of a straight, unmyelinated ending of a sensory nerve fiber, surrounded by concentric lamellas of connective tissue. When pressure is applied, pacinian corpuscle is compressed. This compression causes change in shape of corpuscle which opens the sodium channel. Sodium ions enter the interior of the core fiber leading to depolarizing potential.

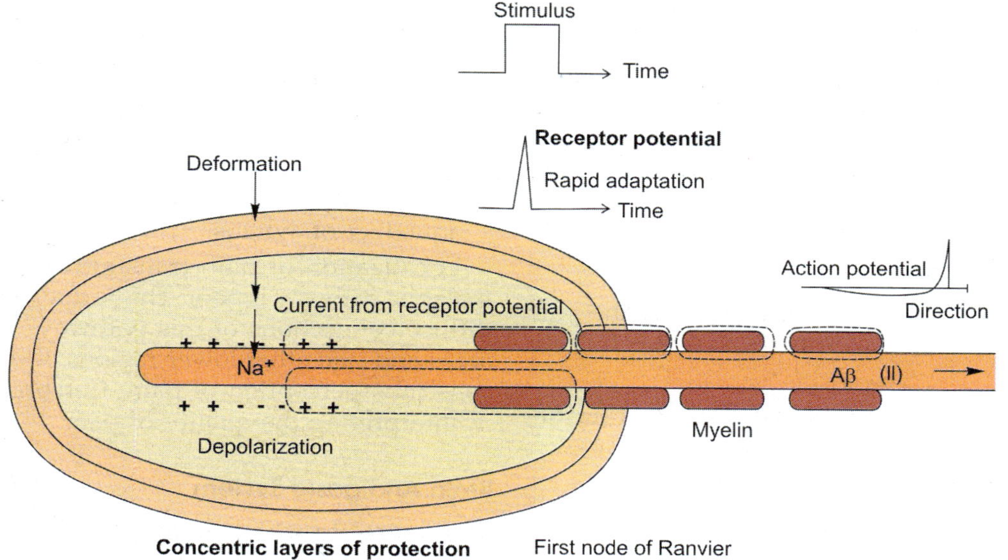

Fig. 11.15: Pacinian vibration detector

11

100. PHYSIOLOGY OF PAIN

Pain is defined as an unpleasant sensation. It is protective in nature as it causes the individual to react to remove the pain stimulus.

Types of Pain

There are two types of pain:

1. Fast pain
2. Slow pain

Fast Pain

- It is felt within about 0.1 second after a pain stimulus is applied.
- It is also known as sharp pain, pricking pain, acute pain and enteric pain. It is felt when a needle is struck into the skin, cut with knife, etc.

Slow Pain

It begins only after 1 sec or more and then increases over many seconds to minutes. It is also known as slow burning pain, aching pain, throbbing pain and chronic pain.

PAIN RECEPTORS

The pain receptors are free nerve endings. They are widely distributed in superficial layer of skin and internal tissues like periosteum, arterial walls, joint surfaces and the falx and tentorium in the cranial vault.

Types of Pain Stimuli

There are three types of stimuli that excite the pain receptors:

1. Mechanical
2. Chemical: Bradykinin, serotonin, histamine, substance P
3. Thermal

Tissue ischemia, muscle spasm and tissue damage can also produce pain.

11

Dual Pathways for Pain Transmission

There are two pathways to transmit two types of pain:

1. Fast pain pathway
2. Slow pain pathway

Fast Pain Pathway (Neospinothalamic Tract)

Type A δ pain fibers transmit mainly mechanical and acute thermal pain. They terminate in lamina I (Lamina marginalis) of the dorsal horns and excite second order neurons. They give rise to long fibers that cross immediately to the opposite side in the spinal cord through the anterior commissure and then ascend to the brain in the antrolateral column. A few fibers terminate in the reticular formation of brainstem. But most of the fibers go to thalamus terminating in basal complex along with tract of Goll and Burdach.

Glutamate which is an excitatory neurotransmitter is secreted in the spinal cord by nerve fibers of this pathway. The fast pain can be localized more accurately in different parts of the body.

Slow Pain Pathway (Paleospinothalamic Pathway)

This is a much older system which transmits pain from the type C pain fibers. These fibers terminate in lamina II and III of dorsal horns which together are called substantia gelatinosa. The fibers cross to the opposite side and ascend in the anterolateral pathway. Substance P is the neurotransmitter released by these fibers. Only a few fibers terminate in the thalamus. Most of the fibers go to the following areas:

1. The reticular nuclei of the brainstem
2. Tectum of the midbrain
3. The periaqueductal gray region surrounding the aqueduct of sylvius.

Localization of pain transmitted by paleospinothalamic pathway is poor. This is due to multisynaptic diffuse connections of this pathway. The brainstem areas and the other lower regions of the brain cause conscious perception of pain. Cerebral cortex helps in interpreting the quality of pain.

Brain Analgesia System

The degree to which a person reacts to pain varies enormously. This is because the brain has an endogenous pain control system called analgesia system.

Analgesic Pathway (Fig. 11.16)

This consists of descending fibers. The fibers arise from frontal lobe of cerebral cortex and

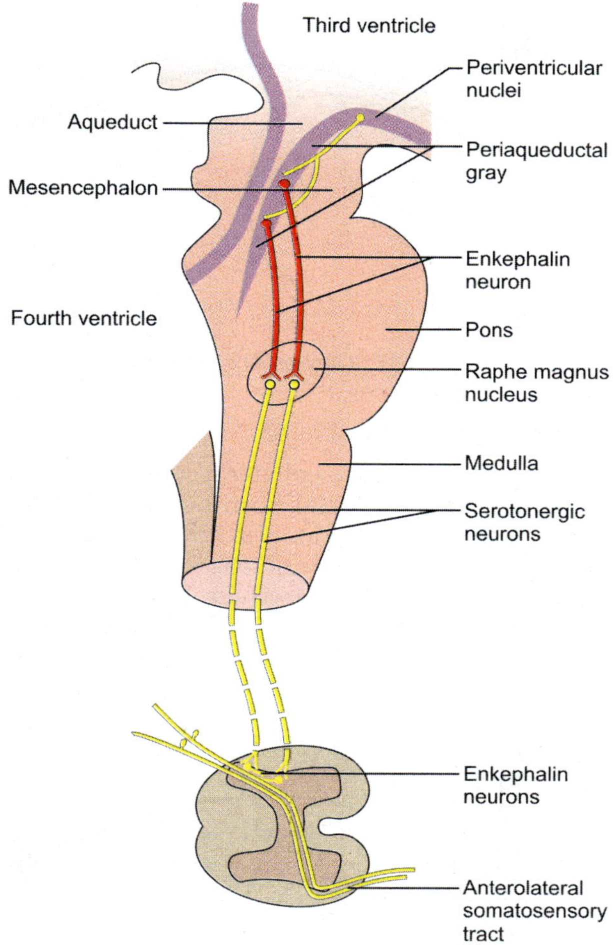

Fig. 11.16: Analgesic pathway

hypothalamus. They terminate in periaqueductal gray and periventricular areas of the midbrain and pons surrounding aqueduct of sylvius and portions of third and fourth ventricles. The fibers from here descend to raphemagnus nucleus and nucleus reticularis paragigantocellularis in the pons and medulla. The fibers from here descend through lateral white column of the spinal cord and synapse in a pain inhibitory complex located in the dorsal horn of the spinal cord. At this point the analgesia signals can block the pain before it is relayed to the brain.

Neurotransmitter of Analgesia Pathway

The neurotransmitters released by the fibers of analgesic pathway are serotonin and opiate receptor substances namely enkephalin and endorphin.

Gate Control Theory

This was postulated by Melzack and Waller in 1965. According to this theory the pain stimuli transmitted by afferent pain fibers are blocked by the gate mechanism located at the posterior gray horn of spinal cord.

Mechanism

When pain receptor is stimulated the touch receptors are also stimulated simultaneously.

When all these impulses reach the spinal cord through the posterior nerve roots, the large A δ fibers increase the substantia gelatinosa activities and block the impulse transmission from the C fibers to the spinothalamic tract. The effect may be by presynaptic inhibition.

The enkephalins released by the brain analgesic fibers cause presynaptic and postsynaptic inhibition of the synapses of A δ and C fibers in the posterior horn. This inhibition is effective for several minutes and even hours.

Visceral Pain

Normally, the viscera are insensitive to various forms of stimuli. For instance the intestine can be cut, torn or pinched without any sensation. But when there is an inflammation of the viscera it can produce diffuse pain. It is poorly localized.

Causes for Visceral Pain

1. Ischemia
2. Overdistension of a hollow viscus like urinary bladder, gall bladder, etc.
3. Obstruction in a hollow viscus-like intestine
4. Spasm of hollow viscus or duct
5. Chemical stimuli: Ruptured gastric or duodenal ulcer causes leakage of proteolytic acid contents into the peritoneal cavity causing chemical damage and severe pain.

Insensitive Viscera

A few visceral areas are almost completely insensitive to pain. They include parenchyma of the liver and the alveoli of the lungs.

Referred Pain

Irritation or inflammation of a viscus produces pain which is felt not in the viscus but in some somatic structure away from it. This is called referred pain.

Examples:
1. Referral of cardiac pain to the inner aspect of the left arm.
2. Pain in the tip of the shoulder caused by irritation of the central portion of the diaphragm.
3. Pain in the testicle due to distension of the ureter.
4. Inflamed appendix: Pain at the umbilicus.

Mechanism of Referred Pain

Dermatomal Rule

According to dermatomal rule, pain is referred to a structure that developed from the same embryonic segment or dermatome from which the pain producing structure is developed. For example, during embryonic development, the diaphragm migrates from the neck region to its adult location between the chest and the abdomen and takes its nerve supply, the phrenic nerve, with it. Phrenic nerve enters the spinal cord at the same level where the afferent from the tip of shoulder enter. Similarly, the heart and the arm have the same segmental origin.

Convergence Theory (Fig. 11.17)

According to this theory, somatic and visceral afferents converge on the spinothalamic neurons in the spinal cord. Since, somatic pain is much more common than visceral pain, the brain has learned that activity arriving in a given pathway is caused by a pain stimulus in a particular somatic area. When the same pathway is stimulated by activity in visceral efferents, the signal reaching the brain is no different and the pain is projected to the somatic area.

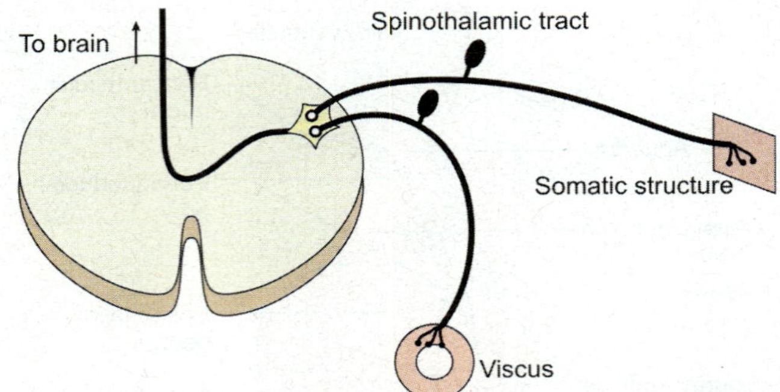

Fig. 11.17: Convergence theory

Facilitation Theory (Fig. 11.18)

According to this theory, collateral connections from visceral afferents to dorsal horn neurons receiving pain impulses from somatic structures could provide a pathway by which the increased activity in the visceral afferents could produce EPSPs and thus increase the excitability of the neurons from somatic structures. Minor activity in somatic afferents could cause continuous pain.

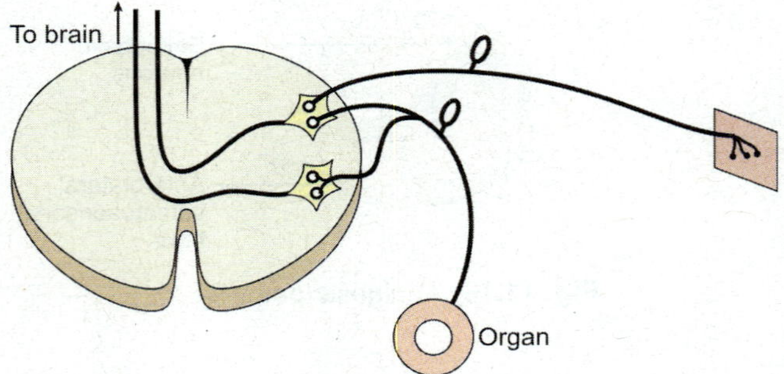

Fig. 11.18: Facilitation theory

101. THE SPINAL CORD

The spinal cord is the downward continuation of medulla oblongata. It is about 45 cm long and extends from C_1 to the lower end of L_1.

Coverings

1. Dura mater
2. Arachnoid membrane
3. Pia mater.

The coverings of brain also continue in spinal cord. Below L_1, the spinal cord rapidly narrows to a cone shape termination called conus medullaris. A slender non-nervous filament called filum terminale extends from conus medullaris downwards up to the level of S_2.

Segments of Spinal Cord (Fig. 11.19)

Spinal cord is made up of 31 segments

Cervical segments	=	8
Thoracic segments	=	12
Lumbar segments	=	5
Sacral segments	=	5
Coccygeal segment	=	1

Spinal Nerves

The segments of spinal cord correspond to 31 pairs of spinal nerves

Cervical spinal nerves	=	8
Thoracic spinal nerves	=	12
Lumbar spinal nerves	=	5
Sacral spinal nerves	=	5
Coccygeal spinal nerve	=	1

Nerve Roots

Each spinal nerve is formed by anterior (ventral) root and posterior (dorsal) root. Both roots on either side leave the spinal cord and pass through the corresponding intervertebral foramina. The first cervical spinal nerve passes through the foramen between occipital bone and 1st vertebra called atlas.

Bell-Magendie Law

Dorsal roots are sensory and ventral roots are motor.

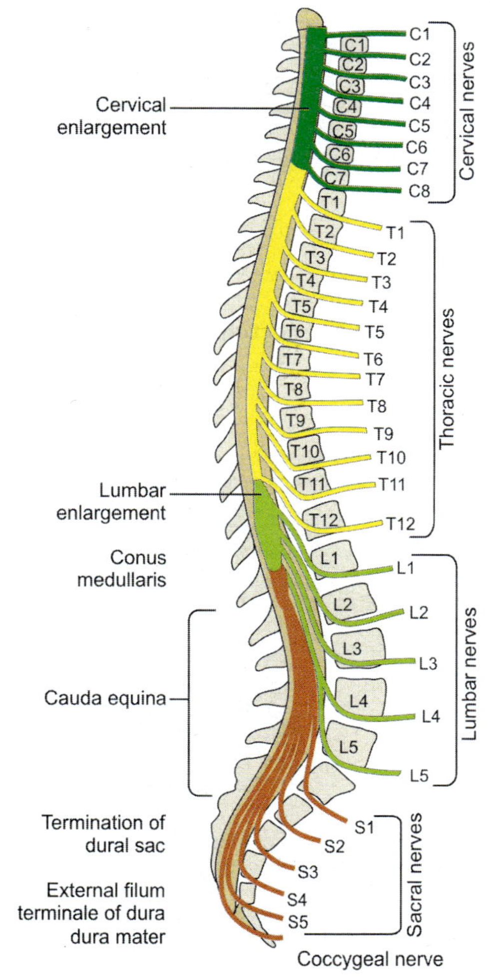

Fig. 11.19: Segments of spinal cord and spinal nerves

Structure of Spinal Cord (Fig. 11.20)

The spinal cord is incompletely divided into two lateral halves by posterior median septum and the anterior median sulcus (fissure). It has central gray matter surrounded by white matter. The gray matter is 'H' shaped in the center of which lies the central canal filled with CSF. The lateral halves are connected by anterior and posterior gray commissures.

Gray Matter of Spinal Cord (Fig. 11.21)

Gray matter of spinal cord is a collection of nerve cells.

Each half of gray matter has:

1. Anterior horn (ventral)

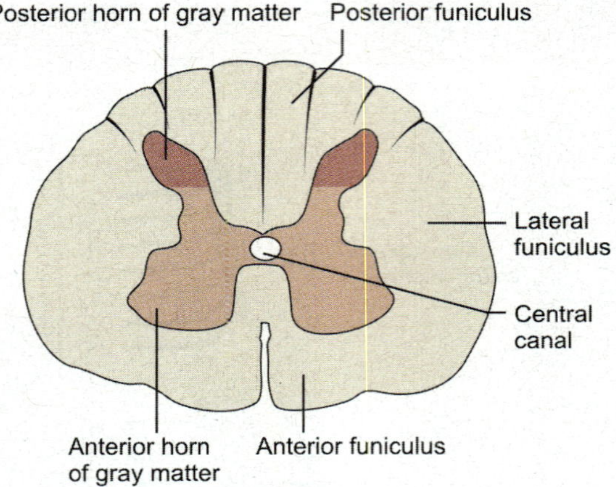

Fig. 11.20: Section of spinal cord

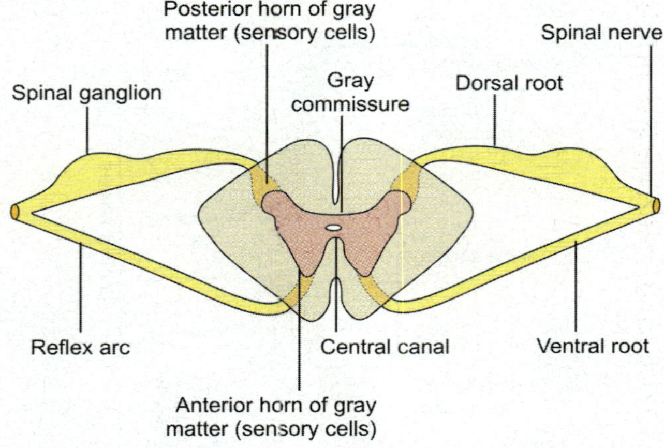

Fig. 11.21: Cross-section of the spinal cord

2. Lateral horn
3. Posterior horn (dorsal)

Gray matter has two types of multipolar neurons:

1. Golgi type I neurons
2. Golgi type II neurons

11

Golgi Type I Neurons

They are found in anterior horn and have long axons which form long tracts in spinal cord.

Golgi Type II Neurons

These neurons have short axons and are found in posterior horns. They form intersegmental connections.

Nuclei in Gray Matter

1. *Nuclei in Posterior Gray Horn*

The posterior horn contains the nuclei of sensory neurons which receive impulses from receptors. There are four types of sensory neurons:

a. Marginal nucleus
   Found in the tip of posterior gray horn in all levels of spinal cord.
b. Substantia gelatinosa of Rolando
   Found at the apex of posterior gray horn in all levels of spinal cord.
c. Chief sensory nucleus
   Located ventral to substantia gelatinosa.
d. Clarke's column
   - Oldest neurons in the spinal cord
   - Occupies basal portion of posterior horn
   - Found in segments from C8 to L3 only.

2. *Nuclei in the Lateral Gray Horn*

- These neurons are called intermediate lateral column of cells. They give rise to sympathetic preganglionic fibers.
- Present in segments from T1 to L2.

3. *Nuclei in Anterior Gray Horn*

Contain lower motor neurons. They are of three types:

1. *Alpha motor neurons:* Large neurons and axons of these neurons supply skeletal muscle fibers.
2. *Gamma motor neurons:* Smaller neurons and supply muscle spindle.
3. *Renshaw cell*
   - Smaller inhibitory neuron
   - Transmits inhibitory signal to the surrounding motor neuron. This is called lateral inhibition which helps in suppressing the tendency for the signals to spread laterally.

Interneurons (Fig. 11.22)

- Present in all areas of gray matter.
- About 30 times as numerous as anterior motor neurons.
- Small highly excitable capable of firing as rapidly as 1500 times per second.
- Synapse with anterior motor neurons also.
- Most of the descending signal synapse with interneurons first where they are appropriately processed and then passed on to anterior motor neurons.

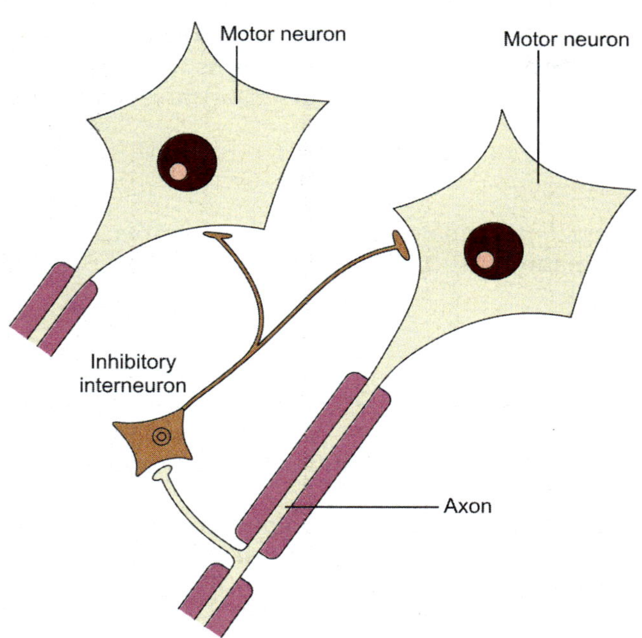

Fig. 11.22: Interneuron

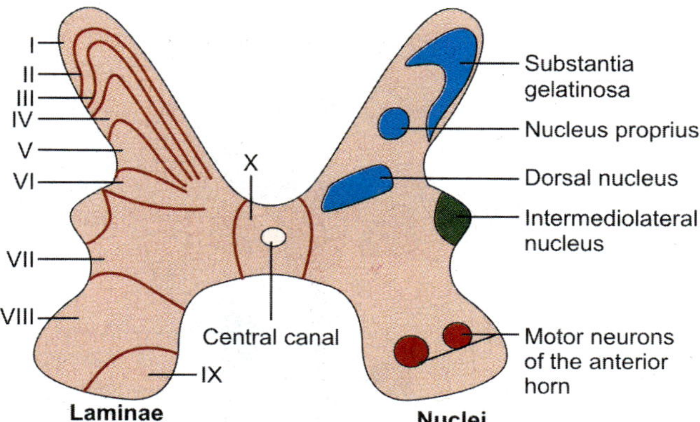

Fig. 11.23: Laminae

Laminae (Fig. 11.23)

The neurons of gray matter are distributed in laminae or layers. This was identified in 1950 by Burke Rexed. He identified 10 laminae which are known as Rexed laminae based on histological characters.

Laminae	*Equivalent*
I	Posterior marginal nucleus containing T cells
II	Substantia gelatinosa of Rolando
III	Nucleus proprius
IV	Nucleus proprius
V	T cells
VI and VII	Intermediolateral neurons and dorsal nucleus
VIII and IX	Anterior horn neuron
X	Gray matter around the central spinal canal

White Matter of Spinal Cord

White matter is formed by the bundles of nerve fibers. The band of white matter lying in front of anterior gray commissure is called the anterior white commissure. The gray horns divide the white matter into three columns:

i. Anterior white column
ii. Lateral white column
iii. Posterior white column.

TRACTS

Definition

A tract is a bundle of nerve fibers located in the CNS.

Types

1. *Ascending tracts:* Which carry sensory information to the brain.
2. *Descending tracts:* Which carry motor information from the brain to the periphery.

Ascending Tracts

The tracts are formed by two or more groups of neurons (Fig. 11.24).

Ascending tracts	
White column	*Tract*
Posterior white column	a. Fasciculus gracilis
	b. Fasciculus cuneatus
	c. Comma tract of Schultz
Lateral white column	d. Lateral spinothalamic tract
	e. Dorsal spinocerebellar tract
	f. Ventral spinocerebellar tract
	g. Spinoreticular tract
	h. Spinotectal tract
	i. Spino-olivary tract
	j. Spinovestibular tract
Anterior white column	k. Antrior spinothalamic tract

Fasciculus gracilis (tract of Goll) and fasciculus cuneatus (tract of Burdach).

Fasciculus gracilis is situated medially and fasciculus cuneatus is located laterally in the posterior column.

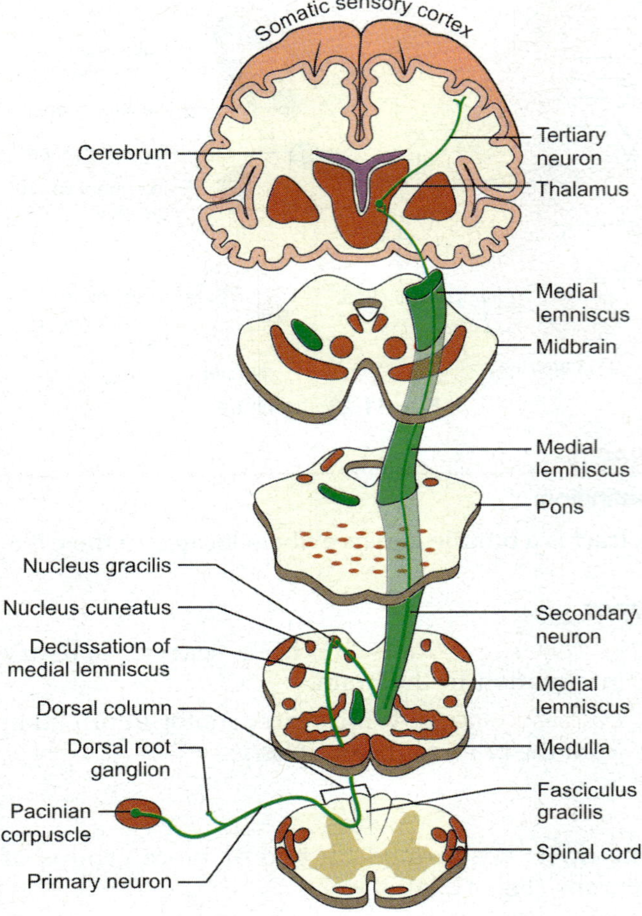

Fig. 11.24: Ascending tracts

Origin

The cell body or the first order neuron is in the dorsal root ganglion.

Course

After entering the spinal cord, the fibers ascend in the posterior white column of the same side. Fibers carrying sensation from the lower half of the body occupy the medial half and form the fasciculus gracilis and sensation from the upper half of the body occupy the lateral half and form the fasciculus cuneatus. The fibers synapse in nucleus gracilis and nucleus cuneatus in the medulla oblongata. The cells of these nuclei form second order neurons. The axons of these neurons form internal arcuate fibers. They cross to opposite side forming sensory decussation. They ascend through pons and midbrain as medial lemniscus. Hence, this tract is also known as dorsal column—medial lemniscal system. The medial lemniscus terminates in ventral posterolateral nucleus of thalamus. The third order neurons originate here. The fibers from here ascend to sensory area of cerebral cortex.

Termination

The tracts terminate in somatosensory area I and II (Brodmann areas 3, 1, 2 and superior wall of Sylvian fissure).

Functions

The tracts carry the following sensations:
1. Fine touch
2. Tactile localization (ability to locate the area of touch with closed eyes)
3. Two point discrimination (ability to recognize two point of stimuli with closed eyes)
4. Stereognosis (ability to recognize the known objects with closed eyes)
5. Vibration
6. Proprioception: Joint position and movement
7. Pressure.

Comma Tract of Schultz

- Situated between tracts of Goll and Burdach.
- Contains short descending tract.
- Function is to establish intersegmental communication and to form short reflex arc.

SPINOTHALAMIC TRACTS (ANTEROLATERAL SYSTEM) (Fig. 11.25)

There are two tracts in this system:
1. Lateral spinothalamic tract
2. Ventral spinothalamic tract

1. Lateral Spinothalamic Tract (Fig. 11.26)

Origin

The first order neuron is located in the dorsal root ganglion.

Course

The fibers on entering spinal cord synapse with marginal nucleus and substantia gelatinosa of Rolando. The axons of these cells cross to the opposite side and ascend in the lateral column. At the lower part of the medulla, the fibers of lateral spinothalamic tract form spinal lemniscus along with fibers of anterior spinothalamic tract. The fiber pass through

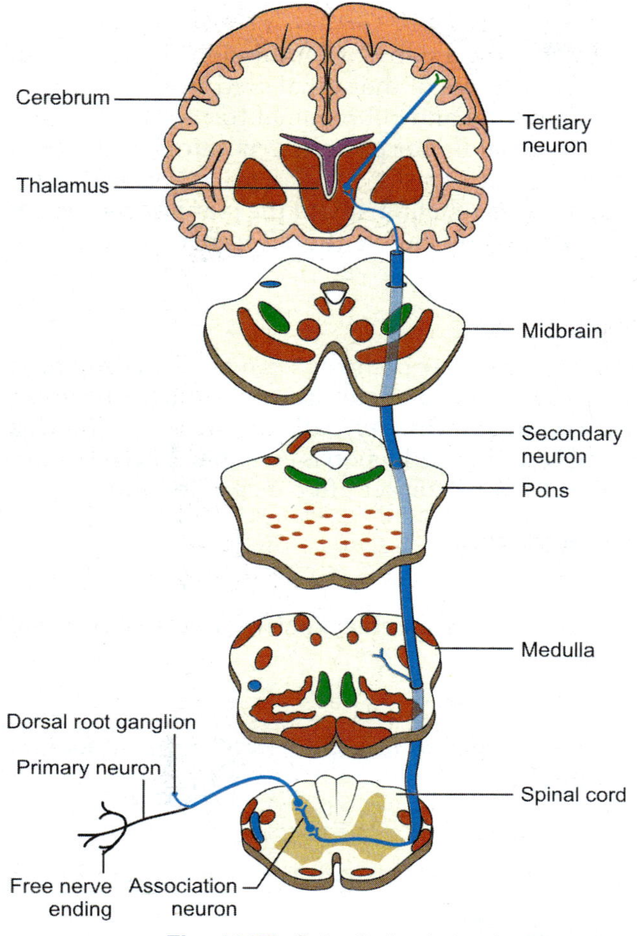

Fig. 11.25: Spinothalamic tract

the pons and midbrain and terminate in the ventral posterolateral nucleus of thalamus. The third order neuron originate here.

Termination

The tracts terminate in somatosensory area I and II.

Functions

The tract carries the following sensation:
- Pain
- Temperature
- Tickle and itch
- Sexual sensation.

Anterior Spinothalamic Tract

Origin

The first order neuron is located in the dorsal root ganglion.

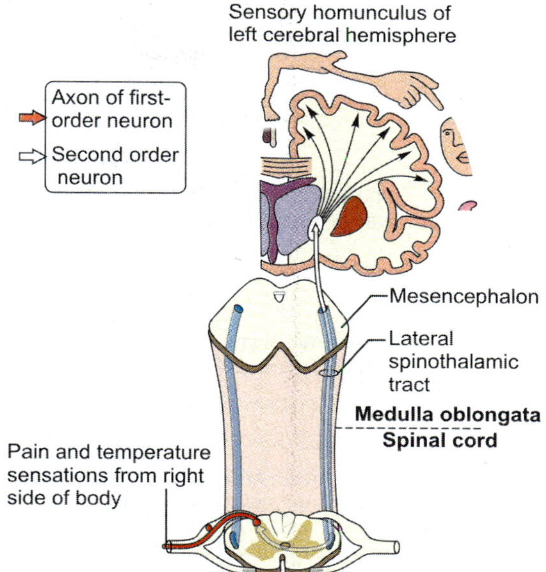

Fig. 11.26: Lateral spinothalamic tract

Course

It has the same course as that of lateral spinothalamic tract. But the first order neurons end in the chief sensory nucleus in the spinal cord.

Termination

The tracts terminate in somatosensory area I and II.

Function

It carries the sensation of crude touch.

Tract of Lissauer

This tract is a component of lateral spinothalamic tract. The first order neurons enter the spinal cord via dorsal nerve root. These fibers ascend or descend a short distance between the tip of posterior gray horn and the periphery of the spinal cord before ending in the cells of substantia gelatinosa of Rolando. This short tract is known as tract of Lissauer.

Dorsal Spinocerebellar Tract (Fig. 11.27)

Origin

It takes origin from Clarkes column of cells in the posterior gray horn.

11

Course

The fibers ascend in the lateral column through medulla, pons and midbrain and enter the cerebellum through inferior cerebellar peduncle.

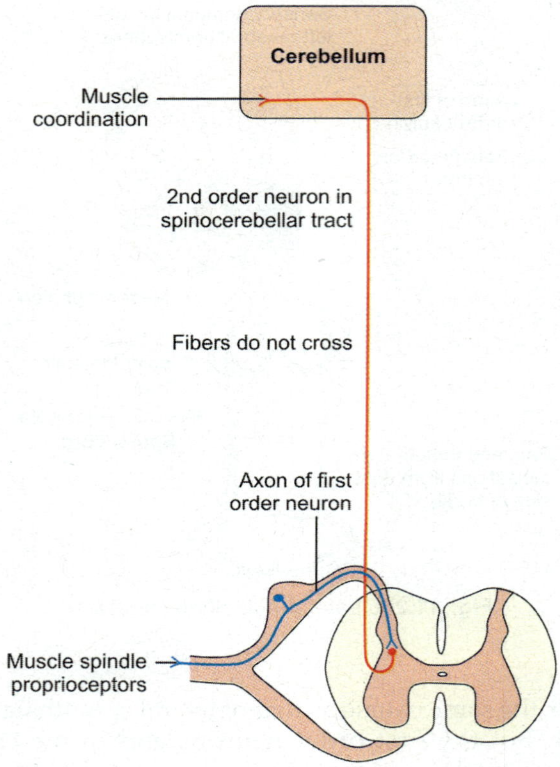

Fig. 11.27: Spinocerebellar tract

Termination

It terminates in the anterior lobe of cerebellum.

Functions

It carries the sensations from muscle spindle, Golgi tendon organ, large cutaneous receptors and joint receptors. All these signals apprise the cerebellum of the momentary status of the following:

1. Muscle contraction
2. Degree of tension on the muscle tendons
3. Position and rate of movements of the parts of the body
4. Forces acting on the surfaces of the body.

2. Ventral Spinocerebellar Tract (Gower's Tract)

Origin, course and termination are same as that of dorsal spinocerebellar tract. The main differences are:

1. This tract enters the cerebellum through superior cerebellar peduncle.
2. It contains both crossed and uncrossed fibers.

Functions

This tract takes a copy of motor signals arriving in the anterior horns of the spinal cord from:

1. Corticospinal and rubrospinal tracts
2. The internal motor pattern generators in the cord itself.

It tells the cerebellum about the planned motor act. This feedback is called the efference copy of the anterior horn motor drive.

Significance

The spinocerebellar pathways can transmit impulses at velocities up to 120 meter/second, which is the most rapid conduction in any pathway in the CNS. This extremely rapid conduction is essential for cerebellum to correct the motor act after many attempts.

Spinotectal Tract

Origin

The fibers arise from chief sensory nucleus in spinal cord.

Termination

The fibers terminate in superior colliculus of tectum in midbrain.

Function

This tract is concerned with spinovisual reflex.

Spinoreticular Tract

Origin

The fibers arise from intermediolateral nucleus.

Termination

The fibers terminate in the reticular formation of brain- stem.

Function

This is concerned with consciousness and awareness.

Spino-olivary Tract

Origin of this tract is not specific. Fibers terminate in the olivary nucleus of medulla oblongata. It is concerned with proprioception.

Spinovestibular Tract

The fibers of this tract arise from all the segments of the spinal cord and terminate in the lateral vestibular nucleus. It is also concerned with proprioception.

DESCENDING TRACTS

They carry motor impulses from the brain to the periphery. They are of two types:
1. Pyramidal tract
2. Extrapyramidal tract

Pyramidal Tract (Corticospinal Tract) (Fig. 11.28)

It is the longest motor tract present only in higher animals and man.

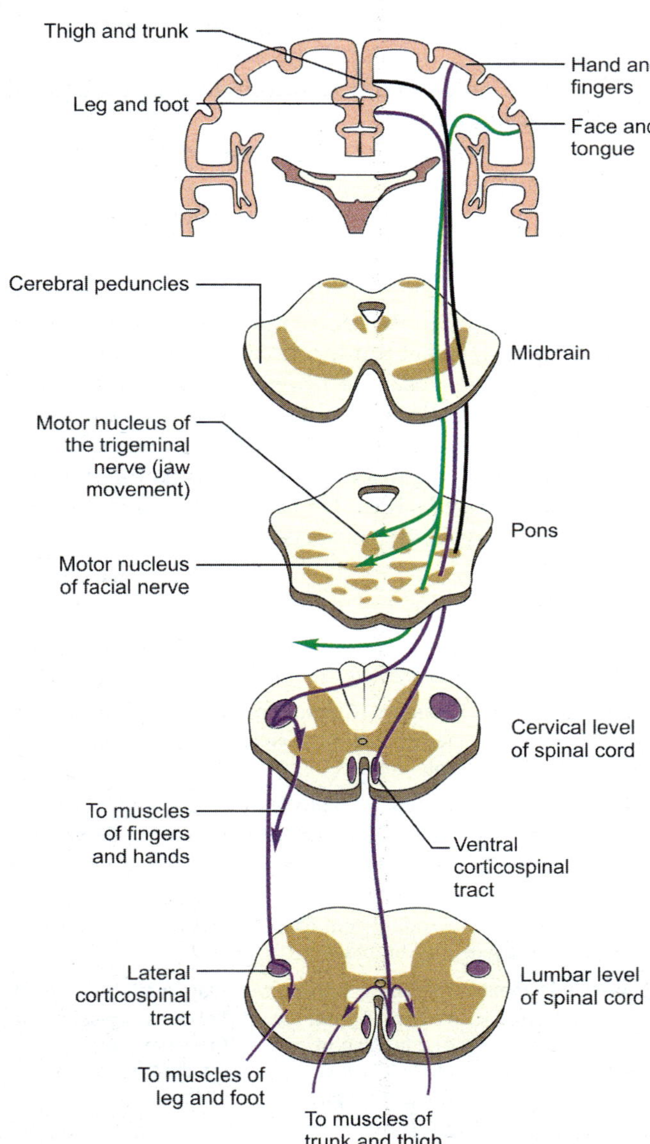

Fig. 11.28: Spinothalamic pathway

Origin

- 30% of the fibers arise from the Betz cells or pyramidal cells in primary motor cortex.
- 30% from premotor and supplementary motor cortex.
- 40% from somatosensory cortex.

Nerve Fibers

There are about 1 million fibers. Of these only 36,000 fibers are fast conducting and have a diameter of more than 10 micrometer and take origin from Betz cells. Rest of the fibers are less than 10 micrometer in diameter.

Course

Corona Radiata

After taking origin the nerve fibers descend in the form of fan-like structure through the white matter of cerebral cortex. The fan-like structure is called corona radiata.

Internal Capsule

The tract occupies the genu and anterior 2/3rds of the posterior limb of the internal capsule.

Midbrain

The fibers pass through pes pedunculi or basis pedunculi which lies ventral to the substantia nigra. The fibers occupy the middle 3/5ths of pes pedunculi.

Pons

On entering the pons, the tract splits into number of bundles due to crossing of pontocerebellar fibers. At the lower border of pons, the fibers again form a compact bundle.

Medulla

The compact bundle of fibers bulges anteriorly close to the midline forming pyramid. Hence, it is known as pyramidal tract (Fig. 11.29). In the lower part of medulla about 80% of fibers cross to the opposite side. This is called as motor decussation. The remaining 20% of fibers descend on the same side. The crossed fibers form the lateral corticospinal tract and the uncrossed fibers form the anterior or direct corticospinal tract.

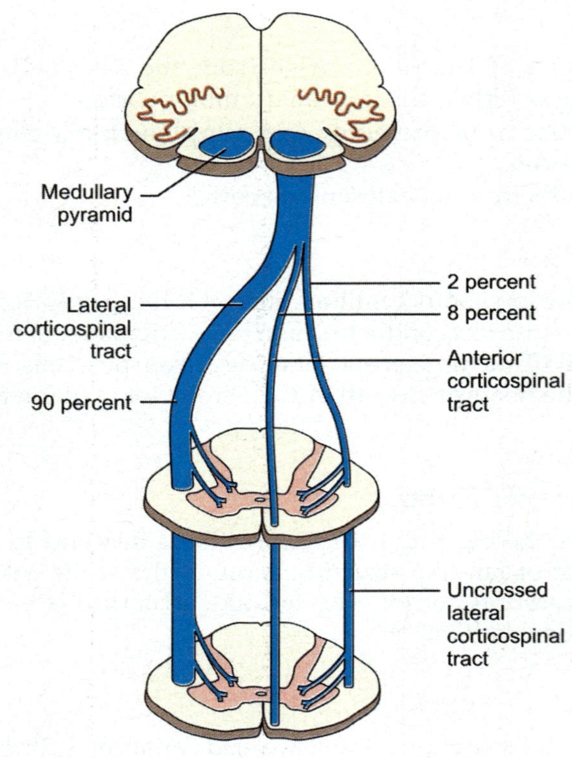

Fig. 11.29

Termination

The fibers of this tract terminate in the anterior motor neurons and interneurons of the different segments of spinal cord.

Upper Motor Neuron

The neurons giving origin to the fibers of pyramidal tract are called upper motor neurons.

Lower Motor Neurons

The anterior motor neurons in the spinal cord and their axons are called lower motor neurons.

Distribution of Pyramidal Fibers

- 55% cervical segments
- 20% thoracic segments
- 25% lumbar segments

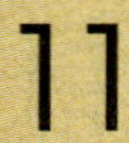

Functions

Myelination of pyramidal tract is completed 18 months afterbirth. Hence, it becomes fully functional only at that time.

- It is concerned with fine, discrete and skilled voluntary movements
- It facilitates muscle tone
- Anterior corticospinal tract controls gross voluntary movements like walking, climbing, etc.

Effects of Lesions of Pyramidal Tracts at Different Levels

1. *Cerebral cortex:* Monoplegia on contralateral side
2. *Corona radiata:* Monoplegia
3. *Internal capsule:* Contralateral hemiplegia
4. *Midbrain:* Contralateral hemiplegia and ipsilateral 3rd nerve palsy
5. *Pons:* Contralateral hemiplegia and ipsilateral 7th nerve palsy
6. *Medulla:* Contralateral hemiplegia and ipsilateral 12th nerve palsy
7. *Upper level of spinal cord:* Respiratory paralysis and quadriplegia
8. *Thoracic and spinal segments:* Paraplegia

Corticobulbar Tract

This tract arises from the motor cortex and in analogous to the pyramidal tract but terminates on the cell bodies of the cranial nerves. The fibers descend along with the pyramidal tract and cross to the opposite side throughout the brainstem to synapse with cranial nuclei. This tract acts as an upper motor neuron for the 3rd, 4th, 5th, 6th, 7th, 9th, 10th, 11th and 12th cranial nerves. In bulbar paralysis, these nerves are affected.

Differences between UMNL and LMNL

	Upper motor neuron lesion	*Lower motor neuron lesion*
Paralysis	Paralysis of movements rather than of muscles (paresis)	Muscles, individual or groups paralysed
Tone	Increased: Muscles hypertonic spasticity (clasp–knife type of rigidity)	Decreased: Muscles hypotonic, flaccidity
Deep reflexes, e.g. knee jerk, ankle jerk	Exaggerated: Clonus may be present	Diminished or absent
Superficial reflexes a. Plantar reflex	Extension with dorsi-flexion of great toe and fanning of outer four toes (Babinski sign)	Plantar reflex is normal flexor response (but if the innervation is affected it may be absent
b. Abdominal reflex	Absent	Present (if innervation is intact)

Contd.

Contd.

	Upper motor neuron lesion	Lower motor neuron lesion
Wasting of muscles	Only slight due to disuse	Marked wasting due to atrophy
Electrical reactions of degeneration	No reaction of degeneration (electrical reactions normal)	Reaction of degeneration is present

Extrapyramidal Tracts

The descending tracts of the spinal cord other than pyramidal tract are called extrapyramidal tracts.

- Rubrospinal tract
- Tectospinal tract
- Vestibulospinal tract
- Reticulospinal tract
- Olivospinal tract

Rubrospinal Tract

Origin

It takes origin from the magnocellular division of red nucleus in midbrain. Red nucleus receives fibers from motor cortex, collaterals from corticospinal tract, basal ganglia, cerebellum and reticular nuclei.

Course

After taking origin from red nucleus, the fibers cross to the opposite side and descend in the spinal cord in the lateral white column along with lateral corticospinal tract.

Termination

The fibers terminate on the interneurons which in-turn synapse with anterior motor neurons in the spinal cord.

Function

Along with lateral corticospinal tract, it is responsible for controlling the distal muscles that are concerned with fine and skilled movements.

Tectospinal Tract

Situation

This tract is situated in the anterior white column of the spinal cord.

Origin

The fibers originate from superior colliculus of midbrain.

Course

After taking origin from the superior colliculus, the fibers cross the midline and descend in the lateral white column.

Termination

The fibers terminate in the anterior motor neurons directly or via interneurons in the spinal cord.

Functions

It is responsible for the movement of the head in response to visual and auditory stimuli.

Vestibulospinal Tract

There are two divisions in this tract:

1. Medial vestibulospinal tract
2. Lateral vestibulospinal tract.

Medial Vestibulospinal Tract

Situation: This is located in the anterior white column of the spinal cord.

Origin: The fibers originate from the medial vestibular nucleus in medulla oblongata.

Extent: Fibers extend up to thoracic segments of spinal cord.

Course: The fibers descend in the anterior white column of the spinal cord. All the fibers are uncrossed.

Termination: The fibers terminate in anterior motor neurons of spinal cord.

Function: It is concerned with movements of head, neck and eyes during rotational movements.

Lateral Vestibulospinal Tract

Situation: This tract occupies the anterior part of lateral white column of spinal cord.

Origin: This tract originates from lateral vestibular nucleus (Deiters nucleus) in medulla.

Extent: The fibers are present throughout the spinal cord.

Course: The fibers descend in the lateral column of the spinal cord. A few fibers cross to the opposite side.

Termination: The fibers terminate in anterior motor neurons of the spinal cord.

Function: This tract is concerned with the postural adjustments during linear accelaratory movements of the body.

Reticulospinal Tract

Situation: This tract is located in anterior white column. There are two divisions in this tract.

1. Pontine reticulospinal tract
2. Medullary reticulospinal tract.

Pontine Reticulospinal Tract

Origin: This tract arises from reticular nuclei in the pons.

Termination: The tract crosses to the opposite side and terminates in the anterior motor neurons.

Function: The pontine reticular nuclei are highly excitatory. This tract is facilitatory tract to antigravity muscles.

Medullary Reticulospinal Tract

Origin: This tract arises from reticular nuclei in the medulla oblongata.

Termination: This tract has both crossed and uncrossed fibers. The fibers terminate in anterior motor neurons.

Functions: This tract is inhibitory to the antigravity muscles. This tract along with pontine reticulospinal tract controls the following:

- Muscle tone of antigravity muscles
- Posture and equilibrium.

Olivospinal Tract

Situation: This is located in the lateral white column.

Origin: This tract takes origin from inferior olivary nucleus in medulla oblongata.

Termination: The fibers terminate in the anterior motor neurons of the spinal cord.

Function: The exact function is not known. It may be involved in reflex movements arising from proprioceptors.

Differences between pyramidal tract and extrapyramidal tract

	Pyramidal tract	*Extrapyramidal tract*
Development	New system	Old system
Myelination	Starts at birth and is completed by second year of life	Starts before birth
Synapses involved	One or two	Polysynaptic
Function	Controls fine, skilled movements	Controls gross movements
Conduction rate	Slow	Fast
Control of body parts	Upper limb shows more pyramidal control	Lower limb shows more extrapyramidal control
Control over types of muscle	Mainly flexor muscles	Mainly extensor muscles
Nature of fibers	Only facilitatory fibers are present	Both facilitatory and inhibitory fibers are present

DYSFUNCTION OF SPINAL CORD

It can be classified into four types:

1. Complete transection
2. Incomplete transection
3. Hemisection
4. Diseases of spinal cord

Complete Transection of Spinal Cord

This may occur due to injuries like gun shot injuries, accident and occlusion of blood vessels. At the moment of section, the subject feels he is cut into two and the lower half of the body is not there. There is immediate and permanent loss of sensation, and voluntary movements below the level of lesion. The higher centers are unaffected, so his mind is clear. But all the parts of the body below the level of the lesion are deprived of all activity. The effects can be divided into three stages:

1. Stage of spinal shock
2. Stage of reflex activity
3. Stage of reflex failure

Stage of Spinal Shock

Spinal shock is due to sudden removal of impulses from the higher centers which normally reinforce the spinal centers. Higher the animal in the phylogenetic scale, longer is the duration of the spinal shock. In the frog it lasts for a few minutes, in the dog a few hours, in monkey a few days and in man a few weeks.

1. The muscle tone is lost and the muscles are completely paralyzed. If the lesion is in the cervical region, it results in quadriplegia. If it is in the mid-thoracic region, paraplegia results.
2. All the reflexes both superficial and deep are lost. Anal reflex may be present.
3. All sensations are lost below the lesion. There is a band of hyperesthesia just above the level of lesion.

4. Autonomic changes:
   - Blood pressure falls if the lesion is at or above the level of T_1. If it is below L_2 segment, BP is not affected
   - Heart rate decreases. Pulse becomes weak and thready
   - Sweat secretions are abolished. The skin is cold and dry
   - Muscles of bladder and rectum are also paralyzed.

   After an interval of about 1–3 weeks, the conditions pass onto stage II.

Stage of Reflex Activity

This is due to the recovery of isolated spinal centers.

1. Muscle tone returns first in the smooth muscle, next in the blood vessel and later in the skeletal muscle.
2. Among the skeletal muscles, it first occurs in the flexor muscles and later in the extensors. As the patient is in the bed, the lower limbs are drawn up in the flexed position. This is called paraplegia in flexion.
3. The first reflex to appear is Babinski sign and is followed by flexor reflexes and later Knee jerk and ankle jerk return.
4. The limbs cannot support the weight of the body.

Mass Reflex

Scratching or any unpleasant stimulus like pinching or pricking of the skin of the lower limbs or abdominal wall, the following responses occur:

1. Flexor spasm of the both lower limbs and spasm of abdominal wall
2. Profuse sweating of the region below the level of lesion.
3. Evacuation of bladder and rectum.

   Mass reflex is actually an exaggeration of normal flexion reflex.

Stage of Reflex Failure (Stage of Degeneration)

The spinal cord below the level of lesion degenerates. The general condition of the patient starts deteriorating. Infection of urinary tract may occur. Breakdown of skin over pressure points leads to bed sores (decubitus ulcer), which gets infected due to poor circulation and the ulcers do not heal. Prolonged immobilization of the patient leads to protein depletion. Excessive calcium removal from bone and hypercalcemia lead to formation of renal stones and renal failure.

The reflexes, including mass reflex disappear. The duration of this stage is short and is followed by death.

Incomplete Transection of Spinal Cord

Three stages are seen:

1. Stage of Spinal Shock

Same as complete transection.

2. Stage of Reflex Activity

If the transection is incomplete involving the corticospinal tract but leaving some fibers of the vestibulospinal tract or reticulospinal facilitatory tract intact, tone returns to extensor muscles. Limbs lie in a position of extension of the hips and knee and toes are drawn up. This is known as paraplegia in extension.

- The deep tendon reflexes are exaggerated. Babinski's sign is positive.
- There is no mass reflex
- In the upper limb, some resistance is offered when the arm is flexed passively. If the forearm is flexed forcefully, the resistance to flexion is abolished suddenly leading to quick flexion of arm. This is called Phillipson's reflex or clasp knife reflex.

3. Stage of Reflex Failure

Same as complete transection.

Hemisection of Spinal Cord

The lesion involving one lateral half of the spinal cord is called hemisection. It can occur due to injury to the spinal cord. There is a clincal condition similar to the hemisection of spinal cord called as Brown-Sequard syndrome.

Brown-Séquard Syndrome (Figs 11.30 and 11.31)

Causes

It may occur as a result of compression of spinal cord by a tumor or damage to the cord, usually at midthoracic level.

Clinical Manifestations

I. Changes Above the Level of Lesion

A band of cutaneous hyperesthesia is seen on the same side of lesion corresponding to the distribution of the next higher sensory nerves. This is due to the irritation of the sensory nerves.

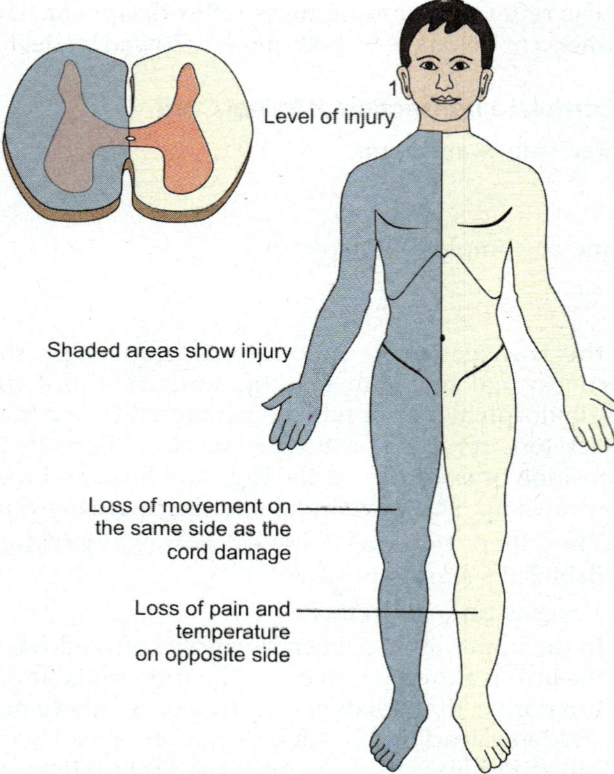

Fig. 11.30: Brown-Séquard syndrome

II. *Changes at the Level of Lesion*

On the same side

Sensory changes

There is complete anesthesia due to destruction of posterior nerve roots.

Motor changes: Lower motor neuron type of lesion is seen.

- Flaccid paralysis
- Wasting of muscles
- All reflexes are lost
- Vasomotor tone is lost

On the opposite side

Sensory changes

- Loss of pain, temperature and crude touch sensations because the crossed spinothalamic tracts are affected.
- Other sensations are preserved as tracts of Goll and Burdach are intact.

Motor changes: No motor changes are seen.

III. *Changes below the Level of Lesion*

On the same side

Sensory changes

The following sensations carried by the tracts of Goll and Burdach are lost:

- Fine touch
- Tactile localization
- Two point discrimination
- Vibration
- Joint position
- Stereognosis

Motor changes: Upper motor neuron type of lesion is seen

- Muscle tone increases leading to spastic paralysis
- Rigidity of the limb
- Superficial reflexes are lost

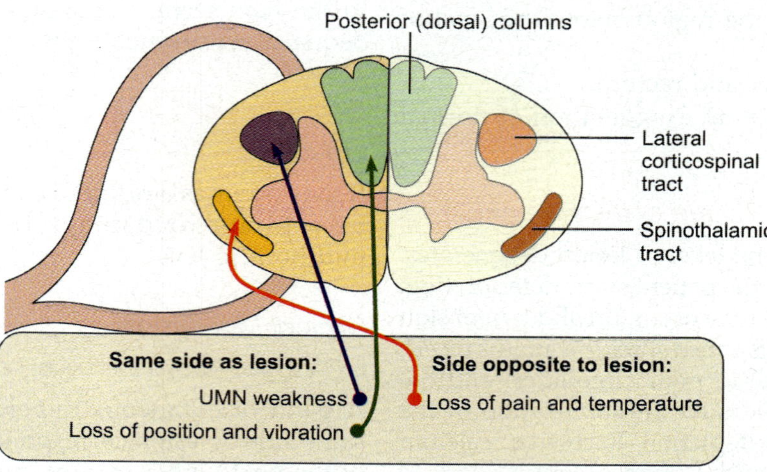

Fig. 11.31: Brown-Séquard syndrome of spinal cord hemisection

- Deep reflexes are exaggerated
- Babinski sign is positive.

On the opposite side

Sensory changes

Loss of pain, temperature and crude touch sensation as the crossed spinothalamic tracts are lost.

Motor changes

No change

Some Diseases of Spinal Cord

Syringomyelia

It is a disorder characterized by presence of fluid filled cavities in spinal cord.

Cause

It is due to overgrowth of neuroglial cells in spinal cord followed by cavity formation. It begins in the gray matter near the central canal of spinal cord. Later it involves the white matter too. Lower cervical and upper thoracic regions are mostly affected.

Features

- If the disease is only around the central canal, there is loss of pain, temperature and crude touch sensations. It is due to lesion in fibers crossing in the anterior gray commissures, but fine touch sensation is preserved as posterior column is intact. This is called dissociated anesthesia.
- If the disease extends to posterior gray horn, all the sensations are lost.
- When the anterior gray horn is involved, flaccid paralysis of muscle occurs. Later, pyramidal and extrapyramidal tracts are also involved. This leads to spastic paraplegia.

Tabes Dorsalis

It is a slowly progressive nervous disorder affecting both sensory and motor functions of spinal cord.

Cause

It is due to degeneration of posterior nerve roots. Hence tracts of Goll and Burdach, spinothalamic tracts and spinocerebellar tracts are affected. It occurs in syphilis.

Features

Sensory Changes

- At the onset of the disease, there is exaggeration of pain sensation. Later all the sensations are lost.
- Loss of pain sensation leads to trophic ulcers and deformity of joints. Painless destruction of joints called Charcot's joints may occur.

Reflexes

All the reflexes, both superficial and deep reflexes are lost.

Voluntary Movements

There is an incoordination of voluntary movements due to absence of information from muscles, tendons and joints.

Gait becomes ataxic. The patient walks with legs apart and raises the leg and stamps it down forcibly. This is called stamping gait.

Urinary Bladder

Micturition reflex is lost if the disease involves sacral segments. The bladder becomes atonic and it is called tabetic bladder.

102. INTERNAL CAPSULE

Internal capsule is a thick curved band of afferent and efferent fibers connecting cerebral cortex with brain- stem and spinal cord (Fig. 11.32).

Situation

It occupies the space between thalamus and caudate nucleus medially and the lentiform nucleus laterally. Superiorly, it fans out as corona radiata which contains the descending fibers of pyramidal tract.

Divisions

It has:

- Anterior limb
- Genu
- Posterior limb
- Caudal part

Anterior Limb

- Lies between head of the caudate and lentiform nucleus.
- Contains anterior thalamic radiation and fronto-pontine tract.

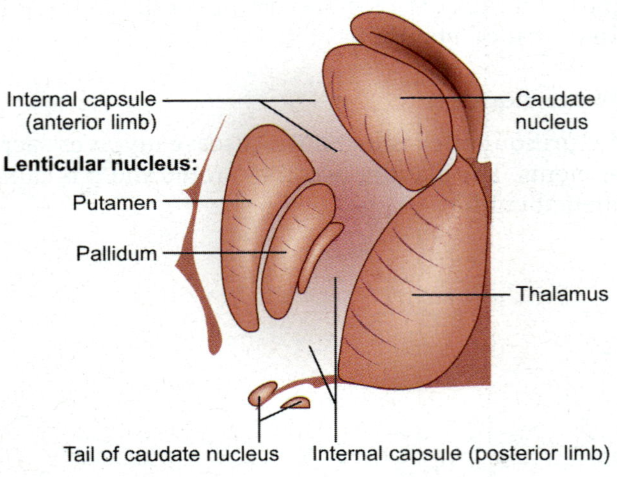

Fig. 11.32: Internal capsule

Genu

- Connects anterior and posterior limbs.
- Contains corticobulbar tract.

Posterior Limb

- It is longer than anterior limb, situated between thalamus medially and lentiform nucleus laterally.
- Contains corticospinal tract, superior thalamic radiation and frontopontine tract.

Caudate Part

It has two divisions:

Retrolentiform

- Lies behind lentiform nuclei.
- Consists of optic radiation, posterior thalamic radiation and corticopontine fibers.

Sublentiform

- Lies beneath posterior part of lentiform nucleus.
- Consists of auditory radiations, inferior thalamic radiation and corticopontine fibers.

Blood Supply

Internal capsule is supplied by the branches of middle, anterior and posterior cerebral arteries.

Applied Physiology

- Lesion in anterior limb causes widespread disability in motor and sensory functions.
- Lesion in genu causes paralysis of cranial nerves.
- Lesion in posterior limb causes.
  - Contralateral hemianesthesia (loss of sensation in opposite side of the body)
  - Contralateral hemihyperesthesia (abnormal sensation in opposite side of the body)
  - Hemiplegia
  - Lesion in caudal portion causes contralateral hemianesthesia, hemianopia and deafness.

103. BASAL GANGLIA

INTRODUCTION

Basal ganglia are scattered subcortical gray nuclear masses present at the base of the cerebral hemisphere (Fig. 11.33).

Components

1. Caudate nucleus ⎤ Corpus striatum
2. Putamen ⎦
3. Globus pallidus (pallidum)] Lenticular nucleus
4. Subthalamic nucleus (body of Luys)
5. Substantia nigra.

Phylogenetic Classification

1. Neostriatum

Caudate nucleus and putamen which are of recent origin constitute neostriatum.

2. Paleostriatum

Globus pallidus which is older and primitive constitutes paleostriatum. It is called pallidum as it looks pale (pallid).

Caudate Nucleus

- It is comma shaped brand of gray matter.
- It consists of head, body and tail.
- Tail ends in close relation to amygdaloid body.

Putamen

- It is dark in color.
- It is in outer part of lenticular nucleus and is separated from pallidum by a white fibrous band.

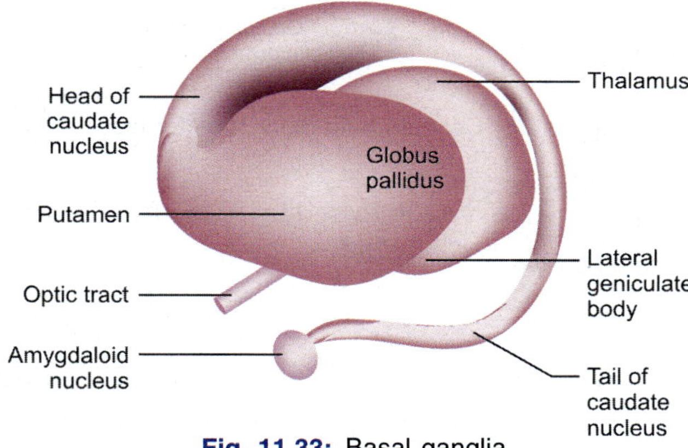

Fig. 11.33: Basal ganglia

Globus Pallidus (GP)

- It is the inner paler region of lenticular nucleus.
- It is divided into GP interna and GP externa by internal lamina of white matter.

Subthalamic Nucleus of Luys

It is biconvex mass of gray matter situated lateral to red nucleus and dorsal to substantia nigra in the midbrain.

Substantia Nigra

It is a sheet of neurons containing a dark pigment neuromelanin. It also contains high level of copper. It is divisible into two parts:

1. *Pars compacta:* It is the dorsal part of substantia nigra. It contains dopaminergic and cholinergic neurons.
2. *Pars reticularis:* It is the ventral part and contains GABA-ergic neurons.

CONNECTIONS

Afferent Connections

1. *Corticostriate projection:* Afferents from all 4 lobes of the cerebral cortex.
2. *Thalamostriate fibers:* Fibers from centromedian nucleus of thalamus to the striatum.

Intranuclear Connections

Nigrostriatal projection:

- Constitutes fibers from the pars compacta of the substantia nigra to the striatum.
- Releases dopamine which is an inhibitory neurotransmitter.

GABA-ergic Inhibitory Projection

Constitutes

a. Fibers from corpus striatum to pars reticulata of substantia nigra and globus pallidus (both internal and external segments).
b. Fibers from external globus pallidus to subthalamic nucleus.
c. Fibers from subthalamic nucleus project to substantia nigra and internal and external segments of globus pallidus and secrete glutamic acid.

11

Efferent Connections

1. From globus pallidus → thalamus → prefrontal and premotor cortex.
2. From pars reticulata of substantia nigra → thalamus.

FEEDBACK CIRCUIT

There are two important circuits in basal ganglia. They are:

1. Putamen circuit
2. Caudate circuit

1. Putamen Circuit (Fig. 11.34)

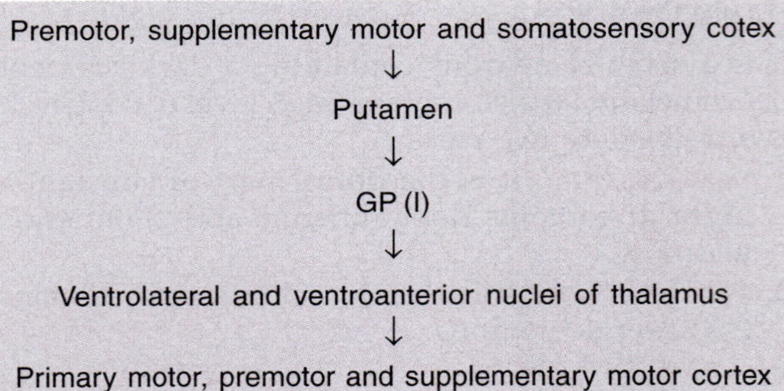

2. Caudate Circuit (Fig. 11.35)

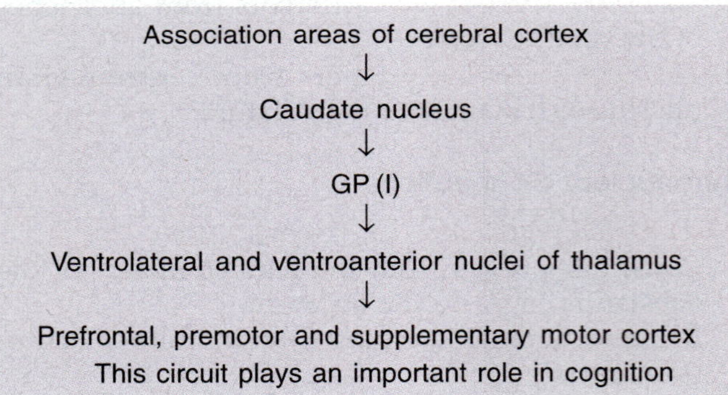

Neurotransmitters

- *Dopamine:* Released by fibers from substantia nigra to caudate nucleus.
- *GABA:* Released by fibers at corpus striatum and substantia nigra.
- *Acetylcholine:* Released by fibers from cerebral cortex to striatum.
- *Glutamate:* Released by fibers from cerebral cortex to striatum.

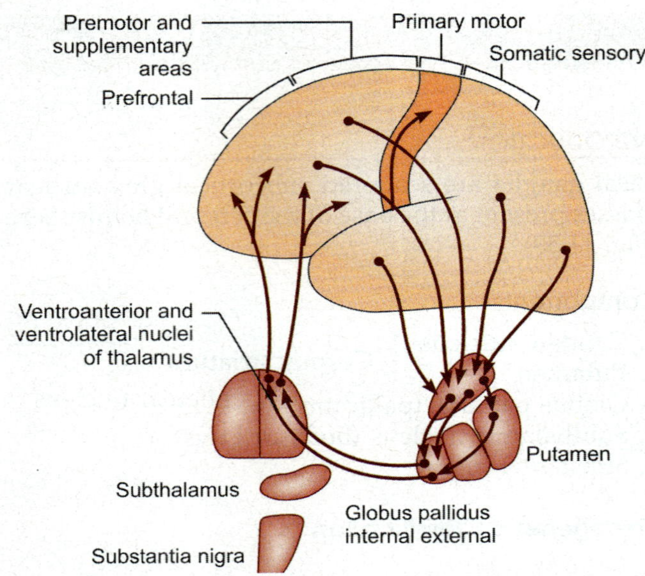

Fig. 11.34: Putamen loop (sensorimotor loop)

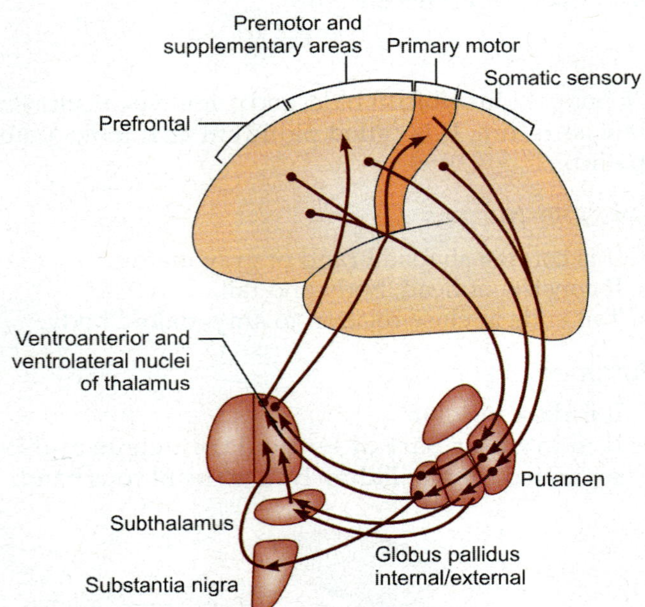

Fig. 11.35: Caudate loop (sensorimotor loop)

- Substance p
- Enkephalins

} Released by fibers from globus pallidus

Functions

1. Planning and programming of movements by preventing oscillations and afterdischarge in the motor system.

2. Cognition: Means thinking processes of brain. Caudate nucleus plays an important role in cognitive control of motor activity.
3. Inhibition of stretch reflex throughout the body by stimulation of caudate nucleus.
4. Basal ganglia suppress the unwanted movements by their inhibitory effect.
5. They control the automatic associated movements like swinging of arms while walking and gestures during speech.
6. They also have a role in regulation of posture.

Applied Physiology

1. *Parkinson's disease:* Also known as paralysis agitans or shaking palsy, is a slow progressive degenerative disorder described originally by James Parkinson and is named after him.

Site of Lesion

Pars compacta of substantia nigra and nigrostriatal dopaminergic fibers.

Causes

Corpus striatum is normally under the inhibitory influence of dopaminergic pathway from substantia nigra. When there is lesion in substantia nigra, the corpus striatum is released from the inhibition and there is an imbalance between excitation and inhibition in basal ganglia.

Parkinsonism can occur due to:

- Viral encephalitis.
- Treatment with drugs like phenothiazine and reserpine.
- Head injury.
- Idiopathic (cause unknown)

Clinical Manifestations

Parkinson's disease is characterized by:

1. Rigidity of the muscles of the body.
2. Involuntary tremor.
3. Akinesia.

1. Rigidity

Stiffness of the muscles in limbs due to hypertonia as a result of removal of inhibitory influence on gamma motor neuron.

- Both flexors and extensors are affected.
- Passive movement of an extremity meets with a resistance like bending a lead pipe and is called lead-pipe rigidity.
- Sometimes there is a series of "catches" during passive movement called cogwheel rigidity is also present.

2. Tremor

- Involuntary rhythmic oscillatory movements of the distal parts of the limbs.
- Present at rest but disappears during activity (resting tremor).
- Occurs at a rate of 4–6 cycles/second.
- The thumb moves rhythmically over the index and middle fingers. So, called pill rolling movement.

3. Akinesia

- Difficulty in initiating movements.
- Begins as bradykinesia (slowing of movements) and progresses.
- Face becomes expressionless (mask-like face).
- Loss of automatic and associated movements like swinging of arms while walking.
- Shuffling or festinant type of gait is seen.

Management

1. L-dopa is given to these patients as dopamine does not cross the blood–brain barrier.

   It is converted to dopamine which restores the normal balance between inhibition and excitation in the caudate nucleus and putamen.
2. L-deprenyl

   This drug inhibits monoamine oxidase (MAO), which is responsible for destruction of dopamine that is released in basal ganglia. It can be combined with L-dopa.

Surgical

1. Transplantation of dopamine secreting cells, obtained from the brains of aborted fetuses into the caudate nuclei and putamen has been used to treat Parkinson's disease. However, the cells do not live for more than a few months.
2. Because abnormal signals from the basal ganglia to the motor cortex cause abnormal movements in Parkinson's disease, these signals can be blocked surgically. The surgical lesions made in the ventrolateral and ventroanterior nuclei of thalamus do

bring about success but also sometimes serious neurological damage.

HUNTINGTON'S DISEASE

- Hereditary disorder; inherited as an autosomal dominant disorder.
- The abnormal gene is located in chromosome 4.
- Onset is usually between 30 and 50 years of age.
- There is a loss of intrastriatal GABA-ergic and cholinergic neurons in basal ganglia.
- Characterized by chorea (rapid, involuntary, dancing movements), hypotonia, progressive dementia followed by death.
- No effective treatment is available at present.

Chorea

- Rapid, involuntary 'dancing' movements due to lesion in putamen.

Hemiballismus

- sudden, flailing movements of an entire limb due to lesion in subthalamus.

Athetosis

- Spontaneous, continuous, writhing movements of a hand, an arm, the neck or the face.
- Due to lesion in globus pallidus.

WILSON'S DISEASE

- Autosomal recessive disorder of copper metabolism.
- The plasma level of the copper-binding protein ceruloplasmin is low, leading to copper intoxication.
- There is severe degeneration of lenticular nucleus.
- Excess copper is deposited in the liver, brain, kidneys and in the eyes.
- Also known as hepatolenticular degeneration.
- Fatal if not treated early.

104. CEREBELLUM

Introduction

cerebellum has been called a silent area of the brain because electrical excitation of the cerebellum does not cause any conscious sensation and rarely causes any motor movements but removal of cerebellum causes the body movements to become abnormal.

Physiological Anatomy

The cerebellum lies dorsal to the brainstem in the posterior cranial fossa. It is connected to the brainstem on each side by three peduncles.

1. Inferior cerebellar peduncle (restiform body) to the medulla.
2. Middle cerebellar peduncle (branchium pontis) to pons.
3. Superior cerebellar peduncle (branchium conjunctivum) to midbrain.

11

Cerebellum has a central vermis and large cerebellar hemisphere on both sides. Each cerebellar hemisphere is divided into many divisions.

a. *Anatomical Divisions* (Fig. 11.36)

Anatomically, cerebellum is divided into three lobes by two deep fissures.

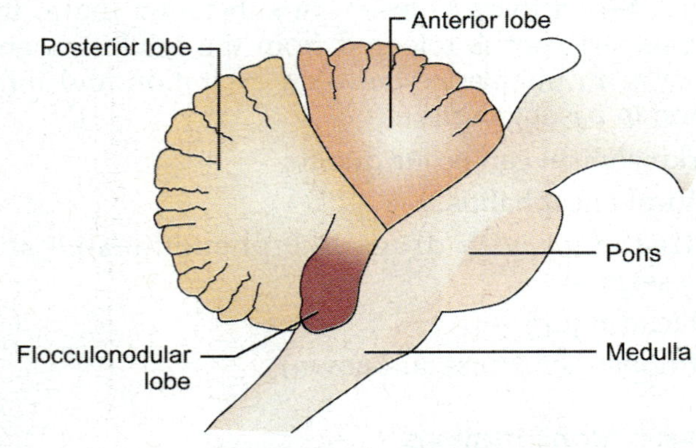

Fig. 11.36: Cerebellum

1. Anterior lobe
2. Posterior lobe
3. Flocculonodular lobe.

Flocculonodular lobe is the oldest of all the portions of the cerebellum.

b. *Phylogenetic Divisions* (Fig. 11.37)

This is based on development of lobes of cerebellum at different times during evolution.

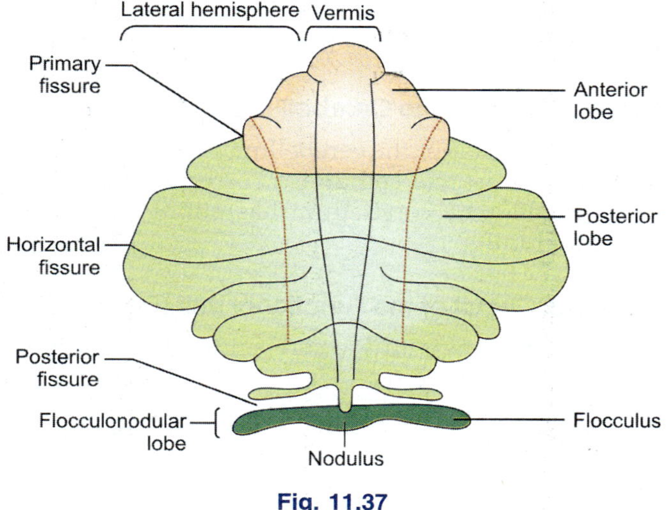

Fig. 11.37

- Archicerebellum
  - The oldest part of cerebellum.
  - Includes flocculonodular lobe.
- Paleocerebellum
  - Evolved next to archicerebellum.
  - Includes anterior lobe and some parts of posterior lobe.
- Neocerebellum
  - The last to evolve.
  - Includes remaining parts of posterior lobe.

c. *Functional Division* (Fig. 11.38)

Functionally, cerebellum is divided into three parts:

1. *Vestibulocerebellar*

- Includes flocculonodular lobe and adjacent parts of the vermis.
- Concerned with bodys equilibrium movements.

2. *Spinocerebellum*

- Includes most of the vermis of the posterior and anterior cerebellum and the intermediate zones on both sides of the vermis.
- Concerned with coordination of movements of the distal portions of the limbs, especially the hands and fingers.

3. *Cerebrocerebellum*

- Consists of large lateral zones of the cerebellar hemisphere.
- Concerned with planning of the next sequential movement a fraction of second in advance while the current movement is still being executed.

Histological Organization

The cerebellum has an external cortex separated by white matter from the cerebellar nuclei.

Cerebellar Cortex (Fig. 11.39)

It is extensively folded on itself constituting folia, i.e. leaf like parts. Cerebellar cortex is about 17 cm wide and 120 cm long. It consists of three layers:

- External molecular layer
- Middle Purkinje cell layer
- Internal granular layer.

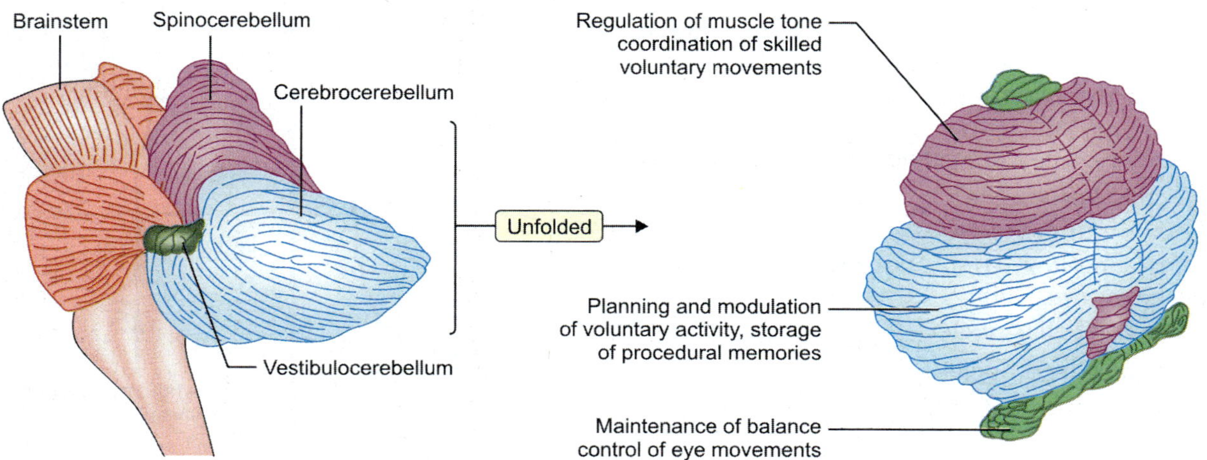

Fig. 11.38: Functional division of cerebellum

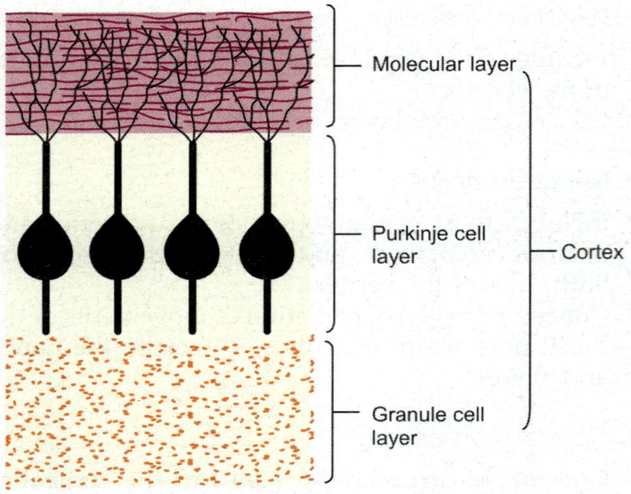

Fig. 11.39: Cerebellar cortex

1. Molecular Layer

There are two types of neurons present in this layer. They are:

1. Stellate cells
2. Basket cells.

2. Purkinje Cell Layer

Purkinje cells are the biggest neurons in the body. They have extensive dendrites which extend throughout the molecular layer. Their axons form the only output from the cerebellar cortex to the deep cerebellar nuclei.

3. Granular Cell Layer

This layer contains granule and Golgi cells.

- *Granule cells* are small and numerous in number.
  - Each cell sends an axon to molecular layer, where the axon bifurcates to form a 't'. The branches of 't' are straight and run long distances. They are called parallel nerve fibers.
- *Golgi cells:* Large cells
  - Less in number
  - Form inhibitory connections with the dendrites of the granule cells
  - Deep cerebellar nuclei.

There are four deep nuclei:

1. Dentate
2. Globose
3. Emboliform
4. Fastigial.

The globose and the emboliform nuclei are sometimes lumped together as the interpositus nucleus.

Functional Unit of the Cerebellum

A functional unit of the cerebellum includes a single, very large Purkinje cell and a corresponding deep nuclear cell. The cerebellum has about 30 million functional units.

Neuronal Circuit of the Functional Unit (Fig. 11.40)

The afferent inputs to the cerebellum are mainly of two types. They are:

- Climbing fibers
- Mossy fibers.

Climbing Fibers

- Originate from the inferior olivary nucleus of the medulla.
- There is about one climbing fiber for about 5 to 10.

Purkinje Cells

- Each climbing fiber on entering cerebellar cortex, sends branches to deep nuclear cells, ascends to the molecular layer and makes about 300 synapses with soma and dendrites of each Purkinje cell.
- The action potential of these fibers shows a strong spike followed by a trail of weakening secondary spikes. This is called complex spike.

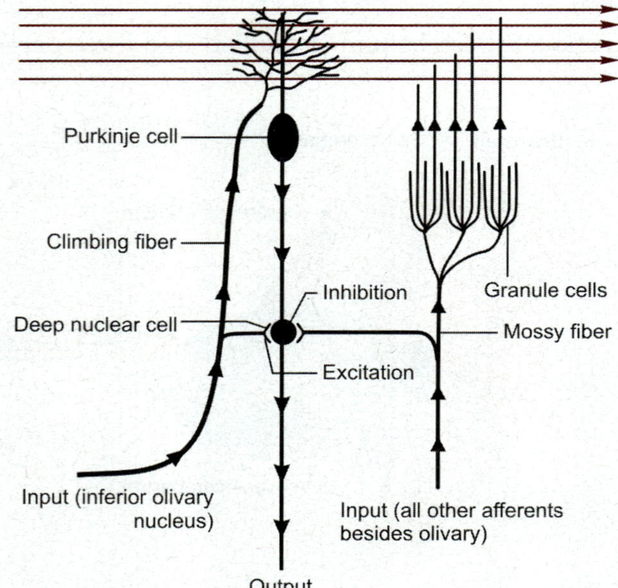

Fig. 11.40: Functional unit of cerebellum and neuronal circuit

Mossy Fibers

- Include all the other fibers that enter the cerebellum from higher center, brainstem and spinal cord.
- On entering cerebellar cortex, they send collaterals to deep nuclei and synapse with granule cells. In turn, granule cells send very small axons to the molecular layer where they divide and form parallel nerve fibers. There are many millions of parallel nerve fibers because there are some 500–1000 granules cells for each Purkinje cell.
- The action potential of these fibers is called simple spike.

Connections of the Cerebellum

Afferent Connections

The afferents to the cerebellum can be broadly classified into two types:
1. Afferents from other parts of the brain.
2. Afferents from the periphery.

Afferents from Other Parts of the Brain

1. *Corticopontocerebellar pathway*
   - Originates in motor, premotor and somatosensory cortex.
   - Passes by way of pontine nuclei to the lateral divisions of cerebellar hemispheres.
2. *Olivocerebellar pathway*
   - Originates from inferior olivary nucleus of medulla to all parts of the cerebellum.
   - Inferior olivary nucleus, in turn, is excited by fibers from motor cortex, basal ganglia, reticular formation and spinal cord.
3. *Vestibulocerebellar pathway*
   - Originates in the vestibular apparatus and brainstem vestibular nuclei.
   - Terminates in flocculonodular lobe and fastigial nucleus of cerebellum.
4. *Reticulocerebellar pathway*
   - Originates in reticular formation of brainstem.
   - Terminates in vermis.

Afferents from the Periphery

1. *Dorsal spinocerebellar tract*
   - Enters the cerebellum through the inferior cerebellar peduncle.
   - Terminates in the vermis and intermediate zones of the cerebellum on the same side of its origin.
   - Carries signals mainly from muscle spindles, Golgi tendon organs, tactile receptors and joint receptors.
   - Inform the cerebellum about the momentary status of muscle contraction, degree of tension in the tendons, position and rate of movement of the parts of the body and forces acting on the surface of the body.
2. *Ventral spinocerebellar tract*
   - Enters the cerebellum through superior cerebellar peduncle.
   - Terminates on both sides of the cerebellum.
   - Tells the cerebellum which motor signals have arrived at the anterior horns of the spinal cord. This feedback is called the efference copy of the anterior horn motor drive.
3. *Cuneocerebellar tract*
   - Carries proprioceptive impulses from the arm and neck muscles.
   - Enters the cerebellum through inferior cerebellar peduncle.
   - Terminates in flocculonodular lobe and uvula.

Efferent Connections

There are three major efferent pathways:
1. From vermis of the cerebellum
   - Fastigial nucleus → pons and medulla.
   - Concerned with maintenance of posture and equilibrium.
2. From intermediate zone
   Interposed nucleus → ventrolateral and ventroanterior nuclei of thalamus → midline nuclei of thalamus → basal ganglia → red nucleus → reticular formation of brainstem.
   - Helps to coordinate the reciprocal contraction of agonist and antagonist muscles of hands and fingers.
3. Lateral zone → dentate nucleus → ventrolateral and ventroanterior nuclei of thalamus → cerebral cortex.

Concerned with coordination of sequential motor activities initiated by the cerebral cortex.

Functions of the Cerebellum (Fig. 11.41)

1. Control of Posture and Equilibrium

Vestibulocerebellum is responsible in controlling balance between agonist and antagonist muscle contractions of the spine, hips and shoulders during rapid changes in body positions. During control of equilibrium, the information from the periphery of the body and the vestibular apparatus is used to provide anticipatory correction of postural motor signals for maintaining equilibrium during rapid motion.

11

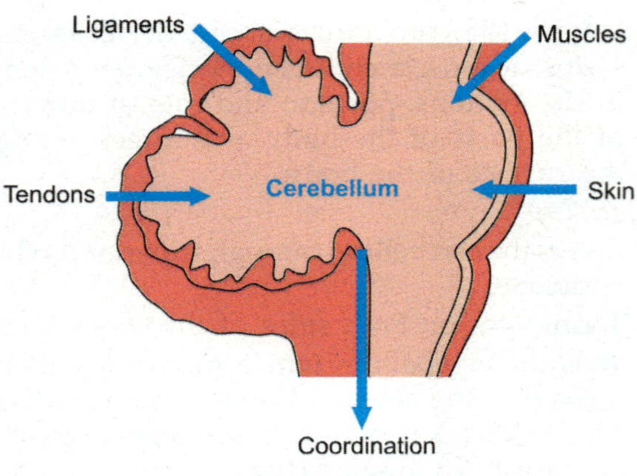

Fig. 11.41

2. *Comparator Function*

The intermediate zone of each cerebellar hemisphere receives two types of information, when a movement is performed:

1. Information from motor cortex and red nucleus telling about the intended sequential plan of movement for the next a few fractions of a second.
2. Information from the peripheral parts of the body telling cerebellum what actual movements result.

   The intermediate zone compares these signals and the corrective signals are sent by the deep nuclear cells to motor cortex and red nucleus. Which in-turn control the movements of the distal parts of the limbs.

3. *Damping action:* All the movements of the body are pendular in nature. For instance, when an arm is moved, a momentum develops. This momentum must be overcome before the movement can be stopped. Because of mementum, all the pendular movements have tendency to overshoot. But, an intact cerebellum stops the movement precisely at the intended point and prevents the overshoot. This is the basis of damping system provided by cerebellum.
4. *Control of ballistic movements:* Rapid movements of the body like movements of the eye, in which the jump from one position to the next when reading occurs so rapidly that it is not possible to receive feedback information either from the periphery to the cerebellum or from the cerebellum back to the motor cortex before the movements are over. These movements are called ballistic movements. The entire movement is preplanned and set into motion to go a specific distance and then to stop. Cerebellum is absolutely essential for the automatism of ballistic movements.
5. *Control of muscletone:* Cerebellum facilitates the muscletone of both axial msucles and distal limb muscles.
6. *Control of complex movements:* Cerebrocerebellum plays an important role in planning and timing of sequential movements, helping in smooth progression of movements.
7. *Learning motor act:* Cerebellum is concerned in the coordination of a motor task when it is performed again and again. Climbing fibers of the inferior olivary nucleus is responsible for producing long-term modification in the sensitivity of the Purkinje cells, thus making the motor task perfect.

11

Cerebellar Dysfunction

1. *Asynergia:* This means lack of coordination of voluntary movements.
2. *Dysmetria (pastpointing):* When a movement is attempted to touch an object with a finger, it overshoots the mark and lands beyond the object. This is due to failure to terminate the movement on time.
3. *Dysdiachokinesia:* It is inability to perform alternate movements rapidly, like rapidly alternating pronation and supination of the forearm.
4. *Intention tremor:* This is oscillatory movement that occurs only during a voluntary movement but absent at rest.
5. *Dysmetria:* The speech is slurring or scanning due to lack of coordination among the muscles of phonation.
6. *Hypotonia:* Lesion in the deep cerebellar nuclei causes decreased tone of the peripheral body musculature on the side of lesion.
7. *Rebound phenomenon:* When the patient is asked to move his forearm, with resistance applied by the observer and if the resistance is suddenly withdrawn, the forearm of the patient moves rapidly and bangs on his face. This is due to inability to stop the movement on time.
8. *Decomposition of movement:* The patient is unable to perform actions that involve stimultaneous motion at more than one joint at a time. This phenomenon is known as decomposition of movement.
9. *Gait:* The patient has wide-based unsteady, "drunken gait".
10. *Nystagmus:* It is the tremor of the eyeballs that occurs when one attempts to fixate the eyes on a scene.

105. THALAMUS

Introduction

The diencephalon consists of two parts (Fig. 11.42):
1. Thalamus
2. Hypothalamus

Thalamus is a large, egg-shaped, ovoid mass of gray matter having groups of nuclei. There are two thalami, one on each side of the midline. They are connected in their rostral portions by an intermediate mass and the caudal parts are separated by corpora quadrigemina.

THALAMIC NUCLEI

Functional Classification

On development and topographic grounds, thalamus can be divided into three parts:
1. The epithalamus
2. The ventral thalamus
3. The dorsal thalamus

1. *Epithalamus*

It consists of pineal body and habenular complex. It has connections to the olfactory system.

2. *Ventral Thalamus*

It is a thin sheet of cells present between the external medullary lamina and the posterior limb of internal capsule.

3. *Dorsal Thalamus*

It is divided into two groups:
1. Nuclei that project diffusely to the whole neocortex.
   a. Midline b. Intralaminar

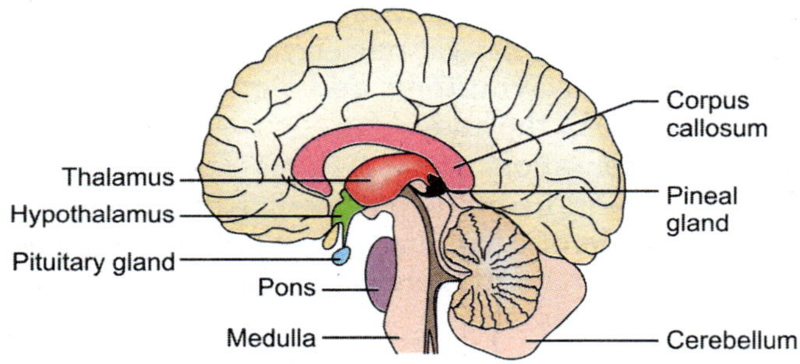

Fig. 11.42

2. Nuclei that project to special areas.

a. Special Sensory Relay Nuclei which Include

1. Medial geniculate body (MGB) and Lateral geniculate body (LGB)

Medial geniculate body (MGB)	Lateral geniculate body (LGB)
↓	↓
Relay auditory impulses to auditory cortex	Relay visual impulses to visual cortex

2. Ventrobasal nuclei which relay somesthetic information to posterior central gyrus.

b. Nuclei Concerned with Efferent Control Mechanism

1. Many nuclei concerned with motor functions which receive input from basal ganglia and cerebellum and project to motor cortex.
2. Anterior nuclei which receive afferents from mammillary bodies that project to limbic cortex.

Neuroanatomic Classification (Fig. 11.43)

Thalamus is divided into three groups by the internal medullary lamina consisting of white matter.

a. Lateral Group

Ventral group	*Dorsal group*
a. Ventral anterior	a. Pulvinar
b. Ventral lateral	b. Lateral posterior
c. Ventral posterior	c. Lateral dorsal
d. Medial geniculate body	
e. Lateral geniculate body	

b. Medial Group of Nuclei

They contain:
- Centromedian nuclei
- Dorsomedial nuclei
- Midline nuclei

c. Anterior Group of Nuclei

They are enclosed by the bifurcation of the internal medullary lamina.

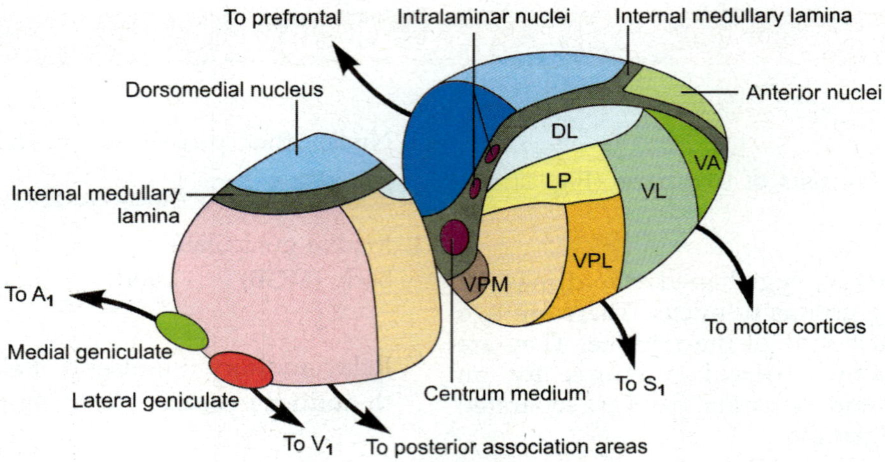

Fig. 11.43

Connections of the Thalamus

Midline nucleus	Globus pallidus, hypothalamus, cerebral cortex, reticular formation, midbrain.	Cerebral cortex, basal ganglia	Center for integrating crude visceral and somatic sensation
Intralaminar nuclei	RAS, trigeminal lemniscus, basal ganglia	Cerebral cortex, putamen, caudate nucleus	1. Integrates somatic and visceral sensory impulses 2. Responsible for altering effects of RAS
Medial nuclei • Anterior • Dorsomedial	Mammillary body	Cingulate gyrus of limbic cortex	Recent memory and emotions
Lateral mass			
Dorsolateral nucleus	Thalamic nuclei, parietal lobe	Cerebral cortex	Speech and complex integrated functions
Postero lateral nucleus	Parietal lobe	Parietal lobe	Association of sensations
Anterior ventral nucleus	Globus pallidus	Putamen, caudate nucleus, premotor cortex.	Integration of motor functions.
Lateral ventral nucleus	Dendate nucleus, red nucleus, globus pallidus	Premotor cortex, motor cortex, putamen	Proprioception and voluntary motor functions
Posterior ventral nucleus	Spinal cord, trigeminal nucleus	Sensory cortex, hypothalamus	Relay somatosensory and sensory impulses
Pulvinar	Parietal, occipital, temporal lobe	Cerebral cortex	Integrates auditory, visual and socratic information
MGB	Auditory tracts	Auditory cortex	Hearing
LGB	Optic tract	Visual cortex	Vision

Functions of Thalamus

1. *Relay center:* Thalamus functions as a relay center for almost all the sensations. The sensory information is processed, filtered and modulated and sent to cerebral cortex through thalamocortical fibers. It also acts as a relay center for motor signals from motor cortex, basal ganglia and cerebellum and modulates their activity.
2. *Arousal and alertness:* Thalamus plays an important role in arousal and alertness reactions along with RAS.
3. It is responsible for subcortical perception of sensation, e.g. pain.
4. *Memory:* Thalamus plays a role in short-term memory and emotions.
5. *Sleep:* It is an integrating center for sleep.
6. It also plays a role in language function (speech).

Applied Physiology

Thalamic Syndrome

Blockage due to thrombosis of thalamogeniculate branch of posterior cerebral artery damages postero ventro and posterolateral nuclei resulting in thalamic syndrome. The symptoms and signs occur on the opposite side of the body.

1. Loss of sensation
2. *Asteriognosis:* Inability to recognize the shape, size and texture of a familiar object with closed eyes due to lesion in the connection with the posterior parietal cortex.
3. *Sensory ataxia:* Due to loss of conscious proprioception.

4. *Thalamic phantom limb:* Inability to locate the parts of the body and position of a limb and the patient searches in the air to locate them.
5. *Amelognosia:* An illusion that the person feels that there is no limb at all due to loss of position sense.
6. *Thalamic over reaction:* The person feels spontaneous pain and the threshold for pain is very much reduced. The person develops unpleasantness even for touch and cold sensations. Sometimes he feels pain even in the absence of pain stimulus. This is due to overactivity of medial nuclei which escapes the lesion.
7. *Thalamic hand:* Abnormal posture of the hand characterized by flexion at wrist with hyper extension of fingers.
8. *Involuntary movements*
   - *Athetosis:* Slow writhing and twisting movements.
   - *Chorea:* Quick jerky dancing movements.
   - *Intentional tremors:* Tremor occurs while attempting to do any voluntary movements.
9. *Emotional instability:* The person may go into unprovoked laughing or crying.
10. *Disturbance in sleep:* Wakefulness cycle.
11. *Loss of recent memory.*

106. HYPOTHALAMUS

Physiological Anatomy

Hypothalamus is a diencephalic structure situated below the thalamus. It extends from optic chiasm anteriorly to mammillary body posteriorly.

Nuclei of Hypothalamus

Hypothalamic nuclei are divided into three groups:
1. Anterior or preoptic group
2. Middle or tuberal group
3. Posterior or mammillary group.

HYPOTHALAMIC NUCLEI (Fig. 11.44)

Nuclei of Hypothalamus

1. *Anterior Group*

- Preoptic nucleus
- Paraventricular nucleus
- Anterior nucleus
- Supraoptic nucleus
- Suprachiasmatic nucleus.

2 *Middle Group*

- Dorsomedial nucleus
- Ventromedial nucleus
- Lateral nucleus
- Arcuate (tuberal) nucleus.

3. *Posterior Group*

- Posterior nucleus
- Mammillary body.

Connections of Hypothalamus

Afferent Connections

1. *Limbic System*

- *Medial forebrain bundle:* From limbic cortex to preoptic nucleus, lateral nucleus and mammillary body.
- *Stria terminalis:* From amygdala to preoptic nucleus.
- *Fornix:* From hippocampus to mammillary body.
- *Corticohypothalamic fibers:* From areas 6 and 8 of cerebral cortex to supraoptic and paraventricular nuclei of hypothalamus.

2. *Brainstem*

From reticular formation of brainstem to diffuse areas of hypothalamus.

3. *Thalamus*

Thalamohypothalamic fibers extend from dorsomedial and midline nuclei of thalamus to hypothalamus.

4. *Basal Ganglia*

Pallidohypothalamic fibers extend from lenticular nucleus (putamen and globus pallidus) to hypothalamus.

5. *Retina*

Retinohypothalamic fibers connect optic chiasm with suprachiasmatic nucleus of hypothalamus.

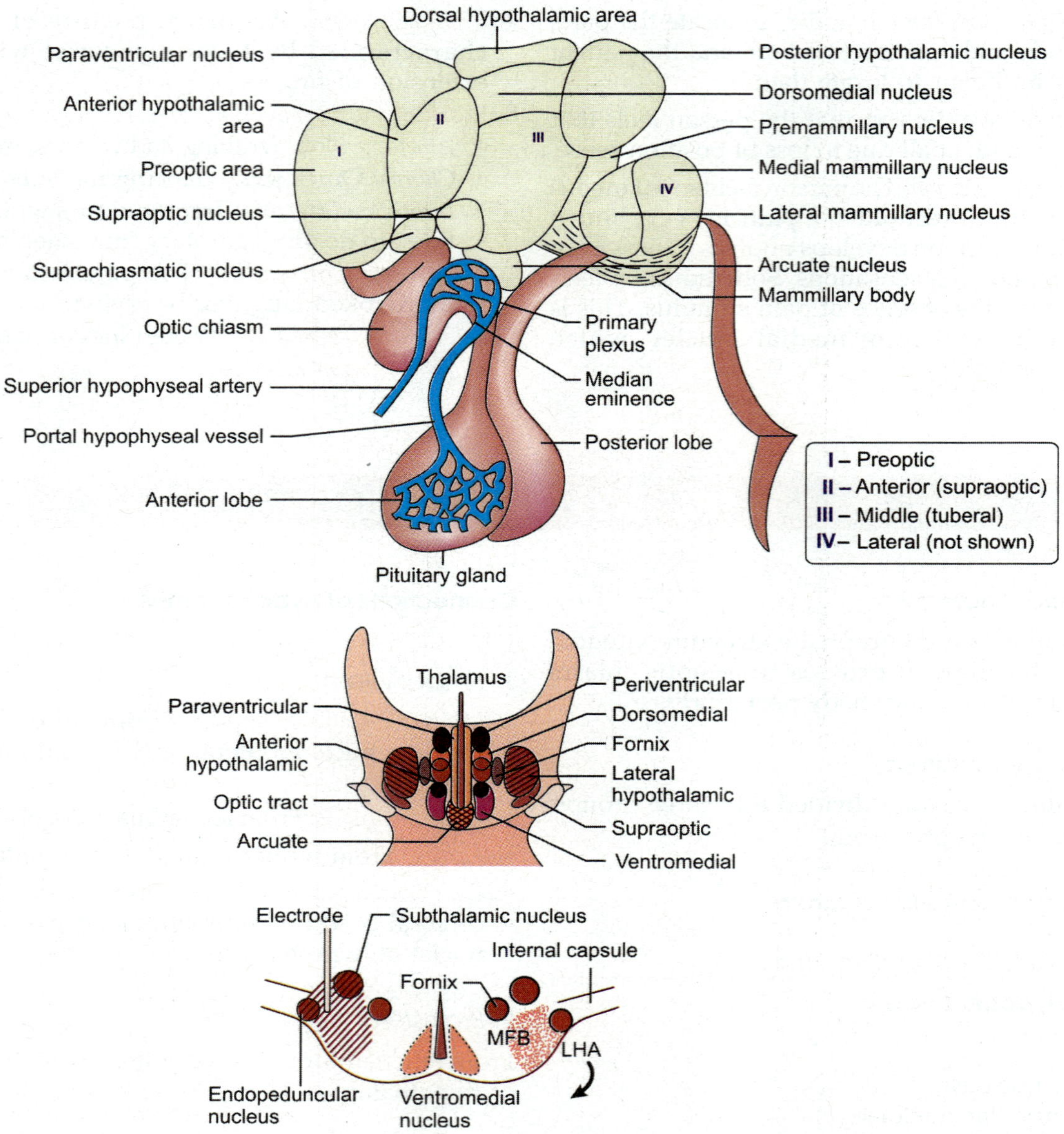

Fig. 11.44: Nuclei of hypothalamus

Efferent Connections

1. Mammillothalamic tract from mammillary body to anterior thalamic nuclei.
2. Mammillotegmental tract from mammillary body to the tegmental nuclei of midbrain.
3. Hypothalamic-hypophysial tract from supraoptic and paraventricular nuclei of hypothalamus to posterior pituitary (Fig. 11.45).
4. Periventricular fibers from posterior, supraoptic and tuberal nuclei of hypothalamus pass through periventricular gray matter to reticular formation in brainstem, dorsomedial nucleus of thalamus and frontal lobe.

Functions of Hypothalamus (Fig. 11.46)

1. Regulation of Body Temperature

Hypothalamus acts as a thermostat in our body to maintain a constant body temperature (37°C). Anterior hypothalamus is concerned with heat loss and posterior hypothalamus is concerned with heat production.

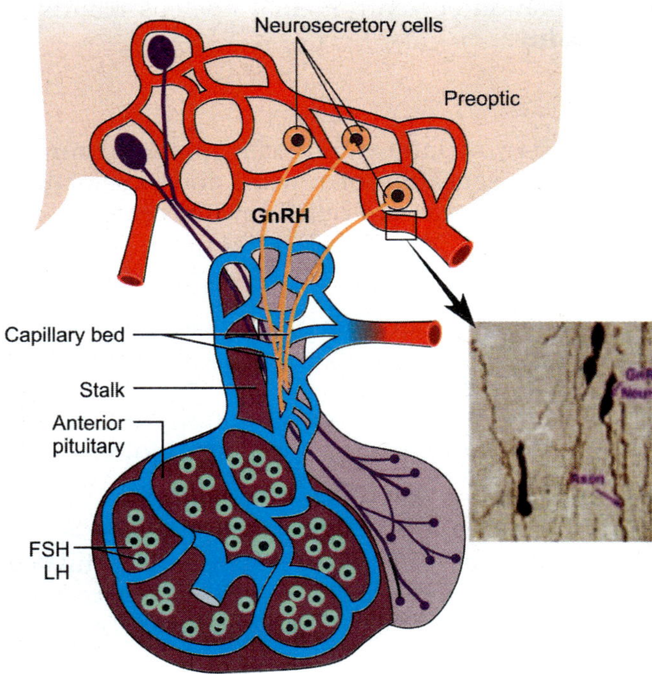

Fig. 11.45: Hypothalamic-hypophyseal axis

2. *Endocrine Function*

Anterior Pituitary

Hypothalamus releases following factors to control the secretion of hormones by anterior pituitary:

- Growth hormone releasing hormone (GHRH)
- Growth hormone inhibiting hormone (GHIH)
- Thyrotropin releasing hormone (TRH)
- Corticotropin releasing hormone (CRH)
- Gonadotropin releasing hormone (GnRH)
- Prolactin inhibitory hormone (PIH).

Posterior Pituitary

Antidiuretic hormone (ADH) and oxytocin secreted by supraoptic and paraventricular nuclei of hypothalamus. They are transported through hypothalamohypophysial tract into posterior pituitary to be stored and released.

Adrenal Medulla

Stimulation of dorsomedial and posterior hypothalamic nuclei produce increased adrenal medullary secretion of catecholamine.

3. *Control of Circadian Rhythm*

Certain physiological processes in our body occur regularly in cycles of 24 hours. This is called circardian rhythm (circa=around the day). The suprachiasmatic nucleus of hypothalamus plays an important role in setting the biological clock by its connection with retina via retinohypothalamic fibers.

4. *Control of Food Intake*

There is a feeding center in the lateral hypothalamus and a satiety center in the ventromedial nucleus. These two centers regulate food intake.

There are four main hypotheses about the mechanisms involved in the control of food intake.

a. *Lipostatic Hypothesis*

This states that adipose tissue produces a humoral signal that is proportionate to the amount of fat which acts on the hypothalamus to decrease food intake and increase energy output. The hormone is called leptin.

b. *Gut Peptide Hypothesis*

This postulates that food in the GIT causes the release of some polypeptides which act on the hypothalamus to inhibit food intake.

c. *Glucostatic Hypothesis*

This states that increased glucose utilization in the hypothalamus produces a sensation of satiety.

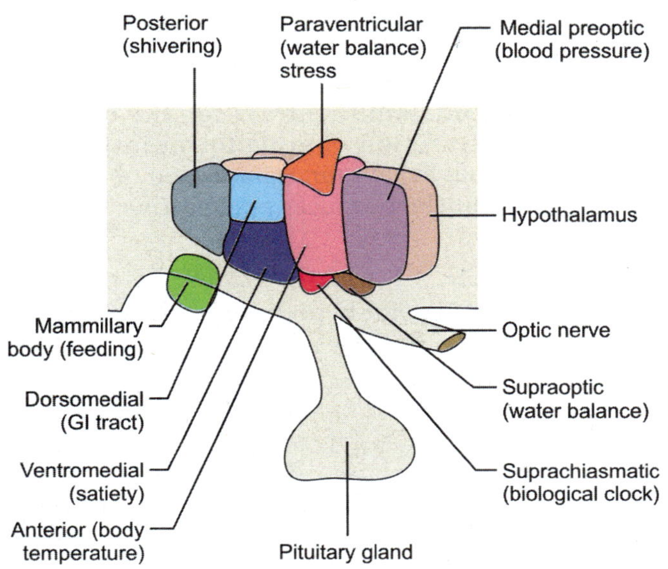

Fig. 11.46: Functions of hypothalamus

d. *Thermostatic Hypothesis*

This states that a fall in body temperature below a given set point stimulates appetite and a rise above the set point inhibits appetite.

5. *Regulation of Water Balance of the Body*

Hypothalamus regulates the body fluids by following mechanisms:

a. There are osmoreceptors in the supraoptic nucleus of hypothalamus which are sensitive to changes in the osmolarity of ECF and plasma. When there is excess water loss, the increase in plasma and ECF osmolarity stimulates osmoreceptors which in-turn increases ADH secretion. ADH increases water reabsorption from renal tubules. On the other hand, in water loading, the fall in plasma and ECF osmolarity inhibits osmoreceptors and ADH secretion. This decreases renal reabsorption of water and restores water balance.
b. *Thirst mechanism:* There is a thirst center in the lateral hypothalamus. Increase in ECF osmolarity stimulates this center and promotes water drinking.

6. *Control of Autonomic Nervous System*

'Hypothalamus may be called as the head ganglion of ANS' were the words by Sherrington. The posterior and lateral nuclei control the sympathetic nervous system. Anterior nuclei were thought to be parasympathetic control center but now it is concluded that there is no specific parasympathetic center.

7. *Control of Sexual Functions*

By means of gonadotropin releasing hormone (GnRH), hypothalamus influences the onset of puberty and secretion of gonadotropins. It also influences sexual behaviour. Stimulation of anterior and posterior nuclei produces sexual drive.

8. *Control of Emotions*

a. Stimulation of lateral hypothalamus increases the anger and rage (intense anger).
b. Stimulation of ventromedial nucleus results in placidity.

Reward Centers

Stimulation of lateral and ventromedial nuclei produces a sensation of reward and satisfaction. Hence, these nuclei are called reward centers.

Punishment Centers

Stimulation of a thin zone of periventricular nuclei and periaqueductal nuclei produces unpleasant sensations like fear, pain, terror, defense, escape reactions and other elements of punishment. Hence, these nuclei are called as punishment centers.

9. *Influences on Sleep*

The existence of a sleep center has been postulated in the posterior hypothalamus. It is concerned with the diurnal rhythm of sleep and wakefulness.

10. *Relation to Stress*

During stress, corticotropin releasing hormone (CRH) is released by hypothalamus which causes release of ACTH from anterior pituitary. ACTH releases glucocorticoids from adrenal cortex to tackle the stress.

Applied Physiology

Lesions in various nuclei of hypothalamus can produce the following diseases:

1. *Narcolepsy:* Irresistable desire to sleep during work.
2. *Cataplexy:* Sudden loss of muscle tone during emotions resulting in falling of the subject to the ground.
3. *Anorexia nervosa:* Person is afraid of gaining weight, reduces food intake and may starve to death.
4. *Bulimia:* A recurrent episode of over eating followed by self-induced vomiting with fear of gaining weight.

107. CEREBRAL CORTEX

Introduction

There are two cerebral hemispheres separated by a deep vertical fissure. The separation is complete anteriorly and posteriorly. But in the middle, the two hemispheres are joined by a band of commissural fibers called corpus callosum. The cerebrum is made up of outer thinner gray matter called cerebral cortex and inner thicker white matter.

Cerebral cortex is characterized by depressions called sulci (singular-sulcus) and elevations called gyri (singular-gyrus).

Histology of the Cerebral Cortex

There are six layers in cerebral cortex.

1. *Molecular or Plexiform Layer*

This layer is the most superficial layer containing a few fusiform cells.

2. *External Granular Layer*

This layer consists of large number of small, round or polygonal cells closely packed together. Their dendrites pass to outer layer and axons enter the deeper layers.

3. *Outer Pyramidal Layer*

It consists of medium sized pyramidal cells in the outer part and larger pyramidal cells in the deeper portion.

4. *Internal Granular Layer*

This layer contains stellate shaped cells. There are plenty of horizontal fibers seen as outer line of Baillarger. This band is prominent in the calcarine cortex where it is referred to as line of Gennari.

5. *Internal Pyramidal Layer*

This layer consists of pyramidal cells of graded sizes. It is well-developed in motor cortex. The pyramidal cells in this region are otherwise known as Betz cells. It also contains cells of Martinotti. The cells of this layer give rise to pyramid, corticopontine and corticorubral fibers.

6. *Fusiform Cell Layer*

This layer is composed of closely packed small spindle shaped cells.

Neocortex (Isocortex, Neopallium)

The major portion of the cerebral cortex that has all six layers is called neocortex.

Allocortex

The remaining part of the cerebral cortex that has less than six layers is called allocortex. It is present in limbic system.

Lobes of the Cerebral Cortex (Fig. 11.47)

The cerebral cortex can be divided into four lobes by three deep sulci or fissures:

1. *Frontal lobe:* In front of central sulcus
2. *Parietal lobe:* Between central sulcus and parieto-occipital sulcus
3. *Occipital lobe:* Behind parieto-occipital sulcus
4. *Temporal lobe:* Below the Sylvian fissure.

BRODMANN AREAS

Brodmann area is a region of cerebral cortex defined on the basis of organization of cells. There are about 50 Brodmann areas. They were originally described by Korbinian Brodmann.

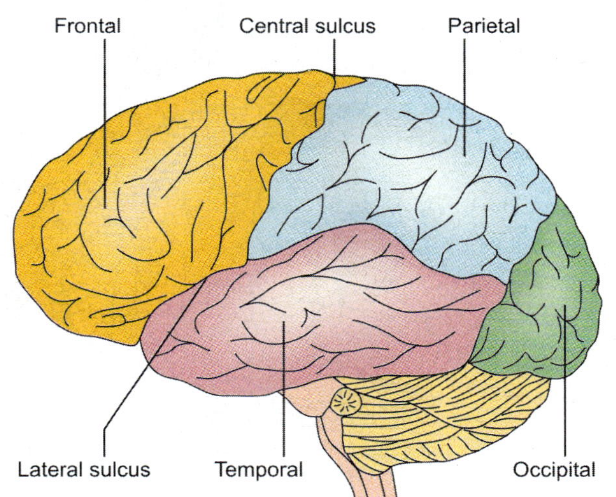

Fig. 11.47

11

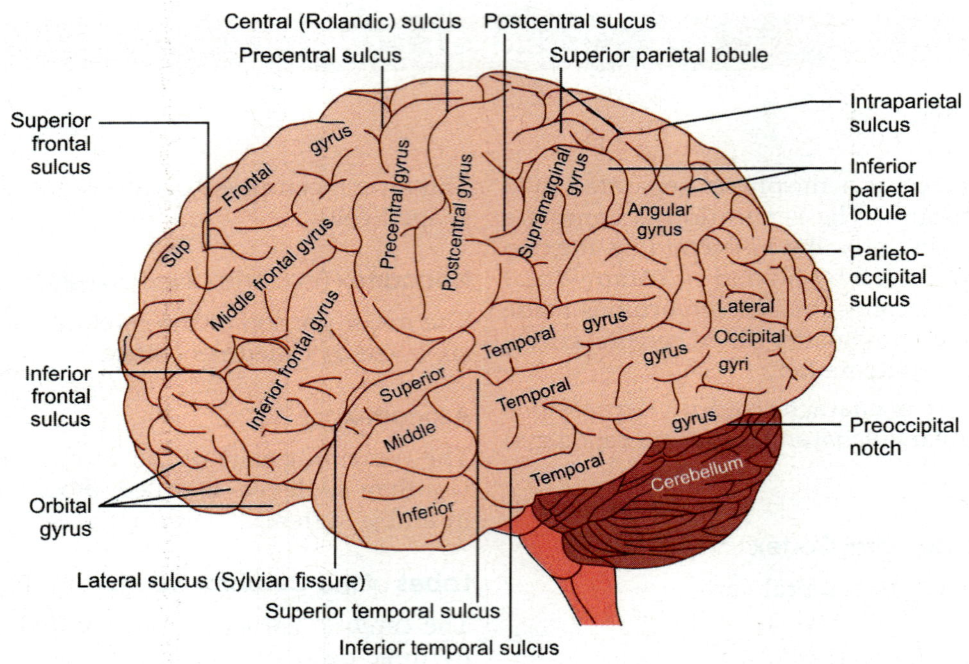

Fig. 11.48

Frontal Lobe (Fig. 11.48)

It is divided into two parts:

- Precentral cortex
- Prefrontal cortex

Precentral Cortex

This is the area in the lip of central sulcus, whole of precentral gyrus and posterior portions of superior, middle and inferior frontal gyri. This is further divided into three areas:

1. Primary motor area (Fig. 11.49)
2. Premotor area
3. Supplementary motor area.

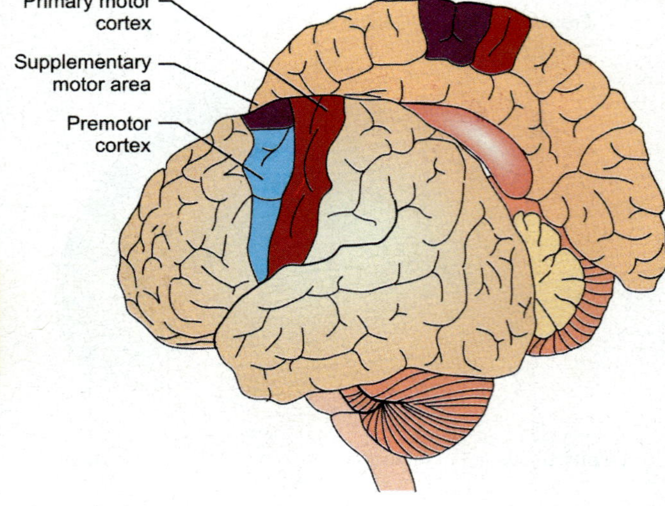

Fig. 11.49

Primary Motor Area (Area 4, Motor Cortex)

It includes precentral gyrus and the adjoining lip of central sulcus. This area is rich in giant pyramidal cells called Betz cells.

Motor homunculus: The muscles of the body are represented in this area. The order of representation is from medial to lateral surface in toes, ankle, knee, hip, trunk, shoulder, arm, elbow, wrist, hand, fingers, and face (Fig. 11.50). This representation is called motor homunculus. The features of the representation are:

- It is contralateral
- Inverted except for the face
- Area depends upon the functional significance and not on the size of the part.

Function of area 4: This is the higher center for voluntary movements.

Area 4s: It is called suppressor area. It forms a narrow strip anterior to area 4. It suppresses the movements elicited from area 4. It also projects to basal ganglia and is concerned with inhibition of stretch reflexes.

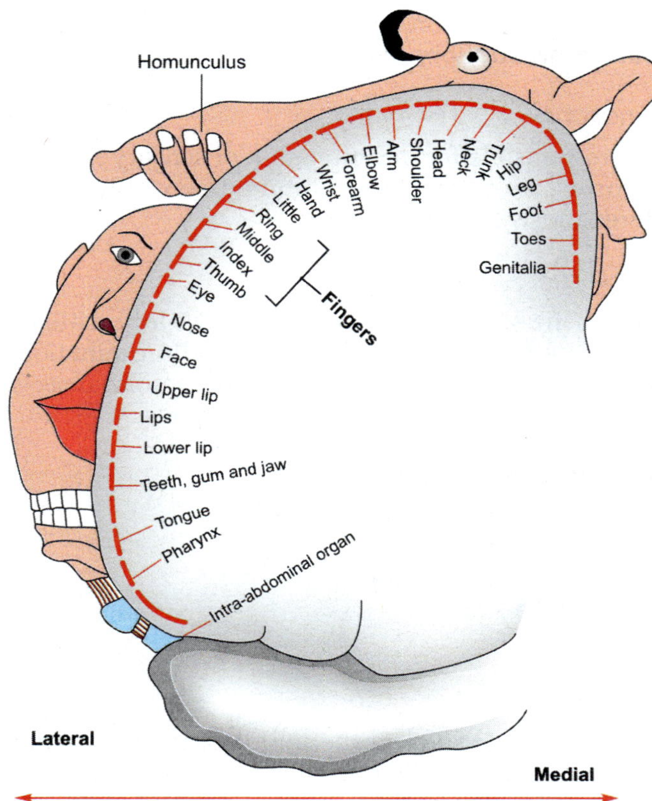

Fig. 11.50: Somatomotor map

Premotor Area

It is situated in front of area 4 and 4s. Fibers from this area project to area 4 and basal ganglia. It gives fibers to the pyramidal tract.

Function: It is concerned with coordination of movements initiated by area 4.

Supplementary Motor Area

It lies on the medial surface of the hemisphere in front of areas 4 and 6. It projects to motor cortex.

Function: It provides a background for fine, complex movements from the motor cortex.

Other Areas

Area 8: It is called frontal eye field. It lies anterior to area 6 in middle frontal gyrus. It receives fibers from occipital cortex (areas 18 and 19) and projects to the oculomotor nuclei in the brainstem.

Function: It is concerned with movement of the head and eyes towards the objects to be seen.

Area 44 (Broca's Area)

This area is present in the left hemisphere (dominant hemisphere) of right handed persons and vice versa. It is situated in inferior frontal gyrus.

Function: It is the motor area for speech.

Prefrontal Cortex

It is the anterior part of the frontal lobe in front of areas 6, 8 and 44. It includes structures on the lateral, medial and orbital surfaces. Areas present here are 9–14, 23, 24, 32 and 45–47.

Connections

Afferents

- Dorsomedial nucleus of thalamus
- Hypothalamus
- Hippocampus

Efferents

- Thalamus
- Hypothalamus
- Caudate nucleus
- Tegmentum of midbrain
- Reticular formation

Functions

It forms the center for higher functions like emotion, learning and memory.

It plays an important role in planning complex motor activities.

FRONTAL LOBE SYNDROME

The lesion in the prefrontal cortex may be due to trauma or tumor. The changes are mainly in personality and behavior.

Features

1. Distractability: Difficulty in fixing attention
2. Inability to solve complex problems
3. Lack of initiative
4. Impairment in recent memory
5. Inability to realize the seriousness of a situation and a general sense of well-being (euphoria).
6. Loss of love or responsibility for the family
7. Emotional instability
8. Increased appetite, tremors and bladder control impairment may also occur.

PARIETAL LOBE

It extends from central sulcus and merges with occipital lobe behind and temporal lobe below. It has three important areas:

1. Somatosensory area I
2. Somatosensory area II
3. Somesthetic association area.

Somatosensory Area I (Primary Sensory Cortex)

This includes areas 3, 1 and 2.

Sensory Homunculus

The different sensory areas of the body are represented in this primary sensory area (post central gyrus). The representation is contralateral except for the face which is bilaterally represented. It is also inverted except for the face as the representation in motor area. The toes are represented in lowest part of medial surface, legs at the upper border of the hemisphere and knee, thigh, hip, trunk, upper limb, neck and face from above downwards. This representation is called sensory homunculus. Those parts of the body which are more used for acquiring sensory information have a larger area of representation as they have more receptors.

Functions

- It is the area for perception and integration of cutaneous and kinesthetic sensations.
- It is concerned with movements of head and eyeball.
- It is also concerned with recognition of discrimination features like tactile sensations, two point discrimination, etc.

Somatosensory Area II

This area lies in the upper wall of Sylvian fissure below the face area of somesthetic area I. It receives sensory impulses from somesthetic area I and thalamus.

Functions

11

The exact function is not clear. It probably receives crude sensations and vibration sense from the pacinian corpuscle.

Somesthetic Association Area

This area is situated posterior to post-central gyrus above the auditory cortex and in front of visual cortex. It has two areas, area 5 and 7. It receives sensory information from sensory area I, thalamus, visual and auditory cortex.

Functions

It is responsible for interpretation of sensory signals. It forms the center for combined sensations like stereognosis.

Applied Physiology

Lesion in sensory areas in parietal lobe causes impairment of tactile localization and discrimination. It also leads to inability to recognize familiar objects with eyes closed. It is called astereognosis.

Temporal Lobe (Fig. 11.51)

There are three areas in the lobe:

1. Auditory areas 41, 42
2. Area for equilibrium
3. Wernicke's area

1. Auditory Areas Include Areas 41, 42, and Wernicke's Area (Area 22)

Area 41: It is located in the middle part of superior temporal gyrus partly buried in Sylvian fissure. It is concerned with perception of frequency intensity and direction of sound.

Area 42: It is located immediately below and surrounding area 41. This area also perceives sound.

Wernicke's Area (Area 22) (Fig. 11.52)

It occupies superior temporal gyrus. This is called area of intelligence. It is concerned with comprehension of both spoken and written words.

Area for Equilibrium

This area is in the posterior part of the superior temporal gyrus. It is concerned with maintenance of equilibrium of the body.

Connections of Temporal Lobe

It is connected with:

- Thalamus
- Hypothalamus
- Amygdala
- Hippocampus
- Pyriform cortex
- Frontal lobe
- Occipital lobe
- Cranial nuclei II, IV and VI

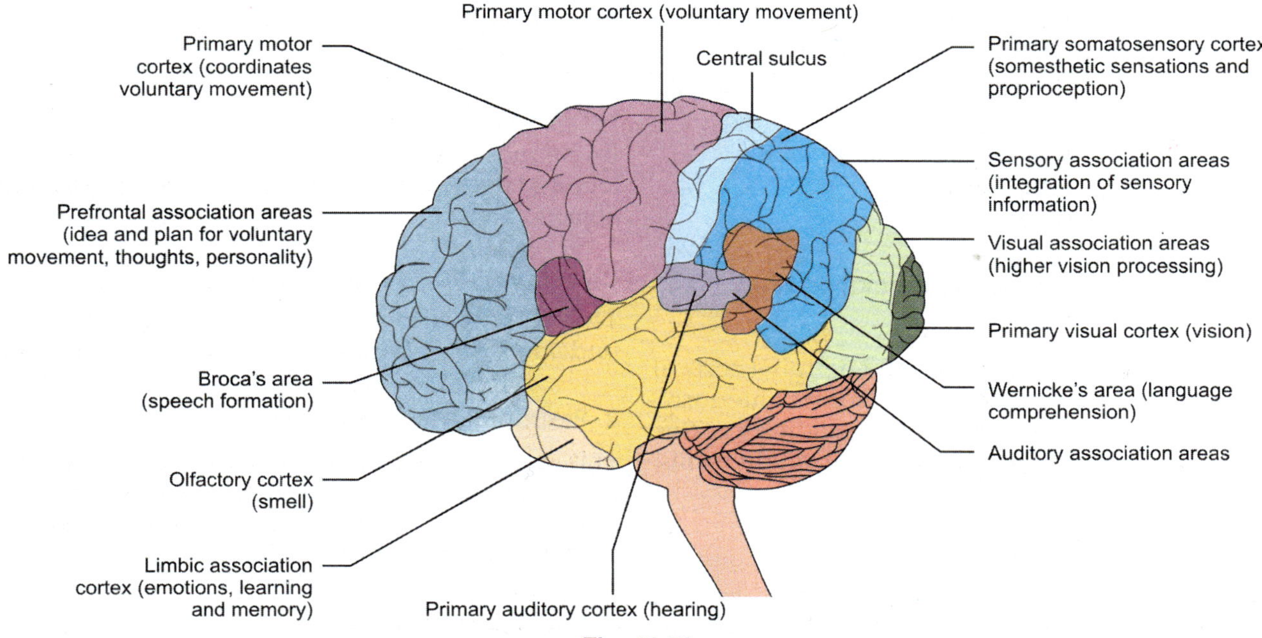

Fig. 11.51

KLUVER-BUCY SYNDROME

It is also known as temporal lobe syndrome. Bilateral lesion in temporal lobe causes this syndrome.

Features

There is placidity and loss of fear:
- Hypersexuality not only to opposite sex but also to same sex
- Extreme curiosity about everything
- Tendency to place everything in mouth
- Dreaming state
- Impairment of recent memory
- Aphasia

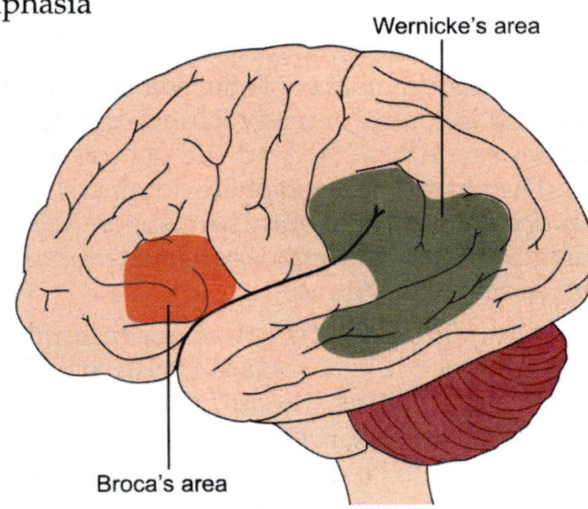

Fig. 11.52

Occipital Lobe

This contains visual areas 17,18 and 19.
- *Area 17:* Primary visual cortex
- *Area 18:* Visual association areas
- *Area 19:* Occipital eye field

Connections

It receives afferents from lateral geniculate body of thalamus. It sends efferents to lateral geniculate body and superior colliculus.

Functions

- *Area 17* is concerned with perception of visual impulses.
- *Area 18* is concerned with interpretation of visual impulses.
- *Area 19* is concerned with movement of eyes.

Applied Physiology

Unilateral lesion in the visual cortex leads to hemianopia. Bilateral lesion leads to complete blindness.

ASSOCIATION AREAS

There are some areas of cerebral cortex that do not fit into rigid categories of primary and secondary motor and sensory areas. These areas are called association areas because they receive and analyze signals from multiple areas of motor and sensory cortex and also from subcortical structures.

There are three important association areas (Fig. 11.53):

- Parieto-occipitotemporal association area
- Prefrontal association area
- Limbic association area.

1. Parieto-occipitotemporal Association Area

Situation

It is located in the large parietal and occipital cortical space bounded by somatosensory cortex anteriorly, the visual cortex posteriorly, and the auditory cortex laterally. This area has some functional subdivisions:

a. *Area of Analysis of the Spatial Coordination of the Body*

An area beginning in the posterior parietal cortex and extending into the superior occipital cortex provides continuous analysis of the spatial coordination of all parts of the body and of the surroundings of the body. This area receives visual sensory information from the posterior occipital cortex and somatosensory information from parietal cortex. From all this information, it computes the coordination of the visual, auditory and body surroundings.

b. *Area for Initial Processing of Visual Language (Reading)*

This area lies posterior to the Wernicke's area in the anterolateral region of the occipital lobe. This area feeds visual information conveyed by words read from a book into Wernicke's area. This is called angular gyrus.

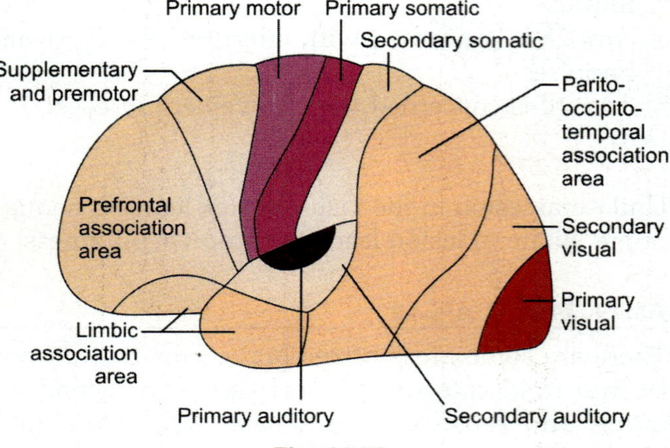

Fig. 11.53

This area is needed to make meaning out of visually perceived words.

c. *Area for Naming Objects*

In the most lateral portions of the anterior occipital lobe and posterior temporal lobe in the area for naming objects.

d. *Area for Recognition of Faces*

This area is situated on the medial side of the undersurface of both occipital and temporal lobes.

2. Prefrontal Association Area

This area functions in close association with the motor cortex to plan complex patterns and sequences of motor movements. It is also essential to carry out thought processes in the mind.

3. Limbic Association Area (Fig. 11.53)

This area is found in the anterior pole of the temporal lobe in the ventral portion of the frontal lobe and in the cingulate gyrus. It is concerned with behavior, emotions and motivation.

Applied Physiology

Lesions in area for face recognition leads to a condition called prosophenosia or prosopagnosia. The subject is unable to recognize the known persons by looking at them, though he can identify them from their voices.

Acalculia: Lesions in frontoparietal areas can cause inability to solve mathematical problems. This is called acalculia.

CEREBRAL DOMINANCE

It is defined as the dominance of one cerebral hemisphere over the other in control of cerebral function. It is related to handedness. About 90% of the people are right handed. They have left hemisphere dominant which is called as dominant or categorical hemisphere. It controls the analytical process and language related functions like speech, reading and writing.

The right hemisphere is called representational hemisphere since it is associated with artistic and visuospatial functions like judging the distance, determining the direction, etc. Lesion in the dominant hemisphere leads to language disorders and lesion in representational hemisphere causes only mild effects like astereognosis.

108. RETICULAR FORMATION

Definition

Reticular formation consists of a diffuse aggregation of neurons interconnected by a network of nerve fibers.

Location

Reticular formation is situated in the central portion of brainstem. It extends downwards into spinal cord and upwards into thalamus and hypothalamus. There are about 50–98 nuclear masses which are all interconnected.

Reticular formation is absolutely essential for life because it includes the various centers like respiratory center, deglutition center, vomiting center, cardiovascular center, etc.

Connections

Afferents

1. Spinal cord via spinoreticular tract.
2. Collateral fibers from all ascending tracts like:
   - Optic pathway
   - Auditory pathway
   - Olfactory pathway
   - Taste pathway
   - Anterolateral column
   - Dorsal-column medial-lemniscal pathway.
3. Cerebellum (cerebelloreticular).
4. Basal ganglia.
5. Tectum (superior and inferior colliculi).
6. Neocortex—corticoreticular fibers from sensory, motor, orbital, preorbital, parietal and temporal lobes, cingulate gyrus and collaterals from corticofugal fibers.
7. Limbic system including amygdala and hippocampus.

Efferents

1. Cerebral cortex.
2. Thalamus, subthalamic nuclei and hypothalamus.
3. Red nucleus, substantia nigra and tectum in midbrain.
4. Cerebellum.
5. Cranial nerve nuclei in brainstem.
6. Spinal cord.

Neurotransmitters Involved in Activation of Brain

- *Norepinephrine:* Released from locus ceruleus situated at the juncture between pons and the midbrain.
- *Dopamine:* Released from substantia nigra in basal ganglia.
- *Serotonin:* Released from raphe nuclei situated in the middle of pons and medulla.
- *Acetylcholine:* Released from gigantocellular neurons in the reticular area.

Functions of Reticular Formation

Based on the function, reticular formation along with its connections are divided into two systems:

1. Ascending reticular activating system (ARAS).
2. Descending reticular activating system (DRAS).

Ascending Reticular Activating System

ARAS is also called as reticular activating system (RAS).

Location

It is a complex polysynaptic pathway which extends from the lower pons through midbrain and thalamus and projects throughout the cerebral cortex. Throughout its course, it receives afferents from all ascending pathways (Fig. 11.54).

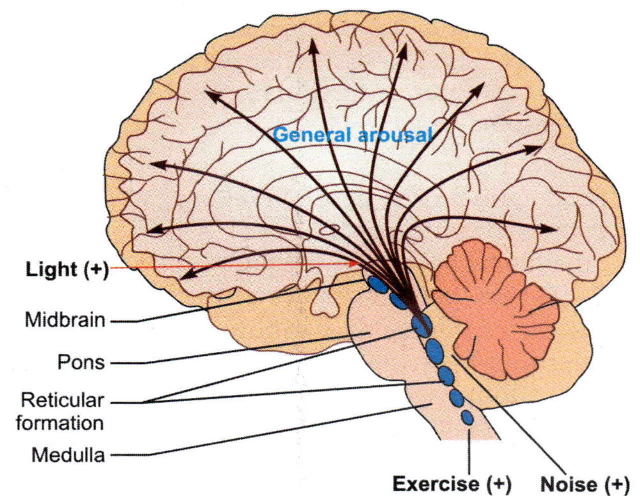

Fig. 11.54: Reticular activating system (RAS)

11

Mechanism of Action of RAS

The impulses of all sensations ascend to cerebral cortex through two channels.

1. *Classical or specific sensory pathways:* These are the pathways which transmit the sensory impulses from receptors to cerebral cortex via thalamus.
2. *Nonspecific sensory pathways:* All the sensory pathways send collaterals to ARAS which is a multisynaptic relay system. These collaterals project to different areas of ARAS. ARAS in-turn sends impulses to all areas of cerebral cortex.

Functions of ARAS

1. ARAS is responsible for arousal, alertness and wakefulness. RAS can also be activated from cortex, especially from orbitofrontal cortex, superior- temporal gyrus, cingulate gyrus, sensory and motor cortex. This is responsible for the alert responses during emotions and muscular work.
2. It influences learning and memory.
3. It plays an important role in development of conditioned reflex.

Descending Reticular System

Descending reticular system includes the fibers that descend from reticular formation in brainstem to spinal cord as reticulospinal tracts. This system has two divisions:

1. Descending facilitatory reticular system (DFRS).
2. Descending inhibitory reticular system (DIRS).

Descending Facilitatory Reticular System

Reticular formation sends facilitatory fibers to extra-pyramidal tracts. The vestibular nuclei also produce facilitatory influence to spinal motor neurons via vestibulospinal tracts.

Functions

1. It maintains muscle tone by exciting gamma motor neurons in spinal cord.
2. It maintains posture and equilibrium.
3. It facilitates the movements of the body.
4. It is the center for facilitation of the autonomic functions such as cardiovascular functions, respiration, gastrointestinal function and body temperature (vegetative functions).

11

Descending Inhibitory Reticular System

Location

The ventromedial part of the medulla is the site of the bulbar inhibitory reticular system. This area is under the influence of the inhibitory areas of the cerebral cortex and caudate nucleus of the basal ganglia. The anterior lobe and paramedian lobules of cerebellum also project via fastigial nucleus to the medullary region and reinforces the inhibitory influence upon the spinal neurons.

Functions

1. It decreases the muscle tone by inhibiting the gamma motor neuron.
2. It is responsible for smooth voluntary movements.
3. It controls the reflex movements.
4. It is the center for inhibition of several autonomic and visceral functions like cardiovascular function, respiration, etc.
5. It modulates the pain transmission.
6. It acts as a filter which allows only important sensory information to the centre.

The signals passing through the thalamus are of two types

1. One type is rapidly transmitted action potential that excites the cerebrum for only a few milliseconds. They originate from large neurons in reticular formation in brainstem.
2. The second type of excitatory signals originate from large numbers of small neurons in brainstem reticular area. They pass to thalamus through small slowly conducting fibers. The excitatory effect produced by these fibers persist for many seconds to a minute or more. These signals are important for controlling long-term background excitability of the brain.

Neurotransmitters involved in activation of brain

1. *Norepinephrine:* Released from locus ceruleus situated at the juncture between pons and the mid-brain.
2. *Dopamine:* Released from substantia nigra in basal ganglia.
3. *Serotonin:* Released from raphe nuclei situated in the middle of pons and medulla.
4. *Acetylcholine:* Released from gigantocellular neurons in the reticular area.

109. LIMBIC SYSTEM

Definition

Limbic system is a complex system of cortical and subcortical structure that forms a ring around the brainstem. Limbic = border. Earlier it was called as rhinencephalon (Fig. 11.55).

Histology

The limbic cortex is the phylogenetically oldest part of the cerebral cortex. Histologically it consists of three layers.

1. *Allocortex*

- It has only three layers
- Surrounds the hilum of the hemisphere, e.g. hippocampus.

2. *Juxtallocortex*

- Lies between allocortex and neocortex
- It has 3 to 6 layers
- For example, cingulate gyrus and insula.

3. *Neocortex*

- It has 6 layers
- The most highly developed type
- The greatest development is seen in humans.

Components

1. Hypothalamus
2. Thalamus
3. Septal nuclei
4. Paraolfactory area
5. Hippocampus
6. Amygdala
7. Orbitofrontal cortex
8. Subcallosal gyrus
9. Cingulate gyrus
10. Parahippocampal gyrus
11. Olfactory nuclei.

Connections

1. *Fornix*

It includes fibers from hippocampus, uncus and amygdala (Fig. 11.56).

2. *Medial Forebrain Bundle*

Extends from the septal and orbitofrontal regions to the brainstem reticular formation through the middle of hypothalamus.

3. *Papez Circuit*

This was described by James Papez. Hippocampus is connected to mammillary bodies of hypothalamus via fornix. Mammillary bodies are connected to anterior thalamic nucleus via mammillothalamic tract. Anterior thalamic nucleus projects into cingulate gyrus through medial thalamocortical fibers. Cingulate gyrus is in-turn connected to hippocampus. Papez circuit plays an important role in memory.

Functions of Limbic System

1. *Behavior and emotion:* Hippocampus, amygdala and hypothalamus play an important role in emotions.

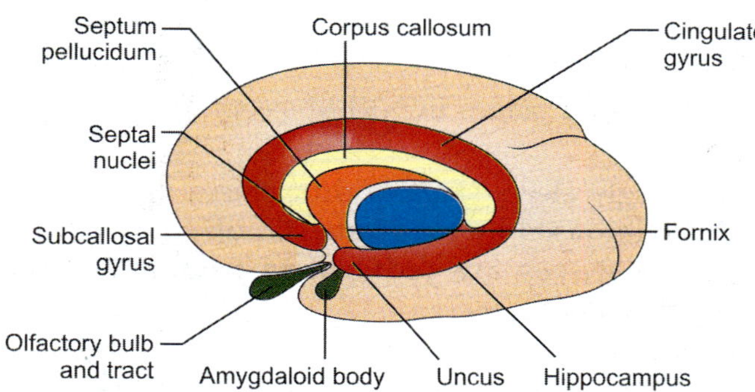

Fig. 11.55: Limbic structures

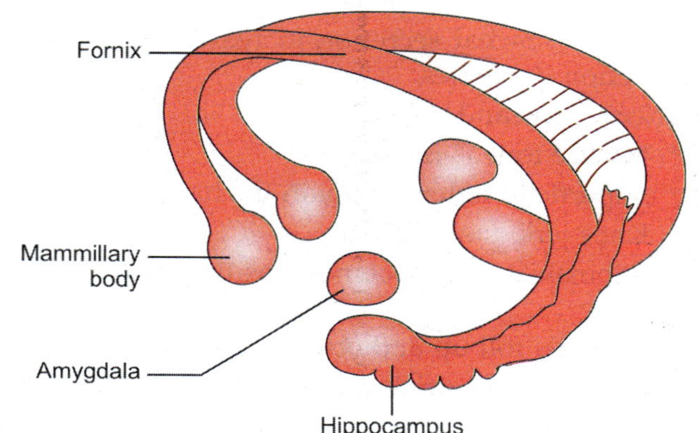

Fig. 11.56: Fornix

11

Amygdala has been called "the window" through which the limbic system sees the place of the person in the world.

2. *Memory:* Hippocampus plays a key role in consolidation of long-term memories. It provides the drive that causes translation of short-term memory in to long-term memory.
3. *Autonomic functions:* Hypothalamus is involved in control of heart rate, blood pressure, GIT movements, etc.
4. *Olfaction:* The pyriform cortex and amygdala form the olfactory centers.

110. SLEEP

Definition

Sleep is defined as a state of unconsciousness from which a person can be aroused by sensory or other stimuli.

Physiological Changes during Sleep

1. *Cardiovascular system:* Heart rate, cardiac output, vasomotor tone and blood pressure decrease.
2. *Respiratory system:* Respiratory rate, tidal volume, and pulmonary ventilation decrease. Cheyne-Stokes type of periodic breathing may occur.
3. GIT
   - Salivary secretion decreases.
   - Gastric juice secretion either remains unaltered or increases.
   - Contraction of empty stomach is more.
4. *Blood volume:* Increases resulting in dilution of plasma leading to a decrease in plasma volume.
5. *Excretory system:* Urine volume decreases but phosphate and specific gravity increases resulting in formation of concentrated urine.
6. *BMR:* Decreases by 10–15%
7. *Secretions:* Sweat secretion increases but lacrimal secretion decreases.
8. Muscle tone and reflexes
   - Muscle tone is reduced
   - Superficial reflexes remain unchanged
   - Knee jerk is abolished
   - Babinski's sign becomes positive during deep sleep
   - Eyeballs roll up and outwards
   - Pupils are constricted and light reflex is retained.
9. *Brain:* Brain shows electrical activity during sleep which can be recorded as waves.

11

Types of Sleep

Sleep is of two types:

1. Nonrapid eye movement (NREM) sleep or slow wave sleep.
2. Rapid eye movement (REM) sleep.

NREM Sleep

This is the sleep that occurs during the first hour after going to sleep. This is exceedingly restful.

Features

- Decrease in peripheral vascular tone.
- 10–30% decrease in blood pressure, respiratory rate and BMR.
- Though this is called "dreamless sleep", dreams, sometimes night mares do occur, but usually they are not remembered because the consolidation of dreams in memory does not occur. So when awakened, the person does not remember the dream.

Physiological Significance

During NREM sleep, there is pulsatile release of growth hormone and gonadotropins from the pituitary.

Stages of NREM Sleep

There are four stages in NREM sleep:

Stage 1

- Very light sleep, stage of drowsiness
- Easily aroused by moderate stimuli
- Alpha waves are reduced in frequency and amplitude.

Stage 2

Light sleep, further lack of sensitivity to stimuli, characterized by appearance of sleep spindles. These are bursts of regular waves (frequency 14 Hz per second) which are due to reverberating activity between the thalamus and cerebral cortex.

Stage 3

- Medium sleep, sleep spindles disappear
- Superimposed by δ waves (frequency 1–2 Hz per second).

Stage 4

- Deep sleep
- Arousal occurs only with vigorous stimuli
- Slow high voltage δ waves occur.

REM Sleep

This is the type of sleep associated with rapid conjugate movements of eyeballs.

Features

1. Appears on the average of every 90 min, each lasting for about 5–30 min.
2. Usually, associated with active dreaming.
3. Though it is difficult to arouse the person during REM sleep, people usually awaken spontaneously in the morning during an episode of REM sleep.
4. Skeletal muscle tone is markedly reduced.
5. Heart rate and respiratory rate become irregular due to dreams.
6. It is characterised by bursts of saccadic eye movements which are small, jerky movements of the eyeball.
7. As the brain waves become desynchronized, this is also called as desynchronized sleep.
8. The brain is highly active in REM sleep. The metabolism of the brain increases by 20%. EEG shows pattern of brain waves similar to those that occur during wakefulness. So, REM sleep is called as paradoxical sleep as it is a paradox that a person can still be asleep despite marked activity in brain.
9. It is necessary for mental well-being.
10. REM sleep is characterised by large phasic potentials, in groups of 3–5, that originate in pons and pass through lateral geniculate body to occipital cortex. These are called pontogeniculo-occipital spikes (PGO).

Theories of Sleep

Several theories have been proposed to explain the cause of sleep.

Differences between NREM sleep and REM sleep

NREM sleep	*REM sleep*
Occupies 75% of the sleep	Occupies 25% of the total sleep
Serotonin is the main neurotransmitter	Noradrenaline and acetylcholine are the neurotransmitters
No rapid movements of eyeball	Rapid movements of eyeball are present
Dreams are not remembered pulse, BP, respiratory rate are reduced and stable	Dreams can be recalled pulse, BP, respiratory rate increase and are irregular
Brain activity and oxygen consumption are reduced	Brain activity and oxygen consumption are increased
Muscle twitching absent	Muscle twitching present

1. *Passive theory:* An earlier theory of sleep which stated that the excitatory areas of upper brainstem, the reticular activating system fatigued during the waking day time and resulted in sleep. But it was proved to be untrue as sleep is caused by an active inhibitory process.
2. *Cerebral ischaemic theory:* According to this theory, sleep is produced by ischemia to cerebral cortex. This explains the drowsiness after food intake during which blood flow to splanchnic area increases and causes relative cerebral ischemia.
3. *Pavlov's theory:* This was proposed by Pavlov. According to him sleep is a special manifestation of condition reflex. This explains rocking movements of the cradle and lullaby producing sleep in children.
4. *Kleitman's theory:* Reduction of the muscle tone and less number of afferent impulses inactivate the cerebral cortex resulting in sleep.
5. *Biochemical theories*
   - *Lactic acid:* Sleep may be due to accumulation of lactic acid during fatigue.
   - *Hypnotoxin:* There may be a hypnotoxin liberated from the brain tissue producing sleep.

Sleep Centers

Stimulation of specific areas of the brain can produce sleep.

1. Raphe nuclei—thin sheet of special neurons located in the midline of the lower half of the pons and medulla. Nerve fibers from these nuclei secrete serotonin.
2. Nucleus tractus solitarius
   This nucleus is situated in medulla and pons.

3. Locus ceruleus
   - Situated in pons
   - Concerned with REM sleep
   - Noradrenaline is the neurotransmitter.
4. Suprachiasmatic area of hypothalamus
5. Diffuse nuclei of thalamus

   Neurotransmitters involved in sleep:
   - Muramyl peptide
   - Serotonin
   - Noradrenaline ⎤
   - Acetylcholine ⎦ REM sleep.

Genesis of NREM Sleep

NREM sleep is produced by two factors:

1. Reticular activating system (RAS): It is concerned with alertness and wakefulness. RAS is inhibited by descending pathways from the preoptic area of hypothalamus and diagonal band of Broca. This abolishes the wakefulness.
2. Activation of sleep centers in the brain.

Genesis of REM Sleep

REM sleep is produced by two factors:

1. Discharge of norepinephrine from the neurons located in the pontine reticular formation and raphe nucleus.
2. Discharge of acetylcholine from the neurons in the locus ceruleus of pons.

Cycle between Sleep and Wakefulness

The exact mechanism of the cycle between sleep and wakefulness is not known. The following possible mechanism has been suggested.

When sleep centers are not activated, the reticular activating system is released from inhibition and becomes spontaneously active. This excites both the cerebral cortex and the peripheral nervous system which send positive feedback signals back to RAS. Thus, once wakefulness begins, it has a natural tendency to sustain itself because of this positive feedback signals.

After the brain remains activated for many hours, the neurons in the RAS become fatigued. The positive feedback cycle between reticular nuclei and cerebral cortex fades away. Sleep centers take over leading to rapid transition from wakefulness back to sleep.

This theory may explain the rapid transition from sleep to wakefulness and from wakefulness to sleep.

Applied Physiology

Sleep disorders:

1. *Insomnia:* It is defined as the subjective problem of insufficient or nonrestorative sleep, despite an adequate oppurtunity for sleep. In short, it is inability to sleep. It occurs at one time or another in almost all adults. It can be persistent in many medical conditions.
2. *Somnambulism (sleep walking):* It occurs mostly in children and may last for several minutes. Such individuals walk with their eyes open and avoid obstacles, but when awakened, they cannot recall the episode as it occurs during slow wave sleep.
3. *Nocturnal enuresis:* This is involuntary voiding of urine occuring during sleep at night.
4. *Narcolepsy:* This is a disease characterized by episodic sudden loss of muscle tone and an irresistable urge to sleep during daytime activities.

111. ELECTROENCEPHALOGRAM (EEG)

Introduction

Electroencephalogram is the graphical record of summated potentials of the cerebral cortex. German psychiatrist Hans Berger analyzed the EEG waves systematically and is called the 'Father of modern electroencephalography'.

Method of Recording

EEG can be recorded by placing the electrodes on the scalp and connecting them via suitable amplifier to a cathode ray oscilloscope.

Electrocorticogram (ECoG) is the recording obtained by placing the electrodes directly on the pial surface of cerebral cortex.

WAVES OF EEG (Fig. 11.57)

1. Alpha rhythm
   - Rhythmical waves which can be recorded when a person is awake but at rest with eyes closed.
   - Frequency of 8–12 Hz
   - Amplitude of 50–100 μV
   - Most marked in parieto-occipital area.
2. Beta rhythm
   - Faster rhythm with desynchronized waves.
   - It has a frequency of 18–30 Hz.
   - It has an amplitude of 5–10 μV.
   - It can be recorded during mental activity and alertness.
3. Theta rhythm
   - Usually recorded in children and during early sleep.
   - It has a frequency of 4–8 Hz.
   - It has an amplitude of 10 μV
4. Delta rhythm
   - It has a frequency of 1–4 Hz.
   - It has an amplitude of 20–200 μV.
   - It can be recorded during deep sleep and in infancy.
   - It can also be recorded in conditions like brain tumour, epilepsy and increased intracranial tension.

ALPHA BLOCK

When attention is focused on something or if the person opens his eyes during recording, the alpha rhythm is replaced by fast, irregular low voltage waves. This phenomenon is called alpha block, indicating arousal or alerting response. It is also called desynchronization as it represents breaking up of synchronized neural activity necessary to produce regular waves.

ORIGIN OF BRAIN WAVES

- Many thousands or even millions of neurons in the brain, fire synchronously and the potentials are summated together to produce the waves.
- Alpha waves result from spontaneous feedback oscillations in the thalamocortical system and reticular activating system.
- Delta waves occur when cerebral cortex is released from the activating influences of the thalamus and other lower centers.

USES OF EEG

1. Localization of lesion in the brain–presence of a tumor or blood clot can be identified.
2. Useful in diagnosis of epilepsy.

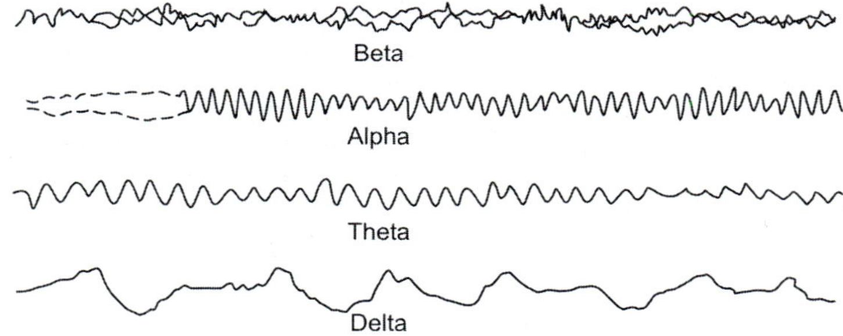

Fig. 11.57: EEG waves

11

3. A flat EEG indicates inactive state of cerebral cortex (coma).
4. Useful in differentiating between organic and functional disorders of brain.

EPILEPSY

Epilepsy (also called seizures) is characterized by uncontrolled excessive activity of either one part or all of the central nervous system.

Types

Epilepsy can be classified into three major types:
1. Grandmal epilepsy
2. Petitmal epilepsy
3. Focal epilepsy

Grandmal Epilepsy

This is characterized by extreme neuronal discharges in all areas of the brain. It produces tonic convulsions of the entire body, followed by alternating tonic and spasmodic muscle contractions called tonic-clonic seizures. The person usually bites his tongue. There is involuntary urination and defecation during the seizures.

It lasts from a few seconds to 3 to 4 minutes. It is also characterized by post seizure depression of the entire nervous system. The person remains in stupor for one to many minutes after the attack. It is followed by severe fatigue and the person sleeps for hours together.

EEG shows high voltage, high-frequency discharges over the entire cortex.

Factors that can initiate an epileptic attack: There is a strong hereditary predisposition for grandmal epilepsy. The other factors are:
1. Strong emotional stimuli
2. Alkalosis caused by overbreathing
3. Drugs
4. Fever
5. Loud noises
6. Flashing lights

11

Grandmal attack stops because of two factors
1. Neuronal fatigue
2. Active inhibition by inhibitory neurons.

Petitmal Epilepsy

It is characterized by 3 to 30 seconds of unconsciousness (or diminished consciousness) during which time the person has twitches like contractions of muscles usually in the head region, especially blinking of the eyes. This is followed by return of consciousness and reception of previous activities. Hence, it is also known as absence syndrome or absence epilepsy.

It begins during late childhood and disappears by the age of 30. Occasionally, petitmal epileptic attack can initiate a grandmal attack. EEG shows typical spike and dome pattern of waves. This epilepsy involves thalamocortical brain activating system.

Focal Epilepsy

Focal epilepsy can involve any part of the brain, cerebral cortex or brainstem.

Causes

Any localized organic lesion can cause focal epilepsy.
1. Scar tissue in brain that pulls the adjacent neuronal tissue.
2. A tumor that compresses an area of the brain.
3. A destroyed area of brain tissue.
4. Congenital causes.

Jacksonian Epilepsy

This is a form of focal epilepsy. The muscle contractions begin in the mouth region marching progressively downwards to the legs but sometimes marching in the opposite direction. This is due to spread of localized reverberatory circuits over the motor cortex.

Psychomotor Seizure

This is a form of focal epilepsy characterized by following features:
1. A short period of amnesia
2. An attack of abnormal rage
3. Sudden attack, discomfort or fear
4. A moment of incoherent speech.

This seizure frequently involves parts of the limbic system such as amygdala, septum and portions of temporal cortex. Surgical excision of the focus prevents the future attacks.

112. PROPRIOCEPTORS

Proprioception is the perception of joint position and joint movement. In simple words, it can be referred as sensation of body position.

Receptors

The important receptors concerned in the proprioception are muscle spindle and Golgi tendon organ. They are called as proprioceptors. However, mechanoceptors like Pacinian corpuscles, Ruffini end organ, Krause end bulb and Merkel's disc present in the ligaments and skin covering the joints also participate in proprioception. They are also called as kinesthetic receptors.

Muscle Tone

Tone in the skeletal muscle is defined as a state of partial contraction of the muscle. It is due to low frequency, asynchronous discharge of impulses from motor neurons. Different groups of muscle fibers contract in relays and only a portion of the muscle fibers are active at any moment. The active groups intermingle with inactive groups scattered throughout the muscle. So, groups of fibers have alternate periods of rest and activity. Thus, tone is maintained without fatigue.

In man, the antigravity muscles exhibit the greatest degree of tone. These muscles are the retractors of the neck and extensors of the back and of knee and ankle joints. When these muscles are completely relaxed, as in an unconscious person, the body collapses to the floor. When standing erect, gravity tends to cause flexion at the hip, knee and ankle. If there is any tendency to give way, it is instantly corrected by stretch reflexes which make the lower limbs into rigid pillars.

Stretch Reflex

The fundamental basis of muscle tone is the stretch or myotatic reflex. The receptor organ concerned with the stretch reflex is the muscle spindle.

MUSCLE SPINDLE—LOCATION IN THE MUSCLE

Muscle Spindle (Fig. 11.58)

Structure

Each spindle is 3 to 10 mm long. It consists of 3–12 specialized musce fibers enclosed in a spindle shaped fusiform fibrous sheath and hence it is called muscle spindle. These are called intrafusal fibers.

The fibrous sheath is attached to the glycocalyx of the surrounding large extrafusal skeletal muscle fibers.

Each intrafusal muscle fiber has no actin or myosin filaments. Hence, this central portion does not contract when the ends do. Instead it functions as a sensory receptor.

Types of Intrafusal Fibers

There are two types:

1. *Nuclear bag fibers*
   - One to three in each spindle.
   - The central portion of the receptor has an expanded bag like structure containing numerous nuclei.

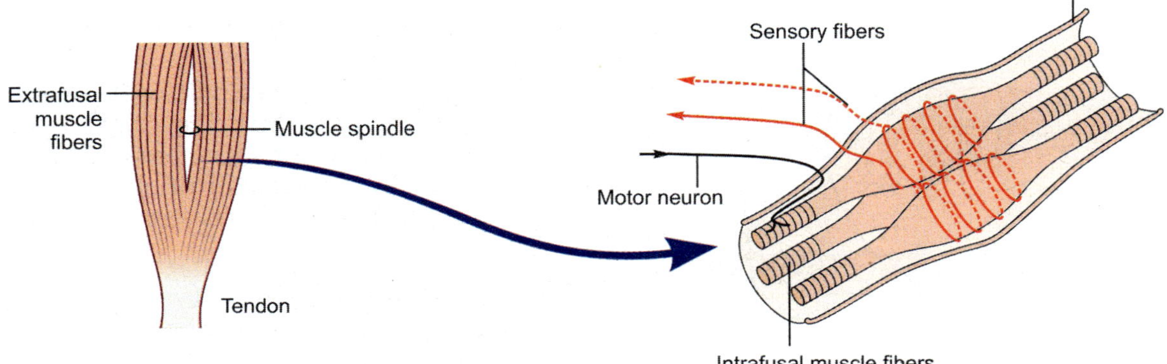

Fig. 11.58

2. *Nuclear chain fibers*
   - Three to nine in each spindle.
   - The nuclei are arranged in a chain throughout the receptor area.

NERVE SUPPLY OF MUSCLE SPINDLE (Fig. 11.59)

Nerve Supply

Sensory Innervation

1. Primary ending or annulospiral ending
   - Encircles the central portion of each intrafusal fiber
   - Type Ia fiber
   - About 17 µm in diameter
   - Transmits sensory signals to the spinal cord at a velocity of 70 to 120 meters/sec
   - Excited by both nuclear bag and nuclear chain fibers.
2. Secondary ending or flower spray ending
   - Innervates the receptor region on one or both sides of the primary ending
   - Type II fibers
   - About 8 µm in diameter
   - Encircles the intrafusal fibers in the same way as Ia but spreads-like branches on a bush
   - Excited only by nuclear chain fiber.

Motor Innervation

1. Gamma efferent fibers

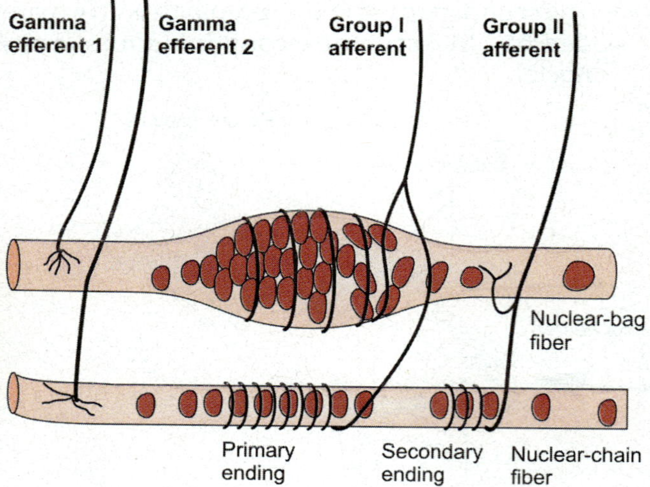

Fig. 11.59: Nerve supply

There are two types:

a. Gamma dynamic (d)
   - Excites the nuclear bag intrafusal fiber
   - Brings about dynamic response of the muscle spindle.

b. Gamma static (s)
   - Excites the nuclear chain intrafusal fiber
   - Brings about static response of the muscle spindle.

2. Alpha efferent fibers
   - Type A alpha nerve fibers
   - Innervates the extrafusal skeletal muscles.

Excitation of Muscle Spindle

Muscle spindle can be stimulated in two ways:
- Lengthening the whole muscle stretches the midportion of the spindle and excites the receptor.
- Even if the length of the entire muscle does not change, contraction of the end portions of the spindles intrafusal fibers stretches the midportion of the spindle and therefore excites the receptor.

Response of the Muscle Spindle

Static Response

When the receptor portion of the muscle spindle is stretched slowly, the number of impulses transmitted from both the primary and the secondary endings increases in proportion to the degree of stretching and this continues for several minutes. This is called static response.

Dynamic Response

When the length of the spindle receptor increases suddenly, only the primary ending is stimulated. This is called dynamic response. This occurs while the length is actually increasing.

Normally, the muscle spindle emits sensory nerve impulses continuously. Stretching the muscle spindle increases the rate of firing whereas shortening the spindle decreases the rate of firing. Muscle spindle detects the muscle length and changes in muscle length.

MUSCLE STRETCH REFLEX

Whenever a muscle is stretched suddenly, excitation of the spindle causes reflex contraction of the large skeletal muscle fibers of the stretched muscle.

Neuronal Circuitry of Stretch Reflex
(Monosynaptic Pathway)

Type Ia fiber in muscle spindle
↓
Dorsal root of spinal cord
↓
Anterior horn of the gray matter
↓
Motor fibers from anterior motor neurons
↓
Large extrafusal fibers of the same muscle
↓
Muscle contraction

Types of Stretch Reflex

There are two components:

1. Dynamic stretch reflex: It is excited by sudden potent dynamic signal from primary sensory endings of muscle spindle caused by rapid stretch or unstretch.
2. Static stretch reflex: It is elicited by the continuous static receptor signals transmitted by both primary and secondary endings. It continues for a long time.

Function of Stretch Reflex

- Stretch reflex prevents the oscillation or jerkiness of body movements. This is a damping or smoothing function.
- Muscle spindle stabilizes the body position during tense motor action.
- As the muscle spindles are more dense in antigravity muscles, they dampen the movements of the different body parts during walking and running.

ALPHA-GAMMA LINKAGE

Whenever signals are transmitted from the motor cortex or any other area of the brain to the alpha motor neurons, the gamma motor neurons are stimulated simultaneously. This is called coactivation of alpha and gamma motor neurons or α–γ linkage. This causes both the extrafusal skeletal muscle fibers and the muscle spindle intrafusal muscle fibers to contract at the same time. This maintains the proper damping function of the muscle spindle.

Golgi Tendon Reflex (Fig. 11.60)

Receptor

The Golgi tendon organ is an encapsulated sensory receptor through which muscle tendon fibers pass.

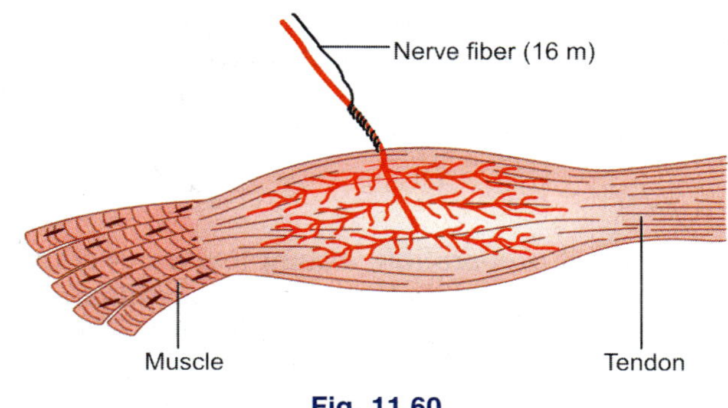

Fig. 11.60

About 10 to 15 muscle fibers are usually connected to each Golgi tendon organ.

Tendon Reflex

Signals from the tendon organ are transmitted through large, rapidly conducting Type Ib nerve fibers. These fibers transmit the signals both into local areas of the cord and after synapsing in the dorsal horn of the cord, through spinocerebellar tracts into cerebellum. The local cord signal excites a single inhibitory interneuron that inhibits the anterior motor neuron. This local circuit directly inhibits the individual muscle without affecting adjacent muscles.

Lengthening Reaction
(Inverse Stretch Reflex and Autogenic Inhibition)

When the tension on the muscle becomes extreme, the inhibitory effect from the tendon organ can be so great that it leads to a sudden reaction in the spinal cord that causes instant relaxation of the entire muscle. This is called lengthening reaction. This is a protective mechanism to prevent the tearing of muscle or avulsion of the tendon.

Polysynaptic Reflexes

Experimental Animal Preparations

All these reflexes can be well demonstrated in experimental animal preparations:

1. *Spinal animal:* A transverse section is made in the medulla below the vestibular nuclei or between the medulla and the spinal cord or in the upper most segments of the spinal cord. The animal is kept alive by the artificial ventilation. Initially there is a complete loss of tone in all the muscles, followed by some return of tone more in flexors and less in extensors. Gamma motor neuron activity is depressed.

2. *Thalamic animal:* A transverse section is made between corpus striatum and thalamus. Thalamus is intact and removed from the influence of cerebral cortex.

Decerebrate Animal

In this animal preparation, a complete transection is made in the brainstem between superior colliculi and vestibular nuclei. Sherrington studied the effects by making a midcollicular section, i.e. between superior and inferior colliculi in cats. The resulting pattern of spasticity is called decerebrate rigidity.

Decerebrate Rigidity (Figs 11.61 and 11.62)

- Respiration continues
- Cardiovascular reflexes are intact. Deep tendon reflexes are exaggerated. Righting reflexes are lost. All the other reflexes are present.
- Muscle tone: There is a marked increase in the tone of both extensors and flexors, but chiefly of the extensors.

  When the animal is lying on its side, the head is drawnback, the limbs are extended, lower jaw held up and neck extended. It is difficult to alter the position of the limbs and hence it is termed as rigidity. When the animal is placed upon its feet, the limbs support the weight of the body. The animal stands stiffly with back arched, tail lifted up and neck extended. This was described by Sherrington as 'caricature of the standing position'.

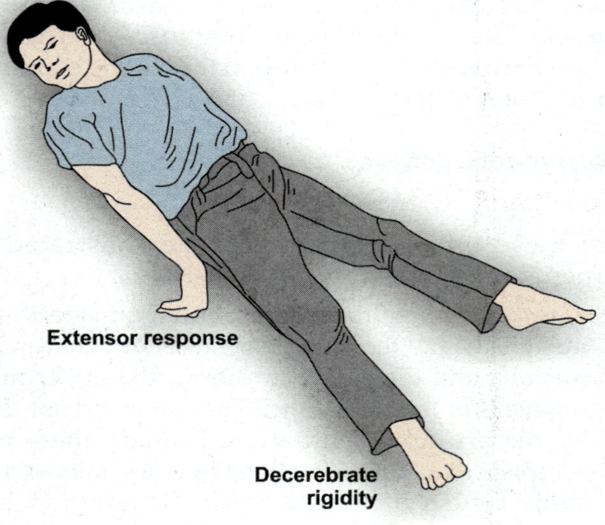

Fig. 11.61: Decerebrate rigidity

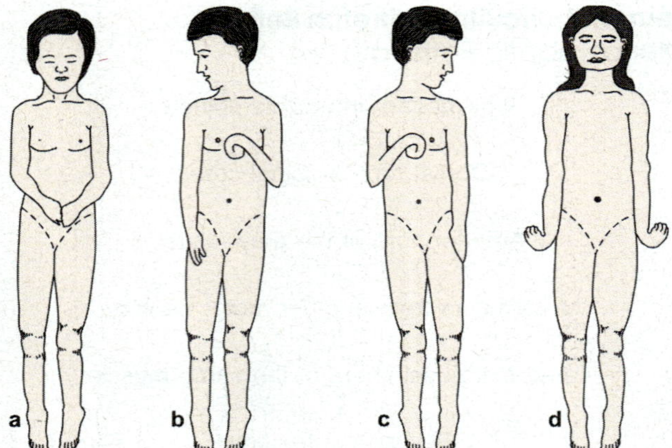

Figs 11.62a to d: (a to c) Decortication in humans; (d) true decerebrate rigidity

Mechanism of Decerebrate Rigidity

Decerebrate rigidity is refered as a 'release phenomenon', i.e. release from the suprabulbar inhibitory influences. The stretch reflexes are facilitated by impulses from pontine recticular formation which is spontaneous. The inhibitory impulses to stretch reflexes come from medullary reticular formation which is not spontaneous, but is driven by fibers from cerebellum, cerebral cortex and basal ganglia.

When the brainstem is transected at the superior border of the pons, the inhibitory areas that drive the reticular inhibitory area are removed, but discharge of the facilitatory area continues. Hence, gamma efferent discharge is increased and stretch reflexes become hyperactive.

Figures 11.62a to d show the effects of decerebration and decortication. Decortication is destruction of cerebral cortex leaving red nucleus and basal ganglia intact. The effects are similar to decerebration except that hypertonia in upper limb is in flexors and degree of tone is influenced by the position of the head. The rubrospinal and tectospinal systems play an important role in modifying the pattern of paralysis in upper limb. The tonic neck and labrynthine reflexes are superimposed on the hypertonicity.

Polysynaptic Reflexes

These reflexes are best demonstrated in a spinal animal.

Flexor Reflex (Figs 11.63a and b)

In a spinal animal, any type of cutaneous sensory stimulus from a limb causes the flexor muscles of the limb to contract, there by withdrawing the limb from the stimulating object. This is called flexor reflex.

This interneuron excites motor neuron causing muscular contraction

Brain

Spinal cord

Motor neuron

This muscle causes withdrawal from source of pain

Axon of sensory neuron (pain)

Cross section of spinal cord

a

This interneuron excites motor neuron causing muscular contraction

Brain

Spinal cord

Motor neuron

This muscle causes withdrawal from source of pain

Axon of sensory neuron (pain)

Cross section of spinal cord

b

Figs 11.63a and b

Flexor reflex is elicited most powerfully by stimulation of pain endings by painful stimuli (Fig. 11.64). Hence, it is also called as nociceptive reflex or pain reflex.

If some part of the body other than one of the limbs is painfully stimulated, that part will be withdrawn from the stimulus. The reflex may not be confined to flexor muscles. This is called the 'withdrawal reflex or withdrawal response'.

The pathway of the flexor withdrawal reflex comprises:

1. Nociceptors
2. Afferent nerves from the receptors which enter the spinal cord via the posterior nerve roots
3. Reflex center in spinal cord and is made up of synapses of several interneurons in several segments of spinal cord
4. Efferent fibers from the anterior motor neuron
5. Effector organ, i.e. the flexor muscles of that limb.

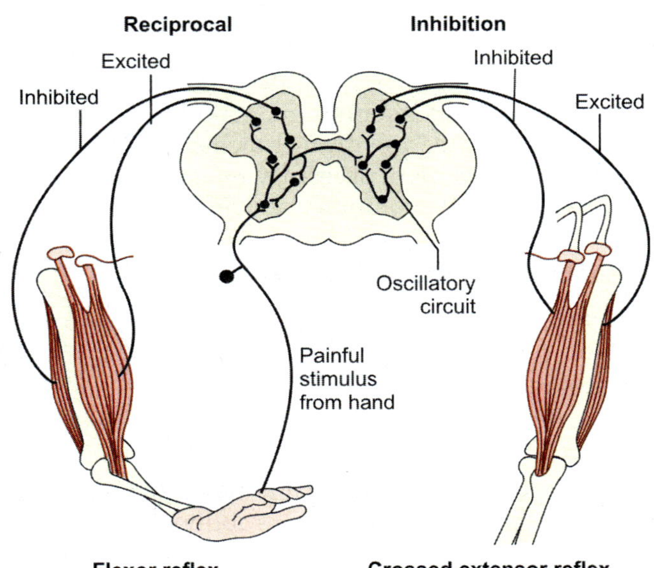

Fig. 11.64

Crossed Extensor Reflex

About 0.2 to 0.5 second after a stimulus elicits a flexor reflex in one limb, the opposite limb begins to extend. This is called crossed extensor reflex (Fig. 11.64). Extension of the opposite limb can push the entire body away from the object causing the painful stimulus in the withdrawn limb. When the interneurons excite the ipsilateral flexor motor neurons, collaterals from these neurons cross to opposite side and cause excitation of the contralateral extensor motor neurons.

113. POSTURE AND EQUILIBRIUM

Definition

Posture is the position of the body in relation to the environment. Equilibrium includes maintenance of posture and maintenance of steadiness during movements such as walking.

Maintenance of posture is a reflex phenomenon which does not require conscious effort. Muscle tone and hence stretch reflex are the basic phenomena for maintenance of posture.

POSTURAL REFLEXES

Postural reflexes are the reflexes which maintain posture and equilibrium. The components of a postural reflex are:

1. The afferent pathways arising from eyes, vestibular apparatus and proprioceptors.
2. The efferent pathways are to alpha motor neurons which supply the skeletal muscles.
3. The integrating centers are located at different levels extending from spinal cord to cerebral cortex. Postural reflexes not only maintain the body in an upright balance position, but also provide the constant adjustment necessary to maintain a stable background for voluntary activity.

Classification of Postural Reflexes

They are divided into two types:

1. Static reflexes
2. Statokinetic reflexes

11

Static Reflexes

Static reflexes are the posturtal reflexes that maintain posture at rest. They are further subdivided into four groups.

1. Local static reflexes
2. General static reflexes
3. Segmental static reflexes
4. Attitudinal reflexes

Local Static Reflexes

Local static reflexes or the supporting reactions support the body in different positions against gravity and also protect the limbs against the hyperextension or hyperflexion. They are of two types:

1. Positive supporting reaction
2. Negative supporting reaction.

Positive supporting reaction: These are the reactions which help to fix the joints and make the limbs rigid like pillars, so that limbs can support the weight of the body against gravity. It is brought about by the simultaneous contractions of both extensors and flexor muscles and other opposing muscles. The impulses for these reflexes arise from proprioceptors present in the muscles, joints and tendons and pressure receptors in skin of the sole.

Negative supporting reaction: These are the reactions which include relaxation of the muscles and unfixing of the joints to enable the limbs to be flexed and move. These occur during stepping movements.

General Static Reflexes

These are called righting reflexes because they help to maintain an upright position of the body. They are divided into five types:

1. Labyrinthine righting reflexes acting on the neck muscles
2. Neck righting reflexes acting on the body
3. Body righting reflexes acting on the head
4. Body righting reflexes acting upon the body
5. Optical righting reflexes.

Labyrinthine righting reflexes acting on the neck muscles: If a blind folded thalamic rabbit (cortex is removed with intact thalamus) is suspended from the pelvis with the head down, the head turns until it assumes a normal position in space. The maintenance of the head in the new position is due to labyrinthine reflexes acting on the neck muscles. Turning the body of the rabbit into different positions is followed by compensatory movements of the head. After the labyrinth is extirpated, suspension of the animal as before fails to produce the compensatory movements in the head. The head-hangs like that of a dead animal.

Neck righting reflexes acting on the body: When the blind folded thalamic rabbit is laid on its side, the head assumes the normal position by the labyrinthine reflexes. Contraction of the neck muscles which rotates the head sets up proprioceptive impulses, which through a center in the upper cervical cord, rotates the body and brings it into normal relation with the head.

Body righting reflexes acting on the head: When a labyrinthectomized animal is laid on its side, due to asymmetrical stimulation of the receptors of the side of the body which has contact with the surface of the table, the position of the head is corrected.

Body righting reflexes acting on the body: When thalamic animal is laid down on the table on its side with the head held down to the table to eliminate labyrinthine and neck righting reflexes, the body attempts to right itself by raising the lower parts. It is because of the impulses from the exteroceptors on that side of the body acting on the body itself.

Optical righting reflexes: A labyrinthectomized animal held in air can orient the position of the head through retinal impulses. The receptors are in the retina and the center is in the occipital cortex. Hence it is absent in the blindfolded or thalamic animal.

Center for righting reflexes: The center for the first formed righting reflexes is in the red nucleus in the midbrain. The center for the optical righting reflexes is in the occipital lobe of the cerebral cortex.

Segmental Static Reflexes

These reflexes are very essential for walking. During walking, in one leg, the flexors are active and the extensors are inhibited. On the opposite leg, the flexors are inhibited and the extensors are active. This is known as crossed extensor reflex. It is due to reciprocal inhibition and the neural mechanism responsible for this reflex is called Sherrington reciprocal innervation. These reflexes can be demonstrated in a spinal animal. The centers for these reflexes are situated in the spinal cord.

Statotonic or Attitudinal Reflexes

They develop according to the attitude of the body. They are of two types:

- Tonic labyrinthine and neck reflexes acting on the limbs.
- Labyrinthine and neck reflexes acting upon the eyes.

Tonic labyrinthine and neck reflexes acting on the limbs: These reflexes decrease or increase the tone of the skeletal muscles of the limbs according to the position of the head. They are best studied in decerebrate animal. The receptors are in vestibular apparatus. Whenever, the position of the head is altered, the receptors present in the labyrinth are stimulated and generate impulses. The impulses are also generated from the neck muscles when the position of the head is altered. The impulses from the labyrinth produce the same effect on the four timbs. But the impulses from neck muscles cause opposite effects in the forelimbs and hind limbs. These reflexes are very effective on the extensor muscles. When the head is dorsiflexed, all the four limbs are extended maximally. When the head is ventriflexed, all the four limbs are flexed.

In a labyrinthectomized animal, where only neck reflexes are operated, dorsiflexion of the head causes extension of the forelimbs and flexion of hind limbs.

The centers for these reflexes are in the upper cervical region.

Tonic labyrinthine and neck reflexes acting upon the eyes: When the head moves in one direction, these reflexes bring about compensatory movement of the eyeball in the opposite direction to enable vision to be fixed properly on an object in the field.

When the head is moved down, the tone in the superior recti and inferior oblique is increased and tone of the inferior recti and superior oblique is reduced so that eyeballs move upwards. When the head is turned to one side, a corresponding compensatory movement of the eyes occur.

When the head is turned to oneside the eyes elevate outward or inward in relation to the head. The eyes are moved in a direction opposite to that of the head movement. It is because of external and internal recti.

Then centers for the statotonic reflexes are present in the medulla oblongata.

Statokinetic Reflexes

These are postural reflexes that maintain posture during movements. They are concerned with angular (rotatory) and linear movements. The vestibular apparatus is responsible for these reflexes.

114. VESTIBULAR APPARATUS

Introduction

The labyrinth or inner ear is a complex structure comprising an auditory portion, the cochlea concerned with hearing and a nonauditory portion called the vestibular apparatus. Vestibular apparatus is concerned with the function of equilibrium and posture.

Vestibular Apparatus (Fig. 11.65)

It consists of:

- Three bony semicircular canals
- Vestibule

Semicircular canals: The semicircular canals are the tubular structures placed at right angles to each other. They are three in number:

1. Anterior canal
2. Posterior canal
3. Lateral or horizontal canal

The anterior and posterior canals are situated vertically. The lateral canal is situated in horizontal plane.

When the head is tilted forward at an angle of 30 degree, the lateral canals of both sides are at horizontal plane parallel to earth with the convexities directed outward and a little backward. The anterior canals are at vertical plane and directed forward and outward at 45 degree. The posterior canals are also at vertical plane, but directed backwards and outward at 45 degree. Hence, the plane of position of anterior canal of one side is parallel to the plane of posterior canal of opposite side (Fig. 11.66).

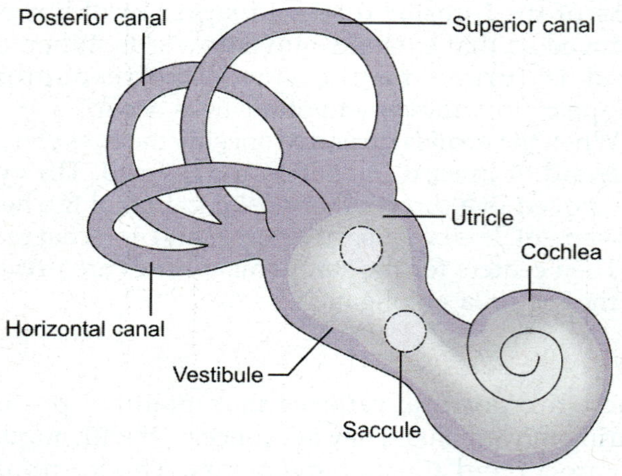

Fig. 11.65: Vestibular apparatus

Ampulla

There are two ends for each semicircular canal. One end is narrow and the other end is dilated. This dilatation is called ampulla. This contains the receptor organ of semicircular canals known as crista ampullaris.

The cristae contain a ridge covered by tall columnar sensor hair cells, each having a number of long stiff hairs which project into a gelatinous material. This is called cupular terminalis or cupula. Between the hair cells, are some supporting or sustentacular cells. The apex of each hair cell has a cuticular plate. From this plate, about 50–70 cilia arise which are called stereocilia. Each stereocilia is attached at its tip to the neighboring taller one by a fine process called tip link. All the stereocilia are held together by tiplinks. One of the cilia is very tall and it is called as kinocilium.

Vestibule or Otolith

Vestibule is formed by utricle and saccule. Utricle communicates with saccule through utriculosaccular duct and saccule communicates with the cochlear duct. Utricle and saccule are referred to as otolith or otolith organs because they contain crystals of calcium carbonate called otoconia or otoliths. The hairs project into a gelatinous structure which contains otoconia.

Receptors in Utricle and Saccule

The receptor organ in otolith organ is called macula. Macula is also covered by a gelatinous membrane called otolith membrane. The stereocilia and kinocilium of each hair cell are embedded in otolith membrane. Otolith membrane contains otoconia.

Macula is situated in horizontal plane in utricle. Hence, the cilia from the hair cells are in vertical direction whereas macula is situated in vertical plane in saccule and the cilia are in horizontal direction.

Nerve Supply to Vestibular Apparatus

The nerve impulses from the hair cells of crista ampullaris and maculae are transmitted to medulla oblongata through the vestibular division of vestibulocochlear nerve (VIII cranial nerve). The cell bodies of this nerve are the bipolar cells in the Scarpa's

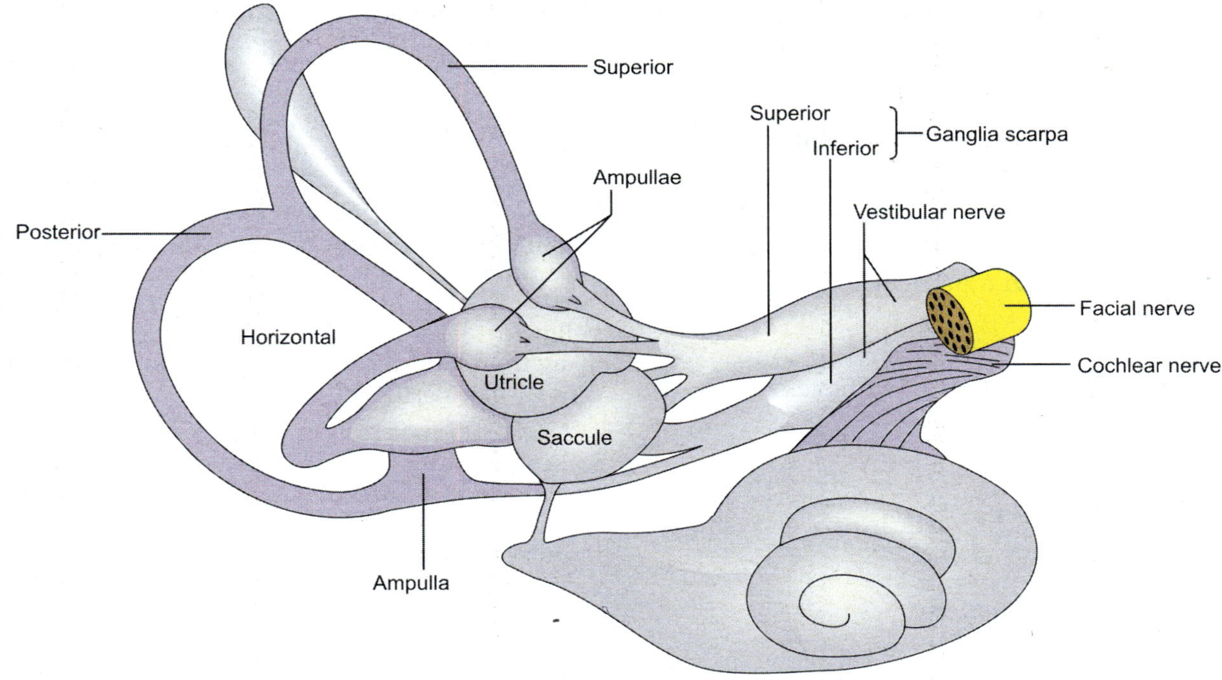

Fig. 11.66

(vestibular) ganglion. The peripheral processes connect with the sensory hair cells in the cristae of the semicircular canals and the macula of the utricle and saccule. The central processes enter the medulla oblongata and end in vestibular nuclei. Some fibers go directly to the cerebellum.

There are four vestibular nuclei in the medulla oblongata viz. superior, inferior, lateral and medial nuclei. Most of the primary vestibular fibers reaching superior and medial nuclei come from crista ampullaris of semicircular canals. Lateral vestibular nucleus receives the fibers mostly from maculae of otolith organ. Inferior vestibular nucleus receives fibers from both crista ampullaris and maculae. Some neurons in vestibular nuclei send efferent fibers back to the hair cells. These fibers provide tonic inhibition of hair cells.

The axons of the vestibular nuclei form four tracts:

1. Vestibulo-ocular tract
2. Vestibulospinal tract
3. Vestibuloreticular tract
4. Vestibulocerebellar tract.

Vestibulo-ocular Tract

Fibers from superior, medial, and inferior vestibular nuclei terminate in the nucleus of III, IV, and VI cranial nerves. This forms vestibulo-ocular tract. This tract is concerned with movements of eyeballs in relation to the position of the head.

Vestibulospinal Tract

Fibers of this tract descend from lateral vestibular nucleus. This tract is concerned with reflex movements of head and body during postural changes.

Vestibuloreticular Tract

This tract includes the fibers from vestibular nuclei to reticular formation of brainstem. These fibers are concerned with facilitation of muscle tone.

The membranous labyrinth is filled with a fluid called endolymph. It is a clear fluid resembling ICF. It has more potassium ions.

Vestibulocerebellar Tract

This tract consists of fibers from all the four vestibular nuclei to cerebellum. This is concerned with coordination of movements according to body position.

Fluids in the Labyrinth

The membranous labyrinth is filled with a fluid called endolymph. It is a clear fluid resembling ICF. It has more potassium ions and less sodium ions. Between the membranous labyrinth and the bony wall is the perilymph which is similar to ECF or CSF.

Mechanism of Action of Vestibular Apparatus

Semicircular Canals

Semicircular canals are concerned with angular (rotatory) acceleration. Each semicircular canal is sensitive to rotation in a particular plane.

Superior Canal

Gives response to rotation in transverse axis, e.g. nodding the head while saying yes-yes.

Horizontal Canal

Responds to rotation in vertical axis, e.g. shaking the head while saying 'no-no'.

Posterior Canal

Responds to rotation in the vertical plane in which the head is rotated from shoulder to shoulder.

At the beginning of the rotation, the receptors are stimulated by the movements of endolymph inside the semicircular canals. The receptors are stimulated only at the beginning and end of the rotation, not during rotation at a constant speed.

When the person rotates the head in clockwise direction in horizontal plane, the horizontal canal moves in clockwise direction. But the inertia of the fluid makes it to remain stationary. This phenomenon causes relative displacement of endolymph in the direction opposite to that of the rotation of the head, i.e. the fluid is pushed in anticlockwise direction. So, fluid flows from the duct towards the ampulla in right horizontal canal and in the left, it moves away from the ampulla.

The movement of the endolymph bends the cupula. When cupula moves towards the ampulla, the stereocilia of the haircells are pushed towards kinocilium leading to stimulation of hair cells. When cupula moves away from ampulla, the stereocilia are pushed away from kinocilium and haircells are not stimulated.

11

At the beginning of rotation in clockwise direction in horizontal plane, the hair cells at ampulla of horizontal canal in right ear are stimulated. But the hair cells in horizontal canal of left ear are not stimulated. Rotation in anticlockwise direction stimulates the hair cells in ampulla of horizontal canal in left ear only.

Electrical Potential in Hair Cells

The resting membrane potential of hair cells is about –60 mV. The movements of stereocilia of hair cells towards kinocilium causes opening of potassium channels. This causes K^+ influx from endolymph causing depolarization and results in receptor potential. This potential is nonpropagative. Depolarization of hair cells causes them to release a neurotransmitter which generates action potential in nerve fibers which surrounds the hair cells. The neurotransmitter is believed to be glutamate. Movements of stereocilia away from kinocilium causes hyperpolarisation of hair cells by closing the ion channels.

Under normal resting conditions the nerve fibers leading from the hair cells transmit continuous nerve impulses at a rate of 100 per second. When the stereocilia are bent towards the kinocilium, the impulse traffic increases. Conversely, bending the cilia away from the kinocilium decreases the impulse traffic. Therefore, as the orientation of the head in space changes and the weight of the stataconia bends the cilia, appropriate signals are transmited to the brain to control equilibrium.

Function of Otolith Organ

This is concerned with linear acceleration. Utricle responds during horizontal acceleration and saccule responds during vertical acceleration.

Function of the Utricle

The utricle responds to horizontal acceleration or deceleration like a sensation we feel while in a car speeding up or slowing down. When the body moves forward, the otoconia fall back in otolith membrane and pull the cilia of hair cells backwards. This stimulates the hair cells which send impulses to vestibular, cerebellar and reticular centers. These centers in turn send instructions to various muscles to maintain equilibrium of the body during the forward movement.

Function of the Saccule

Saccule provides information during vertical acceleration like the sensation we feel while in an elevator moving up or down. While climbing up, the otoconia move down by pulling the cilia downwards. It stimulates the hair cells, which in turn send information to the brain centers to bring about necessary adjust-ments.

Applied Physiology

I. *Nystagmus*

Nystagmus is the rhythmic oscillatory involuntary movements of the eyeball. It is a reflex phenomenon which helps in visual fixation while the body rotates.

Vestibulo-ocular Reflex (VOR)

When rotation starts, the eyes move slowly in a direction opposite to the direction of rotation, maintaining visual fixation. This is called vestibulo-ocular reflex. When the limit of this movement is reached, the eyes quickly snap back to a new fixation point and then again move slowly in the other direction. The slow component is initiated by impulses from the labyrinth. The quick component is triggered by the center in the brainstem.

Types

There are three types of nystagmus:
1. *Horizontal:* The eyes move in the horizontal plane.
2. *Vertical:* The eyes move vertically when the head is tipped sidewise during rotation.
3. *Rotatory:* Nystagmus occurs when the head is tipped forward.

Nystagmus in Pathological Condition

Nystagmus is seen in:
1. Cerebellar lesions
2. Lesions of brainstem
3. Lesions in labyrinth

II. *Motion Sickness*

Any form of travel where there is irregular motion can induce motion sickness.

Clinical manifestations
- Nausea
- Vomiting
- Sweating
- Pallor
- Changes in blood pressure
- Headache
- Vertigo

They are produced by the excessive vestibular stimulation. They are probably due to reflexes mediated via vestibular connection in the brainstem and the flocculonodular lobe of the cerebellum.

III. *Menier's Disease*

This is characterized by vertigo, tinnitus (ringing in the ear) and impairment of hearing. The disease is localized with the labyrinth. It is caused by overdistension of cochlear duct due to disturbed fluid balance in the labyrinth.

115. HIGHER FUNCTIONS OF THE NERVOUS SYSTEM

Higher functions of the nervous system include learning, memory, judgment, language and other functions of the mind. All these intellectual functions of the mind require intact, functioning cerebral cortex.

LEARNING

Learning is defined as the process by which new information is acquired.

Types of Learning

There are two types of learning:
1. Nonassociative learning
2. Associative learning.

Nonassociative Learning

In this type of learning, the organism learns about single stimulus. It is based on two factors:
- Habituation
- Sensitization

Habituation

This is a form of learning in which a neutral stimulus is repeated many times. The first time it is applied, it evokes a reaction. This is called the orientation reflex or "what is it?" response. However, it evolves less and less electrical response as it is repeated. Hence, the subject ignores the stimulus. This is called habituation.

Sensitization

A repeated stimulus produces a greater response if it is coupled one or more times with an unpleasant or a pleasant stimulus. The mother who sleeps through different sounds around her is not disturbed by these sounds. But she wakes up promptly when her baby cries. This because she is sensitized to the crying sound of her baby.

11

Associative Learning

Here, the organism learns about the relation of one stimulus to another stimulus. A classic example of associative learning is a conditioned reflex.

Conditioned Reflex

A conditioned reflex is a reflex response to a stimulus that previously elicited little or no response, but acquired by repeatedly pairing the stimulus with another stimulus that normally produces a response.

There are two types of conditioned reflex:
1. Classical conditioned reflex
2. Instrumental conditioning.

Classical Conditioned Reflex

This was studied extensively by Pavlov in dogs. In Pavlov's experiments, the salivation normally induced by placing meat in the mouth of dog was studied. A bell was rung just before the meat was placed in the dog's mouth and this was repeated a number of times until the animal would salivate when the bell was rung, although no meat was placed in its mouth. The meat placed in the mouth was the unconditioned stimulus (US), the stimulus that normally produces a particular innate response. The conditioned stimulus (CS) was the bell ringing. After CS and US had been paired many times, the CS produced the response, evoked by US. The CS should precede the US for conditioned reflex. This is called classic conditioning.

A number of somatic, visceral and neural changes can be made to occur as conditioned reflex responses. Conditioning of visceral responses is called biofeedback.

Internal Inhibition

If the CS is presented repeatedly without the US, the conditioned reflex eventually dies out. This process is called extinction or internal inhibition.

External Inhibition

If the animal is disturbed by an external stimulus immediately after the CS is applied, the conditioned response may not occur.

Instrumental Conditioning

There are two types in this:
1. Escape and avoidance conditioning
2. Operant conditioning

Escape and Avoidance Conditioning

In this method, the CS is paired with an unpleasant US. For example, the CS is a light glowing and the US is electric shock. The animal learns that after a light is shown there would be electric shock. It can avoid it by pressing a bar.

Operant Conditioning

This is a form of conditioning in which the animal is taught to perform some task in order to obtain a reward or avoid punishment.

MEMORY

Definition

Memory is defined as the retention and storage of the information that can be recalled.

Types of Memory

Physiologically, memory is classified into two types:
1. Explicit memory
2. Implicit memory

Explicit Memory

- This is also called as declarative or recognition memory.
- This is associated with conciousness or at least awareness.
- It involves hippocampus and medial temporal lobe.

It is divided into two types:
1. Episodic Memory
   Memory for events.
2. Semantic memory
   Memory for words, rules and language.

Implicit Memory

- This is called as nondeclarative or reflexive memory.
- It does not involve awareness.
- It includes skills, habits and conditioned reflexes.

Memory is also classified as:
1. Short-term memory
2. Intermediate long-term memory
3. Long-term memory.

Short-term Memory

Recalling of events or material that happened very recently is short-term memory or recent memory, e.g. memory of 7 to 10 numerals in a telephone number for a few seconds to a few minutes.

Intermediate Memory

These memories may last for many minutes or even weeks. They will be lost unless the memory traces are activated enough to become permanent long-term memories.

Mechanism of Intermediate Long-term Memory

Facilitation

Between two synaptic terminals where one terminal is from sensory neuron which synapses with a neuron to be stimulated is called sensory terminal. The other terminal is a presynaptic ending that lies on the surface of the sensory terminals and it is called facilitator terminal.

When the sensory terminal is stimulated repeatedly without stimulation of facilitator terminal, signal transmission is good at first, but becomes less and less intense with repeated stimulation. This phenomenon is called habituation.

If a painful stimulus excites the facilitator terminal at the same time that the sensory terminal is stimulated, then the transmission becomes stronger and stronger. It will remain strong for even up to three weeks.

Steps Involved in Facilitation

1. Stimulation of the facilitator presynaptic terminal at the same time that the sensory terminal is stimulated causes release of serotonin at the synapse.
2. Serotonin acts on serotonin receptors in the sensory terminal membrane. This activates the enzyme adenyl cyclase inside the membrane and results in cyclic AMP formation.
3. Cyclic AMP activates a protein kinase that causes phosphorylation of a protein which is a potassium channel in the sensory terminal membrane. This blocks the potassium conductance through the channels. This block can last for minutes to even several weeks.
4. Lack of potassium conductance causes prolonged action potentials in the synaptic terminals because flow of potassium ions out of the terminals is necessary for rapid recovery from the action potential.
5. The prolonged action potential causes prolonged activation of the calcium channels leading to calcium influx into sensory synaptic terminals. These calcium ions release neurotransmitter which facilitates synaptic transmission.

Long-term Memory

Any thought process which is stored and can be recalled after days or several years is called long-term or permanent memory.

Mechanism of Long-term Memory

This memory is due to long-term potentiation of the synapses involved. The hyperexcitable state of the synapse that develops following application of a tetanising current to presynaptic afferents may last for few days to few months. This is called long-term potentiation. This causes physiological and structural changes in the synapse.

Memory Engram

It is a process by which the memory is facilitated and stored in brain. It is also called as memory trace.

Physiological Changes

- Changes in the gene expression in the postsynaptic neuron.
- Increase in the synthesis and release of excitatory neurotransmitters.
- No (nitric oxide) released from the postsynaptic endings reaches the presynaptic terminal and enhances the release of neurotransmitters.

Structural Changes

- Increase in vesicle release sites for secretion of transmitter substance.
- Increase in number of transmitter vesicles released.
- Increase in number of presynaptic terminals.
- Changes in the structure of the dendritic spines that permit transmission of stronger signals.

Consolidation of Memory

For short-term memory to be converted to long-term memory, it must be consolidated. For this, the short-term memory should be activated repeatedly so that it will initiate chemical, physical and anatomical changes in the synapses that are responsible for long-term memory. This process requires 5 to 10 minutes for minimal consolidation and 1 hour or more for strong consolidation. During this period, consolidation of memory will not take place if disturbed by:

- Electric shock
- Deep general anesthesia
- Convulsions

Rehearsal of the same information again and again in the mind accelerates the transfer of short-term memory into long-term memory.

Disorders of Memory

Amnesia

Loss of memory is known as amnesia. It is of two types:

1. *Anterograde Amnesia*
   - It is the inability to establish new long-term memories.
   - It occurs due to lesion in hippocampus.
2. *Retrograde Amnesia*
   - Failure to recall recent events is called retrograde amnesia.
   - It occurs in lesion of thalamus.

ALZHEIMER'S DISEASE

It is a progressive neurodegenerative disease. It is characterized by short-term memory loss followed by loss of cognitive function and death in middle age. It accounts for 50–60% of senile dementia.

Early changes include atrophy of hippocampus and entorhinal cortex. There is loss of cholinergic neurons in the cerebral cortex and nucleus basalis of Meynert.

The characteristic histological features are intracellular neurofibrillary tangles and extracellular senile plaques of beta amyloid substance.

There is evidence that cardiovascular disease caused by hypertension and atherosclerosis may play a role in Alzheimer's disease.

SPEECH

Definition

Speech is one of the communicating means in which one's thoughts are expressed by production of articulate sounds with meaning.

Mechanism of Speech

Speech is a coordinated act. It involves three components:

1. Sensory input
   - From the receptors
2. Interpretation center
   - Includes visual and auditory association areas, angular gyrus and Wernicke's areas

3. Motor output
   - Includes Broca's areas, premotor cortex, motor cortex, cerebellum and basal ganglia.

Development of Speech

Speech develops in two ways:

First Stage

This stage is the association of certain words through visual, auditory, tactile and other sensations. This gets stored in the memory and the words are learnt.

Second Stage

During this stage, new neuronal circuits are established between auditory area and the motor area tha control the muscles of articulation. The child attempts to pronounce the learnt words.

Speech Centers

The following centers participate in speech production:

1. *Auditory association area (area 42):* This area interprets the meaning of sounds heard.
2. *Visual association area (area 18 and 19):* This area interprets the meaning of written material or symbols.
3. *Wernicke's area (area 22):* This is concerned with comprehension of visual and auditory information.
4. *Angular gyrus:* This area lies immediately behind Wernicke's area. It is concerned with interpretation of visual information.
5. *Broca's area (area 44):* This is motor area for speech.

Speech in Response to Heard Words (Fig. 11.67)

The various steps involved in communication through speech in response to hearing are:

1. Reception of sound signals by primary auditory area 41.
2. Interpretation of the words in Wernicke's area.
3. Wernicke's area decides the choice and sequence of words to be spoken.
4. This information is transmitted from Wernicke's area to Broca's area via arcuate fasiculus.
5. Activation of Broca's area for word formation.
6. Broca's area transmits appropriate signals to motor cortex which in-turn sends motor signals to muscles of phonation.
7. Speech is produced.

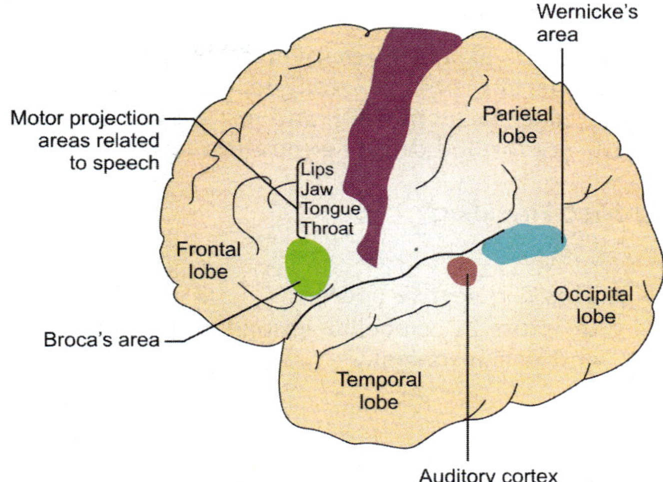

Fig. 11.67

Speech in Response to Written Words (Fig. 11.68)

The steps involved are:

1. Visual impulses reach primary visual cortex area 17
2. Impulses from here reach areas 18 and 19
3. From these areas, signals go to angular gyrus where interpretation of visual information occurs
4. From angular gyrus signals go to Wernicke's area, where comprehension of the signal occurs
5. Wernicke's area decides the choice and sequence of words to be spoken
6. From Wernicke's area, signals go to Broca's area
7. From Broca's area, signals go to cortex and speech is produced.

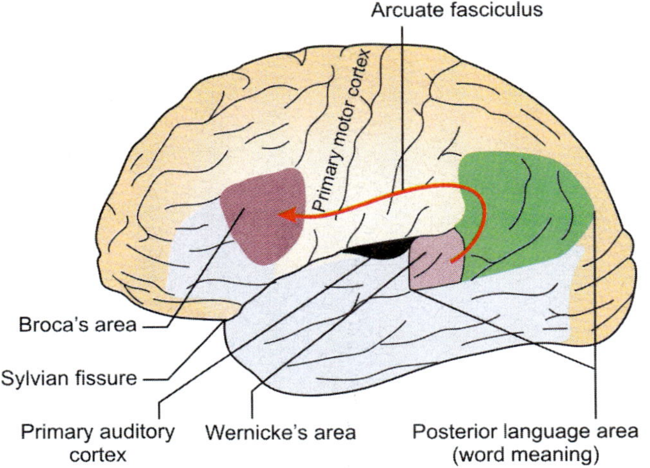

Fig. 11.68

11

Voice Production

The anatomical structures involved in voice production are larynx, pharynx, tongue, teeth, cheek, lips , palate, nose, facial muscles and respiratory muscles. Words are formed during expiration.

Applied Physiology

I. *Dysarthria*

- This is defective speech
- It occurs in cerebellar lesions, bulbar paralysis and parkinsonism.

II. *Aphasia*

Inability to express the ideas that is not due to defects of vision or hearing or to motor paralysis is called aphasia. It is caused by embolism or thrombosis of a cerebral blood vessel.

Types

1. *Fluent aphasia*

   The person talks excessively but he fails to comprehend the meaning of spoken or written words. The lesion is in Wernicke's area.

2. *Nonfluent aphasia*
   - Speech is slow and the words are hard to come out.
   - Lesion is in Broca's area.

3. *Conduction aphasia*
   - The person can speak relatively well but cannot put the words together.
   - The lesion is in and around the auditory cortex.

4. *Global aphasia*
   - It is also known as complete aphasia
   - Speech is scanty
   - Writing is abnormal.

   There are extensive lesions involving speech areas in the frontal, parietal and temporal lobes.

III. *Dyslexia*

- Comprehension of written language is affected.
- In children, it interferes with the learning of academic skills and mathematics.
- The lesion is in angular gyrus.

116. CEREBROSPINAL FLUID

Anatomy

The brain and the spinal cord are surrounded by three membranes. They are:

1. Dura mater
2. Arachnoid mater
3. Pia mater

Dura Mater

It is the outermost membrane and made up of tough fibrous tissue. It has two layers, outer endosteal layer which is attached to cranial bones and inner meningeal layer.

Arachnoid Mater

It is the middle membrane. There is a small potential space between dura and arachnoid mater called subdural fluid which is filled with a thin layer of fluid.

Pia Mater

It is the innermost membrane which is closely attached to brain and spinal cord. The space between pia mater and arachnoid mater is known as subarachnoid space which contains CSF. At some places, subarachnoid space shows dilatations called cisternae, e.g. cisterna magna, cisterna pontin, cisterna basalis.

CSF

It is a clear, colorless fluid that circulates through ventricles of brain, subarachnoid space and central canal of spinal cord.

Site of Formation (Fig. 11.69)

It is produced by choroid plexus of lateral, third and fourth ventricles. Some amount is also formed by ependymal cells that line the ventricles.

Mechanism of Formation

It is formed partly by active secretion and partly by ultrafiltration.

Rate of Formation

550 ml/day

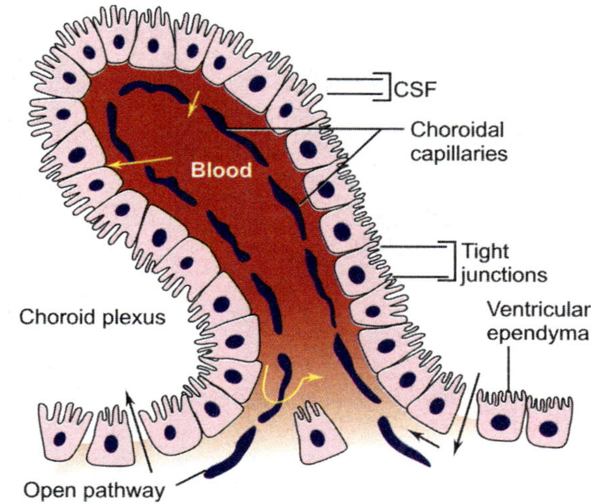

Fig. 11.69: Site of formation of CSF

Normal volume is 150 ml. This CSF turns over about 3.7 times a day.

Substance	*CSF*	*Plasma*
Na^+ mEq/kg H_2O	147	150
K^+ mEq/kg H_2O	2.9	4.6
Mg^{2+} mEq/kg H_2O	2.2	1.6
Ca^{2+} mEq/kg H_2O	2.3	4.7
Cl^- mEq/kg H_2O	113	99
HCO_3 mEq/L	25.1	24.8
Protein mg/dl	20	6000
Glucose mg/dl	64	100
pH	7.3	7.4
Osmolality mOsm/kg H_2O	289	289

Circulation of CSF (Fig. 11.70)

The CSF formed in lateral ventricles flows into the 3rd ventricle through foramen of Monroe. From 3rd ventricle it flows into 4th ventricle through aqueduct of Sylvius. From here it flows into subarachnoid space through foramen of Magendie and foramen of Luschka. From here 80% is absorbed through the arachnoid villi into veins and primary the cerebral venous sinuses. About 20% enters spinal veins by diffusion.

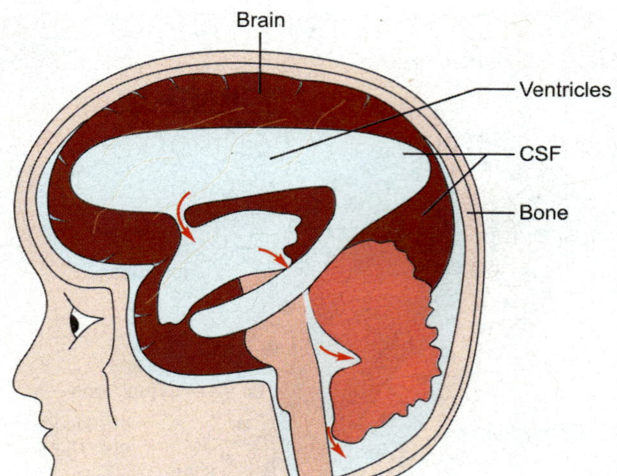

Fig. 11.70: Circulation of CSF

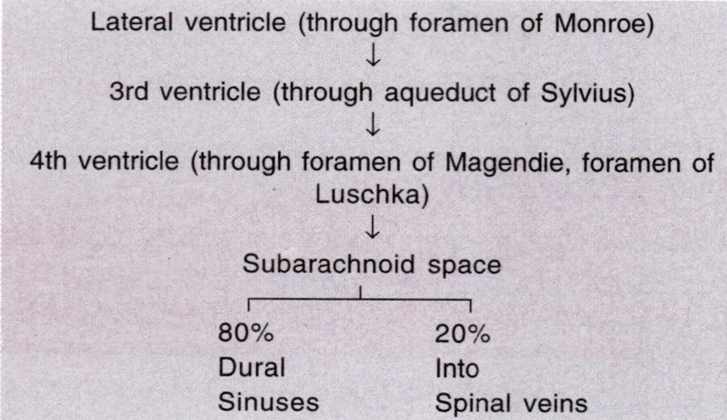

Mechanism of Absorption

It is by a passive mechanism and is controlled by two forces:

1. *Hydrostatic Pressure*

For CSF, it ranges from 180 to 200 mm water where pressure is negative in dural sinuses. The pressure gradient causes filtration of the CSF into the dural sinuses.

2. *Colloidal Osmotic Pressure*

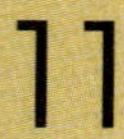

Colloidal osmotic pressure of venous blood is about 25 mm Hg where as in CSF it is almost nil. This facilitates absorption of CSF into the venous blood.

Functions of CSF

1. It acts as a cushion around the brain. If there is a head injury, the impact of the blow is distributed all over the brain. So, CSF acts as a shock absorber.
2. It helps in maintaining a constant internal volume of cranium.
3. It serves as lymph as there is no lymphatic system in the brain.
4. It acts as a medium through which nutritive and waste substances are exchanged between brain tissues and blood.

Applied Physiology

Hydrocephalus

It means excess water in cranial vault. It is a condition where there is accumulation of CSF leading to increased intracranial tension and compression of brain. It may be due to decreased absorption as in block or increased formation as in inflammation of brain. It is of two types:

1. *Internal/noncommunicating hydrocephalus:* It is due to accumulation of CSF in ventricular system. The block may be in 3rd or 4th ventricle or aqueduct of Sylvius.
2. *External/communicating hydrocephalus:* CSF accumulates in subarachnoid space due to inflammation of meninges or thrombosis in dural sinuses.

Management

A silicone tube shunt is surgically done all the way from one of the brain ventricles to the peritoneal cavity to drain the excess fluid where it can be absorbed into the blood.

Lumbar Puncture

CSF can be collected by lumbar puncture or cistern puncture needle is introduced through intervertebral disc between L_3 and L_4 into subarachnoid space and CSF is collected.

Uses of Lumbar Puncture

1. To collect CSF for diagnostic purposes.
2. To inject drug for spinal anesthesia.
3. To measure CSF pressure.

Abnormal CSF

- Subarachnoid hemorrhage—blood is present.
- Viral meningitis—protein is increased.
- TB meningitis—protein is increased, but glucose and chloride levels are low.
- High CSF pressure causes edema of optic disc and this is called papilledema.

117. BLOOD–BRAIN BARRIER (BBB)

In 19th century, Paul Ehrlich, a great Austrian chemist noted that a dye like tryptan blue when injected into an animal and if the animal is subsequently killed, all tissues were found stained except the brain. He suggested that there is a barrier between blood and brain. This is called blood–brain barrier.

Formation of BBB (Fig. 11.71)

The tight junctions in the endothelial cells of the brain capillaries supported by astrocyte act as BBB. The expanded foot processes of astrocytes incompletely cover the capillaries. The pericytes play an important role in formation and maintenance of tight junctions and structural stability of the barrier.

At birth, BBB is not fully mature. Functional maturation is completed by 1–2 years afterbirth. That is why in severely jaundiced infants, the bile pigments damage the basal ganglia causing kernicterus.

Movement of Substances Across BBB

The movement of substances across the BBB is dependent on the following factors:

- Size of the molecule
- Lipid solubility
- Protein binding
- pH of the body fluids.

Substances which can pass through BBB

- O_2
- CO_2
- H_2O
- Glucose
- Anesthetic gases like nitrous oxide and ether
- Steroid hormones.

Substances which cannot pass through BBB

- Pro teins
- Protein bound forms

Functions of BBB

1. Maintain a constant chemical environment around the neurons.
2. Protects the brain from endogenous and exogenous toxins in the blood.
3. Prevents the escape of neurotransmitters into the general circulation.

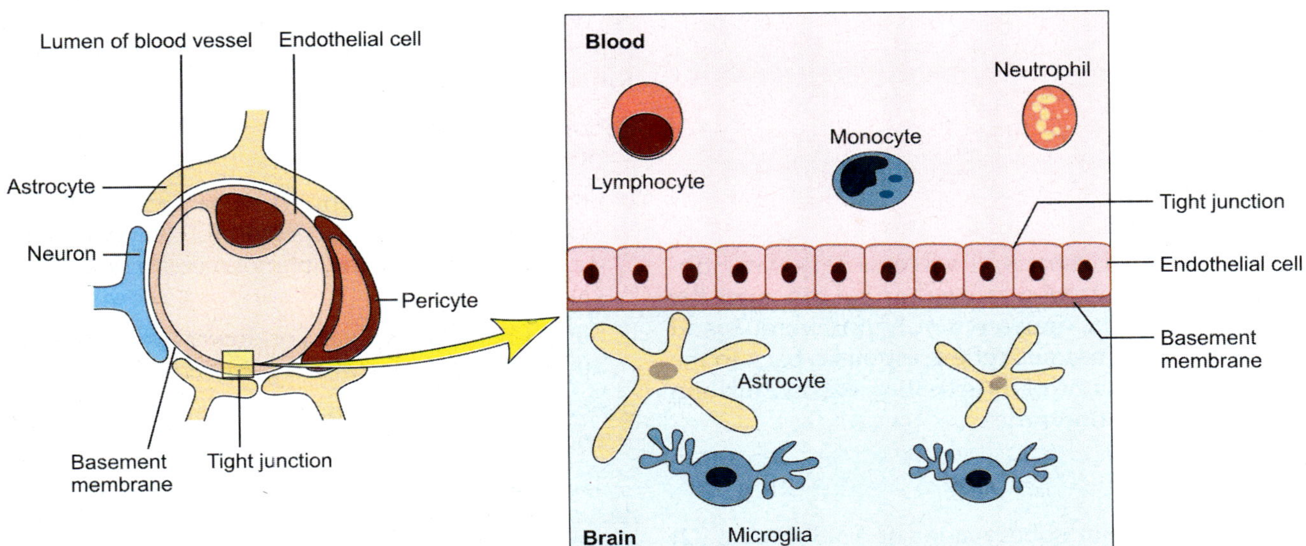

Fig. 11.71: Formation of blood–brain barrier

BLOOD–CSF BARRIER

It is the barrier between blood and CSF that exists at the choroid plexus. It does not allow some substances to pass through it.

Applied Physiology

1. Adequate knowledge about BBB helps the physician in the selection of drugs in management of meningitis and encephalitis.
2. BBB breaks down in areas of injury, infection or tumor.

Circumventricular Organs

The structures which lie outside BBB are called circumventricular organs. They are:

- Posterior pituitary
- Area postrema
- Organum vasculosum of lamina terminalis (OVLT)
- Subfornical organ (SFO)
- Median eminence
- Pineal gland.

118. AUTONOMIC NERVOUS SYSTEM (ANS)

Introduction

The portion of the nervous system that controls most visceral functions of the body is called autonomic nervous system (Fig. 11.72). The characteristic feature of ANS is the rapidity and intensity with which it can change visceral functions. Within 3 to 5 seconds, it can increase the heart rate twice the normal. Sweating can begin within seconds and the bladder can be emptied involuntarily within seconds.

Control by Higher Centers

ANS is activated by centers in the following areas:

1. Spinal cord
2. Brainstem
3. Hypothalamus
4. Cerebral cortex
5. Limbic cortex

Visceral Reflexes

ANS operates by means of visceral reflexes. Subconscious signals from a visceral organ can enter the autonomic ganglia, brainstem or hypothalamus and then return subconscious reflex responses back to the visceral organ to control its activities, e.g. micturition reflex and defecation reflex.

11

Divisions of ANS

There are two major subdivisions of ANS (Fig. 11.72)

1. Sympathetic nervous system
2. Parasympathetic nervous system.

These two systems communicate with enteric nervous system (ENS) in the gastrointestinal tract. ENS in sometimes called as third division of ANS.

Sympathetic Nervous System

Sympathetic nervous system is made up of:

- Preganglionic neurons
- Postganglionic neurons.

Preganglionic Neurons

The sympathetic nerve fibers take origin from the intermediolateral horn of gray matter in spinal cord from T_1 to L_2 segments. They come out of the spinal cord via anterior root and end in the following ways:

a. Some fibers end in paravertebral sympathetic chain of ganglia.
b. Some fibers pass through these ganglia without synapsing and end in the peripheral collateral ganglia, e.g. superior mesenteric, inferior mesenteric and celiac ganglia.
c. Some fibers pass upward or downward in the chain and synapse in one of the ganglia of the chain.
d. Some fibers pass through the splanchnic nerve and end in adrenal medulla.

This is called thoracolumbar outflow of sympathetic nervous system. These fibers from their origin up to the ganglia are called preganglionic fibers.

The preganglionic nerve fibers are usually short and synapse with postganglionic neurons.

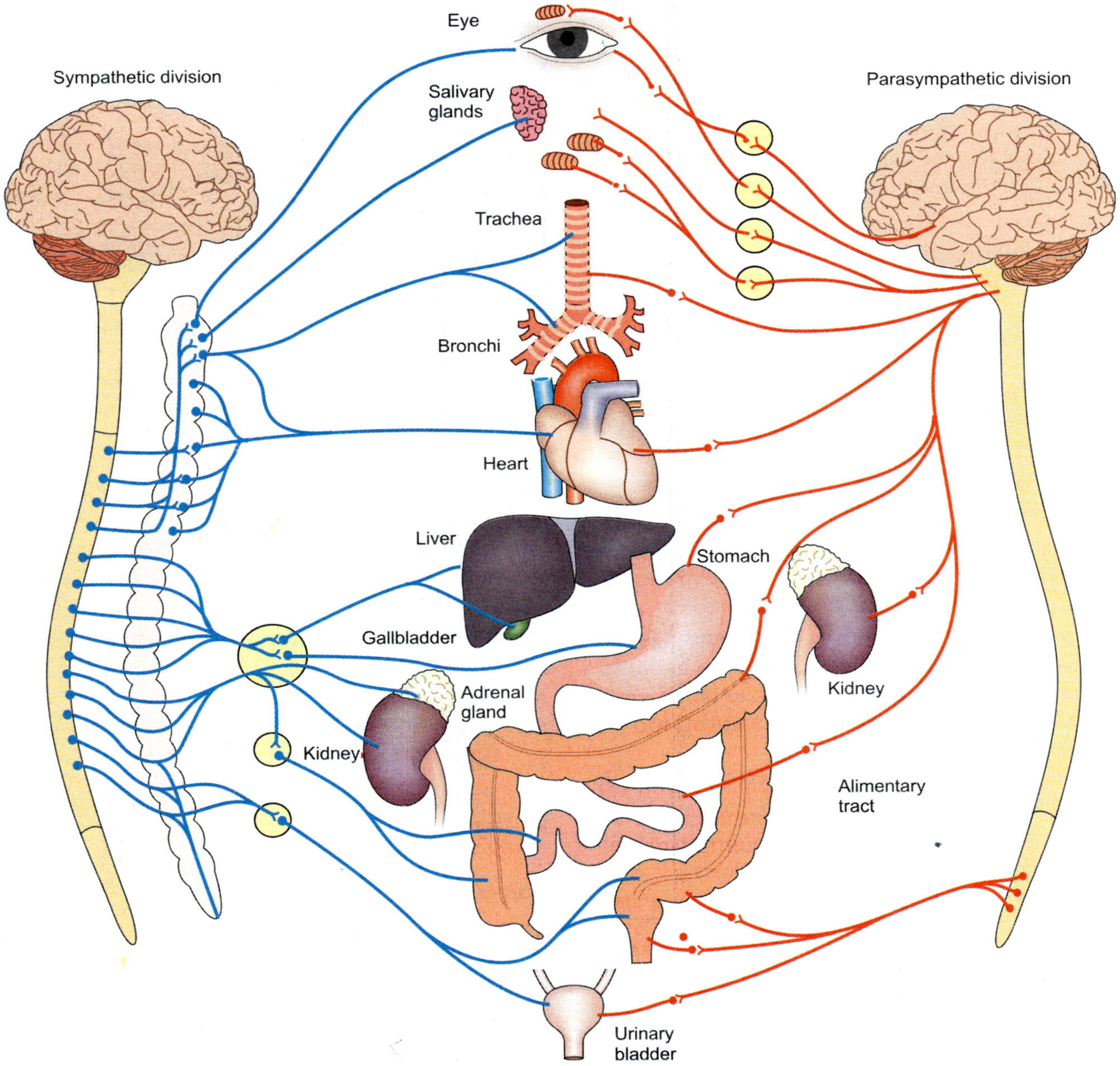

Fig. 11.72: Autonomic nervous system

Postganglionic Neurons

They are present in the peripheral sympathetic ganglia. The axons of these neurons are called post-ganglionic nerve fibers. These fibers are long and supply the target organs.

In adrenal medulla, the postganglionic neurons are modified into secretory cells called pheochromocytes which store noradrenaline and adrenaline.

Parasympathetic Nervous System

It also has two types of neurons:

1. Preganglionic neurons
2. Postganglionic neurons.

Preganglionic Neurons

Parasympathetic fibers arise from nuclei of cranial nerves III, VII, IX and X and from sacral segments of spinal cord. This is called craniosacral outflow.

Cranial division

The preganglionic neurons are present in:

1. Edinger-Westphal nucleus
2. Superior salivary nucleus
3. Inferior salivary nucleus
4. Dorsal nucleus of vagus

These ganglia are present near the target organs.

Sacral division

The preganglionic neurons are present in the lateral horns of sacral segments (S_2, S_3 and S_4). Preganglionic fibers come out through the anterior root and form nerve erigentis or pelvic nerve.

Postganglionic Neurons

Postganglionic neurons of parasympathetic nervous system are present in the target organ itself.

Neurotransmitters of ANS

Acetylcholine is the parasympathetic transmitter and norepinephrine is the sympathetic transmitter.

Acetylcholine

It is secreted by:

- All preganglionic autonomic nerve endings
- Postganglionic parasympathetic nerve endings
- Postganglionic sympathetic fibers to blood vessels of skeletal muscles, sweat glands and piloerector muscles of the hair
- Preganglionic fibers supplying adrenal medulla.

Synthesis

It is synthesized in the nerve endings from choline and acetylCoA and stored in the vesicles.

$$\text{AcetylCoA} + \text{choline} \xrightarrow[\text{(CAT)}]{\text{choline acetyl transferase}} \text{acetylcholine}$$

Release and Metabolism

Once acetylcholine is secreted by the nerve endings, it persists in the tissue for a few seconds. Then it is split into acetate and choline by the enzyme acetylcholinesterase that is bound with collagen and glycosaminoglycans in the local connective tissue and neuromuscular junctions. The choline is transported back into the terminal nerve ending for resynthesis of new acetylcholine.

Receptors of Acetylcholine (Fig. 11.73)

There are two types of acetylcholine receptors:

- Nicotinic
- Muscarinic

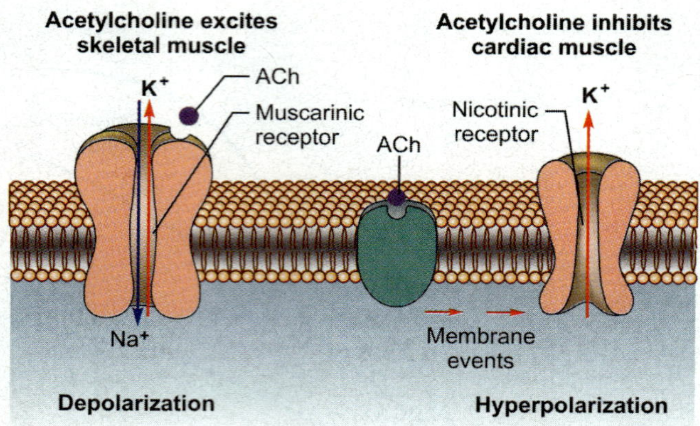

Fig. 11.73: Acetylcholine receptors

Nicotinic Receptors

They are present in:

- Autonomic ganglia
- Neuromuscular junction and brain.

Muscarinic Receptors

There are five types of muscarinic receptors found in following organs:

M_1 : Brain

M_2 : Heart

M_3 : Smooth muscle

M_4 : Pancreas, smooth muscle

M_5 : Uncertain

Norepinephrine

Synthesis of norepinephrine begins in the axoplasm of the terminal nerve endings of adrenergic fibers but is completed inside the secretory vesicles. The steps are the following:

1. Tyrosine → $\xrightarrow{\text{hydroxylase}}$ → dopa
2. Dopa → $\xrightarrow{\text{decarboxylation}}$ → dopamine
3. Transport of dopamine into the vesicles
4. Dopamine → $\xrightarrow{\text{hydroxylation}}$ → norepinephrine
5. Norepinephrine → $\xrightarrow{\text{methylation}}$ → epinephrine.

After synthesis, norepinephrine is removed from the secretory site in three ways

1. Reuptake into the adrenergic nerve endings themselves by an active process.
2. Diffusion into the surrounding body fluids and blood.

3. Destruction by tissue enzymes (monoamine oxidase (MAO) and catechol-O-methyl transferase (COMT).

Receptors of Norepinephrine

There are two types of adrenergic receptors:

1. Alpha
   - α_1
   - α_2
2. Beta
   - β_1
   - β_2
   - β_3

Norepinephrine excites mainly alpha receptors and excites beta receptors to a lesser extent. Epinephrine excites both types of receptors equally. Therefore, the relative effects of norepinephrine and epinephrine on effector organs are determined by the types of receptors in the organs. If they are all beta receptors, epinephrine will be more effective than norepinephrine.

Receptors and their Location

Alpha 1	Smooth muscle of blood vessels, dilator papillae, sphincters of GIT, urinary bladder, salivary glands, sweat glands
Alpha 2	Pancreatic acini, platelets, some blood vessels
Beta 1	Cardiac muscle, JG cells, adipose tissue
Beta 2	Smooth muscle in bronchi, coronary blood vessels, skeletal blood vessels, liver, ciliary muscle
Beta 3	Brown adipose tissue

Effects of sympathetic and parasympathetic stimulation on specific organs

Organ	*Effect of sympathetic stimulation*	*Effect of parasympathetic stimulation*
Eye:		
Pupil	Dilated	Constricted
Ciliary muscle	Slight relaxation (far vision)	Constricted (near vision)
Glands:		
Nasal Lacrimal Parotid Submandibular Gastric Pancreatic	Vasoconstriction and slight secretion	Stimulation of copious secretion (containing many enzymes for enzyme-secreting glands
Sweat glands:	Copious sweating (cholinergic)	Sweating on palms of hands
Apocrine glands:	Thick, odoriferous secretion	None
Blood vessels:	Most often constricted	Most often little or no effect
Heart:		
Muscle	Increased rate Increased force of contraction	Slowed rate Decreasedforce contraction (especially of atria)
Coronaries	Dilated (β_2); constricted (α)	Dilated
Lungs:		
Bronchi	Dilated	Constricted
Blood vessels	Mildly constricted	Dilated
Gut:		
Lumen	Decreased peristalsis and tone	Increased peristalsis and tone
sphincter	Increased tone (most times)	Relaxed (most times)
Liver:	Glucose released	Slight glycogen synthesis
Gallbladder and bile ducts:	Relaxed	Contracted
Kidney:	Decreased output and renin secretion	None
Bladder:		
Detrusor	Relaxed (slight)	Contracted
Trigone	Contracted	Relaxed
Penis:	Ejaculation	Erection
Systemic arterioles:		
Abdominal viscera	Constricted	None
Muscle	Constricted (adrenergic α) Dilated (adrenergic β_2) Dilated (cholinergic)	None
Skin	Constricted	None
Blood:		
Coagulation	Increased	None
Glucose	Increased	None
Lipids	Increased	None
Basal metabolism:	Increased up to 100%	None
Adrenal medullary secretion:	Increased	None
Mental activity:	Increased	None
Piloerector muscles:	Contracted	None
Skeletal muscle:	Increased glycogenolysis Increased strength	None
Fat cells:	Lipolysis	None

Anabolic and Catabolic Systems

Parasympathetic nervous system favors digestion and absorption of food and helps to save energy. Hence it is called as anabolic nervous system.

Sympathetic nervous system causes glycolysis and lipolysis depleting the energy stores. Hence, it is called as catabolic nervous system.

Functions of ANS

1. Controls the activity of smooth muscle and cardiac muscle through many visceral reflexes.
2. Controls secretion from exocrine and endocrine glands.
3. Plays an important role in homeostasis.

Role in Stress

During stress, the subject requires higher amounts of energy substrates like glucose and free fatty acids which are brought about by glycogenolysis and lipolysis. More O_2 is supplied to the necessary muscles. All these changes prepare the subject for fight or flight. These changes are brought about by activation of sympathetic nervous system during any stress which inturn activates adrenal medulla to release catecholomines. This occurs when hypothalamus is activated by fear or severe pain. These reactions together constitute alarm or stress response. The entire sympathetic nervous system discharges simultaneously as a complete unit, a phenomenon called mass discharge. The effects are the following:

1. Increased BP.
2. Increased blood flow to active muscles and less blood flow to organs such as GIT and kidneys that are not needed for rapid motor activity.
3. Increased rate of cellular metabolism throughout the body.
4. Increased blood glucose concentration.
5. Increased glycolysis in the liver and muscle.
6. Increased muscle strength.
7. Increased mental activity.
8. Increased rate of blood coagulation.

Control of ANS by Higher Centers

11

1. *Spinal cord:* It has limited control over ANS as section of spinal cord results in fall in BP.
2. *Brainstem:* Brainstem especially medulla oblongata is responsible for tonic activities of ANS.
3. *Hypothalamus:* Hypothalamus is considered as head ganglion of ANS by Sherrington.
4. Cerebral cortex.

PHARMACOLOGY OF ANS

Drugs that Act on Adrenergic Effector Organs

Drugs that have the same effects throughout the body as sympathetic stimulation are called sympatho-mimetic or adrenergic drugs, e.g. epinephrine, methoxamine.

Drugs that Release Norepinephrine from Nerve Endings

For example, ephedrine, tyramine, amphetamine.

Drugs that Block Adrenergic Activity

1. Blocker of synthesis and storage of norepinephrine
   Reserpine
2. Blocker of norepinephrine release
   Guanethidine
3. Receptor blockers
   α_1 blocker : Prazosin
   α_2 blocker : Yohimbine
   β_1 blocker : Metoprolol
   β_2 blocker : Butoxamine.

Drugs that Act on Cholinergic Effector Organs

Drugs that produce typical parasympathetic effects are called parasympathomimetic drugs, e.g. pilocarpine, methacholine.

Anticholinesterase Drugs

Some drugs do not have a direct effect on parasympathetic effector organs but potentiate the effects of naturally secreted acetylcholine at the parasympathetic endings. They act by inhibiting acetylcholinesterase, thus preventing rapid destruction of acetylcholine. These drugs are called anticholinesterase drugs, e.g. neostigmine, physostigmine and ambenonium.

Antimuscarinic Drugs

These drugs block the action of acetylcholine at the muscarinic receptors. They do not affect the nicotinic action of acetylcholine, e.g. atropine, homatropine, scopolamine.

Ganglionic Blocking Drugs

These drugs block the impulse transmission at the autonomic ganglia of both sympathetic and parasympathetic systems, e.g. hexamethonium, pentolinium.

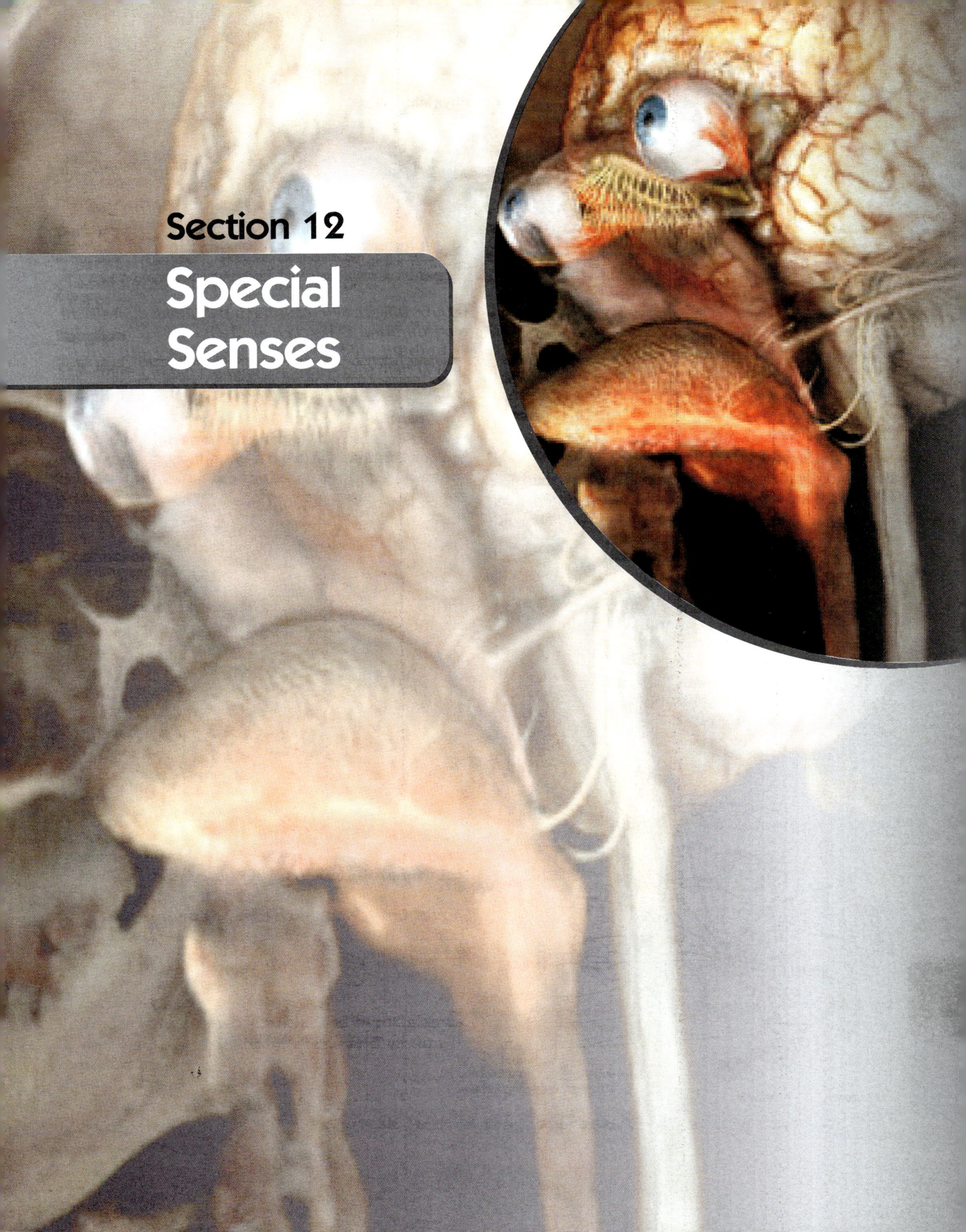

Section 12

Special Senses

119. VISION

PHYSIOANATOMY OF THE EYE

The eye is the organ of vision (Fig. 12.1). It is enclosed on a bony socket called orbit. Between the orbit and eyeball several structures are present namely:

1. Voluntary muscles
2. Connective tissue
3. Fat
4. Lacrimal gland.

These structures are separated from the eyeball by the Buck's fascia.

The eye has three layers

1. Outer fibrous coat consisting of sclera and cornea.
2. Middle vascular and pigmented coat called uvea which consists of the iris, ciliary body and choroid.
3. Inner nervous coat called retina.

Sclera

It is the outer protective layer. It forms the posterior 5/6 of the outer coat. It is smooth and white in color. The lamina cribrosa is the exit point of the optic nerve. The anterior 1/6 is modified to form the transparent cornea.

The cornea is the first and most important refractive medium of the eye. It is made up of five layers from outside inwards.

1. The stratified layer of squamous epithelium
2. The basal layer of epithelial cells (Bowman's membrane)
3. The stromal layer (substantia propria)
4. The basal lamina of endothelial cells (Descemet's membrane)
5. The layer of endothelial cells.

The junction of the sclera with the cornea is called the limbus (sclerocorneal junction). The Schlemm's canal is located here.

The cornea is transparent, avascular, and dehydrated. It is richly supplied with branches of the trigeminal nerve. Hence it is sensitive to pain.

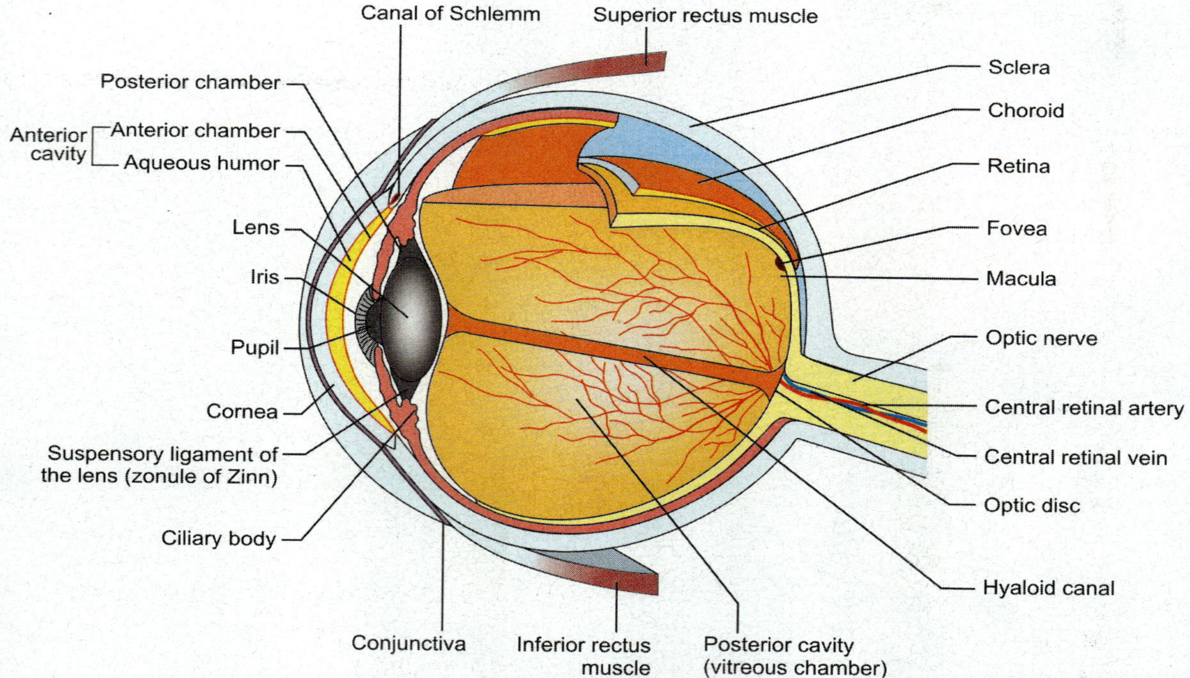

Fig. 12.1: Physioanatomy of the eye

The Uveal Tract

Lies interior to the sclera and consists of the iris, ciliary body and the choroid.

Iris

Iris is situated in front of the lens. It is pigmented and encloses a central aperture called the pupil. It contains two muscles that control the papillary movements namely:

1. The sphincter pupillae: A circular bundle running around the papillary margin.
2. The dilator pupillae arranged radially near the root of the iris.

Nerve supply: The sphincter pupillae are supplied by parasympathetics through branches of the oculomotor nerve.

The dilator pupillae is supplied by the sympathetic from cervical sympathetic ganglia.

The iris regulates the amount of light falling on the lens. Together with the lens it forms a circular diaphragm which partitions the eye into anterior and posterior chambers.

Ciliary Body

It has an outer part and an inner part. The outer part is made up of smooth muscle called ciliary muscle. It contains both circular and longitudinal muscle fibers which arise from a common ciliary tendon, running circumferentially around the eyeball. The inner part is the ciliary process which is highly vascular and secretes the aqueous humor.

Choroid

It is the posterior 2/3 of the uveal layer. It is pigmented and extremely vascular layer in contact with the sclera. On the inner side it is covered by a thin elastic membrane the membrane of Bruch. Beneath the membrane of Bruch is a plexus of choriocapillaries.

The Lens

It is a crystalline biconvex structure situated behind the iris. It is enclosed by a capsule which is suspended from the ciliary body by the suspensory ligament of the lens. At their lateral ends the suspensory ligaments are attached to the ciliary body. When the ciliary muscles contract, the tension on the suspensory ligaments eases and the anterior surface of the lens bulges. The lens is made up of ribbon-like transparent fibers arranged in concentric lamellae. Its central part consists of older cells and its periphery contains younger cells. As age advances the lens loses water and becomes hard and it loses its ability to change shape. This is called presbyopia. The center of the lens also becomes opaque resulting in cataract.

Retina

It is the innermost light sensitive coat of the eye. It extends from the optic disc posteriorly to the limbus behind the ciliary body anteriorly. It ends in an irregular margin called ora serrata. It is made up of 10 layers (Fig. 12.2). They are (from outside to inside):

1. Pigment cell layer
2. Layer of rods and cones
3. Outer limiting membrane
4. Outer nuclear layer
5. Outer plexiform layer
6. Inner nuclear layer
7. Inner plexiform layer
8. Layer of ganglion cells
9. Layer of optic nerve fibers
10. Inner limiting membrane.

1. Pigment Cell Layer

Single layer of hexagonal epithelial cells. It extends from periphery of optic disc to ora serrata and continues into ciliary epithelium. The basal part of the cell contains the nucleus while the apical portions project between rod and cone processes as microvilli. The cytoplasm contains mitochondria, endoplasmic reticulum and melanin. Melanin absorbs light and prevents its back reflection thus preventing blurring of vision. The pigment cell layer has phagocytic function. It ingests and digests fragmented tips of the outer segments of the rods and cones. It also stores large quantities of vitamin A which is exchanged back and forth through the cell membrane of the outer segments of rods and cones (Fig. 12.3).

2. Layer of Rods and Cones

It contains the outer and inner segments of the rods and cones.

3. Outer Limiting Membrane

It is a thin membrane formed of processes of glial cells called Müller cells. They bind the nervous layers together and give physical support to the retina.

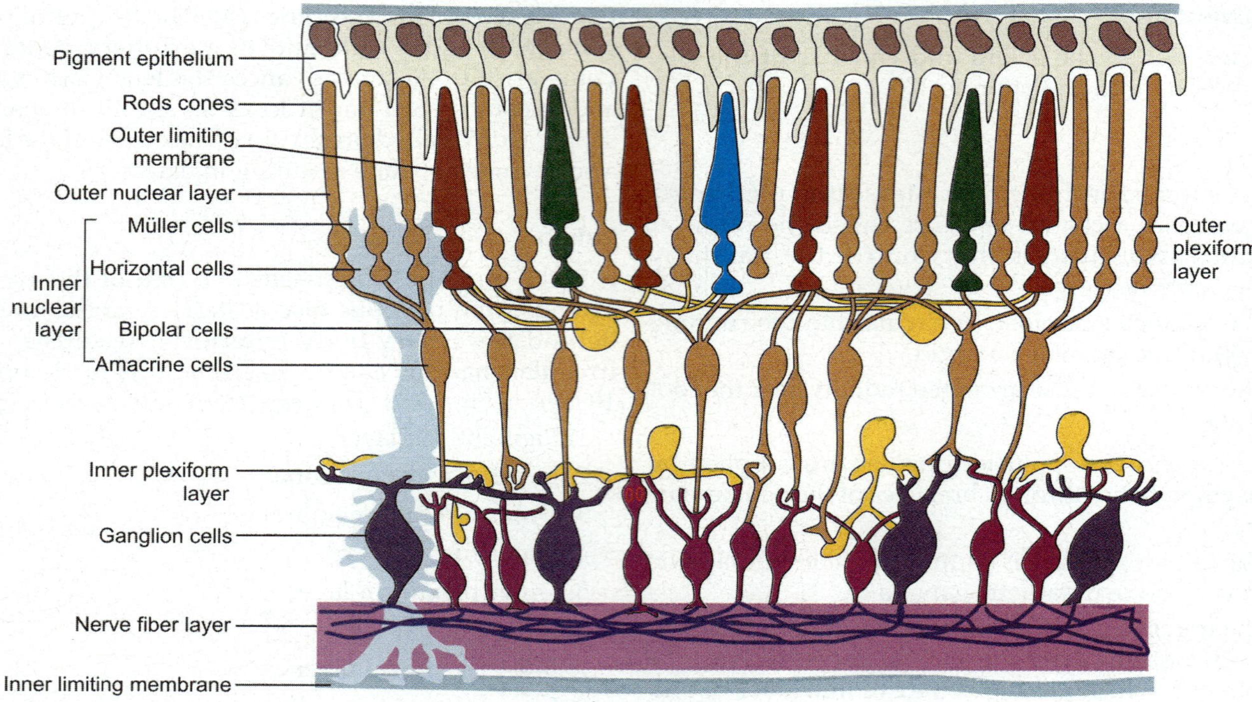

Fig. 12.2: Structure of retina

4. Outer Nuclear Layer

It contains the cell bodies of rods and cones which contains the nucleus. The cytoplasm also contains mitochondria, endoplasmic reticulum and ribosomes. The inner portion synapses with the bipolar and horizontal cells.

5. Outer Plexiform Layer

It is made up of connections of the processes of bipolar cells and horizontal cells with the fibers of the rods and cones.

6. Inner Nuclear Layer

It is made up cell bodies of bipolar cells, horizontal cells, amacrine cells and glial cells of Müller. The bipolar cells are of three types: rod, flat and midget. The rod bipolar cells connect with groups of rod fibers. The flat bipolar cells connect with several cones. Midget bipolar cells connect with single cone. The axons of the horizontal cells run horizontally and connect rod and cone fibers with one another and function as association fibers. The amacrine cells are of 29 types. They have no axons and have polarity in the opposite direction. They connect ganglion cells to one another in the inner plexiform layer.

7. Inner Plexiform Layer

It is made up of synapses of dendrites of ganglion cells with the processes of the bipolar cells. A giant ganglion cell connects with a few rod and flat bipolar cells. Midget ganglion cells connect with single midget bipolar cell.

8. Layer of Ganglion Cells

It contains one layer of cell bodies of the optic nerve fibers. They are of different sizes and shapes ranging from giant to small midget cells. The large cells are (M) magna cells and small cells are (P) parvo cells.

9. Layer of Optic Nerve Fibers

It made up of axons of ganglion cells. They turn sharply from their origin and converge towards the optic disc to form the optic nerve. The axons are unmyelinated and are surrounded by the processes of neuralgia cells.

10. Inner Limiting Membrane

It is a thin basement membrane that separates the nerve fiber layer from the vitreous humor and is made up of processes of glial cells.

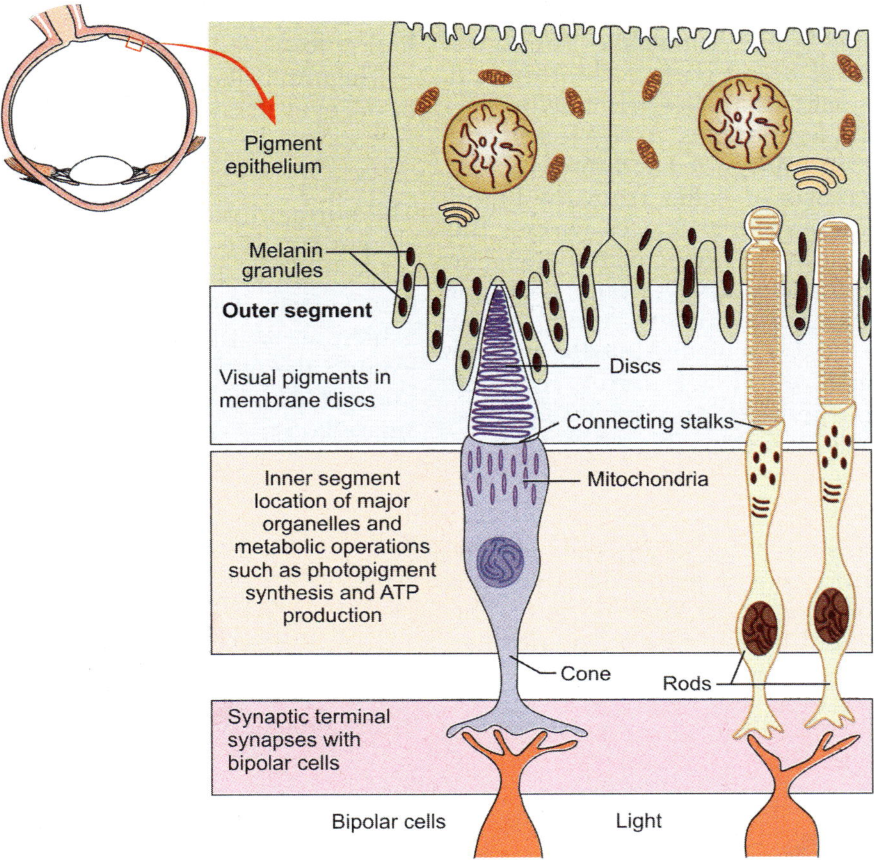

Fig. 12.3: Retinal receptors—rods and cones

Optic Disc (Blind Spot)

Location: 3 mm medial to and a little above the posterior pole of the eyeball.

It has a diameter of 1.5 mm and its circumference is slightly elevated to form optic papilla. All the layers of the retina except optic nerve fibers are absent in this region. Hence, it is totally insensitive to light. So, it is called blind spot. The optic disc is pierced near its center by the central artery of the retina and its accompanying vein.

Macula Lutea (Yellow Spot)

Location: Temporal to the posterior pole of the eyeball 3.5 mm from the outer edge of the optic disc.

It measures 2 mm horizontally and 1 mm vertically. It is yellow in color due to the presence of the pigment xanthophyll. It has a central depression—fovea centralis (0.4 mm in diameter). This portion is very thin as all the elements of the retina including the rods are absent. It contains only cones which are densely packed (35000 cones) the cones in this region are thin and long and each cone is connected to a single midget bipolar cell and single midget ganglion cell. The fovea and the macular region have no blood vessels and nourishment is obtained from the choroid. The fovea is the region of maximal visual acuity.

Chambers of the Eye and Intraocular Fluid

The eye is divided into two chambers by the iris and the lens.

The anterior chamber: Lies between the posterior surface of the cornea and the anterior surface of the iris.

The posterior chamber: Lies between the posterior surface of the lens and retina.

Aqueous Humor

Which lies in front of the lens is a thin watery fluid secreted by the ciliary processes at a rate of 2–3 micro liters/minute. It is produced by active secretion by the epithelium of the ciliary process. Initially sodium is actively transported by the epithelial cells into the intercellular spaces. It drags with it chloride and bicarbonate ions to maintain the electrical neutrality. Severely nutrients like amino acids. Ascorbic acid and glucose are also actively transported or diffused across the epithelium. Osmosis of water from the blood capillaries into the intercellular spaces washes the solution into the anterior chamber of the eye. The aqueous humor thus formed passes through the pupil into the anterior chamber of the eye. From here it escapes through the canal of Schlemm into the anterior ciliary veins. The small veins that lead from the canal of Schlemm into the larger veins contain only aqueous. So, they are called aqueous veins (Fig. 12.4).

Vitreous Humor

It is a hydrated transparent gel lying between the lens and the retina. It contains albumin and hyaluronic acid which is responsible for its high viscosity. The gelatinous mass is held together by a fine fibrillar network composed of greatly elongated proteoglycan molecules.

The intraocular fluid maintains sufficient pressure in the eyeball and keeps it distended.

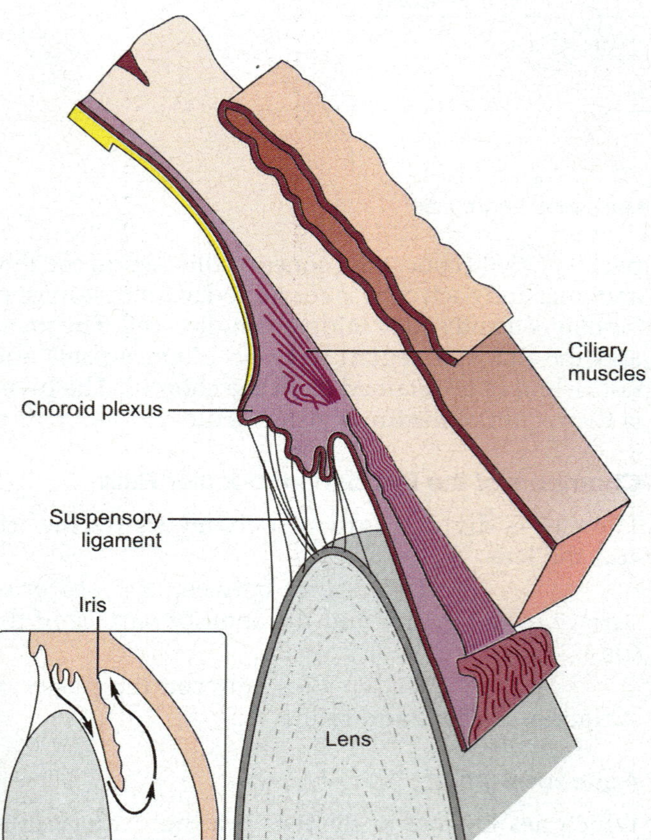

Fig. 12.4: Flow of aqueous humour

Intraocular Pressure (IOP)

The normal intraocular pressure ranges from 12 to 20 mm Hg. The average pressure of 15 mm Hg. It is maintained by the resistance to outflow of aqueous humor from the anterior chamber into the canal of Schlemm. At the normal IOP the amount of fluid leaving the eye through the canal of Schlemm (2.5 microliter/min) equals the inflow of fluid from the ciliary body.

Measurement of IOP

IOP is measured using a tonometer. The cornea is anesthetized and the footplate of the tonometer is placed on its surface. A small force is applied to the central plunger, which causes the part of cornea beneath the plunger to be displaced inwards. The amount of displacement is measured on the scale of the tonometer which is calibrated in terms of IOP.

The Lacrimal Apparatus

It comprises the lacrimal glands which secrete tears and the lacrimal passages which drain the tears into the nasal cavity.

The lacrimal glands secrete tears. The tear film in front of the cornea has three layers. The outermost lipid layer is secreted by the Meibomian glands in the eyelids. It prevents evaporation of the middle aqueous layer. The middle aqueous layer is secreted by the lacrimal gland lubricates the ocular surface and also has antimicrobial action. The innermost mucin layer is secreted by the goblet cells of the conjunctiva. This is necessary for soaking the tears.

Applied Aspects

Glaucoma

Glaucoma is an elevation of intraocular pressure with degenerative changes in the optic nerve. Glaucoma is of two types.

Angle-Closure Glaucoma

The sclera-corneal angle is narrow and therefore easily occludable by the peripheral part of the iris. This causes pooling of aqueous humor which further accentuates the occlusion. This is called appositional closure at the angle resulting in sudden rise in IOP. It can be relieved by making a small hole in the iris (peripheral iridectomy) which allows aqueous to flow freely anteriorly.

Open Angle Glaucoma

The sclera corneal angle is not reduced, but the increase of IOP is due to the increased resistance by the trabeculae to aqueous flow. This may be due to deposition of pigments and polysaccharides in the trabecular meshwork. The exact etiology is unknown, but people with myopia, diabetes, and thyroid disorders are prone to it. Also people with family history of glaucoma also develop this glaucoma commonly called as primary open angle glaucoma.

The treatment in both types of glaucoma comprises immediate reduction in IOP with the help of hyperosmotic agents like mannitol, glycerol, sorbitate or urea which causes shrinkage of the vitreous humor. Intravenous acetazolamide reduces aqueous humor formation.

Medical management is the main line of treatment in open angle glaucoma. Miotics like pilocarpine are useful in both types of glaucoma.

Surgical treatment of open angle glaucoma involves trabeculectomy, i.e. the creation of a fistula between the anterior chamber and the subconjunctival space.

OPTICS OF VISION

The Eye as a Camera

The eye can be compared to a camera. It has a lens system, the pupil which acts as a variable aperture system and the retina which corresponds to the film in the camera.

Reduced Eye

The lens system of the eye has four refractive interfaces:

1. The interface between air and the anterior surface of the cornea.
2. The interface between the posterior surface of the cornea and the aqueous humor.
3. The interface between the aqueous humor and the anterior surface of the lens.
4. The interface between the posterior surface of the lens and vitreous humor.

The refractive index of:
Air: 1
Cornea: 1.38
Aqueous humor: 1.33
Lens: 1.40
Vitreous humor: 1.34

If all the refractive surfaces of the eye are added together and considered to be a single lens, then the optics of the normal can be represented schematically as a 'reduced eye'. In such an eye, a single refractive surface exists with its central point 17 mm in front of the retina and a total refractive power of 59 diopters when the lens is accommodated for distant vision.

Of the 59 diopters of refractive power 2/3 is due to the anterior surface of the cornea and the refractive power of the lens is only 20 diopters. The importance of the lens is that in response to nervous signals from the brain it can greatly increase its curvature and thus provide accommodation.

Image Formation in Retina

The crystalline lens in the eye is biconvex. Hence, light rays from an object produce an inverted and real image on the retina. However, the mind perceives the object in the upright position because the brain is trained to consider an inverted image as normal.

Accommodation

Accommodation is the process by which objects which lie very far away from the eye or close to the eye are brought into focus on the retina by altering the curvature of the lens.

In children the refractive power of the lens can be increased from 20 diopters to about 34 diopters, an increase of 14 diopters. This is done by the suspensory ligaments which are attached radially around the lens and pulls the lens outwards causing the lens to remain flat. The ciliary muscles which contain meridional and circular fibers are located at the lateral attachment of the lens ligament and when they contract it causes the ligaments to relax so that the lens assumes a more spherical shape.

The ciliary muscles are supplied by the parasympathetic through the oculomotor nerve. Stimulation of parasympathetic causes contraction of ciliary muscle and relaxation of lens ligaments, thus increasing the curvature of the lens while viewing near objects.

Errors of Refraction (Fig. 12.5)

Emmetropia

It is normal vision. The eye is emmetropic when parallel light rays from distant objects are brought to focus on the retina when the ciliary muscle is completely relaxed.

Hypermetropia (Far Sightedness)

Occurs due to the eyeball being too short or the lens system being too weak. Hence, parallel rays of light are brought to a focus behind the retina. This can be corrected by using a convex lens which converges the image on the retina.

Myopia (Near Sightedness)

Here the ciliary muscle is completely relaxed so that the light rays coming from distant objects are brought to focus in front of the retina. This may be due to the increase in length of the eyeball or increase in the refractive power of the lens system. This can be corrected using concave lens which diverges the light and brings it to focus on the retina.

Astigmatism (Fig. 12.6)

This is a refractive error of the eye that causes the visual image in one plane to focus at a different distance from that of the plane at right angles. This occurs due to greater curvature of the cornea in one plane of the eye. Since, the curvature of the astigmatic lens along one plane is less than the curvature along the other plane, light rays striking the peripheral portions of the lens in one plane are not bent nearly as the rays striking the peripheral portions of the other plane. Hence, they do not focus on a common focal point.

The accommodative power of the eye can never compensate for astigmatism, because during accommodation the curvature of the eye lens changes approximately equally on both sides. Therefore, astigmatism is corrected using two cylindrical lenses of different strengths placed at right angles to each other.

Presbyopia

When a person grows older, the lens becomes larger thicker and less elastic due to progressive denatura-

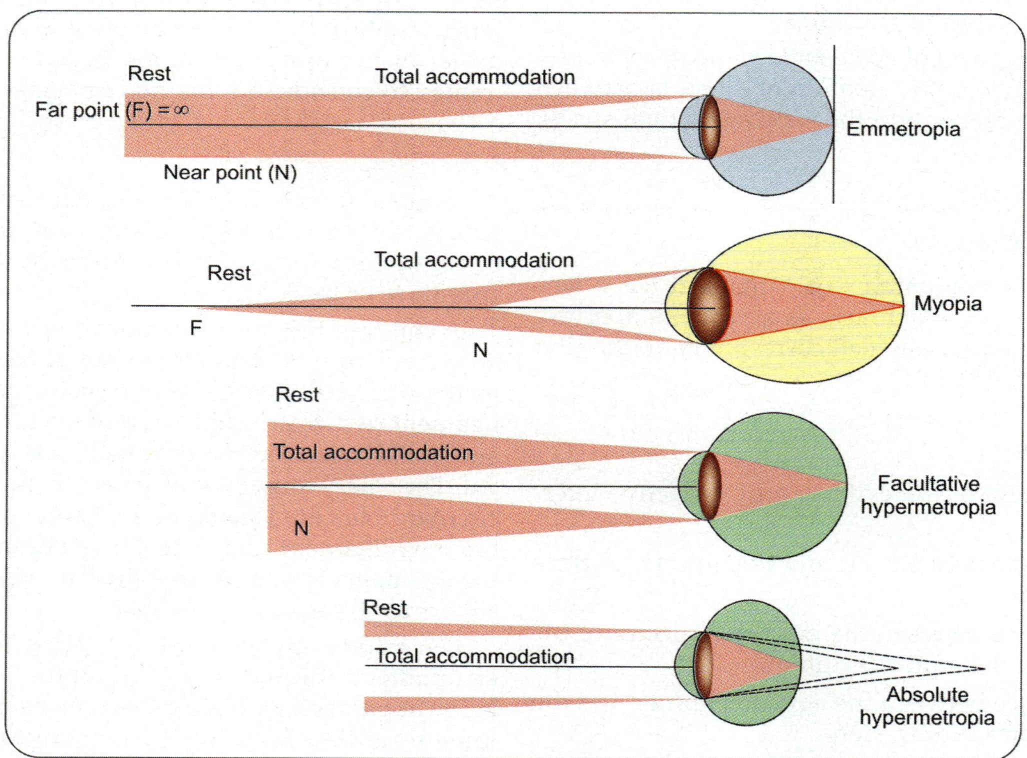

Fig. 12.5: Errors of refraction

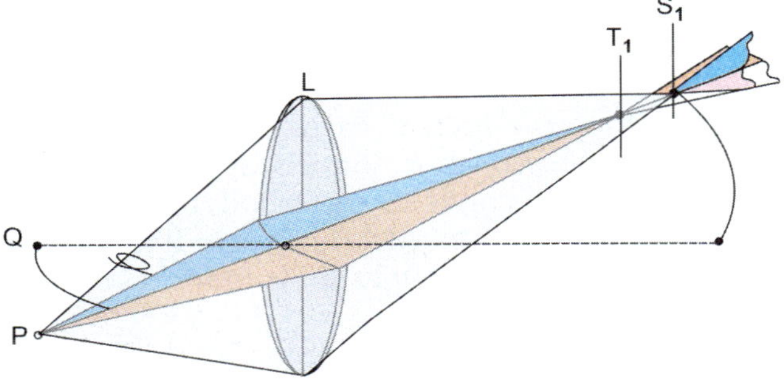

Fig. 12.6: Astigmatism

tion of the lens protein. So, the ability of the lens to change shape decreases with age. The power of accommodation changes from 14 diopters in a child to less than 2 diopters at the age of 45–50 years and to 0 diopters at the age of 70. This condition where the lens remains nonaccommodating is called presbyopia. Here, the eye remains focused permanently at a constant distance. The eye can no longer accommodate for near and far vision. A person with presbyopia must wear bifocal glasses with the upper segment, segment focused for far seeing and the lower segment, segment focused for near-seeing (reading).

Cataract

A cataract is a cloudy or opaque area or areas in the lens. This occurs due to denaturation of the protein fibers in the lens which later coagulate to form opaque areas in the normally transparent lens. When light transmission is greatly obstructed it can be treated by surgical removal of the lens. When the lens is removed a large portion of the refractive power is lost. Hence, the person should wear a powerful convex lens in front of the eye. Nowadays, an artificial plastic lens is implanted in the eye in place of the removed lens.

PHOTOCHEMISTRY OF VISION

The retina is the light sensitive portion of the eye. It contains the rods and cones which are the light receptors. The rods are responsible for black and white vision and vision in the dark, while the cones are responsible for color vision (Fig. 12.3).

Retinal Receptors: Rods and Cones

The total number of rods present in the eye is 120,000,000 and the number of cones is 6,000,000. The rods are narrower and longer than the cones. The outer segment of the cones is conical in shape. The rods have a diameter of 2 to 5 micrometres while the cones have a diameter of 5 to 8 micrometers. In the foveal region the cones are narrower and have a diameter of only 1.5 micrometers.

Structure of Rods and Cones

Each rod and cone is divided into an:

- Outer segment
- Inner segment
- Nucleus
- Synaptic body

Outer Segment

The outer segment is photosensitive and lies between the outer limiting membrane and the pigment cell layer. The light sensitive photochemical found in the rods is rhodopsin and in the cones it is photopsin.

The outer segments are modified cilia made up of regular stacks of flattened saccules or discs composed of membranes. The saccules or discs contain the photosensitive compounds that react to light initiating action potentials in the visual pathway.

In cones the outer segment is formed by infolding of the cell membrane but in the rods the discs are separated from the cell membrane. In the rods the outer segments are being constantly renewed by the formation of new discs at the inner edge of the segment and phagocytosis of the old discs from the outer tip by the cells of the pigment epithelium. Renewal of the outer segment of the cones occurs at multiple sites.

The inner segment contains the nucleus and synaptic body. In the rods the nucleus is smaller and chromatin is more condensed while in cones the nucleus is larger and pale staining.

Phototransduction

The photoreceptor cell has a membrane potential of –40 mV. The potassium channels are located in the inner segment of the photoreceptors while the Na^+ channels are located in the outer segment. The Na^+ K^+ pump is located in the inner segment. The membrane potential is largely due to the outward diffusion of K^+ rather than the inward diffusion of Na^+.

The Na^+ channels are open when no light falls on the photoreceptors. Hence, in darkness Na^+ continuously flows into the outer segment. This is called the dark current. Due to this the photoreceptor remains depolarized in the dark and a steady stream of neurotransmitter (glutamate) is released from its terminals. The neurotransmitter release is mediated through Ca^{++} influx into the synaptic terminal through voltage gated Ca^{++} channels.

When light falls on the retina, the light energy is trapped in the photosensitive pigments present in the photoreceptors and through a series of steps called visual cycle causes the closure of the Na^{+} channels and decrease in the dark current. This hyperpolarizes the photoreceptors to –70 mV and reduces the neurotransmitter output. Phototransduction is a unique example of sensory transduction that is associated with hyperpolarization and decrease in neurotransmitter release from the sensory receptor.

Visual Cycle

Rhodopsin-retinal visual cycle

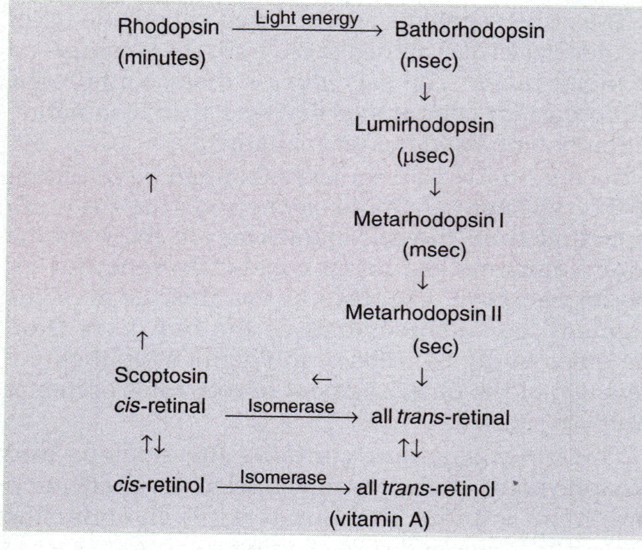

Decomposition of Rhodopsin by Light

The outer segment of the rod that projects into the pigment layer of the retina has a concentration of 40% of the light sensitive pigment rhodopsin or visual purple. The photosensitive pigment (rhodopsin) is composed of a protein moiety called scotopsin and a carotenoid pigment retinal or retinene. This retinal is 11-*cis*-retinal because only the cis form can combine with scotopsin to synthesize rhodopsin.

When light energy is absorbed by rhodopsin it decomposes within a fraction of a second. This is due to the photoactivation of the electrons in the retinal portion of rhodopsin, which converts the *cis* form to all *trans* form. Since the three-dimensional orientation of the all *trans* form does not fit with the orientation of the reactive sites on scotopsin, the all trans form moves away from scotopsin. It gets converted to bathorhodopsin which is extremely unstable and decays in nanoseconds to lumirhodopsin. This then decays in microseconds to metarhodopsin I then in about a milliseconds to metarhodopsin II and finally within seconds it completely splits to form scotopsin and all *trans*-retinal.

Metarhodopsin II is called activated rhodopsin as it excites the electrical changes in the rods. The action potential in the rods help to transmit the visual image in the retina to the central nervous system.

Resynthesis of Rhodopsin

The first stage in the resynthesis is the conversion of all *trans*-retinal to 11-*cis*-retinal. This is catalyzed by the enzyme retinal isomerise and requires metabolic energy. 11-*cis*-retinal formed automatically combines with scotopsin to form rhodopsin, which then remains stable until it is decomposed by light energy again.

Role of Vitamin A in Formation of Rhodopsin

In the visual pathway, some of the all *trans*-retinal gets converted to all *trans*-retinol which is one form of vitamin A. Then all *trans*-retinol gets converted to 11-*cis*-retinol by the enzyme isomerise and this is again converted to 11-*cis*-retinal which combines with scotopsin to form rhodopsin.

Vitamin A is normally present in the cytoplasm of the rods and in the pigment layer of retina. Hence, vitamin A can always form new retinal when needed.

Applied Aspect

Night Blindness

Severe vitamin A deficiency causes night blindness. The amount of retinal and rhodopsin that can be formed is severely depressed so the light available at night is too little to permit adequate vision.

Since a large amount of vitamin A is stored in the liver, deficiency can occur only if vitamin A is not provided in the diet over a long period.

Treatment: Consists of substitution of vitamin A orally. If night blindness develops then intravenous injection can be given.

COLOR VISION

The photochemicals in the cones are exactly the same composition as that of rhodopsin present in the rods.

The only difference is that the protein portion or the opsins called photopsins in the cones are slightly different from the scotopsin in the rods. The color sensitive pigments of the cones therefore are a combination of retinal and photopsin.

There are three primary colors–red, green and blue. Each cone contains pigments of a single primary color. Hence, three types of cones—cones containing blue sensitive pigment, cones with green sensitive pigment and cones with red sensitive pigments are present.

The absorption characteristics of the pigments in the three types of cones show peak absorbencies at light wavelengths of 445, 535 and 570 nanometers, respectively.

Interpretation of Color in the Nervous System

If a monochromatic light with a wavelength of 580 nanometers stikes the eye, it stimulates the red cones to a stimulus of about 99%, the green cones to a stimulus value of 42%, but the blue cones are not stimulated. The nervous system interprets this set of ratios as the sensation of orange. Similarly, monochromatic blue light of wavelength 450 nanometers will stimulated blue cones 97%, green cones 0% and red cones 0% and is interpreted by the nervous system as blue.

Perception of White Light

There is no single wavelength corresponding to white. White is a combination of all wavelength of the spectrum. Equal stimulation of the red, green and blue cones give rise to the sensation of white.

Theories of Color Vision

1. Young-Helmholtz Theory—Trichromatic Theory of Color Vision

This theory was put forth by Thomas Young in 1802 and later modified by Helmholtz. He states that there are three types of cones for the three primary colors each containing a different photochemical substance. Each receptor and photopigment is specifically acted upon by the light of the corresponding color while others have less effect. Thus, monochromatic red light stimulates red sensitive pigments maximally and other cones feebly. The impulses set up are conducted along separate nerve fibers to different nerve cells in the visual cortex. The analysis of color occurs peripherally in the retina and the information is then passed onto the brain for interpretation.

2. Polychromatic Theory of Color Vision—Dominators and Modulators

According to this theory, brightness and color are mediated by separate independent receptors. Brightness is the function of the cones which are sensitive over a wide range of wavelength and are called dominators. Color is the function of cones sensitive to a narrow range of wavelength and is called as modulators. The dominant visual sensation is colorless white or brightness. The modulators with restricted sensitivity modify this dominant sensation and give rise to the sensation of color. According to this theory; the modulators are the mediators of color vision, with the dominators subserving luminosity or brightness.

Defects of Color Vision

Color Blindness

Total color blindness is rare, but defects in the perception of one or more colors is often present. The subject is usually unaware of the defect. The classification of color vision defects is based on the Trichromatic theory. The deficiency may be for one, two, or three primary colors, and the subjects are referred to respectively as monochromats, dichromats and trichromats.

Anomalous Trichromatic Vision

This is one form of partial color blindness. There is no complete blindness for any color but appreciation of one color is less. The anomaly for red is called protanomaly, for green is called deuteranomaly, and for blue (rare) is called tritanomaly.

The defect is detected with an instrument called anomaloscope.

Dichromatic Vision

Here the subject cannot see one primary colors, the corresponding color pigment is missing. Blindness to red color is called protanopia, blindness to green is deuteranopia. These two defects are more common than blindness to blue which is called tritanopia.

Monochromatic Vision (Total Color Blindness)

This is a rare congenital abnormality in which colors are not seen. Genuine monochromats are called red monochromats do not perceive any color and see only white, grey or black and the surroundings appear white which may be tinged with blue as in twilight vision. As the cones are not functioning, foveal vision is absent and visual acuity is impaired. Total color blindness is also called achromasia or achromatopsia.

Importance of Color Vision

In many professions it is necessary to test color vision. For example, people working as signal men, engine drivers, and air crew, it is important for them to identify the colors as the safety of passengers depends on them.

Tests for Color Vision

Holmgren's Wool Test

This depends on matching of different shades of colored wool. The subject is given one type of wool and is asked to pick out the same shade from a large number of colored wool pieces of different shades. A red or green blind person matches pale green with cream, buff, pale brown and straw color. Pink is confused with violet and blue by a protanope, and with shades of green, red and brown by a dueteranope.

Pseudoisochromatic Charts

The most commonly used are Ishihara's charts. This is in the form of a booklet with a series of cards. Spots of different colors and grey are printed to form digits or patterns outlined against the general field. Other spots of confusing colors are also printed on it. The normal eye can detect the figures easily, whereas to the colorblind, it may appear to be another figure or may be indistinguishable from the background (Fig. 12.7).

Edridge Green Color Perception Lantern

Edridge green lantern consists of discs of colored lights which can be varied in size and illumination. The various atmospheric conditions like fog, mist, and rain can be mimicked by using suitable filters and the perception of colored lights can be tested under such conditions.

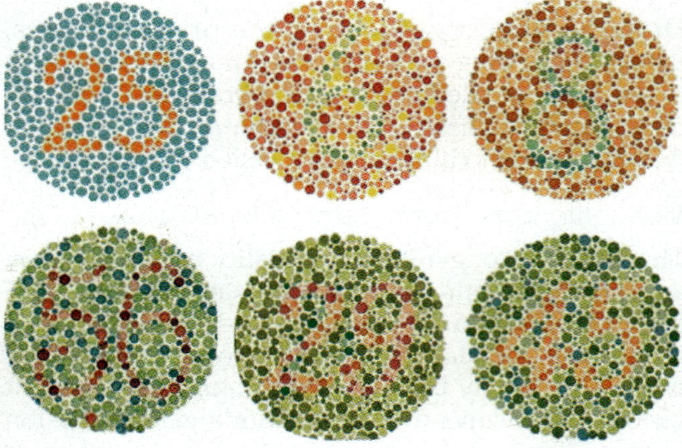

Fig. 12.7: Ishihara's test for colour blindness

Farnsworth 100 Hue Test

It is a simple test in which colored pastel chips are arranged in a color sequence. A color deficient person makes error in arranging the chips.

Spectroscopic Test

The extent of visibility of the spectrum. Identification of the different spectral colors and their positions and regions of maximal luminosity can be determined.

Anomaloscope

It is used to determine the ratio of red and green colors to match yellow.

Adaptation of Eye to Varying Light Intensities

Light adaptation: When a person passes from a dim to a brightly lit environment, the light seems intense until the eyes adapt to the increased illumination. This adaptation occurs over a period of 5 minutes and is called light adaptation. The changes that occur are constriction of the pupil and decreased sensitivity of the retina. The decline is rapid in the first a few minutes and slower for the next 10 minutes. There is bleaching of the visual purple and the neurotransmitter output is zero and no further decrease is possible. This renders the rods useless for signalling bright light, but the neurotransmitter output of the cones gradually increases again even in the presence of bright light. Ca^{++} plays an important role in the recovery of cone sensitivity.

Dark adaptation: If a person spends a considerable amount of time in brightly lit surroundings and then moves to a dim-lit environment, the retina slowly becomes more sensive to light as the individual becomes accustomed to the dark. This increase in visual sensitivity is known as dark adaptation. It is nearly maximal in about 20 minutes. The time required for dark adaptation is the time required for the build up of photopigment stores, which are constantly depleted in bright light. The dark adaptation response has two components. The initial rapid but small rise in visual sensitivity is due to the dark adaptation of cones. A late, slow but large rise in visual sensitivity occurs due to the dark adaptation of rods. It occurs only in the peripheral portions of the retina and not in the fovea, which contains only cones (Fig. 12.8).

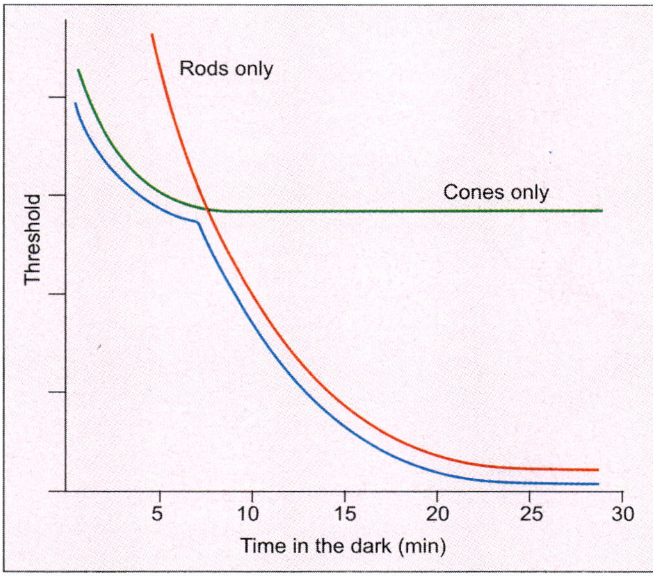

Fig. 12.8

Aircraft pilots taking off into the night sky need to become dark adapted immediately on take-off. Hence, they wear red goggles when on the ground in bright light. Red light is a poor stimulator of rods but it stimulates cones reasonably well. Therefore, pilots wearing red glasses can see in bright light and yet their rods remain dark adapted.

VISUAL PATHWAY (Fig. 12.9)

The visual field is divided into temporal and nasal halves by a vertical line passing through the fixation point. The retina too is divided into nasal and temporal halves by a vertical line passing through the fovea centralis. The retinal receptors (rods and cones) connect with the peripheral processes in the retina.

The central processes of the bipolar cells are the first order neurons and synapse with the dendrites of the ganglion cells in the retina.

The axons of the ganglion cells converge at the optic disc to form the optic nerve. They form the second order neurons. The optic nerve comes out of the orbit and enters into the cranial cavity. The optic nerves of the two sides converge at the optic chiasm situated above the sella turcica. In the optic chiasm fibers of the nasal half of the retina crosses to the opposite side. The fibers from the temporal half do not cross but remain on the same side.

The optic tract is formed by the fibers from the nasal half of the opposite retina and the temporal half of the same side. It passes backwards, and sweeps round the under surface of the cerebral peduncle and divide into lateral and medial roots. The lateral root which contains the visual fibers ends in the lateral geniculate body. The medial root contains fibers for reflexes and ends in the superior colliculus and the pretectal region. Some fibers go to the suprachiasmatic nucleus of the hypothalamus.

The third order neuron rise from the lateral geniculate body as the optic radiation. It passes along the posterior limb of the internal capsule runs backwards in the temporal lobe and ends in the visual cortex in the occipital lobe (striate area).

Cortical visual area: The striate area (area 17-primary visual area) is present in the pole of the occipital cortex and on the medial surface and lips and walls of the calcarine surface. It is concerned with the appreciation of visual sensations.

Parastriate area: (area 18) lies adjacent to the primary visual area and is concerned with the correlation and integration of visual sensation. The area 19 which adjoins the parastriate area is the occipital eye field and it projects to the frontal eye field (area 8) concerned with eye movements.

PUPILLARY REFLEXES (Fig. 12.10)

Light Reflex

When light is shown in one eye, there is simultaneous constriction of the ipsilateral pupil (direct light reflex) and the contralateral pupil (consensual light reflex).

The afferent pathway for the constrictor reflex is:

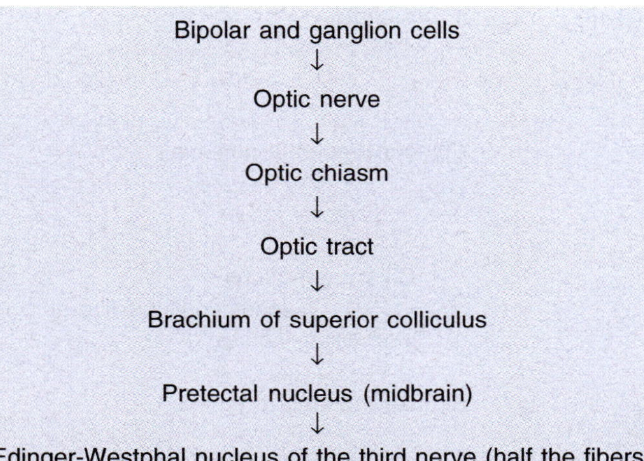

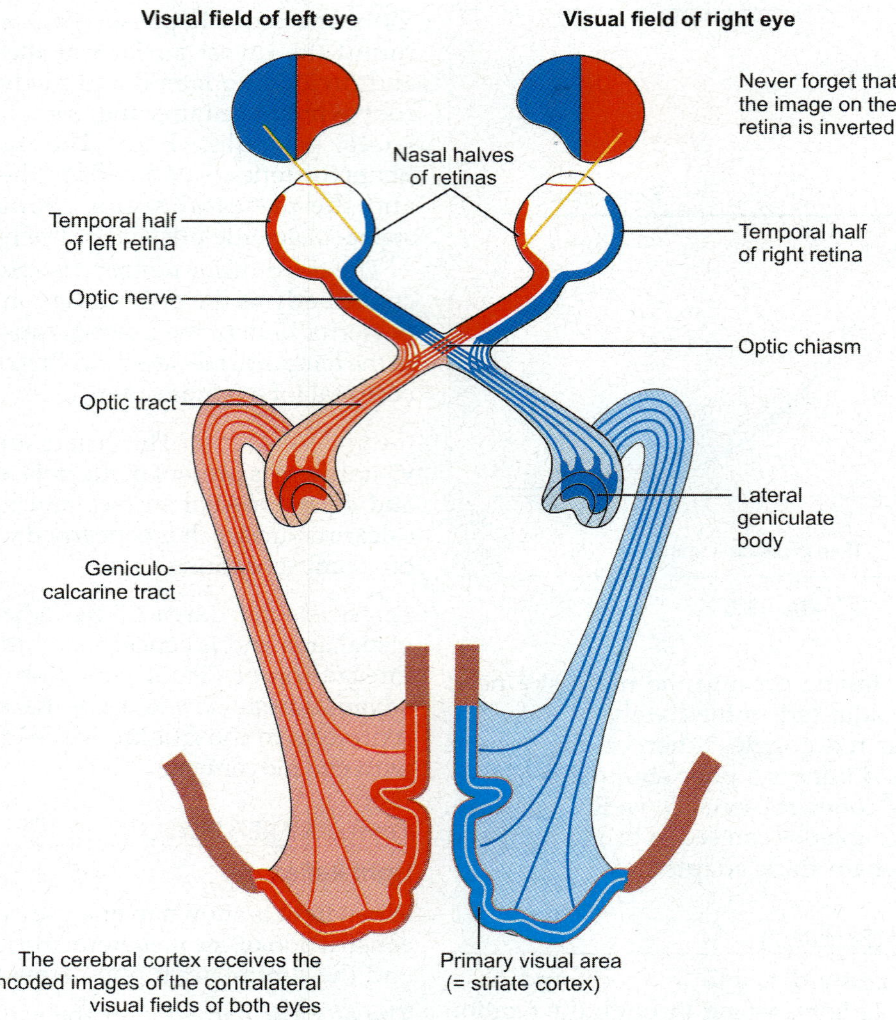

Fig. 12.9: Visual pathway

Efferent Pathway

Edinger-Westphal nucleus
↓
Oculomotor nerve
↓
Ciliary ganglions
↓ (postganglionic fibers)
Short ciliary nerves
↓
Circular muscles to the iris

Pupillary Dilator Pathway

Afferent Pathway

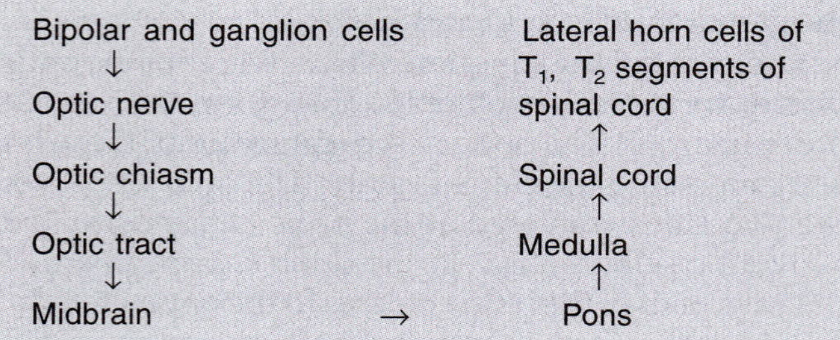

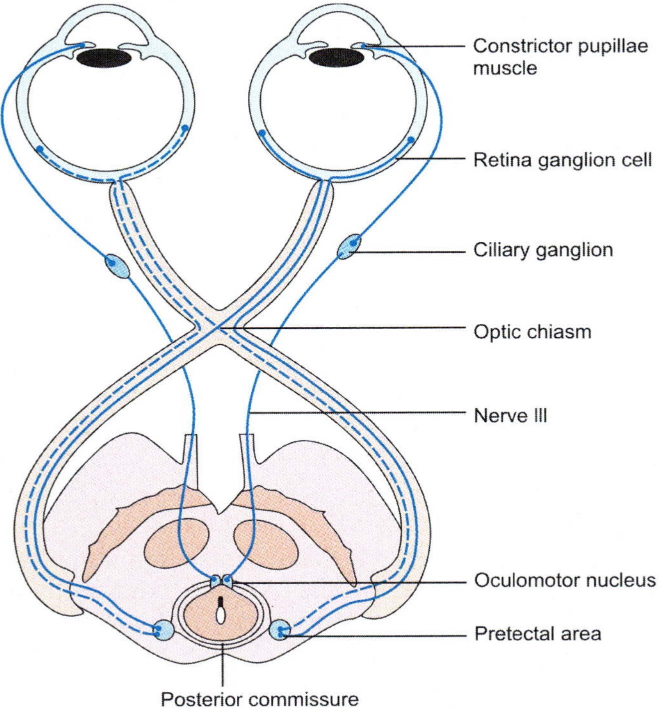

Fig. 12.10: Pupillary reflexes

Efferent Pathway

Lateral horn cells of T_1, T_2 segments of spinal cells cord (preganglion fibers)
↓
Superior cervical ganglion (postganglion fibers)
↓
Plexus around internal carotid artery
↓
Long ciliary nerves (branch of ophthalmic division of trigeminal nerve)
↓
Dilator muscles of iris

Accommodation Reflex or Near Response

It is a three part response that occurs when an individual looks at a near object. It consists of:

1. Contraction of ciliary muscle through the occulomotor nerve as result of which the anterior curvature of the lens increases.
2. Constriction of pupil due to contraction of sphincter papillae. This allows the light to fall only on the center of the lens where the accommodation changes are maximum.
3. Convergence of visual axes due to contraction of medial rectus muscle. This helps in focusing the image of the object on fovea centralis.

Accommodation Pathway

Afferent pathway same as visual pathway up to occipital cortex.

Occipital cortex (area 17)
↓
Frontal eye field (area 8)
↓ via corticonuclear fibers
Edinger-Westphal nucleus (third nerve)
↓
Ciliary muscles, sphincter papillae, medial rectus

Applied Aspect

Argyll-Robertson pupil (AR pupil): It was described by Argyll-Robertson in 1869. The essential features of this condition are:

1. Light reflex both direct and consensual is absent but accommodation reflex is present.
2. Both the pupils are constricted but are of unequal size and papillary margins are irregular.
3. Very little dilatation of the pupil with atropine or painful stimuli.
4. Vision is normal.

It occurs in syphilitic lesions of the central nervous system (e.g. tabes dorsalis).

Effect of Lesions of the Visual Pathway (Fig. 12.11)

The effect of lesions of the visual pathway is described in terms of field of vision (visual field).

Anopia

It is the complete loss of visual field in eye, i.e. blindness.

Hemianopia

It is blindness of half of the visual field.

Homonymous Hemianopia

When the same half of the visual field in both eyes are lost (e.g. loss of right or left half of the visual field of both eyes).

Heteronymous Hemianopia

When different halfs of the visual field are lost in two eyes (e.g. loss of right half of visual field in one eye and the left half of visual field in the other eye) it is of two types—bitemporal and binasal (Fig. 12.11).

Quadrantanopia

When 1/4th of the visual field is lost in one eye.

Scotoma

Loss of central field of vision.

Effects of Lesions

1. *Lesion of the optic nerve:* It can occur due to increase intracranial tension or due to injury to the optic nerve. It results in atrophy of the optic nerve and causes complete blindness and loss of direct light reflex.
2. *Lesion of the optic chiasm:* Occurs due to aneurysm of the internal carotid artery or tumors of the pituitary gland. It causes damage of the fibers from both sides of the nasal half of the retina producing bitemporal hemianopia (heterinymous hemianopia).
3. *Lesion of outer margin of optic chiasm:* Damages the fibers from both sides of the temporal retina causing binasal hemianopia.
4. *Lesion of optic chiasm and its right outer margin:* It damages the fibers from both sides of the nasal retina and that of the right temporal retina and causes blindness in the right eye with temporal hemianopia in the left eye.
5. *Lesion of optic tract:* It causes homonymous hemianopia (loss of same half of the visual field in both eyes).
6. *Lesion of lateral geniculate body or optic radiation:* It causes homonymous hemianopia with normal papillary reaction to light.
7. *Lesion of occipital cortex (area 18):* It produces only discrete quadrantic visual field defects because of specific anatomic arrangement of the optic nerve fibers in the occipital cortex. There is loss of peripheral vision with normal and complete macular vision called macular sparing. This is because the macular representation in the occipital lobe is separate and far greater than the peripheral parts of the retina.

Nystagmus

When a subject's gaze is fixed at a stationary object, the eyeballs are not still, i.e. without motion, there are continuous jerky movements. This is called physiologic nystagmus.

When the image of an object is fixed, it falls steadily on the same point on the retina and the object disappears from the view. This is because of the fact that for continuous visualization of objects, the retinal images must be continuously and rapidly shifted from one receptor to another.

However, when the body is rotated at great speed round a vertical axis, e.g. merry-go-round ride, a

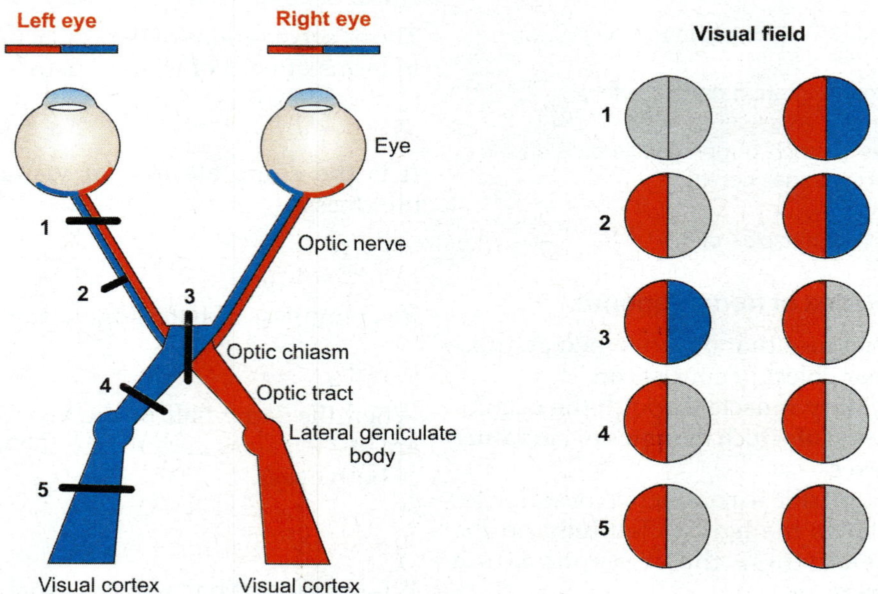

Fig. 12.11: Effect of lesions of the visual pathway

skater performing a spin. There occurs a slow motion of the eyes in the opposite direction to that of the rotation, it is followed by a quick, jerky, binocular 'return' movement in the direction of movement. This sequence is repeated as long as the regular acceleration lasts. This is initiated by the vestibular mechanism and is called occulovestibular nystagmus.

120. SENSE OF HEARING

The sense of hearing, along with vision and olfaction provides vertebrates with the information about events occurring at a distance. Hearing rivals vision as a system of gathering and utilizing high complex environmental information. Even when an animal is asleep, or directing its attention elsewhere, it can still respond to sounds. For example, a mother who is asleep is aware of her babys' slightest movement. The sense of hearing thus serves as a primitive alarm or warning system.

Hearing is the subjective experience of exposure to vibration in the range of about 20 cycles/sec to about 20,000 cycles/sec.

Properties of Sound

Sound is the sensation produced when the longitudinal vibrations of the molecules in the external environment, i.e. alternative phases of condensation and rarefaction of the molecules, strikes the tympanic membrane.

Speed of sound in air is 344 m/sec at 20°C in fresh water, 1450 m/sec at 20°C in sea water. It is still higher in solids. When sound waves pass from one medium to another (e.g. from air to water which has greater acoustical resistance) most of the sound waves are reflected back into the air at the boundary and much less sound energy is transmitted into the water.

Characteristics of Sound

Sound has three qualities:

1. Loudness
2. Pitch
3. Timber or quality

Loudness or Intensity

Depends upon the amplitude of sound waves. The greater the amplitude of sound waves, louder the sound. However, the loudness of sound is what is perceived by the ear. It is not the same as intensity of sound which depends upon sound energy.

Though loudness varies to sound intensity it is modified by other factors such as sensitivity of the ear and distance of the ear from the source of sound, etc.

Pitch

- Depends upon the frequency of waves (CPS or Hz)
- Higher the frequency greater the pitch
- High frequency sounds are shrill
- Low frequency sounds are flat
- Females have higher frequency (250 Hz) than males (120 Hz).

Timber or Quality

It is the property by which one can differentiate between two tones of the same pitch intensity, e.g. a violin and flute. The tone of a vibrating tuning fork is a pure tone.

If a pure tone is superimposed over overtones (additional waves repeated regularly) these waves determine the timber or quality while the frequency of the primary wave determines the pitch, e.g. from a pitch we can differentiate male and female voice, but the timber enables us to recognize a known person or a singer from a voice without seeing them.

Waves which have frequencies which are multiples of the primaries are harmonics or overtones.

If the sound waves have frequencies which are not multiples of the fundamental or primary is called noise.

PHYSIOANATOMY OF THE EAR

External Ear (Fig. 12.12a)

The external ear consists of the pinna the external auditory meatus and auditory canal and ends in the tympanic membrane. The pinna funnels the sound waves to the external auditory canal.

Middle Ear (Fig. 12.12b)

The middle ear is an air filled cavity in the temporal bone that opens through the eustachian tube into the nasopharynx. The tube is usually closed, but during swallowing, chewing and yawning it opens to maintain the air pressure equal on the two sides of the tympanic membrane.

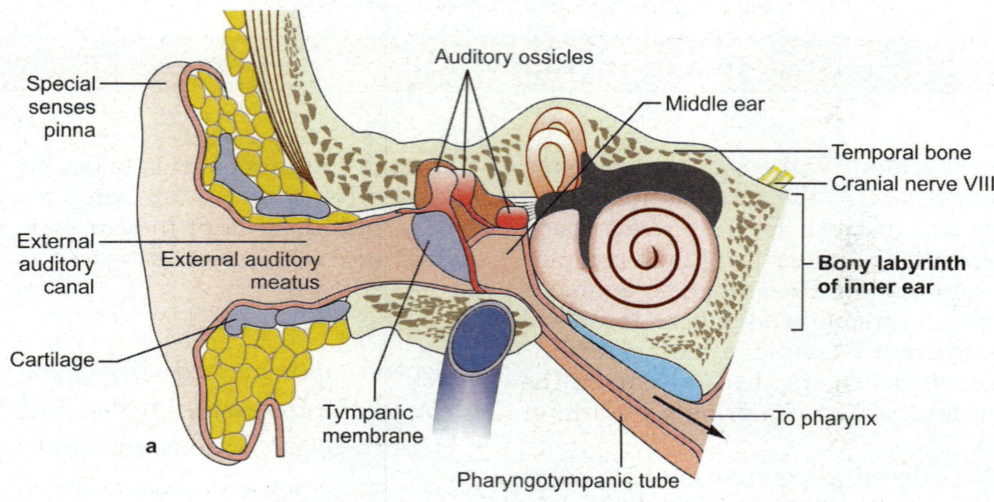

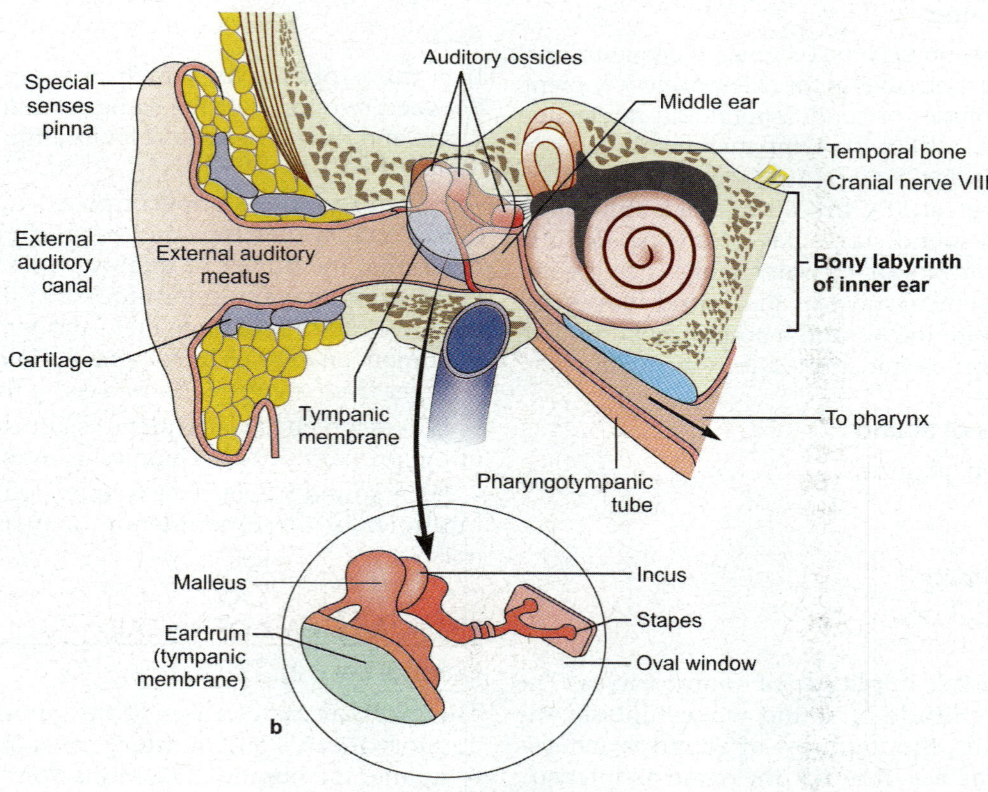

Figs 12.12a and 12b

The middle ear contains three ossicles namely the malleus, incus and the stapes.

Malleus

It is shaped like a hammer. The manubrium or handle of the malleus is attached to the inner side of the tympanic membrane, and its tip is situated in the umbo (shallow funnel) in the center of the tympanic membrane. Its head is attached to the wall of the middle ear. Its short process is attached to the incus.

Incus (Anvil)

It is attached to the malleus on one side and its long process passes downwards to articulate with the head of the stapes.

Stapes (Stirrup)

The head of the stapes articulates with the incus and the footplate is attached by the annular ligament to the walls of the oval window.

The two muscles present in the middle ear are:
1. Tensor tympani
2. Stapedius

The tensor tympani is attached to the neck of the malleus. On contraction it pulls the manubrium of the malleus medially and decreases the vibrations of the tympanic membrane.

The stapedius is attached to the neck of the stapes and posterior wall of the middle ear. On contraction it pulls the footplate of the stapes out of the oval window thus decreasing the vibrations passing onto the inner ear.

Inner Ear

The inner ear or the labyrinth contains the cochlea which is the organ of hearing as well as the vestibular apparatus which is responsible for maintaining the equilibrium of the body. Only the cochlea is discussed here (Fig. 12.13).

Cochlea: The cochlea resembles a snail shell. It is 35 mm long. It is coiled and makes 2 ¾ turns around bony core called modiolus. The inside of the cochlea is divided into three chambers or scalae by two membranes which run throughout its length namely the Basilar membrane and the Reissner's membrane.

The three chambers are:
1. Scala vestibuli (upper)
2. Scala media (middle)
3. Scala tympani (lower)

The scala vestibuli and scala tympani contain perilymph and communicate with each other at the apex of the cochlea through an opening called the helicotrema. At the base of the cochlea the scala vestibule ends at the oval window, which is closed by the footplate of the stapes.

The scala tympani ends at the round window, a foramen on the medial wall of the middle ear closed by the flexible secondary tympanic membrane.

The scala media, the middle chamber is continuous with the membranous labyrinth and does not communicate with the other two scalae.

Organ of Corti (Fig. 12.14)

It is the receptor organ of hearing that generates nerve impulses in response to vibrations of the basillar membrane. The basilar membrane is a fibrous membrane containing 20,000–30,000 basilar fibers. These fibers are stiff elastic and reed-like. The basilar membrane is attached to the bony spiral lamina medially and to the fibrous spiral ligament laterally. The organ of Corti which has the hair cells, the auditory receptors are located on the basilar membrane. It

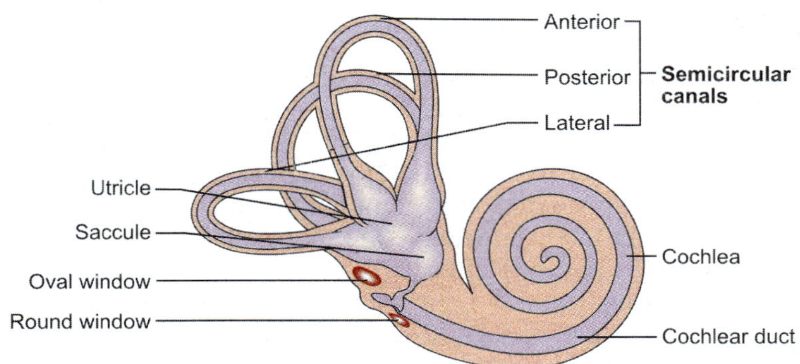

Fig. 12.13: Inner ear

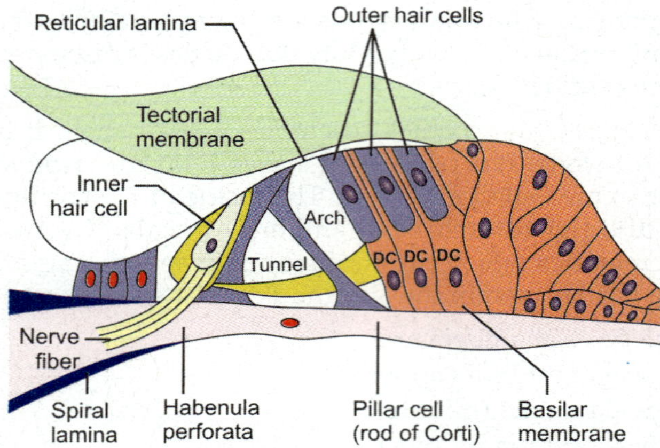

Fig. 12.14: Organ of Corti

extends from the apex to the base of the cochlea in a spiral shape.

The hair cells are arranged on either sides of the tunnel of Corti. The tunnel of Corti is formed by the rods of Corti. There are 4 rows of hair cells: 3 rows of outer hair cells arranged lateral to the tunnel and one row of inner hair cells medial to the tunnel. There are 20,000 outer hair cells and about 3,500 inner hair cells.

The processes of the hair cells pierce the tough reticular lamina which is supported by the rods of Corti. Covering the rows of hair cells is a thin, elastic, viscous tectorial membrane in which the tips of the outer hair cells but not the inner hair cells are embedded.

The inner hair cells are supported by inner phalangeal cells, while the outer hair cells are supported by the Deiter's cells (outer phalangeal cells).

Structure of Hair Cell

Each hair cell is embedded in an epithelium made up of supporting or sustentacular cells, with the basal ends in close contact with the fibers of the afferent neuron. Projecting from the upper end of the hair cells are 30–150 rod shaped processes or hairs. Except in the cochlea one of these the kinocilium, is a true but nonmotile cilium. However, the other processes called Stereocilia are present in all hair cells. They have cores composed of parallel filaments of actin coated with various isoforms of myosin. Towards the kinocilium the stereocilia increase in height. Along the perpendicular axis all the stereocilia have the same height.

The cilia or the stereocilia on the upper surface of the hair cell are 8–12 micrometer in diameter and 4 micrometer in length.

The nerve fibers of the neurons located in the spiral ganglion in the modiolus arborize around the base of the hair cell. 90–95% of afferent fibers innervate the inner hair cells, and only 5–10% innervates the outer hair cell.

Most of the efferent fibers in the auditory nerve terminate on the outer hair cell than on the inner hair cell.

The axons of the afferent nerves that innervate the hair cells unite to form the auditory (cochlear) portion of the VIII cranial nerve.

In the cochlea, tight junctions between the hair cells and the phalangeal cells prevent the endolymph from reaching the base of the cells. However, the basilar membrane is relatively permeable to perilymph in the scala tympani and consequently the tunnel of Corti and the base of the hair cells are bathed in perilymph. Therefore, the cilia are exposed to endolymph while the base is bathed in perilymph.

Perilymph and Endolymph

The perilymph is formed from the plasma and has a composition similar to the ECF. The endolymph is formed in the scala media by the stria vascularis, and has a high concentration of potassium and low concentration of sodium similar to the ICF.

Electrical Response

The membrane potential of the hair cell is –60 mV. When the stereocilia are pushed towards the kinocilium, the membrane potential is decreased to –50 mV. When the processes are pushed in the opposite direction, the hair cell is hyperpolarized. Displacing the processes in a direction perpendicular to the axis produces no change in the membrane potential.

Therefore, depending upon the direction and distance to which the processes are displaced the hair cells generate a depolarizing or hyperpolarizing potential.

Genesis of Action Potential in Afferent Nerve Fibers

The tip of each stereocilia is connected to the side of its higher neighbor by very fine processes called tiplinks. At this junction there are cation channels in the higher processes that are mechanically sensitive. When the shorter stereocilia are pushed towards the higher one, the cation channels are opened and potassium, the most abundant cation in the endolymph and calcium also enters into the cell and causes depolarization. Then the molecular motor in the higher neighbor next moves the channel towards the base, releasing the tension in the tiplink. This causes the channel to close and permits the restoration of the membrane potential to the resting state.

Transmission of Sound Waves in the Ear

The ear converts the sound waves of the external environment into action potentials in the auditory nerve.

The sound waves which reach the tympanic membrane via the external auditory meatus causes the membrane to vibrate. The tympanic membrane has very little inertia and is aperiodic, i.e. it does not have a natural frequency of its own. This is because the middle layer of the tympanic membrane contains circular and radial fibers whose tension varies at different points:

When the sound reaches the tympanic membrane, it acts like a resonator and vibrates at the same frequency as that of the sound.

The handle of the malleus draws the membrane inwards and its apex is below its true center. It also prevents the membrane from continuing to vibrate after the sound waves stop, i.e. it critically dampens the vibrations immediately after the sound ceases.

The movement of the tympanic membrane causes the movement of the handle of the malleus. The malleus rocks on an axis through the junction of the long and short processes, so that the short process transmits the vibrations to the incus. The incus transmits the movement to the head of the stapes. This brings about a to and fro movement of the footplate of the stapes at the oval window like a door hinged to the posterior edge of the window. This sets up vibrations in the fluid in the inner ear.

The ear ossicles function as a lever system which converts the vibrations of the tympanic membrane into movement of footplate of stapes against the perilymph in the scala vestibule of the cochlea. The handle of the malleus forms the long arm and the long process of the incus, the short arm of the lever system.

The footplate of the stapes does not move in a piston like fashion but like a bell crank and it rocks about its posterior pole, the movement being more in the anterior than in the posterior part of the footplate.

When the handle of the malleus moves inwards, the head of the malleus and the greater part of the incus moves outwards, but the long process of the incus and stapes move inwards

This is ossicular conduction and the most important mode of transmission of sound waves in the ear.

Sound waves may be transmitted through the bones of the skull—bone conduction—bypassing the outer and middle ear, the vibrations of the bones causing the movements of the fluid in the inner ear. A large amount of sound energy is lost in this mode of transmission.

Impedance Matching

Sound waves do not readily pass through the media of different acoustical resistances, but are reflected at the boundary between the media. Water has a much greater acoustical resistance than air.

Hence, between the air filled ear and the fluid filled inner ear only a fraction of the sound energy will be transmitted. Also in between the middle and the inner ears there are two windows equally exposed to the sound waves. Hence, very little energy will be transmitted to the fluid in the inner ear due to the inertia and incompressibility of the fluid.

Advantages of Ossicular Conduction

1. It ensures selective delivery of sound energy to one window (oval window) rather than both.
2. It magnifies the pressure on the oval window.

The surface area of the tympanic membrane is about 63 m^2, but that of the foot plate of the stapes is 3.2 mm^2. Hence, the pressure is magnified 20 times.

As the handle of the malleus is about 1.3 times that of the long process of the incus, the pressure is further magnified 1.3 times, the increase being 26 times.

Due to damping and frictional effects the actual increase in pressure is only 10-fold. The amplitude of the waves is correspondingly reduced to 10-fold.

This is referred to as impedance matching. This ensures that a large amount of the sound energy is transmitted to the fluid in the inner ear.

Attenuation Reflex (Tympanic Reflex)

Loud sounds of low frequency cause contraction of the tensor tympani which pulls the handle of the malleus inwards, while the stapedius contracts and pulls the footplate of the stapes out of the oval window, thus restricting the movements of the ossicular chain. This called the attenuation reflex or tympanic reflex.

The attenuation reflex has a long latent period of 40–150 msec. And hence it is unable to protect against intense brief stimulus such as gunshot.

Another function of this reflex is that when a person talks collateral signals are sent to the muscles to reduce his own hearing sensitivity, so that his speech will not over stimulate his hearing mechanism.

Role of Internal Ear (Fig. 12.15)

The movement of the foot plate of the stapes causes vibrations of the perilymph which is transmitted to the endolymph. This brings about an up and down movement of the basilar membrane resulting in rocking movements of the rods of Corti and reticular lamina and shearing movement between the lamina and tectorial membrane.

This causes the bending of the hair cells, whose one end is embedded in the reticular lamina. Bending of the hairs stimulates the hair cells and sets up an action potential which is transmitted by the auditory nerve fibers and auditory pathway to the auditory area in the temporal lobe of the cerebral cortex.

THEORIES OF HEARING

Telephone or Frequency Theory

It was proposed by Rutherford in 1886. According to this theory, the basilar membrane vibrates as a whole, aperiodically at the same frequency as the sound waves (like the diaphragm of the telephone) and sets up nerve impulses of the same frequency. According to this theory, sound analysis is a function of the cerebral cortex and not the cochlea.

Volley Theory

Since the auditory nerve has a large number of fibers, the impulses are transmitted over separate fibers, not synchronously, but as a scattered volley, so that a group of fibers may discharge at a very high frequency.

Resonance Theory

The resonance theory was put forward by Helmholtz in 1863.

According to this theory the cochlea has a series of resonators each responding to a different frequency. The fibers in the basilar membrane were comparable to the strings of a harp, with the shorter fibers at the base responding to higher frequencies, and the longer fibers at the apex responding to low frequencies. But individual resonators could not be identified and the fibers in the basilar membrane were not under tension. So, the resonance theory gave way to place theory.

Place Theory

The entire cochlea is a tuned structure, with different parts of the basilar membrane responding to different frequencies. The basal part of the basilar membrane near the oval window is the narrowest and stiffest

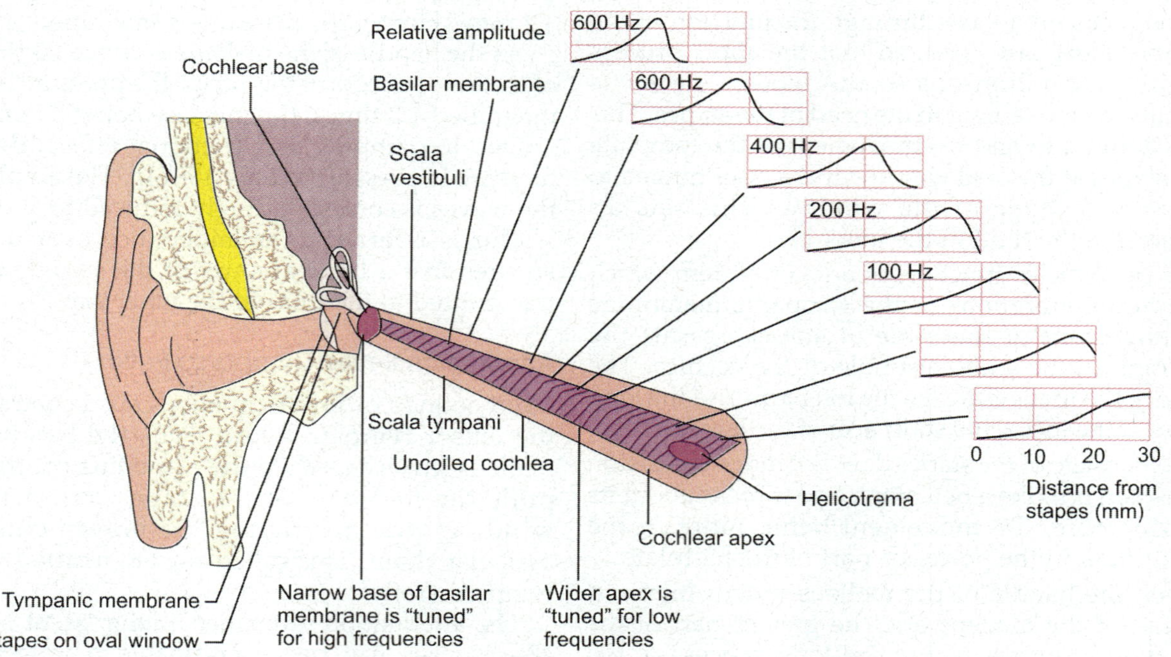

Fig. 12.15

part and responds best to high frequencies, while the apical part near the helicotrema is the widest and most complaint part and responds best to low frequencies.

Analysis of sounds (discrimination of pitch) is thus a function of the cochlea.

Traveling Wave Theory

The movement of the footplate of the stapes sets up a series of traveling waves in the perilymph of the scala tympani which pushes the round window outwards. Movement of the fluid in the scala vestibuli causes displacement of the basilar membrane. The movements of the basilar membrane were studied by von Bekesy using Stroboscopic illumination.

The pattern of vibration of the basilar membrane shows a traveling wave of transverse displacement similar to the waves seen on shaking a piece of rope from one end. The wave starts from the base of the cochlea at high velocity, reaches a maximum and then dies away with rapid reduction in amplitude and velocity. The region of maximum amplitude varies with the frequency of sound waves. The higher frequency waves have maximum amplitude at the base, and low frequency waves at the apex. Hair cells at the region of maximum amplitude are maximally stimulated.

In human cochlea, traveling waves are demonstrable at frequencies of 150 Hz. Below this, the basilar membrane moves more or less as a unit and below 50 Hz, the entire basilar membrane moves as a whole.

ELECTROPHYSIOLOGY OF HEARING

Endocochlear Potential or Endolymphatic Potential

When two electrodes, one inserted into the scala media containing endolymph and the other into the scala vestibule containing perilymph are connected through a suitable amplifier to cathode ray oscilloscope, a steady potential of +50 to + 100 mV is recorded. This is called the endolymphatic potential or endocochlear potential. It is due to the differences in the composition of the endolymph and the perilymph sustained by the metabolic activities of the structures in the stria vascularis.

Ions	*Endolymph*	*Perilymph*	*ECF*	*ICF*
K^+	138	5	5	155
Na^+	15	154	145	12
Cl^-	108	120	110	8
Proteins	15	50	15	60

Genesis of Endolymphatic Potential

The cell membrane separates the two fluid compartments, namely the ECF and ICF having widely different ionic composition with the inside (ICF) being negative to the outside. Similarly, Reissner's membrane separates the two fluids of widely different composition across the membrane.

The endolymphatic potential in the scala media is positive with respect to the perilymph in the scala vestibule. The stria vascularis which covers the lateral wall of the scala media has a high concentration of Na^+ K^+ ATPase. There is also an electrogenic K^+ pump which accounts for the high K^+ concentration of the endolymph. So, the scala media is positive to the scala vestibuli and scala tympani.

Cochlear Microphonic Potentials

The three principal dynamic potentials that accompany sound stimuli delivered to the cochlea are:

1. Cochlear microphonics
2. Positive and negative summation potentials
3. Nerve action potentials in the auditory nerve.

Cochlear Microphonics

They are generated instantaneously by the pattern of vibration of the cochlear partition. Analogous to the function of a microphone, the cochlear microphonic potentials are faithful to the acoustic stimuli with regard to the waveform, frequency and amplitude. This was first discovered by Wever and Bray in 1930 and so it is known as the Wever Bray phenomenon. They are not nerve action potentials and cannot be obtained from the auditory nerve or auditory pathway, but can be recorded by placing an active electrode on or near the cochlea and an indifferent electrode anywhere in the body.

They are the summed activity of many hair cells. It is called microphonic cochlear potentials, because if these potentials are amplified, the loud speaker records the pure tones (i.e. the same frequency and intensity of sounds) fed to the ear.

These potentials are similar to the generator potentials because:

1. They show no latency or refractory period
2. Do not obey the all-or-none law
3. They are resistant to ischemia and anesthesia
4. They do not fatigue
5. Follow stimulus rates in excess of that followed by auditory neurons.

The cochlear microphonic potentials are produced by the transformation of mechanical energy into electrical energy. Like the endolymphatic potentials they are also altered by the movement of the basilar membrane and show linear relationship to the magnitude of basilar membrane displacement. Cochlear microphonics are preliminary to the nerve responses and boost receptor excitation.

Summating Potentials

Positive summating potentials are due to bending of the hair cells. Negative summating potential have their origin in the nerve.

Action Potentials of Auditory Nerve Fibers

The processes of the hair cells project into the endolymph (in the scala media) whereas the bases are bathed in the perilymph. The Reissner's membrane is impermeable to Na^+ and K^+, whereas the basilar membrane is freely permeable to these ions. In addition, the reticular lamina is a barrier to diffusion. Therefore, the perilymph from the scala tympani diffuses across the relatively permeable basilar membrane into the tunnel of Corti and the bases of the hair cells.

Hair cell depolarization initiates the release of neurotransmitter (glutamate) that activates the receptor sites on the terminals of the afferent neuron in the base of the hair cell and causes the generation of action potential in the neuron.

95% of the neurons in the cochlear nerve are the afferents originating in the inner hair cells, while the remaining 5% originate from the outer hair cells. The cell body of these neurons are located in the spiral ganglion inside the modiolus.

Auditory Pathway (Fig. 12.16)

The cochlea nerve terminates tonotopically, i.e. in an orderly sequence representing the various frequencies

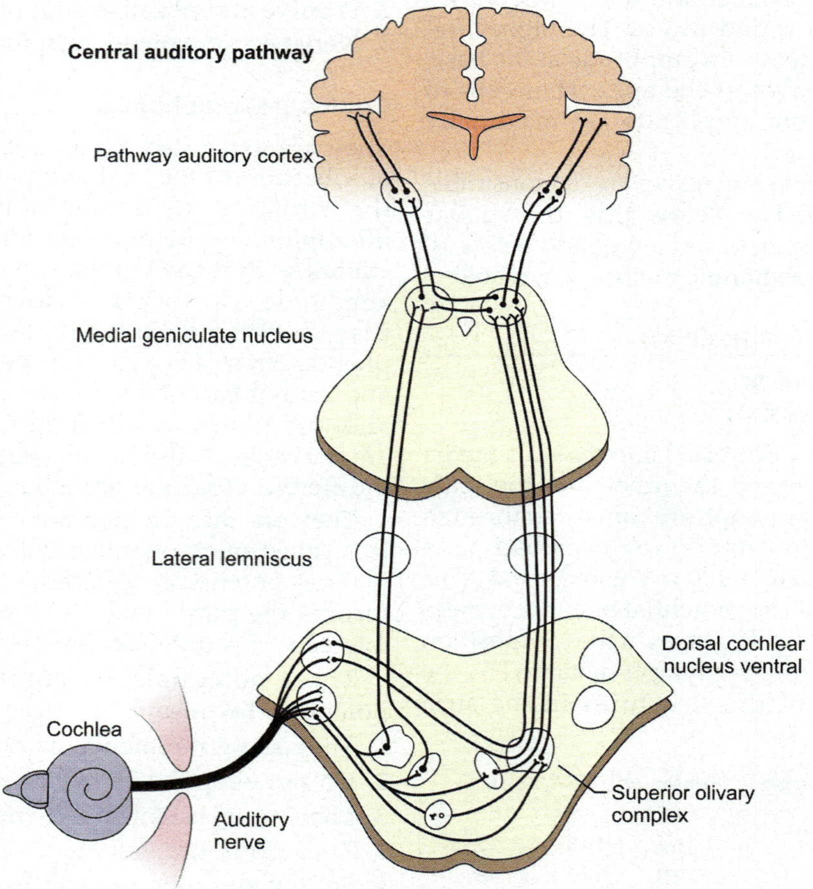

Fig. 12.16: Auditory pathway

in the cochlea nucleus in the medulla. The fibers of the cochlear nuclei form the second order and pass to the superior olivary nuclei which receive input from both ears.

From each olivary nucleus, fibers ascend in the lateral lemniscus to project to the ipsilateral inferior colliculus and from there to the medial geniculate body of the thalamus.

From the medial geniculate body, auditory fibers project to the primary auditory cortex (area 41).

Primary Auditory Cortex (Area 41) (Fig. 12.17)

It lies in the superior portion of the temporal lobe in the floor of the lateral cerebral sulcus. There is an orderly tonotopic representation the anterior part receives impulses from the apex of the cochlea (low frequency) and the posterior part of the gyrus receives impulses arising from the base of the cochlea (high frequency).

Auditory Association Areas (Areas 22, 21, 20)

Area 22 is the Wernicke's area. It lies in the superior temporal gyrus behind area 41 and 42 in the categorical hemisphere. Its function is comprehension, i.e. interpretation and understanding of auditory and visual information. It processes auditory signals related to speech.

Areas 21 and 20: Lie in the middle and inferior temporal gyrus. Its function is interpretation and integration of auditory impulses.

Applied Aspects

Deafness

It is the inability of an individual to hear, either wholly or partially. It is of two types:

1. Conductive deafness
2. Sensorineural deafness.

Conductive Deafness

It is due to defect in conduction of sound waves in the external and middle ear.

Causes

1. Foreign body or wax in external ear
2. Thickening of tympanic membrane due to repeated infection
3. Otitis media
4. Otosclerosis
5. Blockage of eustachian tube.

Sensorineural Deafness

It is due to defects of internal ear (hair cells) or damage to the neural pathway.

Causes

1. *Aging:* (Presbycusis) is due to gradual loss of hair cells and cortical neurons.
2. *Hereditary:* Congenital deafness occurs as a result of genetic mutation in 0.1% of newborns. Syndromic deafness, i.e. deafness associated with abnormalities in other systems account for 30% and nonsyndromic for 70% of the cases. Examples of syndromic deafness include Pendred's syndrome, Long QT syndrome, Barters' syndrome.
3. Trauma to VIII nerve
4. Hazards of industrial noises
5. Toxic degeneration of VIII nerve due to drugs like injection streptomycin, injection gentamycin and quinine which obstruct the sensitive channels in the stereocilia of the hair cells and cause degeneration of the hair cells.
6. Infections like measles and meningitis
7. *Tumors:* Acoustic neuroma
8. Vascular damage to the medulla—leading to destruction of the auditory pathways.

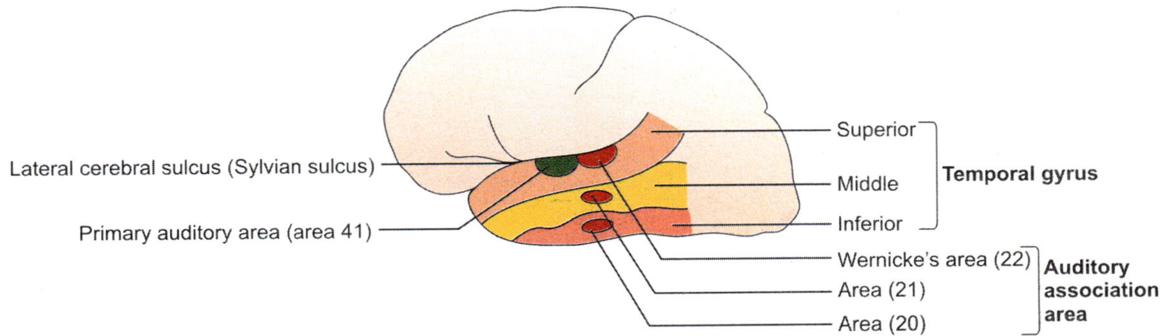

Fig. 12.17: Location of auditory areas

12

Tinnitus: It is a ringing sensation in the ears caused by irritant stimulation of either the internal ear or the auditory nerve.

Tests for Hearing

Tuning fork Tests

Tuning fork tests provide a convenient method of assessing whether the deafness is of the conductive or sensorineural type. The frequency of the tuning fork should be 256 Hz. The vibrations of the tuning fork can be heard in two ways: When the prongs of the tuning fork are held in front of the ear, sound waves pass from air to tympanic membrane and across middle ear to reach the cochlea. This is air conduction.

If the base of the vibrating tuning fork is presses against the mastoid, the vibration is transmitted through the bones of the skull to the cochlea, bypassing the middle ear. This is bone conduction.

Rinne's Test

The base of the vibrating tuning fork is placed on the mastoid process. When the subject is no longer able to hear the sound, the tuning fork is brought to the front of the ear on the same side. A normal subject will still be able to hear the sound, showing that air conduction is better than bone conduction. This is Rinne's positive. A person with conductive deafness has better bone conduction than air conduction and the Rinne's test is said to be negative. In sensorineural deafness air conduction is better than bone conduction, and Rinne's test remains positive.

Weber's Test

The base of the vibrating tuning fork is placed on the vertex of the skull, allowing the sound to be conducted through the bone to both ears. A normal subject hears equally on both sides. If hearing is deficient in one ear, it indicates sensorineural deafness in that ear or conduction deafness in the opposite ear. Bone conduction is better in the ear with conductive deafness because of reduced background noise conducted through air.

Schwabach's Test

Here the examiner compares the bone conduction of the patient with his own, assuming that he himself

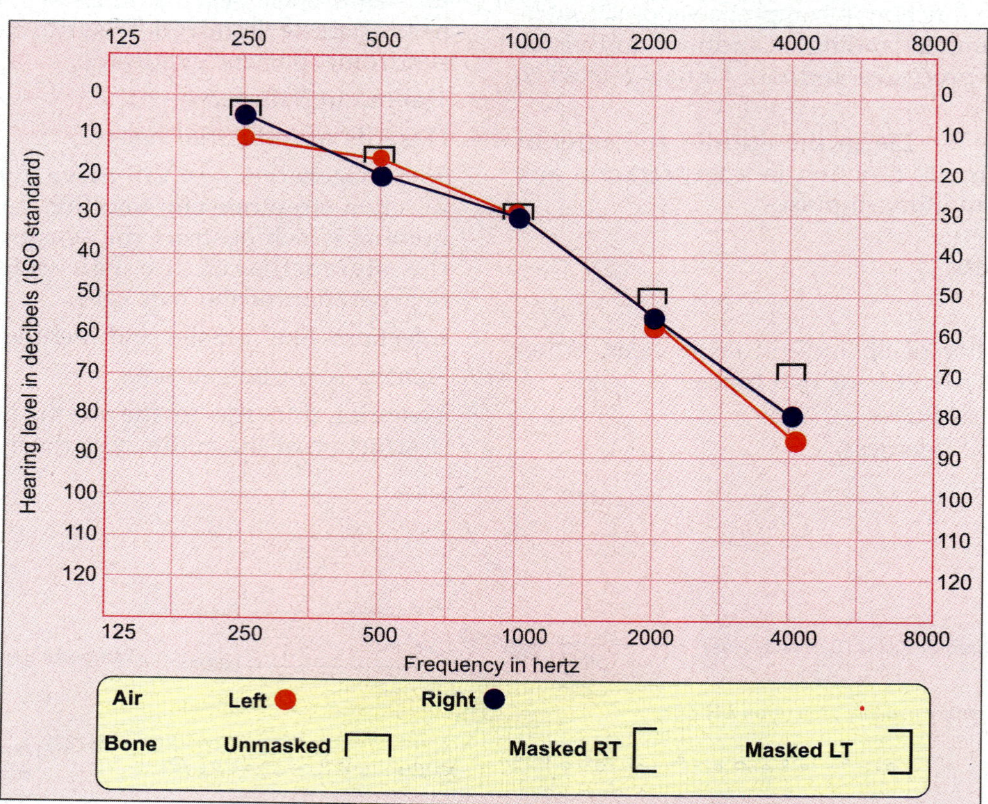

Fig. 12.18

has normal hearing. The base of the vibrating tuning fork is placed first on the mastoid process of the patient until he stops hearing the sound. The examiner then places the tuning fork on his own mastoid. If he still hears the sound, it indicates that the patient has defective bone conduction, probably due to sensorimotor deafness. The reliability of the test is higher if the tragus of the patient and the examiner are kept occluded during the test. This is called absolute bone conduction test or the modified Schwabach test.

Audiometry (Figs 12.18 and 19)

There are different types of audiometric tests like pure tone audiometry and speech audiometry. In pure tone audiometry, a pure tone audiometer delivers tones of variable frequency and intensity. Both air conduction and bone conduction are measured. For each frequency, a series of tone pips are delivered at increasing intensities and the patient is instructed to signal every time he hears a sound. The frequencies tested are at octave steps, i.e. 125, 250, 500, 1000, 2000, 4000, 8000 Hz. Each frequency is tested in the intensity range of 10–120 dB. The results are charted as an audiogram.

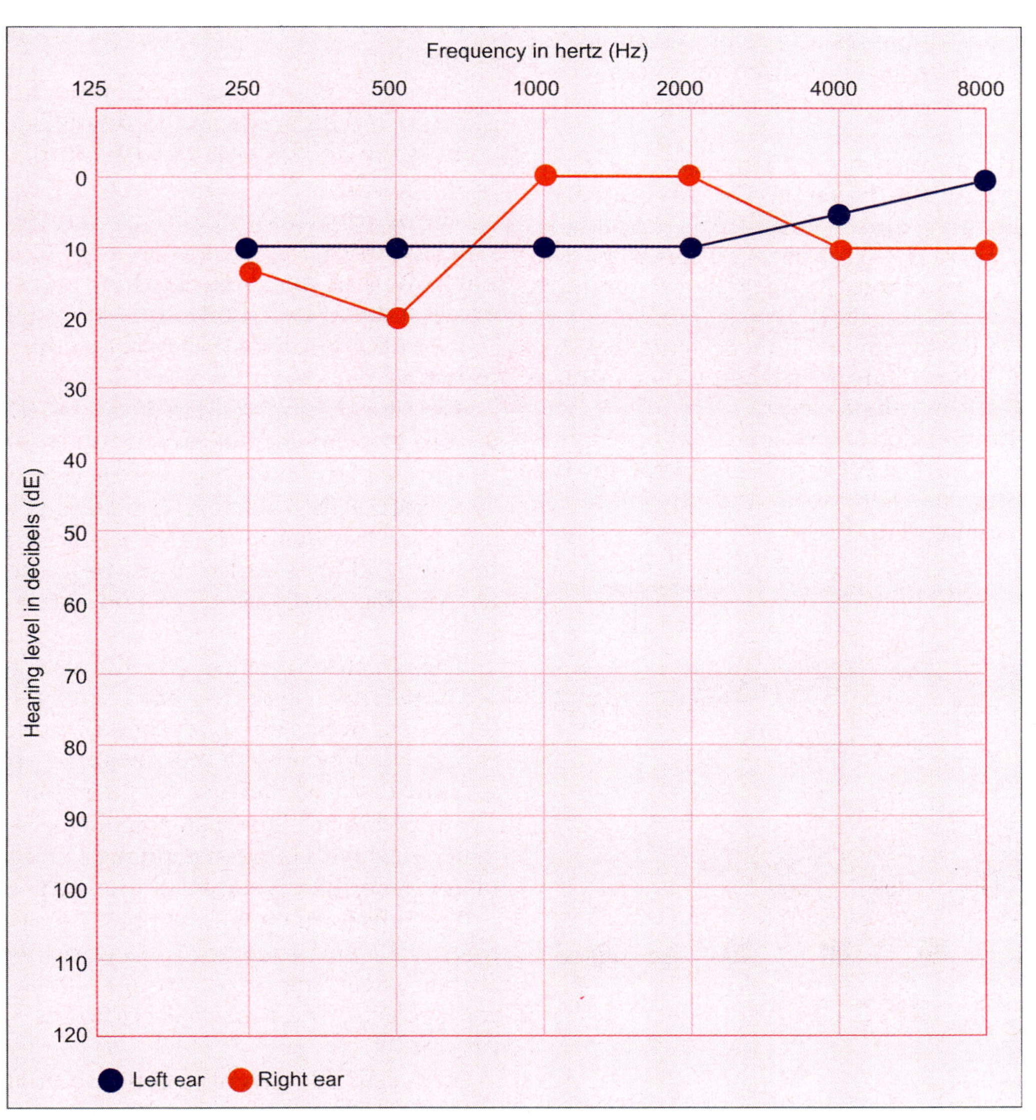

Fig. 12.19

121. SMELL—OLFACTION

Smell and taste are classified under visceral senses because of their close association with GI function.

The flavors of various foods are in large part a combination of their taste and smell. So, food may taste different if one has a cold that depress the sense of smell. Both taste and smell are chemoreceptors that are stimulated by molecules in solution in mucous membrane of nose and saliva in the mouth.

However, anatomically they are different. Smell receptors are distance receptors (telereceptors) and smell pathway does not relay in the thalamus.

The taste pathway passes up the brainstem to the thalamus and project to the postcentral gyrus along with those for touch and pressure sensation from the mouth.

Animals have a much higher perception of smell than man, but man has better vision. An animal in which the sense of smell is acute is known as macrosmatic animals. The area covered by the olfactory membranes large. In microsmatic animals (man) the area is small.

The sense of olfaction is much more acute than the sense of taste. Smell can be perceived in minute quantities and from a distance.

The olfactory stimulus is a chemical stimulus. It is presented as vapors which get dissolved in the secretion of mucous membrane and stimulate the olfactory end organs (Fig. 12.20).

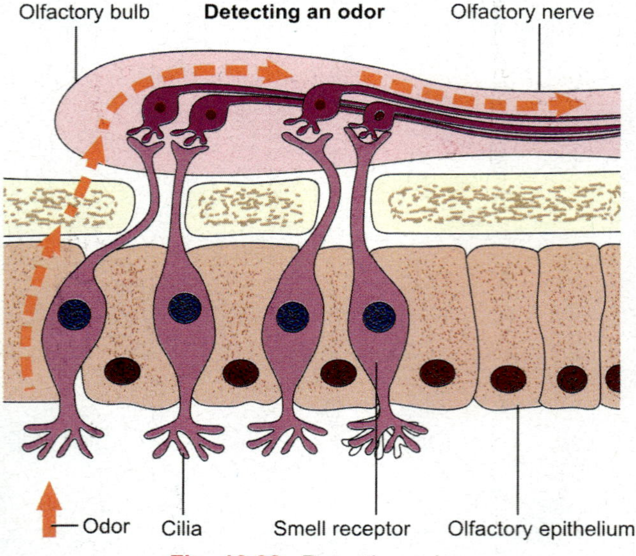

Fig. 12.20: Detecting odor

12

Olfactory Mucous Membrane

Located in the upper part (roof) of the nasal cavity near the nasal septum, covers a small area of 5 cm^2.

It is yellowish in color. Normally, air does not pass directly over the olfactory end organs, but it is supplied with air by eddy currents. This is useful because it prevents the harmful effects of direct impact of cold dry air which may contain noxious vapors.

When a person wants to find out the nature or direction of the smell, he achieves it by sniffing whereby more air is drawn towards the olfactory epithelium.

The olfactory mucous membrane (OMM) contains olfactory receptor cells, supporting cells and progenitor cells (stem cells). There are around 10–20 million receptor cells.

The olfactory receptor cell is a bipolar neuron with two processes.

Each neuron has a short thick dendrite with an expanded end called olfactory rod.

From these rods cilia project to the surface of the mucous.

The cilia are unmyelinated processes 2 μm long and 0.1 um in diameter. Each neuron has 10–20 cilia.

The cilia have receptor sites for odorant molecules. The axon of the olfactory receptors is unmyelinated and passes upwards pierces the cribriform plate of the ethmoid bone and joins the processes of other cell to form the olfactory nerve and enters the olfactory bulb.

The olfactory neurons-like the taste receptors cells are constantly being replaced with a half time of a few weeks unlike other neurons. (The renewal process is regulated by a bone morphogenic protein (BHP) a growth factor exhibiting an inhibitory effect.)

Supporting cells or sustentacular cells are columnar, cylindrical with large oval nucleus and have granules of golden brown (yellowish) pigment.

The cells form tight junctions. The nasal surface has microvilli and they form a continuous epithelial surface except for gaps through which the olfactory rod projects. The proximal portion is a long slender process.

Stem cells or progenitor cells are small conical cells at the base. They give rise to new receptor cells which push the muscles up between the supporting cells and

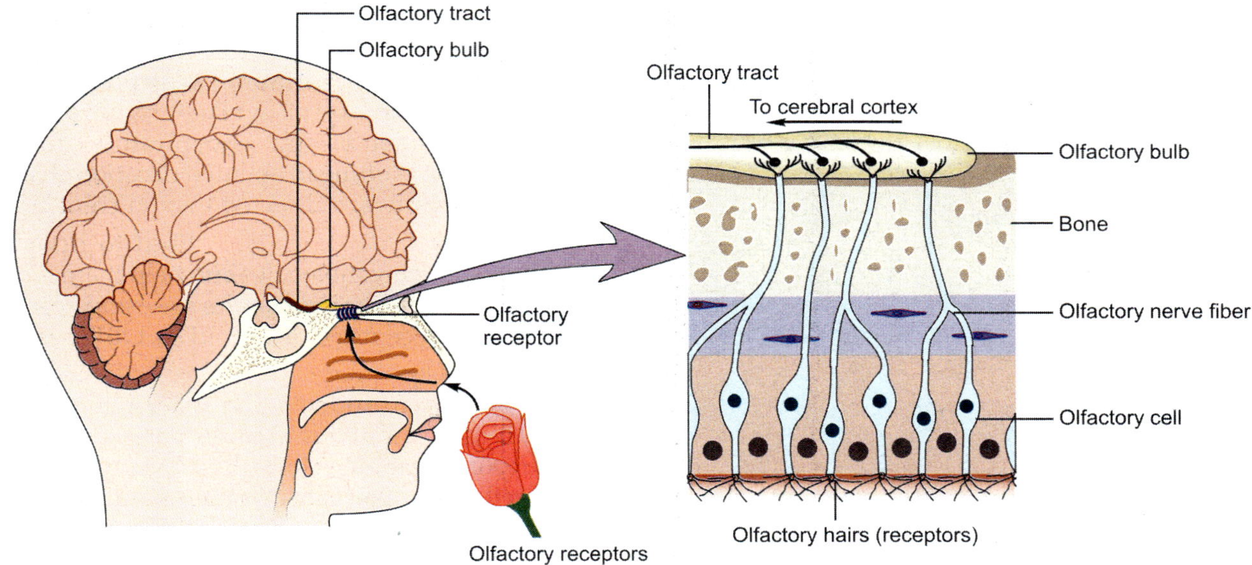

Fig. 12.21: Olfactory receptors

form tight junctions with them. They also replace supporting cells.

Mucus secreting glands called Bowman's gland are present below the basal lamina of the membrane.

Olfactory bulb: In the olfactory bulb, the axons of the receptors contact the primary dendrites of the mitral cells and tufted cells to form the complex globular synapses called olfactory glomeruli (Fig. 12.21).

The tufted cells are smaller than the mitral cells and have thinner axons. But both types send their axons to the olfactory cortex and have the same function.

In addition to mitral cell and tufted cells the olfactory bulbs contain periglomerular cells which are inhibitory neurons connecting one glomerulus to another and granule cells which have no axons and make reciprocal synapses with the lateral dendrites of the mitral and tufted cells.

At these synapses the mitral or tufted cells excites the granule cell synapses by releasing glutamate and the granule side of the synapse in turn inhibits the mitral or tufted cell by releasing GABA.

Olfactory cortex: The axons of the mitral and tufted cells are the second order nervous which from the olfactory tract and ends in the olfactory cortex (Fig. 12.22).

The olfactory cortex is made up of:

- Anterior olfactory nucleus
- Prepyriform area
- Pyriform cortex
- Preamygdaloid cortex
- Amygdaloid nucleus
- Entorhinal cortex

All are parts of limbic cortex

The olfactory tract consists of

- Medial
- Intermediate
- Lateral

} striae

Some fibers cross and so there is bilateral representation.

Axons of mitral cells → lateral and intermediate striae → pyriform lobe (prepyriform area and pyriform cortex) → main olfactory area where discrimination of cell occurs.

Amygdala receives fibers from medial striae and is concerned with emotional response to smell. Olfactory memory is mediated by the entorhinal cortex.

The olfactory bulb receives efferent fibers from ipsilateral and contralateral anterior. Olfactory nucleus which are inhibitory and regulate the activity of the olfactory bulb.

Olfactory Threshold and Discrimination

Olfactory receptors are chemoreceptors and telereceptors. They respond to vapors of volatile substance and should come in contact with the olfactory epithelium after dissolving in the mucus secreted by the Bowman's glands.

12

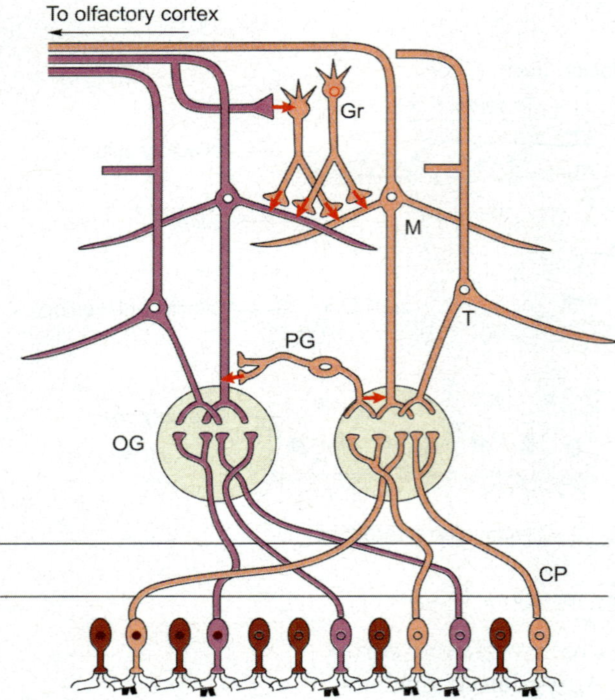

Fig. 12.22: Basic neural circuits in olfactory bulb
OG olfactory glomerulus, CP Cribriform plate, T tufted cell, PG periglomerular cell, M mitral cell, Gr granule cell

1. The olfactory threshold for various substances varies, e.g. methyl mercaptan (garlic): 0.0000004 mg/L in air
   Artificial musk: 0.0004 mg/L in air
   Ethyl ether: 5.83 mg/L in air
2. Olfactory discrimination in humans is remarkable. Up to 10,000 different odors are recognized by humans.
3. The determination of differences in intensity is poor. The concentration of the odor producing substances must be changed by more than 30% before a difference is detected (whereas in case of light intensity 1% change in the intensity of light can be differentiated).
4. The direction of odor can be made out by the slight difference in the arrival time of odor producing molecule in the two nostrils.
5. Odor producing molecules contain 3–20 carbon atoms and molecules with same number of carbon atoms but different structural configuration have different odors.
6. Strong odors have high water and lipid solubility.
7. Different odors have different receptors and more than 1000 different odor receptors have been identified in mice.
8. Once the odor molecule reaches the olfactory receptors it causes depolarization potential. They act through heterotrimeric G protein and via cAMP and adenylyl cyclase. Others act via phospholipase C and phosphatidyl inositol hydrolysis resulting in opening of cation channels causing an inward directed Ca^{++} current.
9. *Odor binding protein (OBP):* Bind to lipophilic odor producing molecules and help them to cross the hydrophilic mucus in the nose and reach the olfactory receptors. An 18 kDA OBP has been isolated.

   Pheromones: In rodents and other mammals the nasal cavity contains another patch of olfactory mucous membrane along the nasal septum which is well-developed called vomeronasal organ. This structure is concerned with the perception of odors that act as pheromones. Its receptors project to the accesory olfactory bulb and from there project to areas in the amygdala and hypothalamus that are concerned with reproduction and ingestive behavior, e.g. pregnancy block in the mice, the pheromones of a male from different strain prevent pregnancy as a result of mating with that male, but mating with a mouse of same strain does not produce blockade.

   Vomeronasal organs are not well-developed in humans although a pit in the amount 1/3 of the nasal septum appears to be the same organ.
10. Sense of smell is more acute in females than males and most acute at the time of ovulation.

Sniffing

The portion of the nasal cavity containing olfactory epithelium is poorly ventilated in humans. Only eddy currents set up reach the olfactory mucous membrane. These are set up by convection as cool air strikes the warm mucosal surface. Sniffing greatly increases the amount of air entering the region by contraction of the lower part of the nares on the septum and deflecting the airstream upwards.

Role of Pain Fibers in the Nose

Naked endings of the trigeminal nerve fibers are present in the olfactory mucous membrane. They are stimulated by irritating substances. These endings are responsible for initiating sneezing, lacrimation, and respiratory inhibition and often reflex responses to nasal irritants.

Adaptation

Continuous exposure to an odor even if it is disagreeable causes the perception of odor to decrease and eventually cease. This is due to adaptation or desensitization. It is mediated by Ca^{++} acting via calmodulin in cyclic nucleotide gated (CNG) ion channels.

Classification of Odors

There are several classifications of odor producing substances. The most complete is the Zwaardemaker classification.

Zwaardemaker Classification

It has nine main divisions with two or more subdivisions:

1. Elthereal (fruits, ethers)
2. Aromatic (camphor, cloves, bitter almond)
3. Fragrant (flowers, perfumes)
4. Ambrosial (musk)
5. Alliaceous (garlic, onion)
6. Empyreumatic (burning of feather, tobacco, roasted coffee)
7. Caprylic (goat odors, sweat, caproic acid)
8. Repulsive (bed bug, belladonna)
9. Nauseating (excreta, decaying meat and vegetables).

Other Classifications

Henings classification: It has six primary smells:

1. Flavour
2. Fruity
3. Foul
4. Burnt
5. Spicy
6. Resinous

Crocker-Henderson system: It has four fundamental smells:

1. Fragrant
2. Acid
3. Burnt
4. Caprylic (goaty)

Test for Sense of Smell

Olfactometer is used for testing the acuity of smell. The commonly used instrument is Zwaardemaker apparatus. It consists of an inner tube and an outer tube. The inner tube is graduated and curved at its upper end and can be drawn to various lengths.

The inner surface of the outer tube is painted with the substance whose smell is to be tested. By varying the length of the inner tube exposed to the air currents of inspired air the threshold of smell can be determined. This only gives a relative value. To obtain the absolute values a known quantity of the substance can be dissolved in a known volume of air and the threshold can be determined by varying the concentration to get the minimum perceptible odor.

Clinical Test for Smell

Three bottles containing oil of clove, oil of peppermint and tincture of asafetida are given to the patient for sniffing and identifying the odor. Each nostril is tested separately.

Abnormalities of Smell

Anosmia: It is the absence or loss of sense of smell. It can occur temporarily due to common cold or mechanical obstruction due to conditions like nasal polyp. Other conditions include:

- Cerebral tumor
- Prolonged use of snuffs
- Irritant fumes
- Fracture of cribriform plate of ethmoid bone.

Hyperosmia: Increase in perception of smell. It is a rare disorder and can occur in hysteria in a menopause and neurasthenia.

Hyposmia: It is the diminished sensitivity to smell. It can occur due to repeated exposure to some odors.

Parosmia: It is the abnormal perception of smell. It can occur in old age and sinusitis.

Kallman's syndrome: It is a single gene mutation characterized by anosmia with hypogonadism.

Deodorant

Offensive human smell is most often due to sweat which undergoes bacterial decomposition. A deodorant contains antibacterial, a masking agent or antiperspirant. It also contains a substance which chemically alters the odoriferous material or a substance which absorbs it.

Aluminum chlorohydroxide acts as an antiperspirant and antibacterial agent. A fatty base is used which has the property of absorbing odor producing substances.

122. TASTE

Taste and smell are visceral senses because of their association with the gastrointestinal function.

Taste Receptors (Fig. 12.23a)

The sense organ for taste is the taste buds. They are located on the anterior surface of the tongue on numerous small projections called papillae. There are four types of papillae:

1. *Fungiform papillae:* They are rounded structures present in large numbers near the tip of the tongue. There are 5 taste buds per fungiform papillae.
2. *Vallate or circumvallate papillae:* They are arranged in a V shape on the back of the tongue. Large vallate papillae located along the sides of the tongue contain up to 100 taste buds.
3. *Filiform or conical papillae:* They are present on the dorsum of the tongue. They do not contain taste buds. Taste buds are also present in the mucosa of the epiglottis, palate and pharynx. There are about 10,000 taste buds totally.

Structure of Taste bud (Fig. 12.23b)

Each taste bud extends the entire thickness of the epithelium. The free surface has an opening called pore canal. Each taste bud is an ovoid cluster of 40–50 epithelial cells. The base receives the branches of the glossopharyngeal and chorda tympani nerves. The apex communicates with the cavity of the mouth by a small pore called the gustatory pore.

There are three types of cells:

1. *Gustatory cells:* Which are bipolar cells with central nucleated cell body. They are the taste receptors. The distal process passes towards apex of the taste bud and ends in a small hairlet which projects into the gustatory pore. The proximal process is more delicate and branched. There are 15–20 gustatory cells in each taste bud (Fig. 12.23c).
2. *Sustentacular or supporting cells:* They are flattened cells with pointed ends. They surround and support the gustatory cells. They also have microvilli which project into the gustatory pore.
3. *Basal cells:* Arise from the epithelium in the floor of the taste bud and they give rise to new receptor cells The receptor cells have a short lifespan of about a week.

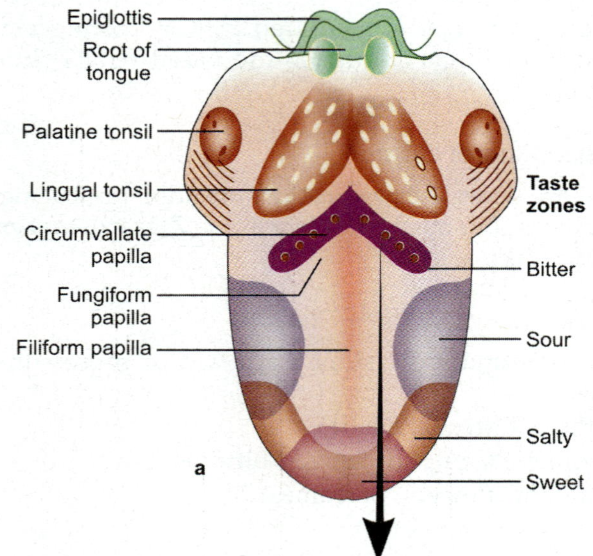

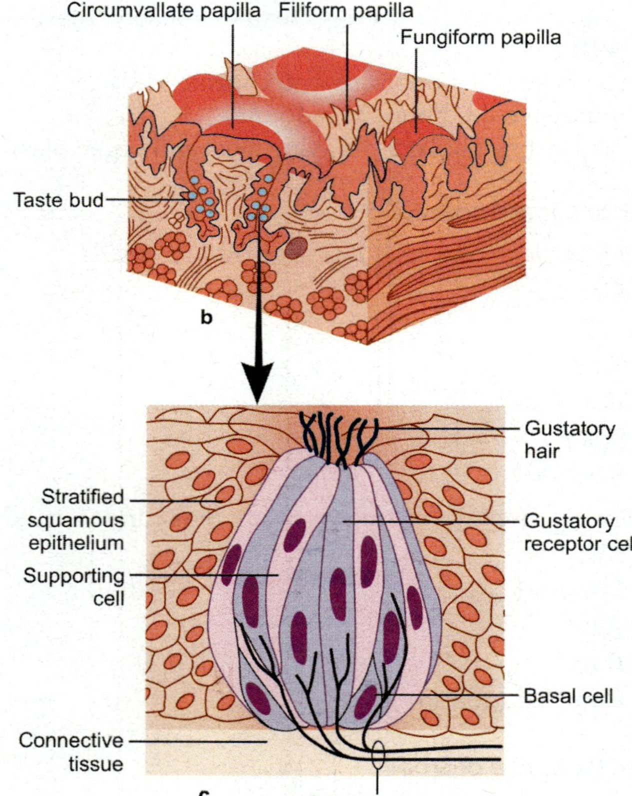

Figs 12.23a to c: **(a)** Location of papillae and taste zones on dorsum of tongue, **(b)** details of papillae, **(c)** taste bud

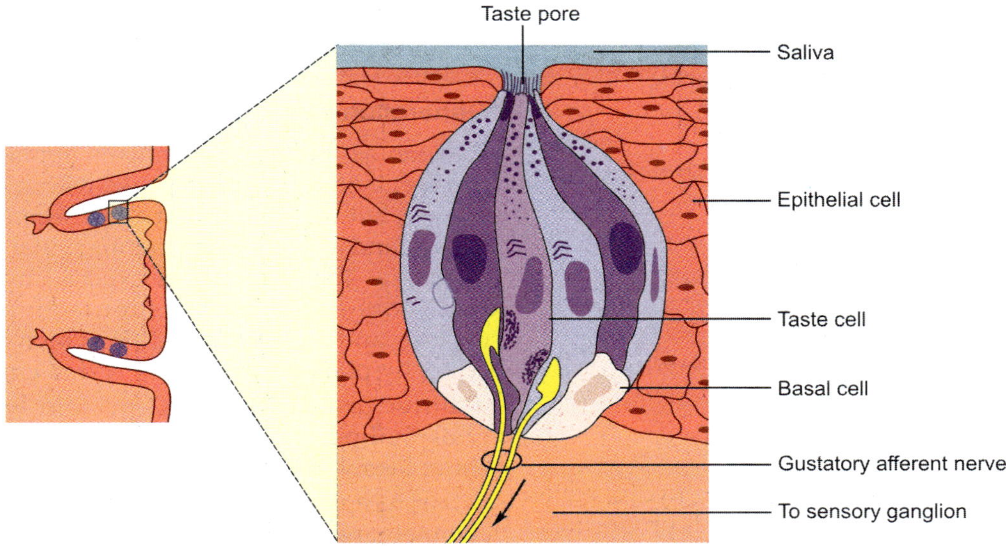

Fig. 12.24: Structure of taste bud

Each taste bud receives several nerve fibers. Hence there is convergence and integration at the level of first order neuron (Fig. 12.24).

Taste Pathway (Fig. 12.25)

The anterior 2/3 of the tongue receives fibers from the chorda tympani branch of the facial nerve and the posterior 1/3 from the glossopharyngeal nerve.

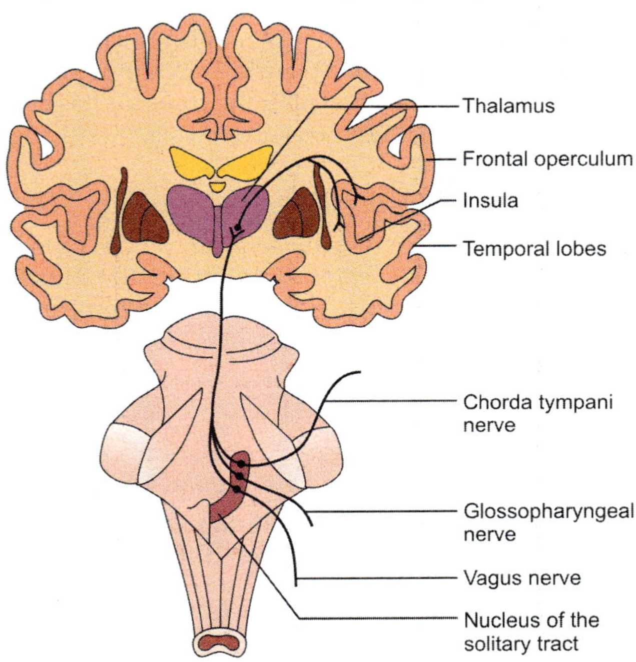

Fig. 12.25: Taste pathway

The vagus supplies the taste receptors in the regions other than the tongue.

The nerve fibers pass to the nucleus of tractus solitarius (NTS) in the medulla. The cell bodies of the second order neurons are located in the NTS. Their axons ascend in the same side to join the medial leminiscus and terminate with nerve fibers from the trigeminal nerve in the posteroventral nucleus of the thalamus.

The third order neurons arise from here and end in the inferior part of the ipsilateral postcentral gyrus (somatosensory area).

Physiology of Taste (Fig. 12.26)

The five basic qualities of taste include:

1. Sweet
2. Salt
3. Sour
4. Bitter
5. Umami

Sweet and salt sensations are felt maximally in the tip of the tongue, sour in the sides and bitter in the back of the tongue.

Substances Producing the Basic Taste Sensations

Salt: This is produced by ionised salts mainly by sodium ions. Salt causes depolarization of the salt receptor cells by influx of sodium ions through the channels and causes release of glutamic acid. The anion contributes to the taste of salt, but the cation modifies it.

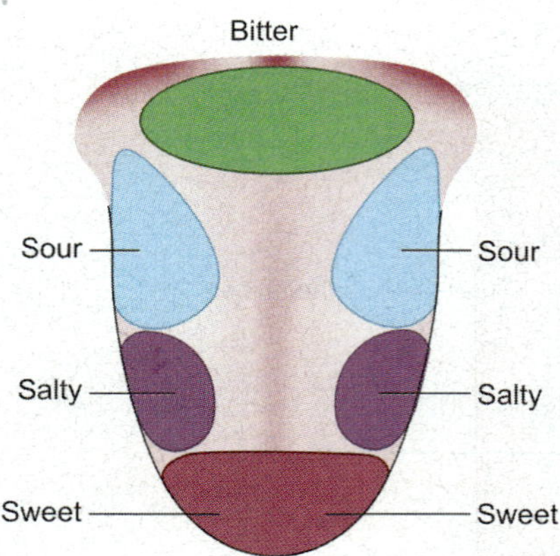

Fig. 12.26: Taste zones

Sour: It is caused by acids, namely by the hydrogen ion concentration. The intensity of the taste is proportional to the logarithm of the hydrogen ion concentration.

Bitter: It is due to alkaloids. Chemical substances like quinine sulfate, strychnine, hydrochloride, morphine, nicotine, caffeine, urea, phenylthiourea, magnesium sulphate produce bitter taste. Bitter taste is due to cations. They act via G protein coupled receptors and phospholipase C to cause release of calcium ions from the endoplasmic reticulum.

Sweet: It is due to organic compounds, e.g. sugar (fructose, sucrose, and maltose). Other substances that produce sweet sensations are polysaccharides, glycerol, chloroform, alcohol, aliphatic aldehydes, and ketones. Some inorganic compounds like beryllium salts, lead acetate and alkalies in high dilution produce sweet taste.

Umami: (Japanese word meaning delicious) is the pleasant taste of food containing L-glutamate, e.g. meat extracts, aging cheese.

Mechanism of Stimulation of Taste Receptors

Receptor Potential

Taste receptors are stimulated only by substances in solution. Solid substances are dissolved by saliva in the mouth. They act on the microvilli of the taste receptors and sets up a generator potential. The mechanism by which the stimulating substances react with the taste villi is by binding of the taste chemical to a protein receptor molecule that lies on the outer surface of the taste receptor. On binding it opens ion channels which allow positively charged sodium ions or hydrogen ions to enter and depolarize the cell. In case of sweet and bitter taste sensation, the receptor protein molecules activate second messenger inside the taste cell, which in-turn causes intracellular chemical changes that elicit the taste signals.

12

Generation of Nerve Impulses by Taste bud

As soon as the taste stimulus is applied, the rate of discharge of nerve fibers peaks within a fraction of a second, but within the next a few seconds adaptation occurs, and a weaker continuous signal is transmitted as long as the taste bud is exposed to the stimulus. Receptors fo sweet sensation activates adenylyl cyclase and increases cAMP, which decreases K^+ efflux by phosphorylation of K^+ ion channels.

Bitter taste activates G protein which acts on phospholipase C and causes release of Ca^{++} from endoplasmic reticulum.

Salt receptors are depolarized by Na^+ entry. These channels are blocked by amoloride. Sour receptors are depolarized by H^+ entry, blocking K^+ channels. The concentration of a substance necessary to stimulate taste receptors varies for different substances.

Substance	*Concentration*
Sucrose	1/200
Sodium chloride	1/400
Dilute HCl	1/15000
Quinine	1/20,000,000

Bitter is the most sensitive taste. The taste of certain substances linger for a long time. This may be due to the persistence of the stimulating agent or the persistence of the sensation after the stimulus has been withdrawn. This is known as aftertaste.

Applied Aspects

Aguesia: It is absence of taste sensation. Loss of taste sensation occurs in lesions involving the chorda tympani, glossopharyngeal nerve and lesions along the taste pathway.

Hypoguesia: It is diminishing in taste sensation. It can occur in common cold.

Dysguesia: It is abnormal taste sensation. Hallucination of taste can occur as aura in temporal lobe epilepsy.

Taste blindness: Some people are taste blind for certain substances especially for different types of thiourea compounds.

A substance used frequently by psychologists for demonstrating taste blindness is phenylthiocarbamide for which 15–30% of people exhibit taste blindness.

Index